# Role of Neuropeptide Receptors in Neuroendocrinology

# Role of Neuropeptide Receptors in Neuroendocrinology

Editor: Gilbert Holmes

MURPHY & MOORE
www.murphy-moorepublishing.com

www.murphy-moorepublishing.com

MURPHY & MOORE

**Cataloging-in-Publication Data**

Role of neuropeptide receptors in neuroendocrinology / edited by Gilbert Holmes.
p. cm.
Includes bibliographical references and index.
ISBN 978-1-63987-496-5
1. Neuropeptides. 2. Neuroendocrinology. 3. Nerve tissue proteins. 4. Neurotransmitters.
5. Endocrinology. 6. Neurology. I. Holmes, Gilbert.
QP552.N39 R43 2022
612.804 2--dc23



Murphy & Moore Publishing,
1 Rockefeller Plaza,
New York City, NY 10020, USA

ISBN 978-1-63987-496-5 (Hardback)

# Contents

# Preface

Neuroendocrinology is a branch of biology which is concerned with the functional and anatomical interactions between the endocrine system and the nervous system. Major neuroendocrine systems are hypothalamic-pituitary-adrenal axis, hypothalamic-pituitary-thyroid axis, hypothalamic-pituitary-gonadal axis and hypothalamic-neurohypophyseal system. Neuropeptide receptors are the G-protein coupled class that comprises of seven transmembrane receptors. Peptides are released into the synaptic cleft and they activate these receptors through high affinity binding and also mediate internal signaling events through cytoplasmic G-protein coupled effector. When these receptors are activated, this inhibits and activates a variety of second messenger systems which results in cell firing, phosphorylation and dephosphorylation events, modulation of membrane threshold and alteration of gene expression. This book covers in detail some existent theories about the role of neuropeptide receptors in neuroendocrinology. It presents researches and studies performed by experts across the globe. Students, researchers, experts and all associated with this field will benefit alike from this book.

This book is the end result of constructive efforts and intensive research done by experts in this field. The aim of this book is to enlighten the readers with recent information in this area of research. The information provided in this profound book would serve as a valuable reference to students and researchers in this field.

At the end, I would like to thank all the authors for devoting their precious time and providing their valuable contribution to this book. I would also like to express my gratitude to my fellow colleagues who encouraged me throughout the process.

**Editor**

# 1

# The physiological role of orexin/hypocretin neurons in the regulation of sleep/wakefulness and neuroendocrine functions

***Ayumu Inutsuka and Akihiro Yamanaka****

*Department of Neuroscience II, Research Institute of Environmental Medicine, Nagoya University, Nagoya, Japan*

***Edited by:***
*Hubert Vaudry, University of Rouen, France*

***Reviewed by:***
*Luis De Lecea, Stanford University, USA*
*Christelle Peyron, CNRS UMR5292, INSERM U1028, France*

****Correspondence:***
*Akihiro Yamanaka, Department of Neuroscience II, Research Institute of Environmental Medicine, Nagoya University, Furo, Chikusa, Nagoya 464-8601, Japan.*
*e-mail: yamank@riem.nagoya-u.ac.jp*

The hypothalamus monitors body homeostasis and regulates various behaviors such as feeding, thermogenesis, and sleeping. Orexins (also known as hypocretins) were identified as endogenous ligands for two orphan G-protein-coupled receptors in the lateral hypothalamic area. They were initially recognized as regulators of feeding behavior, but they are mainly regarded as key modulators of the sleep/wakefulness cycle. Orexins activate orexin neurons, monoaminergic and cholinergic neurons in the hypothalamus/brainstem regions, to maintain a long, consolidated awake period. Anatomical studies of neural projections from/to orexin neurons and phenotypic characterization of transgenic mice revealed various roles for orexin neurons in the coordination of emotion, energy homeostasis, reward system, and arousal. For example, orexin neurons are regulated by peripheral metabolic cues, including ghrelin, leptin, and glucose concentration. This suggests that they may provide a link between energy homeostasis and arousal states. A link between the limbic system and orexin neurons might be important for increasing vigilance during emotional stimuli. Orexins are also involved in reward systems and the mechanisms of drug addiction. These findings suggest that orexin neurons sense the outer and inner environment of the body and maintain the proper wakefulness level of animals for survival. This review discusses the mechanism by which orexins maintain sleep/wakefulness states and how this mechanism relates to other systems that regulate emotion, reward, and energy homeostasis.

**Keywords: orexin, hypocretin, sleep, hypothalamus, optogenetics, neuropeptide**

## INTRODUCTION

The hypothalamus plays a critical role in maintaining energy homeostasis by coordinating behavioral, metabolic, and neuroendocrine responses (Bernardis and Bellinger, 1996). Within this region, the lateral hypothalamic area (LHA) has been regarded as an important center for feeding and arousal because animal models with LHA lesions exhibit hypophagia and decreased arousal that frequently leads to death. Orexin A and orexin B (also known as hypocretin 1 and hypocretin 2) are neuropeptides expressed exclusively by LHA neurons. Orexin-producing neurons (orexin neurons) project their axons throughout the brain (Peyron et al., 1998; Nambu et al., 1999), which suggests that their functions are varied. Remarkably, dense projections of orexin neurons are observed in the serotonergic dorsal raphe nucleus (DR), noradrenergic locus coeruleus (LC), and histaminergic tuberomammillary nucleus (TMN); and all of these nuclei are involved in promoting arousal (Saper et al., 2005). Prepro-orexin knockout mice, orexin receptor knockout mice, and orexin neuron-ablated transgenic mice all show severely defective sleep/wakefulness cycles (Chemelli et al., 1999; Hara et al., 2001; Willie et al., 2003). Consistently, deficiencies of orexin function were found in human narcolepsy (Nishino et al., 2000; Peyron et al., 2000; Thannickal et al., 2000). These findings clearly show the importance of the orexin system in the regulation of sleep/wakefulness. Past studies also revealed roles for orexin neurons beyond feeding and arousal, including autonomic nervous system control (Sellayah et al., 2011; Tupone et al., 2011) and in reward and stress systems (Boutrel et al., 2005; Harris et al., 2005).

In this review, we first discuss the basic biological features of orexins and their receptors, and we then describe the neuronal inputs and outputs of the orexin neurons. Finally, we discuss the various physiological roles of the orexin system, focusing on the regulation of sleep and wakefulness.

## OREXIN AND OREXIN RECEPTORS

In 1998, two groups independently found the same new peptides by using different strategies. Sakurai et al. (1998) used reverse pharmacology to identify ligands of orphan G-protein-coupled

---

**Abbreviations:** AgRP, agouti-related peptide; Arc, arcuate nucleus; BAT, brown adipose tissue; BST, bed nucleus of the stria terminalis; CTB, cholera toxin B subunit; DR, dorsal raphe nucleus; DREADD, designer receptors exclusively activated by designer drugs; FEO, food-entrainable oscillator; GPCRs, G-protein-coupled receptors; ICV, intracerebroventricular; LC, locus coeruleus; LDT, laterodorsal tegmental nucleus; LHA, lateral hypothalamic area; NMDAR, *N*-methyl-D-aspartate receptor; NPY, neuropeptide Y; OX1R, orexin receptor 1; OX2R, orexin receptor 2; PPT, pedunculopontine tegmental nucleus; PTX, pertussis toxin; PVN, paraventricular thalamic nucleus; SCN, suprachiasmatic nucleus; TMN, tuberomammillary nucleus; TTC, C-terminal fragment of tetanus toxin; VLPO, ventrolateral preoptic nucleus; VTA, ventral tegmental area.

receptors (GPCRs). They found a novel family of neuropeptides that binds to two closely related orphan GPCRs. Because the injection of the ligands induced feeding behavior, they named the ligands "orexin" after the Greek word orexis, which means appetite (Sakurai et al., 1998). At the same time, de Lecea et al. (1998) isolated cDNAs selectively expressed within the hypothalamus. Two peptides of the cDNAs showed substantial amino acid sequence homology with the gut peptide hormone secretin, so they named these peptides "hypocretin." They suggested that hypocretins function within the central nervous system as neurotransmitters.

Prepro-orexin polypeptide is proteolysed to produce two orexins, orexin A and orexin B. Orexin A is a 33-amino acid peptide of 3.5 kDa, with an N-terminal pyroglutamyl residue and C-terminal amidation. The four Cys residues of orexin A form two sets of intrachain disulfide bonds. This structure is completely conserved among several mammalian species (human, rat, mouse, cow, sheep, dog, and pig). On the other hand, rat orexin B is a 28-amino acid, C-terminally amidated, linear peptide of 2.9 kDa, which is 46% identical in sequence to rat orexin A. The 3.2 kb fragment of the 5′-upstream region of the human prepro-orexin gene is reported to be sufficient to express genes in orexin-containing neurons (Sakurai et al., 1999; Moriguchi et al., 2002).

*In situ* hybridization of prepro-orexin shows orexin-containing neurons are located in the LHA. Prepro-orexin mRNA was shown to be upregulated under fasting conditions, indicating that these neurons somehow sense the animal's energy balance (Sakurai et al., 1998). Recently, the forkhead box transcription factor Foxa2, a downstream target of insulin signaling, was reported to be involved in this transcriptional regulation (Silva et al., 2009).

Orexin A acts on both orexin receptor 1 (OX1R) and 2 (OX2R), while orexin B selectively acts on OX2R (Sakurai et al., 1998). While orexin neurons are localized within the LHA, they have widespread projections throughout the brain (Peyron et al., 1998; Nambu et al., 1999; **Figure 1**). Therefore, it is important to know the distribution pattern of orexin receptors to identify the functional neuronal network. Marcus et al. (2001) used *in situ* hybridization to demonstrate that OX1R and OX2R differ in distribution. OX1R mRNA was observed in many brain regions including hippocampus, paraventricular thalamic nucleus (PVN), ventromedial hypothalamic nucleus, DR, and LC. OX2R mRNA was prominent in a complementary distribution including the cerebral cortex, hippocampus, DR, and many hypothalamic nuclei including PVN, TMN, and the ventral premammillary nucleus. Among these regions, DR, LC, and TMN are well known to be involved in maintenance of the awake state. Consistently, orexin-deficient mice display a narcolepsy-like phenotype (Chemelli et al., 1999), as do dogs with a mutation preventing the expression of OX2R (Lin et al., 1999). Note that the regions expressing orexin receptors contain several areas of the hypothalamus, including LHA, PVN, and the arcuate nucleus (Arc), which are all strongly implicated in the modulation of feeding.

## SIGNAL TRANSDUCTION SYSTEM OF OREXIN NEURONS

OX1R and OX2R are seven-transmembrane GPCRs, which transmit information into the cell by activating heterotrimeric G proteins. The signal transduction pathways of orexin receptors were examined in cells transfected with OX1R or OX2R. The inhibitory effect of orexin on forskolin-stimulated cyclic adenosine monophosphate (cAMP) accumulation was not observed in

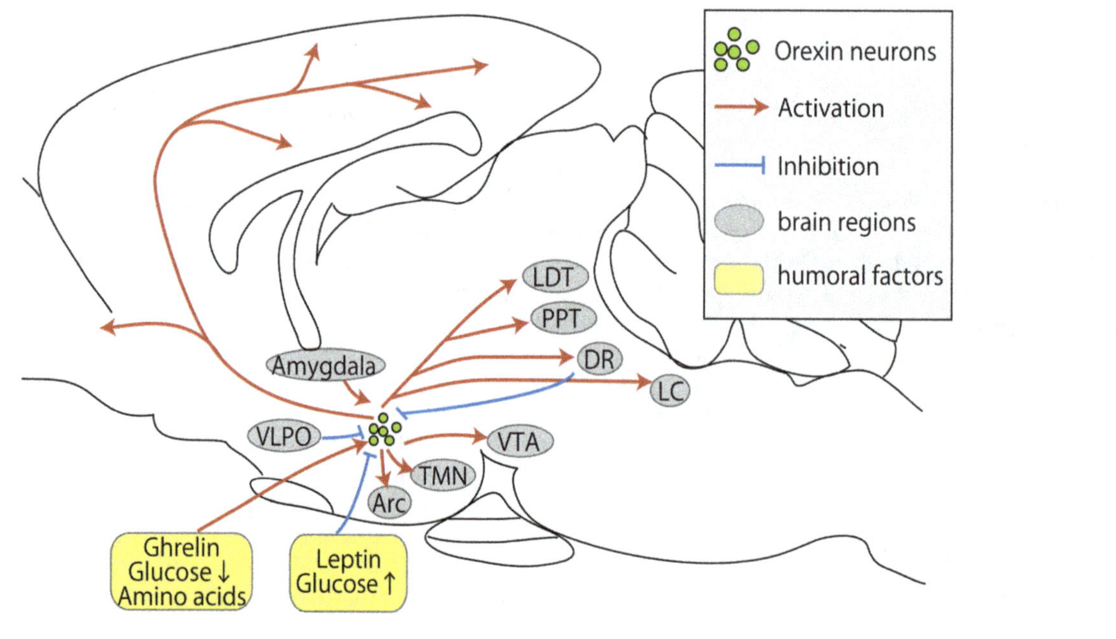


**FIGURE 1 | Schematic representation of inputs and outputs of orexin neurons.** Orexin neurons are found only in the lateral hypothalamic area but project throughout the entire central nervous system. Red arrows show excitatory projections, while blue lines show inhibitory projections. Abbreviations: Arc, arcuate nucleus; DR, dorsal raphe nucleus; LC, locus coeruleus; LDT, laterodorsal tegmental nucleus; PPT, pedunculopontine tegmental nucleus; TMN, tuberomammillary nucleus; VTA, ventral tegmental area; VLPO, ventrolateral preoptic nucleus.

OX1R-expressing cells. In addition, orexin-stimulated elevation in $[Ca^{2+}]i$ in OX1R- or OX2R-expressing cells was not affected by pertussis toxin (PTX) pretreatment. These results suggest that OX1R does not couple to Gi proteins. On the other hand, forskolin-stimulated cAMP accumulation in OX2R-expressing cells was inhibited by orexin in a dose-dependent manner, and this effect was abolished by pretreatment with PTX. These results indicate that OX2R couples to both PTX-sensitive and PTX-insensitive proteins (Zhu et al., 2003). Note that orexin has two independent actions on neuronal activity: activation of noisy cation channels that generate depolarization and activation of a protein kinase C (PKC)-dependent enhancement of $Ca^{2+}$ transients mediated by L-type $Ca^{2+}$ channels (Kohlmeier et al., 2008).

Orexin neurons innervate monoaminergic neurons. In particular, noradrenergic neurons of the LC, dopaminergic neurons of the ventral tegmental area (VTA), and histaminergic neurons of the TMN are activated by orexins (Hagan et al., 1999; Horvath et al., 1999b; Nakamura et al., 2000; Yamanaka et al., 2002). LC neurons exclusively express OX1R, while TMN neurons express OX2R, suggesting that both OX1R and OX2R signaling are excitatory on neurons. Orexin colocalizes with dynorphin (Chou et al., 2001) and glutamate (Abrahamson et al., 2001). It has also been demonstrated that orexin increases local glutamate signaling by facilitation of glutamate release from presynaptic terminals (Li et al., 2002).

## INPUT TO OREXIN NEURONS

### ANATOMICAL ANALYSIS OF NEURONAL INPUT TO OREXIN NEURONS

It has been challenging to study the neuronal afferents to orexin neurons because they are scattered sparsely within the LHA. To address this point, retrograde tracing studies were performed. The non-toxic C-terminal fragment of tetanus toxin (TTC) can be utilized to retrogradely transfer the fused protein to interconnected neurons and transport toward the cell bodies of higher-order neurons (Maskos et al., 2002). Sakurai et al. (2005) generated transgenic mouse lines expressing a fused protein of TTC and green fluorescent protein (GFP) exclusively in orexin neurons by using the promoter of human prepro-orexin. They identified several brain regions including the basal forebrain cholinergic neurons, gamma-aminobutyric acid (GABA)ergic neurons in the ventrolateral preoptic nucleus (VLPO), and serotonergic neurons in the median raphe and paramedian raphe nucleus. Moreover, regions associated with emotion including the amygdala, infralimbic cortex, shell region of the nucleus accumbens, and the bed nucleus of the stria terminalis (BST) were found to innervate orexin neurons.

In addition to TTC, the cholera toxin B subunit (CTB) is also used to retrogradely trace neuronal projections. Yoshida et al. (2006) injected CTB into the LHA and counted every labeled cell in rats. Interestingly, they found strong projections from the lateral septum, preoptic area, BST, and posterior hypothalamus. In addition, they also found that hypothalamic regions preferentially innervate orexin neurons in the medial and perifornical parts of the field, but most projections from the brainstem target the lateral part of the field.

The results of these two papers present slight distinctions. TTC::GFP sometimes labeled regions with no known projections to the orexin field such as the medial septum possibly because of transport to second-order neurons or ectopic expression of the transgene. In addition, the TTC::GFP technique also appears to be less sensitive than conventional retrograde tracers, as it failed to label neurons in the lateral septum or VTA – regions that probably innervate orexin neurons as indicated by anterograde tracing and other retrograde tracing studies (Yoshida et al., 2006; Richardson and Aston-Jones, 2012).

Given that inputs to orexin neurons are so anatomically varied and associated with multiple functions, it might be reasonable to hypothesize the existence of subgroups of orexin neurons. Indeed, anterograde tracers injected into the DR marked the lateral LHA preferentially, while injections into the VMH preferentially stained neurons in the medial LHA (Yoshida et al., 2006). With current technology we cannot only trace neuronal projections but also analyze functional connectivity by utilizing optogenetic and pharmacogenetic tools (Lammel et al., 2012).

### INPUT FROM HYPOTHALAMUS

Previous studies indicated that the LHA is innervated by several hypothalamic regions, and some of these innervations project toward orexin neurons in the LHA. The LHA has long been considered a brain region regulating food intake and body weight. The localization of orexin neurons to the LHA and the functions ascribed to orexin neurons suggest that they may constitute components of a central circuitry controlling energy metabolism. Therefore, it is reasonable to assess their connectivity to other neuronal populations involved in ingestive behaviors. Neuropeptide Y (NPY), produced by specific neurons in the hypothalamic Arc (Allen et al., 1983; Chronwall et al., 1985), was demonstrated to be a prominent inducer of food intake upon central administration (Clark et al., 1984; Stanley and Leibowitz, 1985). Projections to orexin neurons from NPY/agouti-related peptide (AgRP) neurons in the Arc were identified by anatomical studies (Broberger et al., 1998; Elias et al., 1998). Furthermore, orexin neurons express NPY receptors, and direct administration of NPY agonists into the LHA increases Fos-like immunoreactivity in orexin neurons (Campbell et al., 2003). These findings suggest NPY excites orexin neurons; however, electrophysiological analyses showed that direct application of NPY instead reduces spike frequency and hyperpolarizes the membrane potential of orexin neurons (Fu et al., 2004).

### INPUT FROM LIMBIC SYSTEM

Given that depletion of orexin neurons induces the sleep disorder narcolepsy, the limbic system might also provide important projections to orexin neurons. Narcolepsy patients often suffer from an attack called "cataplexy," which is characterized by sudden weakening of postural muscle tone. Cataplexy is often triggered by strong, generally positive emotion while consciousness is preserved during the attack (Honda et al., 1986). This fact implies that orexin neurons may play a role in the physiological responses associated with emotions. Consistently, local injection of orexin into the pedunculopontine tegmental nucleus (PPT) strongly inhibited rapid eye movement (REM)-related atonia in the cat (Takakusaki et al., 2005). Therefore, it is hypothesized that emotional stimuli increase orexin release in the PPT to prevent muscle atonia in wild-type animals.

The innervations from limbic system may mediate emotional arousal and fear-related responses. Prepro-orexin knockout mice showed weaker cardiovascular and locomotor responses to emotional stress in an awake and freely moving condition (Kayaba et al., 2003). Consistently, air jet stress-induced elevations of blood pressure and heart rate were attenuated in conscious orexin/ataxin-3 mice, in which orexin neurons were specifically ablated by expressing neurotoxic protein (Zhang et al., 2006).

### INPUT FROM PREOPTIC AREAS

The preoptic area, especially the VLPO, plays a critical role in non-REM sleep initiation and maintenance (Lu et al., 2002). The VLPO has multiple inhibitory projections to neurons that release wake-promoting neurotransmitters, including histamine neurons in the TMN, noradrenergic neurons in the LC, serotonergic neurons in the DR, and acetylcholinergic neurons (Sherin et al., 1996, 1998; Steininger et al., 2001; Lu et al., 2002).

Neurons in the VLPO fire at a rapid rate during sleep, with attenuation of firing during the awake period. Likewise, neurons in wake-promoting centers fire rapidly during wakefulness and are relatively quiescent during sleep, with the exception of cholinergic neurons, which are divided into two classes of neurons: one is active in both the awake and REM sleep period, and the other is active only in the REM sleep period.

Orexin neurons are strongly inhibited by both a $GABA_A$ agonist, muscimol (Yamanaka et al., 2003b), and a $GABA_B$ receptor agonist, baclofen (Xie et al., 2006). Orexin neurons are also innervated by cells in the VLPO that also contain GABA (Sakurai et al., 2005; Yoshida et al., 2006). These observations suggest that VLPO neurons send GABAergic inhibitory projections to wake-promoting neurons including orexin neurons. This pathway might be important to initiate and maintain sleep.

### INPUT FROM SUPRACHIASMATIC NUCLEUS

Given that sleep/wakefulness is a circadian phenomenon, it is reasonable to consider that orexin neurons receive information from the suprachiasmatic nucleus (SCN), which is the center of the circadian rhythm according the environmental light–dark information. Indeed, the circadian fluctuation of orexin levels in the cerebrospinal fluid (CSF) disappears when the SCN is removed (Deboer et al., 2004). Although direct input to orexin neurons from the SCN appears to be sparse, orexin neurons receive abundant innervations from the BST, supraventricular zone, and dorsomedial hypothalamus (DMH; Sakurai et al., 2005; Yoshida et al., 2006), which receive input from the SCN (Leak and Moore, 2001). This suggests the possibility that orexin neurons receive circadian influences from the SCN via these regions. Note that excitotoxic lesions of the DMH reduce the circadian rhythmicity of wakefulness. The DMH projects to orexin neurons (Chou et al., 2003), although the DMH also projects to multiple brain areas such as the LC and the VLPO that are involved in sleep and wakefulness. In addition, considering that the orexin system is involved in food-entrainable oscillator (FEO; Mieda et al., 2004), the circadian change in the activity of orexin neurons might be regulated by other elements, such as energy balance.

## FACTORS THAT INFLUENCE ACTIVITY OF OREXIN NEURONS

Electrophysiological studies have identified several modulators that regulate activity of orexin neurons. Recordings from transgenic mice expressing GFP in orexin neurons demonstrated that agonists of ionotropic glutamate receptors activated orexin neurons, while glutamate antagonists reduced their activity (Li et al., 2002; Yamanaka et al., 2003b). These results indicate that orexin neurons are tonically activated by glutamate.

Dopamine, noradrenaline, and serotonin (5-HT) hyperpolarize and inhibit orexin neurons via alpha2 and $5\text{-}HT_{1A}$ receptors, respectively (Yamanaka et al., 2003b; Muraki et al., 2004; Li and van den Pol, 2005). Dopamine-induced hyperpolarization is most likely mediated by alpha2-adrenergic receptors since a very high concentration of dopamine is necessary to induce hyperpolarization and also because dopamine-induced hyperpolarization is inhibited by the alpha2-adrenergic receptor antagonist, idazoxan (Yamanaka et al., 2006). However, it is noteworthy that dopamine potentially affects both dopamine receptors and adrenergic receptors, while the dopamine D2 receptor antagonist eticlopride blocks the actions of dopamine on spike frequency and membrane potential (Li and van den Pol, 2005). Thus, dopamine might act through both alpha2-adrenergic receptor and dopamine D2 receptor.

Recently, it was found that orexin itself excites orexin neurons via OX2R (Yamanaka et al., 2010). This suggests that orexin neurons form a positive-feedback circuit through indirect and direct pathways, which results in the preservation of the orexin neuron network at a high activity level and/or for a longer period.

Calcium imaging using transgenic mice in which orexin neurons specifically express yellow cameleon 2.1 showed that neurotensin, sulfated octapeptide form of cholecystokinin, oxytocin, and vasopressin activate orexin neurons, while 5-HT, noradrenaline, dopamine, and muscimol, a $GABA_A$ receptor agonist inhibit these cells (Tsujino et al., 2005). Recently, it was also reported that orexin neurons express glycine receptors throughout adulthood and that glycine inhibits the electric activity of orexin neurons directly and indirectly (Hondo et al., 2011; Karnani et al., 2011b).

Other factors that reportedly influence the activity of orexin neurons include corticotrophin-releasing factor (Winsky-Sommerer et al., 2004), ATP (Wollmann et al., 2005), NPY (Fu et al., 2004), and physiological fluctuations in acid and $CO_2$ levels (Williams et al., 2007). It is noteworthy that the factors that are supposed to be influenced by feeding (such as glucose, ghrelin, and leptin) inhibit the activity of orexin neurons (Yamanaka et al., 2003a). The large variety of factors regulating orexin neuronal activities demonstrates the integral role of orexin neurons in monitoring circadian rhythms, energy balance, and vigilance level.

## REGULATION OF OREXIN NEURONS BY HUMORAL FACTORS

Motivated behaviors such as food-seeking are deeply involved in maintenance of arousal. Orexin neurons are thought to function as the sensor of energy balance. Electrophysiological studies revealed that increasing extracellular glucose concentrations induce striking hyperpolarizations, while decreasing the glucose concentration induces depolarization and increases the frequency of action potentials of orexin neurons (Yamanaka et al., 2003a; Burdakov et al., 2005). Importantly, this mechanism is sufficiently sensitive to respond to physiological fluctuations of glucose concentration induced by normal feeding. Note that other dietary nutrients, amino acids, also activate orexin neurons, and they can suppress the glucose response of orexin neurons at physiological concentration (Karnani et al., 2011a).

In addition, the orexigenic peptide ghrelin activated isolated orexin neurons with depolarization and an increase in action potential frequency (Yamanaka et al., 2003a). In contrast, the strong anorectic factor leptin robustly inhibited orexin neurons, causing hyperpolarization and decreasing the firing rate (Yamanaka et al., 2003a). Notably, insulin exerted no direct effects on orexin neurons. These findings are consistent with the idea that orexin neurons act as a sensor of nutritional status (Sakurai et al., 1998). Indeed, transgenic mice without orexin neurons fail to show fasting-induced arousal (Yamanaka et al., 2003a).

## PHYSIOLOGICAL FUNCTIONS OF OREXIN NEURONS

### FUNCTIONS IN FEEDING BEHAVIORS AND ENERGY HOMEOSTASIS

Orexin neuron-ablated transgenic mice show hypophagia and late-onset obesity (Hara et al., 2001), although the severity of the obese phenotype critically depends on genetic background (Hara et al., 2005). These findings imply a role for orexin in the regulation of energy homeostasis. Although orexins stimulate feeding behavior, they do not slow metabolic rate, which might be expected in a system geared for weight gain. Instead, orexins increase both food intake and metabolic rate (Lubkin and Stricker-Krongrad, 1998). Because animals must be aware and active when they seek and eat food, this function might be important for feeding behavior.

The Arc is attributed to the regulation of feeding behaviors. Orexin neurons densely project to this region (Date et al., 1999; Horvath et al., 1999a). Principal components of the regulating system of feeding behaviors include antagonistic and complementary appetite-stimulating (orexigenic) and appetite-suppressing (anorectic) pathways: NPY/AgRP neurons and proopiomelanocortin (POMC) neurons. It was reported that intracerebroventricular (ICV) injection of orexin induced c-Fos expression in NPY neurons of the Arc (Yamanaka et al., 2000). Therefore, orexin-stimulated feeding may occur at least partly through NPY pathways. However, because NPY antagonist (which completely abolished NPY-induced feeding) only partially abolished orexin-induced feeding in rats, other pathways by which orexin induces feeding might exist. POMC neurons of the Arc are known to suppress appetite, and lack of POMC-derived peptides or electrical silencing of POMC neurons causes obesity. Orexin neurons might affect feeding behavior by inhibiting POMC-expressing neurons (Muroya et al., 2004). Indeed, orexin suppresses action potential firing and hyperpolarizes the membrane potential of POMC neurons in the Arc (Ma et al., 2007).

Intracerebroventricular injection of orexin induces water intake as well as food intake (Kunii et al., 1999). Additionally arginine-vasopressin, also known as antidiuretic hormone, activates orexin neurons via the V1a receptor (Tsunematsu et al., 2008). These results suggest a role for orexin neurons in fluid homeostasis too.

### FUNCTIONS IN SLEEP AND WAKEFULNESS

The roles of orexin neurons in the regulation of sleep and arousal have been reported repeatedly. ICV injection of orexin A or orexin B during the light period increased awake time and reciprocally decreased REM and non-REM sleep time (Hagan et al., 1999; Bourgin et al., 2000; Piper et al., 2000). Sleep fragmentation observed in orexin knockout mice (Chemelli et al., 1999), orexin receptor knockout mice (Willie et al., 2003), and orexin neuron-ablated transgenic mice (Hara et al., 2001) shows us the importance of their physiological functions. Narcolepsy is a sleep disorder characterized by primary disorganization of sleep/wakefulness cycles. It has also been reported that the number of orexin neurons is greatly reduced, and orexin peptide levels in the cerebrospinal fluid are decreased to undetectable levels in narcoleptic patients (Nishino et al., 2000; Peyron et al., 2000; Thannickal et al., 2000). Orexin-ataxin-3 mice are a well known mouse model of narcolepsy. However, in orexin-ataxin-3 mice, orexin neurons are absent from birth, and therefore other neuronal mechanisms might compensate for the function of orexin neurons during development. Indeed, the frequency of cataplexy is not high in these mice. Timing-controlled neuronal ablation models using the tTA-TetO system might overcome this problem.

The activities of monoaminergic neurons in the brainstem and hypothalamus are known to be associated with sleep and awake states. Furthermore, the DR, LC, and TMN monoaminergic neurons express orexin receptors and are densely innervated by orexin neurons. These findings suggest that these regions mediate the effects of orexins. Consistently, noradrenergic neurons of the LC (Hagan et al., 1999), serotonergic neurons of the DR (Brown et al., 2002; Liu et al., 2002), and histaminergic neurons of the TMN (Huang et al., 2001; Yamanaka et al., 2002) have been shown to be activated by orexins. These observations suggest that the activity of these monoaminergic neurons is at least partly regulated by orexins. Orexins also have a strong direct excitatory effect on cholinergic neurons of the basal forebrain (Eggermann et al., 2001), which is hypothesized to play an important role in arousal.

The PPT and the laterodorsal tegmental nucleus (LDT) provide cholinergic afferents to several brain regions and play a pivotal role in the regulation of REM sleep and wakefulness. These regions are also strongly innervated by orexin neurons (Peyron et al., 1998; Nambu et al., 1999). Electrophysiological experiments revealed that the firing rate of cholinergic neurons is increased by orexin A (Burlet et al., 2002). Microinjection of orexin A into the LDT increases awake time and decreases REM sleep time in cats (Xi et al., 2001), and when orexin A is injected into the PPT in cats, an increased stimulus at the PPT is required to induce muscle atonia (Takakusaki et al., 2005). However, it is noteworthy that the LDT/PPT contains other neuronal types beside cholinergic neurons that show activity associated with sleep/wake cycles (Sakai, 2012).

Emerging new studies using optogenetics have revealed the physiological roles of orexin neurons *in vivo*. Direct selective photostimulation of orexin neurons expressing channelrhodopsin2 increases the probability of transition from non-REM or REM sleep to wakefulness (Adamantidis et al., 2007) and activates downstream wake-promoting nuclei such as LC and TMN (Carter et al., 2009). Consistently, it was also shown that direct selective inhibition of orexin neurons expressing halorhodopsin induces non-REM sleep (Tsunematsu et al., 2011). Furthermore, optogenetic stimulation of the LC produces immediate sleep-to-wake transitions, whereas the inhibition causes a decrease in wakefulness (Carter et al., 2010). Recently it was also reported that photoinhibition of LC neurons during the photostimulation of orexin neurons cancels these sleep-to-wake transitions (Carter et al., 2012). These findings indicate that the LC is a major effector of orexin neurons in the regulation of sleep and wakefulness. However, it is noteworthy that LC noradrenergic neurons express only OX1R, and that OX1R knockout mice show only weak fragmentation of sleep and no cataplexy (Mieda et al., 2011).

Recently, not only photo-activated ion channels or ion pumps but also other natural and modified proteins have been used to regulate the activity of specific neuronal circuits *in vivo*. One interesting example is "Designer Receptors Exclusively Activated by Designer Drugs (DREADD)." This method employs modified muscarinic receptors (hM3Dq for excitation and hM4Di for inhibition) that have lost their affinity for endogenous acetylcholine but can be activated by a synthetic ligand, clozapine-N-oxide, which can cross the blood–brain barrier (Armbruster et al., 2007; Alexander et al., 2009). Because stimulation of GPCRs with a specific ligand has a longer effect on cellular signaling than optical stimulation, the DREADD system can facilitate the examination of the chronic effects of modulating the activity of specific neurons. Using this technique, it was reported that the excitation of orexin neurons significantly increased the amount of time spent in wakefulness and decreased both non-REM and REM sleep times and that inhibition of orexin neurons decreased wakefulness time and increased non-REM sleep time (Sasaki et al., 2011). Additionally, melanopsin, a photosensitive G-protein-coupled photopigment, makes it possible to control wakefulness by blue light in a way similar to channelrhodopsin (Tsunematsu et al., 2012).

## FUNCTIONS IN AUTONOMIC NERVOUS SYSTEM

Orexin-deficient mice show lower blood pressure than wild-type littermates (Kayaba et al., 2003; Zhang et al., 2006). Consistently, ICV injection of orexins increases blood pressure and heart rate (Shirasaka et al., 1999), and these effects are abolished by administration of alpha1-adrenergic receptor antagonist, prazosin, or beta-adrenergic receptor antagonist, propranolol. These results suggest that orexins physiologically stimulate the sympathetic nervous system and regulate energy expenditure.

Heat production in brown adipose tissue (BAT) also contributes to body weight regulation through the maintenance of body temperature. Recently Tupone et al. (2011) reported that orexinergic projections to raphe pallidus increase BAT thermogenesis in rat. This finding provides a new mechanism contributing to the disrupted regulation of body temperature and energy metabolism in the absence of orexin. Orexin neuron-ablated transgenic mice show late-onset obesity, although they also show hypophagia (Hara et al., 2001). The regulation of BAT thermogenesis by orexin neurons might account for this phenotype of energy metabolism (Sellayah et al., 2011).

## FUNCTIONS IN REWARD AND STRESS SYSTEMS

To attenuate the symptoms of the sleep disorder, psychostimulants such as amphetamine or methylphenidate are often given to

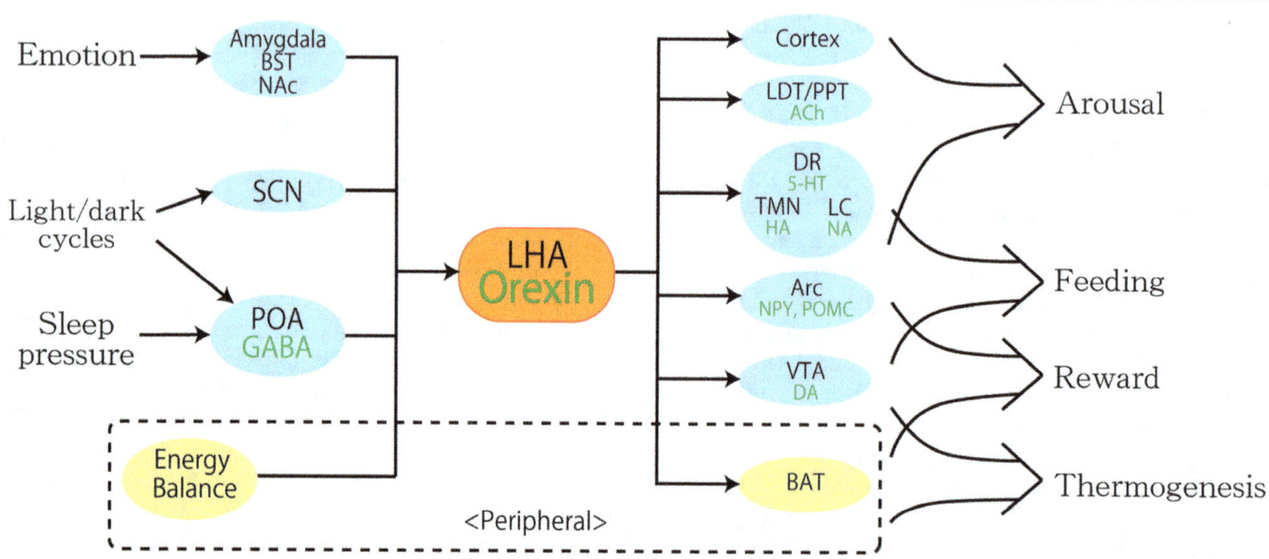


**FIGURE 2 | A schematic diagram to illustrate the integrative physiological roles of orexin neurons.** Orexin neurons regulate various physiological phenomena such as wakefulness, feeding, reward, and thermogenesis. The body energy level influences orexin neuronal activity to coordinate arousal and energy homeostasis. Inputs from the limbic system may be important to regulate the activity of orexin neurons to evoke emotional arousal or fear-related responses. Abbreviations: 5-HT, serotonin; ACh, acetylcholine; Arc, arcuate nucleus; BAT, brown adipose tissue; BST, bed nucleus of the stria terminalis; DA, dopamine; DR, dorsal raphe nucleus; GABA, gamma-aminobutyric acid; HA, histamine; LC, locus coeruleus; LDT, laterodorsal tegmental nucleus; LHA, lateral hypothalamic area; NA, noradrenalin; NAc, nucleus accumbens; NPY, neuropeptide Y; POA, preoptic area; POMC, proopiomelanocortin; PPT, pedunculopontine tegmental nucleus; SCN, suprachiasmatic nucleus; TMN, tuberomammillary nucleus; VTA, ventral tegmental area.

narcolepsy patients. Interestingly, drug addiction hardly occurs in these patients. This finding suggests that the orexin system mediates the establishment of drug addiction. The LHA, where orexin neurons exist, is a brain region historically implicated in reward and motivation, and orexin neurons project to many brain areas including the LC, nucleus accumbens, and VTA (Fadel and Deutch, 2002) that are implicated in behavioral responses to drugs of abuse. Orexin directly activates VTA dopaminergic neurons (Nakamura et al., 2000; Korotkova et al., 2003). ICV or local VTA infusion of orexin drives behavior motivated by either food or drug rewards (Sakurai et al., 1998; Boutrel et al., 2005; Harris et al., 2005).

It was demonstrated that orexin A input to the VTA potentiates *N*-methyl-D-aspartate receptor (NMDAR)-mediated neurotransmission via a PLC/PKC-dependent insertion of NMDARs in VTA dopamine neuron synapses (Borgland et al., 2006). Furthermore, intra-VTA microinjection of an OX1R antagonist abolished a conditioned place preference for morphine (Narita et al., 2006) and locomotor sensitization to cocaine (Borgland et al., 2006). These data indicate that orexin signaling plays an important role in neural plasticity relevant to addiction in the VTA.

## CONCLUDING REMARKS

Although the name orexin is derived from the word orexigenic after its function in feeding, mounting evidence has revealed various physiological roles for orexin other than feeding, such as maintenance of sleep, autonomous regulation, and reward processing. Orexin neurons in the LHA are anatomically well placed to provide a link between the limbic system, energy homeostasis, and brain stem monoaminergic or cholinergic neurons. Like the hypothalamus where orexin neurons exist, orexin neurons themselves monitor various physiological conditions and coordinate various behaviors to respond to environmental change adequately (**Figure 2**). For example, feeding behaviors affect the activity of orexin neurons through changes in concentration of glucose or amino acids, and these changes modulate the vigilance state, regulating aspects of the autonomic nervous system such as blood pressure, heart rate, and thermogenesis at the same time. These findings indicate a critical role for orexin neurons in the regulation of vigilance states, according to internal and external environments, for survival.

By combining viral-mediated tracing, electrophysiology, and optogenetic manipulations, it might be determined that there are several subpopulations of orexin neurons that project to different target areas. For example, the distribution pattern of orexin neurons appears to be divided into two groups: medial and lateral. Some of the input projections to orexin neurons demonstrate a preference between these two areas as well. With new tools to manipulate specific neuronal projections, we can now study physiological differences within the orexin system. These upcoming findings may reveal that discrete functional units underlie the integral role of the orexin system.

## ACKNOWLEDGMENTS

This study was supported by JST PRESTO program and Grant-in-Aid for Scientific Research (B) (23300142), Grant-in-Aid for Scientific Research on Innovative Area "Mesoscopic Neurocircuitry" (23115103) from the Ministry of Education, Culture, Sports, Science and Technology (MEXT) of Japan (Akihiro Yamanaka), and Grant-in-Aid for Young Scientists (B) (24790192) (Ayumu Inutsuka).

## REFERENCES


Abrahamson, E. E., Leak, R. K., and Moore, R. Y. (2001). The suprachiasmatic nucleus projects to posterior hypothalamic arousal systems. *Neuroreport* 12, 435–440.

Adamantidis, A. R., Zhang, F., Aravanis, A. M., Deisseroth, K., and De Lecea, L. (2007). Neural substrates of awakening probed with optogenetic control of hypocretin neurons. *Nature* 450, 420–424.

Alexander, G. M., Rogan, S. C., Abbas, A. I., Armbruster, B. N., Pei, Y., Allen, J. A., et al. (2009). Remote control of neuronal activity in transgenic mice expressing evolved G protein-coupled receptors. *Neuron* 63, 27–39.

Allen, Y. S., Adrian, T. E., Allen, J. M., Tatemoto, K., Crow, T. J., Bloom, S. R., et al. (1983). Neuropeptide Y distribution in the rat brain. *Science* 221, 877–879.

Armbruster, B. N., Li, X., Pausch, M. H., Herlitze, S., and Roth, B. L. (2007). Evolving the lock to fit the key to create a family of G protein-coupled receptors potently activated by an inert ligand. *Proc. Natl. Acad. Sci. U.S.A.* 104, 5163–5168.

Bernardis, L. L., and Bellinger, L. L. (1996). The lateral hypothalamic area revisited: ingestive behavior. *Neurosci. Biobehav. Rev.* 20, 189–287.

Borgland, S. L., Taha, S. A., Sarti, F., Fields, H. L., and Bonci, A. (2006). Orexin A in the VTA is critical for the induction of synaptic plasticity and behavioral sensitization to cocaine. *Neuron* 49, 589–601.

Bourgin, P., Huitron-Resendiz, S., Spier, A. D., Fabre, V., Morte, B., Criado, J. R., et al. (2000). Hypocretin-1 modulates rapid eye movement sleep through activation of locus coeruleus neurons. *J. Neurosci.* 20, 7760–7765.

Boutrel, B., Kenny, P. J., Specio, S. E., Martin-Fardon, R., Markou, A., Koob, G. F., et al. (2005). Role for hypocretin in mediating stress-induced reinstatement of cocaine-seeking behavior. *Proc. Natl. Acad. Sci. U.S.A.* 102, 19168–19173.

Broberger, C., De Lecea, L., Sutcliffe, J. G., and Hokfelt, T. (1998). Hypocretin/orexin- and melanin-concentrating hormone-expressing cells form distinct populations in the rodent lateral hypothalamus: relationship to the neuropeptide Y and agouti gene-related protein systems. *J. Comp. Neurol.* 402, 460–474.

Brown, R. E., Sergeeva, O. A., Eriksson, K. S., and Haas, H. L. (2002). Convergent excitation of dorsal raphe serotonin neurons by multiple arousal systems (orexin/hypocretin, histamine and noradrenaline). *J. Neurosci.* 22, 8850–8859.

Burdakov, D., Gerasimenko, O., and Verkhratsky, A. (2005). Physiological changes in glucose differentially modulate the excitability of hypothalamic melanin-concentrating hormone and orexin neurons in situ. *J. Neurosci.* 25, 2429–2433.

Burlet, S., Tyler, C. J., and Leonard, C. S. (2002). Direct and indirect excitation of laterodorsal tegmental neurons by Hypocretin/Orexin peptides: implications for wakefulness and narcolepsy. *J. Neurosci.* 22, 2862–2872.

Campbell, R. E., Smith, M. S., Allen, S. E., Grayson, B. E., Ffrench-Mullen, J. M., and Grove, K. L. (2003). Orexin neurons express a functional pancreatic polypeptide Y4 receptor. *J. Neurosci.* 23, 1487–1497.

Carter, M. E., Adamantidis, A., Ohtsu, H., Deisseroth, K., and De Lecea, L. (2009). Sleep homeostasis modulates hypocretin-mediated sleep-to-wake transitions. *J. Neurosci.* 29, 10939–10949.

Carter, M. E., Brill, J., Bonnavion, P., Huguenard, J. R., Huerta, R., and De Lecea, L. (2012). Mechanism for Hypocretin-mediated sleep-to-wake transitions. *Proc. Natl. Acad. Sci. U.S.A.* 109, E2635–E2644.

Carter, M. E., Yizhar, O., Chikahisa, S., Nguyen, H., Adamantidis, A., Nishino, S., et al. (2010). Tuning arousal with optogenetic modulation of locus coeruleus neurons. *Nat. Neurosci.* 13, 1526–1533.

Chemelli, R. M., Willie, J. T., Sinton, C. M., Elmquist, J. K., Scammell, T., Lee, C., et al. (1999). Narcolepsy in orexin knockout mice: molecular genetics of sleep regulation. *Cell* 98, 437–451.

Chou, T. C., Lee, C. E., Lu, J., Elmquist, J. K., Hara, J., Willie, J. T., et al. (2001). Orexin (hypocretin) neurons contain dynorphin. *J. Neurosci.* 21, RC168.

Chou, T. C., Scammell, T. E., Gooley, J. J., Gaus, S. E., Saper, C. B., and Lu, J. (2003). Critical role of dorsomedial hypothalamic nucleus in a wide range of behavioral circadian rhythms. *J. Neurosci.* 23, 10691–10702.

Chronwall, B. M., Dimaggio, D. A., Massari, V. J., Pickel, V. M., Ruggiero, D. A., and O'Donohue, T. L. (1985). The anatomy of neuropeptide-Y-containing neurons in rat brain. *Neuroscience* 15, 1159–1181.

Clark, J. T., Kalra, P. S., Crowley, W. R., and Kalra, S. P. (1984). Neuropeptide Y and human pancreatic polypeptide stimulate feeding behavior in rats. *Endocrinology* 115, 427–429.

Date, Y., Ueta, Y., Yamashita, H., Yamaguchi, H., Matsukura, S., Kangawa, K., et al. (1999). Orexins, orexigenic hypothalamic peptides, interact with autonomic, neuroendocrine and neuroregulatory systems. *Proc. Natl. Acad. Sci. U.S.A.* 96, 748–753.

Deboer, T., Overeem, S., Visser, N. A., Duindam, H., Frolich, M., Lammers, G. J., et al. (2004). Convergence of circadian and sleep regulatory mechanisms on hypocretin-1. *Neuroscience* 129, 727–732.

de Lecea, L., Kilduff, T. S., Peyron, C., Gao, X., Foye, P. E., Danielson, P. E., et al. (1998). The hypocretins: hypothalamus-specific peptides with neuroexcitatory activity. *Proc. Natl. Acad. Sci. U.S.A.* 95, 322–327.

Eggermann, E., Serafin, M., Bayer, L., Machard, D., Saint-Mleux, B., Jones, B. E., et al. (2001). Orexins/hypocretins excite basal forebrain cholinergic neurones. *Neuroscience* 108, 177–181.

Elias, C. F., Saper, C. B., Maratos-Flier, E., Tritos, N. A., Lee, C., Kelly, J., et al. (1998). Chemically defined projections linking the mediobasal hypothalamus and the lateral hypothalamic area. *J. Comp. Neurol.* 402, 442–459.

Fadel, J., and Deutch, A. Y. (2002). Anatomical substrates of orexin-dopamine interactions: lateral hypothalamic projections to the ventral tegmental area. *Neuroscience* 111, 379–387.

Fu, L. Y., Acuna-Goycolea, C., and van den Pol, A. N. (2004). Neuropeptide Y inhibits hypocretin/orexin neurons by multiple presynaptic and postsynaptic mechanisms: tonic depression of the hypothalamic arousal system. *J. Neurosci.* 24, 8741–8751.

Hagan, J. J., Leslie, R. A., Patel, S., Evans, M. L., Wattam, T. A., Holmes, S., et al. (1999). Orexin A activates locus coeruleus cell firing and increases arousal in the rat. *Proc. Natl. Acad. Sci. U.S.A.* 96, 10911–10916.

Hara, J., Beuckmann, C. T., Nambu, T., Willie, J. T., Chemelli, R. M., Sinton, C. M., et al. (2001). Genetic ablation of orexin neurons in mice results in narcolepsy, hypophagia, and obesity. *Neuron* 30, 345–354.

Hara, J., Yanagisawa, M., and Sakurai, T. (2005). Difference in obesity phenotype between orexin-knockout mice and orexin neuron-deficient mice with same genetic background and environmental conditions. *Neurosci. Lett.* 380, 239–242.

Harris, G. C., Wimmer, M., and Aston-Jones, G. (2005). A role for lateral hypothalamic orexin neurons in reward seeking. *Nature* 437, 556–559.

Honda, Y., Doi, Y., Ninomiya, R., and Ninomiya, C. (1986). Increased frequency of non-insulin-dependent diabetes mellitus among narcoleptic patients. *Sleep* 9, 254–259.

Hondo, M., Furutani, N., Yamasaki, M., Watanabe, M., and Sakurai, T. (2011). Orexin neurons receive glycinergic innervations. *PLoS ONE* 6:e25076. doi: 10.1371/journal.pone.0025076

Horvath, T. L., Diano, S., and van den Pol, A. N. (1999a). Synaptic interaction between hypocretin (orexin) and neuropeptide Y cells in the rodent and primate hypothalamus: a novel circuit implicated in metabolic and endocrine regulations. *J. Neurosci.* 19, 1072–1087.

Horvath, T. L., Peyron, C., Diano, S., Ivanov, A., Aston-Jones, G., Kilduff, T. S., et al. (1999b). Hypocretin (orexin) activation and synaptic innervation of the locus coeruleus noradrenergic system. *J. Comp. Neurol.* 415, 145–159.

Huang, Z. L., Qu, W. M., Li, W. D., Mochizuki, T., Eguchi, N., Watanabe, T., et al. (2001). Arousal effect of orexin A depends on activation of the histaminergic system. *Proc. Natl. Acad. Sci. U.S.A.* 98, 9965–9970.

Karnani, M. M., Apergis-Schoute, J., Adamantidis, A., Jensen, L. T., De Lecea, L., Fugger, L., et al. (2011a). Activation of central orexin/hypocretin neurons by dietary amino acids. *Neuron* 72, 616–629.

Karnani, M. M., Venner, A., Jensen, L. T., Fugger, L., and Burdakov, D. (2011b). Direct and indirect control of orexin/hypocretin neurons by glycine receptors. *J. Physiol.* 589, 639–651.

Kayaba, Y., Nakamura, A., Kasuya, Y., Ohuchi, T., Yanagisawa, M., Komuro, I., et al. (2003). Attenuated defense response and low basal blood pressure in orexin knockout mice. *Am. J. Physiol. Regul. Integr. Comp. Physiol.* 285, R581–R593.

Kohlmeier, K. A., Watanabe, S., Tyler, C. J., Burlet, S., and Leonard, C. S. (2008). Dual orexin actions on dorsal raphe and laterodorsal tegmentum neurons: noisy cation current activation and selective enhancement of Ca2+ transients mediated by L-type calcium channels. *J. Neurophysiol.* 100, 2265–2281.

Korotkova, T. M., Sergeeva, O. A., Eriksson, K. S., Haas, H. L., and Brown, R. E. (2003). Excitation of ventral tegmental area dopaminergic and nondopaminergic neurons by orexins/hypocretins. *J. Neurosci.* 23, 7–11.

Kunii, K., Yamanaka, A., Nambu, T., Matsuzaki, I., Goto, K., and Sakurai, T. (1999). Orexins/hypocretins regulate drinking behaviour. *Brain Res.* 842, 256–261.

Lammel, S., Lim, B. K., Ran, C., Huang, K. W., Betley, M. J., Tye, K. M., et al. (2012). Input-specific control of reward and aversion in the ventral tegmental area. *Nature* 491, 212–217.

Leak, R. K., and Moore, R. Y. (2001). Topographic organization of suprachiasmatic nucleus projection neurons. *J. Comp. Neurol.* 433, 312–334.

Li, Y., Gao, X. B., Sakurai, T., and van den Pol, A. N. (2002). Hypocretin/Orexin excites hypocretin neurons via a local glutamate neuron-A potential mechanism for orchestrating the hypothalamic arousal system. *Neuron* 36, 1169–1181.

Li, Y., and van den Pol, A. N. (2005). Direct and indirect inhibition by catecholamines of hypocretin/orexin neurons. *J. Neurosci.* 25, 173–183.

Lin, L., Faraco, J., Li, R., Kadotani, H., Rogers, W., Lin, X., et al. (1999). The sleep disorder canine narcolepsy is caused by a mutation in the hypocretin (orexin) receptor 2 gene. *Cell* 98, 365–376.

Liu, R. J., van den Pol, A. N., and Aghajanian, G. K. (2002). Hypocretins (orexins) regulate serotonin neurons in the dorsal raphe nucleus by excitatory direct and inhibitory indirect actions. *J. Neurosci.* 22, 9453–9464.

Lu, J., Bjorkum, A. A., Xu, M., Gaus, S. E., Shiromani, P. J., and Saper, C. B. (2002). Selective activation of the extended ventrolateral preoptic nucleus during rapid eye movement sleep. *J. Neurosci.* 22, 4568–4576.

Lubkin, M., and Stricker-Krongrad, A. (1998). Independent feeding and metabolic actions of orexins in mice. *Biochem. Biophys. Res. Commun.* 253, 241–245.

Ma, X., Zubcevic, L., Bruning, J. C., Ashcroft, F. M., and Burdakov, D. (2007). Electrical inhibition of identified anorexigenic POMC neurons by orexin/hypocretin. *J. Neurosci.* 27, 1529–1533.

Marcus, J. N., Aschkenasi, C. J., Lee, C. E., Chemelli, R. M., Saper, C. B., Yanagisawa, M., et al. (2001). Differential expression of orexin receptors 1 and 2 in the rat brain. *J. Comp. Neurol.* 435, 6–25.

Maskos, U., Kissa, K., St Cloment, C., and Brulet, P. (2002). Retrograde trans-synaptic transfer of green fluorescent protein allows the genetic mapping of neuronal circuits in transgenic mice. *Proc. Natl. Acad. Sci. U.S.A.* 99, 10120–10125.

Mieda, M., Hasegawa, E., Kisanuki, Y. Y., Sinton, C. M., Yanagisawa, M., and Sakurai, T. (2011). Differential roles of orexin receptor-1 and -2 in the regulation of non-REM and REM sleep. *J. Neurosci.* 31, 6518–6526.

Mieda, M., Williams, S. C., Sinton, C. M., Richardson, J. A., Sakurai, T., and Yanagisawa, M. (2004). Orexin neurons function in an efferent pathway of a food-entrainable circadian oscillator in eliciting food-anticipatory activity and wakefulness. *J. Neurosci.* 24, 10493–10501.

Moriguchi, T., Sakurai, T., Takahashi, S., Goto, K., and Yamamoto, M. (2002). The human prepro-orexin gene regulatory region that activates gene expression in the lateral region and represses it in the medial regions of the hypothalamus. *J. Biol. Chem.* 277, 16985–16992.

Muraki, Y., Yamanaka, A., Tsujino, N., Kilduff, T. S., Goto, K., and Sakurai, T. (2004). Serotonergic regulation of the orexin/hypocretin neurons through the 5-HT1A receptor. *J. Neurosci.* 24, 7159–7166.

Muroya, S., Funahashi, H., Yamanaka, A., Kohno, D., Uramura, K., Nambu, T., et al. (2004). Orexins (hypocretins) directly interact with neuropeptide Y, POMC and glucose-responsive neurons to regulate Ca 2+ signaling in a reciprocal manner to leptin: orexigenic neuronal pathways in the mediobasal hypothalamus. *Eur. J. Neurosci.* 19, 1524–1534.

Nakamura, T., Uramura, K., Nambu, T., Yada, T., Goto, K., Yanagisawa, M., et al. (2000). Orexin-induced hyperlocomotion and stereotypy are mediated by the dopaminergic system. *Brain Res.* 873, 181–187.

Nambu, T., Sakurai, T., Mizukami, K., Hosoya, Y., Yanagisawa, M., and Goto, K. (1999). Distribution of orexin neurons in the adult rat brain. *Brain Res.* 827, 243–260.

Narita, M., Nagumo, Y., Hashimoto, S., Khotib, J., Miyatake, M., Sakurai, T., et al. (2006). Direct involvement of orexinergic systems in the activation of the mesolimbic dopamine pathway and related behaviors induced by morphine. *J. Neurosci.* 26, 398–405.

Nishino, S., Ripley, B., Overeem, S., Lammers, G. J., and Mignot, E. (2000). Hypocretin (orexin) deficiency in human narcolepsy. *Lancet* 355, 39–40.

Peyron, C., Faraco, J., Rogers, W., Ripley, B., Overeem, S., Charnay, Y., et al. (2000). A mutation in a case of early onset narcolepsy and a generalized absence of hypocretin peptides in human narcoleptic brains. *Nat. Med.* 6, 991–997.

Peyron, C., Tighe, D. K., van den Pol, A. N., De Lecea, L., Heller, H. C., Sutcliffe, J. G., et al. (1998). Neurons containing hypocretin (orexin) project to multiple neuronal systems. *J. Neurosci.* 18, 9996–10015.

Piper, D. C., Upton, N., Smith, M. I., and Hunter, A. J. (2000). The novel brain neuropeptide, orexin-A, modulates the sleep-wake cycle of rats. *Eur. J. Neurosci.* 12, 726–730.

Richardson, K. A., and Aston-Jones, G. (2012). Lateral hypothalamic orexin/hypocretin neurons that project to ventral tegmental area are differentially activated with morphine preference. *J. Neurosci.* 32, 3809–3817.

Sakai, K. (2012). Discharge properties of presumed cholinergic and noncholinergic laterodorsal tegmental neurons related to cortical activation in non-anesthetized mice. *Neuroscience* 224C, 172–190.

Sakurai, T., Amemiya, A., Ishii, M., Matsuzaki, I., Chemelli, R. M., Tanaka, H., et al. (1998). Orexins and orexin receptors: a family of hypothalamic neuropeptides and G protein-coupled receptors that regulate feeding behavior. *Cell* 92, 573–585.

Sakurai, T., Moriguchi, T., Furuya, K., Kajiwara, N., Nakamura, T., Yanagisawa, M., et al. (1999). Structure and function of human prepro-orexin gene. *J. Biol. Chem.* 274, 17771–17776.

Sakurai, T., Nagata, R., Yamanaka, A., Kawamura, H., Tsujino, N., Muraki, Y., et al. (2005). Input of orexin/hypocretin neurons revealed by a genetically encoded tracer in mice. *Neuron* 46, 297–308.

Saper, C. B., Scammell, T. E., and Lu, J. (2005). Hypothalamic regulation of sleep and circadian rhythms. *Nature* 437, 1257–1263.

Sasaki, K., Suzuki, M., Mieda, M., Tsujino, N., Roth, B., and Sakurai, T. (2011). Pharmacogenetic modulation of orexin neurons alters sleep/wakefulness states in mice. *PLoS ONE* 6:e20360. doi: 10.1371/journal.pone.0020360

Sellayah, D., Bharaj, P., and Sikder, D. (2011). Orexin is required for brown adipose tissue development, differentiation, and function. *Cell Metab.* 14, 478–490.

Sherin, J. E., Elmquist, J. K., Torrealba, F., and Saper, C. B. (1998). Innervation of histaminergic tuberomammillary neurons by GABAergic and galaninergic neurons in the ventrolateral preoptic nucleus of the rat. *J. Neurosci.* 18, 4705–4721.

Sherin, J. E., Shiromani, P. J., Mccarley, R. W., and Saper, C. B. (1996). Activation of ventrolateral preoptic neurons during sleep. *Science* 271, 216–219.

Shirasaka, T., Nakazato, M., Matsukura, S., Takasaki, M., and Kannan, H. (1999). Sympathetic and cardiovascular actions of orexins in conscious rats. *Am. J. Physiol.* 277, R1780–R1785.

Silva, J. P., Von Meyenn, F., Howell, J., Thorens, B., Wolfrum, C., and Stoffel, M. (2009). Regulation of adaptive behaviour during fasting by hypothalamic Foxa2. *Nature* 462, 646–650.

Stanley, B. G., and Leibowitz, S. F. (1985). Neuropeptide Y injected in the paraventricular hypothalamus: a powerful stimulant of feeding behavior. *Proc. Natl. Acad. Sci. U.S.A.* 82, 3940–3943.

Steininger, T. L., Gong, H., Mcginty, D., and Szymusiak, R. (2001). Subregional organization of preoptic area/anterior hypothalamic projections to arousal-related monoaminergic cell groups. *J. Comp. Neurol.* 429, 638–653.

Takakusaki, K., Takahashi, K., Saitoh, K., Harada, H., Okumura, T., Kayama, Y., et al. (2005). Orexinergic projections to the cat midbrain mediate alternation of emotional behavioural states from locomotion to cataplexy. *J. Physiol.* 568, 1003–1020.

Thannickal, T. C., Moore, R. Y., Nienhuis, R., Ramanathan, L., Gulyani, S., Aldrich, M., et al. (2000). Reduced number of hypocretin neurons in human narcolepsy. *Neuron* 27, 469–474.

Tsujino, N., Yamanaka, A., Ichiki, K., Muraki, Y., Kilduff, T. S., Yagami, K., et al. (2005). Cholecystokinin activates orexin/hypocretin neurons through the cholecystokinin A receptor. *J. Neurosci.* 25, 7459–7469.

Tsunematsu, T., Fu, L. Y., Yamanaka, A., Ichiki, K., Tanoue, A., Sakurai, T., et al. (2008). Vasopressin increases locomotion through a V1a receptor in orexin/hypocretin neurons: implications for water homeostasis. *J. Neurosci.* 28, 228–238.

Tsunematsu, T., Kilduff, T. S., Boyden, E. S., Takahashi, S., Tominaga, M., and Yamanaka, A. (2011). Acute optogenetic silencing of orexin/hypocretin neurons induces slow-wave sleep in mice. *J. Neurosci.* 31, 10529–10539.

Tsunematsu, T., Tanaka, K. F., Yamanaka, A., and Koizumi, A. (2012). Ectopic expression of melanopsin in orexin/hypocretin neurons enables control of wakefulness of mice in vivo by blue light. *Neurosci Res.* doi: 10.1016/j.neures.2012.07.005 [Epub ahead of print].

Tupone, D., Madden, C. J., Cano, G., and Morrison, S. F. (2011). An orexinergic projection from perifornical hypothalamus to raphe pallidus increases rat brown adipose tissue thermogenesis. *J. Neurosci.* 31, 15944–15955.

Williams, R. H., Jensen, L. T., Verkhratsky, A., Fugger, L., and Burdakov, D. (2007). Control of hypothalamic orexin neurons by acid and CO2. *Proc. Natl. Acad. Sci. U.S.A.* 104, 10685–10690.

Willie, J. T., Chemelli, R. M., Sinton, C. M., Tokita, S., Williams, S. C., Kisanuki, Y. Y., et al. (2003). Distinct narcolepsy syndromes in Orexin receptor-2 and Orexin null mice: molecular genetic dissection of Non-REM and REM sleep regulatory processes. *Neuron* 38, 715–730.

Winsky-Sommerer, R., Yamanaka, A., Diano, S., Borok, E., Roberts, A. J., Sakurai, T., et al. (2004). Interaction between the corticotropin-releasing factor system and hypocretins (orexins): a novel circuit mediating stress response. *J. Neurosci.* 24, 11439–11448.

Wollmann, G., Acuna-Goycolea, C., and van den Pol, A. N. (2005). Direct excitation of hypocretin/orexin cells by extracellular ATP at P2X receptors. *J. Neurophysiol.* 94, 2195–2206.

Xi, M. C., Morales, F. R., and Chase, M. H. (2001). Effects on sleep and wakefulness of the injection of hypocretin-1 (orexin-A) into the laterodorsal tegmental nucleus of the cat. *Brain Res.* 901, 259–264.

Xie, X., Crowder, T. L., Yamanaka, A., Morairty, S. R., Lewinter, R. D., Sakurai, T., et al. (2006). GABA(B) receptor-mediated modulation of hypocretin/orexin neurones in mouse hypothalamus. *J. Physiol.* 574, 399–414.

Yamanaka, A., Beuckmann, C. T., Willie, J. T., Hara, J., Tsujino, N., Mieda, M., et al. (2003a). Hypothalamic orexin neurons regulate arousal according to energy balance in mice. *Neuron* 38, 701–713.

Yamanaka, A., Muraki, Y., Tsujino, N., Goto, K., and Sakurai, T. (2003b). Regulation of orexin neurons by the monoaminergic and cholinergic systems. *Biochem. Biophys. Res. Commun.* 303, 120–129.

Yamanaka, A., Kunii, K., Nambu, T., Tsujino, N., Sakai, A., Matsuzaki, I., et al. (2000). Orexin-induced food intake involves neuropeptide Y pathway. *Brain Res.* 859, 404–409.

Yamanaka, A., Muraki, Y., Ichiki, K., Tsujino, N., Kilduff, T. S., Goto, K., et al. (2006). Orexin neurons are directly and indirectly regulated by catecholamines in a complex manner. *J. Neurophysiol.* 96, 284–298.

Yamanaka, A., Tabuchi, S., Tsunematsu, T., Fukazawa, Y., and Tominaga, M. (2010). Orexin directly excites orexin neurons through orexin 2 receptor. *J. Neurosci.* 30, 12642–12652.

Yamanaka, A., Tsujino, N., Funahashi, H., Honda, K., Guan, J. L., Wang, Q. P., et al. (2002). Orexins activate histaminergic neurons via the orexin 2 receptor. *Biochem. Biophys. Res. Commun.* 290, 1237–1245.

Yoshida, K., Mccormack, S., Espana, R. A., Crocker, A., and Scammell, T. E. (2006). Afferents to the orexin neurons of the rat brain. *J. Comp. Neurol.* 494, 845–861.

Zhang, W., Sakurai, T., Fukuda, Y., and Kuwaki, T. (2006). Orexin neuron-mediated skeletal muscle vasodilation and shift of baroreflex during defense response in mice. *Am. J. Physiol. Regul. Integr. Comp. Physiol.* 290, R1654–R1663.

Zhu, Y., Miwa, Y., Yamanaka, A., Yada, T., Shibahara, M., Abe, Y., et al. (2003). Orexin receptor type-1 couples exclusively to pertussis toxin-insensitive G-proteins, while orexin receptor type-2 couples to both pertussis toxin-sensitive and -insensitive G-proteins. *J. Pharmacol. Sci.* 92, 259–266.

# 2

# Stress responsiveness of the hypothalamic–pituitary–adrenal axis: age-related features of the vasopressinergic regulation

**Nadezhda D. Goncharova**[1,2]*

[1] Research Institute of Medical Primatology of Russian Academy of Medical Sciences, Sochi, Russia
[2] Sochi State University, Sochi, Russia

**Edited by:**
Hubert Vaudry, University of Rouen, France

**Reviewed by:**
James A. Carr, Texas Tech University, USA
Dóra Zelena, Institute of Experimental Medicine, Hungary

***Correspondence:**
Nadezhda D. Goncharova, Research Institute of Medical Primatology of Russian Academy of Medical Sciences, Veseloye 1, Adler, Sochi 354376, Krasnodarskii Krai, Russia.
e-mail: ndgoncharova@mail.ru

The hypothalamic–pituitary–adrenal (HPA) axis plays a key role in adaptation to environmental stresses. Parvicellular neurons of the hypothalamic paraventricular nucleus secrete corticotrophin releasing hormone (CRH) and arginine vasopressin (AVP) into pituitary portal system; CRH and AVP stimulate adrenocorticotropic hormone (ACTH) release through specific G-protein-coupled membrane receptors on pituitary corticotrophs, CRHR1 for CRH and V1b for AVP; the adrenal gland cortex secretes glucocorticoids in response to ACTH. The glucocorticoids activate specific receptors in brain and peripheral tissues thereby triggering the necessary metabolic, immune, neuromodulatory, and behavioral changes to resist stress. While importance of CRH, as a key hypothalamic factor of HPA axis regulation in basal and stress conditions in most species, is generally recognized, role of AVP remains to be clarified. This review focuses on the role of AVP in the regulation of stress responsiveness of the HPA axis with emphasis on the effects of aging on vasopressinergic regulation of HPA axis stress responsiveness. Under most of the known stressors, AVP is necessary for acute ACTH secretion but in a context-specific manner. The current data on the AVP role in regulation of HPA responsiveness to chronic stress in adulthood are rather contradictory. The importance of the vasopressinergic regulation of the HPA stress responsiveness is greatest during fetal development, in neonatal period, and in the lactating adult. Aging associated with increased variability in several parameters of HPA function including basal state, responsiveness to stressors, and special testing. Reports on the possible role of the AVP/V1b receptor system in the increase of HPA axis hyperactivity with aging are contradictory and requires further research. Many contradictory results may be due to age and species differences in the HPA function of rodents and primates.

**Keywords: hypothalamic–pituitary–adrenal axis, vasopressin, stress, aging, V1b receptors**

## INTRODUCTION

The hypothalamic–pituitary–adrenal (HPA) axis is a key adaptive neuroendocrine system. Regulation of glucocorticoid secretion through adrenocorticotropic hormone (ACTH) is critical to life and essential to maintain the mammalian response to stressor (Pedersen et al., 2001; McEwen, 2007; Lupien et al., 2009). The HPA axis consists of the nucleus paraventricularis hypothalami (PVN), which secretes corticotrophin releasing hormone (CRH) and arginine vasopressin (AVP); the pituitary gland that is sensitive to CRH and AVP, which stimulate ACTH release; the adrenal gland cortex, which secretes the glucocorticoids, mainly cortisol in humans and non-human primates, and corticosterone in rodents, and dehydroepiandrosterone (DHEA) in humans and non-human primates in response to interaction with ACTH. DHEA and its sulfate DHEAS are important regulators of glucocorticoid activity (Yen and Laughlin, 1998; Maninger et al., 2009). The glucocorticoids act on specific receptors present in most peripheral tissues and the brain and trigger the metabolic, immune, neuromodulatory, and behavioral changes needed to cope with the impact of the stressors (Tuckermann et al., 2005; McEwen, 2007; Vegiopoulos and Herzig, 2007). In turn, the glucocorticoids act through the pituitary and limbic structures, especially the hippocampus, in a negative feedback loop to regulate the activity of CRH-producing neurons in the PVN and, thus the entire the HPA axis. The adaptive influence of the HPA axis under stress is realized not only through ACTH and the corticosteroids but also through the hypothalamic neuropeptides CRH and AVP, which are released in the brain, where they are responsible for behavioral and autonomic responses to stress (Bale and Vale, 2004; Roper et al., 2011).

In resting conditions, activity of the HPA axis shows circadian and ultradian changes with pulsatile glucocorticoid secretion that is greater in amplitude during the phase of wakefulness. This leads to higher average levels of glucocorticoids during the day in humans and most other primates and to higher activity of the HPA axis during the night in rodents (Goncharova et al., 2002; Kalsbeek et al., 2010; Russell et al., 2010; Walker et al., 2010). Stress responsiveness of the pituitary–adrenal axis in humans and non-human primates also shows the circadian rhythms with higher stress response in the afternoon and evening, and lower in the morning (Goncharova, 2006; Goncharova et al., 2006a; De Weerth et al., 2007). Rhythmicity in the HPA axis is essential for the normal functioning of the brain and other glucocorticoid responsive organs (Van Cauter et al., 1997; Lupien et al., 2002; Yoshimura et al., 2007; Goncharova et al., 2008a,b).

While the acute stress activation of the HPA axis is critical for life, chronic exposure to stressors leads to its excessive stimulation and hypercortisolemia. Hypercortisolemia plays a pathophysiological role in the development of a variety of stress-related diseases: psychiatric, reproductive, immune, metabolic, and others. It is a major factor in aging and age-related pathology (Chrousos, 2000; de Kloet et al., 2005, 2008; Perez-Neri et al., 2008). While CRH is widely recognized as a major hypothalamic factor controlling the HPA axis activity in resting conditions and under stress, the role of AVP in regulation of the HPA axis remains to be studied. Almost all current data on the role of AVP in regulation of the HPA axis were obtained in experiments on adult rodents. In the available literature, there are no review articles devoted to the role of AVP in the regulation of HPA axis stress responsiveness in aged subjects. In any event, aging is generally characterized by hyperactivation of the HPA axis, breakdown of the circadian rhythm, progressive decline in DHEA and DHEAS production, and high incidence of stress-dependent diseases, including depression, in which AVP production and the corticosteroids are of great importance (Yen and Laughlin, 1998; de Winter et al., 2003; Dinan and Scott, 2005; Kondratova and Kondratov, 2012). This review will focus on the evaluation of the role of AVP in the regulation of stress responsiveness of the HPA axis with emphasis on HPA axis vasopressinergic regulation during healthy aging in rodents as well as in humans and non-human primates.

## MECHANISMS OF HPA AXIS REGULATION

### CORTICOTROPHIN RELEASING HORMONE

Corticotrophin releasing hormone is the main physiological regulator of the HPA axis in basal conditions and in response to most acute stressors (Jacobson et al., 2000; Bale and Vale, 2004; Aguilera, 2011). CRH is a peptide consisting of 41 amino acid residues, which was discovered and sequenced by Vale et al. (1983). It is produced in the medial parvicellular neurons of the PVN, which project to the outer zone of the median eminence. There it is released into the portal system of the pituitary, which reaches the anterior lobe. CRH stimulates ACTH secretion through activation of type 1 CRH receptors (CRHR1) in the pituitary corticotrophs. CRHR1 belongs to the CRH family of G-protein-coupled membrane receptors (GPCRs) (Bale and Vale, 2004; Zorrilla and Koob, 2010).

The collection of CRH-producing neurons (CRH neurons) of the PVN is a key center of the central nervous system, integrating the neuroendocrine effects of stress, and a key part of the HPA axis. On the one hand, the CRH neuron is under the regulatory influence of numerous afferent nerve pathways that carry information about the stressor. In addition, it is regulated by glucocorticoids and it is the central link of the autoregulation mechanism in the HPA axis.

#### *Afferent regulation*

The CRH neuron receives projections from ascending catecholaminergic pathways including noradrenergic projections from the A2 noradrenergic cell group within the nucleus of the solitary tract and the locus ceruleus. It also receives input from areas of the limbic system, notably the bed nucleus of the stria terminalis, the hippocampus, and the amygdala (Herman et al., 1996; Dinan and Scott, 2005). Indirect pathways from the sensory systems in the forebrain through the amygdala and bed nucleus of the stria terminalis may stimulate CRH neurons by activating stimulatory (glutamatergic) or repressing inhibitory ($\gamma$-aminobutyric acid – GABA-ergic) interneurons (Herman et al., 1996; Arvat et al., 2002; Aguilera, 2011). There is also significant evidence in relation to the stimulatory effect of the cholinergic system on CRH secretion implemented through direct and indirect projections from both the basal forebrain and the mesopontine tegmentum (Rhodes and Rubin, 1999; Rubin and Rhodes, 2002).

#### *Glucocorticoid feedback mechanism*

Feedback mechanism plays an essential role in the regulation of CRH production and in limiting the stress response. The central sensors of feedback to the HPA axis are two corticosteroid receptors, the high-affinity mineralocorticoid receptor (MR) and the low-affinity glucocorticoid receptors (GR), which are expressed in the brain and on the corticotrophs of the pituitary (Ratka et al., 1989). GRs are distributed throughout the brain, but mostly in hypothalamic neurons and corticotrophs (Jacobson and Sapolsky, 1991; Funder, 1997), whereas MRs are present in the hypothalamus and in the greatest numbers in the hippocampus (Ratka et al., 1989; Funder, 1997). A significant role of direct inhibition of transcription of pro-opiomelanocortin (POMC) and ACTH secretion by glucocorticoids in the regulation of the HPA axis by a feedback mechanism has been previously demonstrated (Autelitano et al., 1989; Dallman et al., 1994). Development of MR antagonists has enabled demonstration of the important role of glucocorticoid feedback at the suprapituitary level, probably from the hippocampus in regulation of the HPA axis both in animals and humans (Wellhoener et al., 2004; Giordano et al., 2005). The presence of GRs in CRH neurons (Liposits et al., 1987), as well as a demonstrated inhibitory effect of intra-PVN glucocorticoid injection on CRH mRNA, and the reduction in CRH promoter activity in reporter gene assays following incubation with glucocorticoids, give reason to believe that a direct inhibitory effect of glucocorticoids on CRH transcription underlies the central mechanisms of feedback regulation of CRH transcription and desensitization of the HPA axis to stress responses (Kovacs et al., 1986; Sawchenko, 1987; Harbuz and Lightman, 1989; Makino et al., 1995; Fenoglio et al., 2004; Aguilera, 2011).

### ARGININE VASOPRESSIN

#### *Distribution of AVP*

While it is generally accepted that CRH is a critical coordinator of HPA axis function in resting conditions and in response to stress (Aguilera, 1998, 2011; Jacobson et al., 2000; Bale and Vale, 2004), the role of AVP in the regulation of the HPA axis remains a subject of active research. Following its identification in 1954, AVP, a nonapeptide, was considered the principal factor in the regulation of ACTH secretion until the subsequent identification of CRH, which led to the replacement of AVP with CRH as the principle regulator of the HPA axis. Nevertheless, AVP is still considered as an important regulator of the HPA axis (Antoni, 1993; Herman, 1995; Volpi et al., 2004; Aguilera, 2011). In addition, AVP is seen as a hormonal regulator of water homeostasis and has significant effects on vascular tone (Knepper, 1997; Koshimizu et al., 2006). AVP is also believed to regulate circadian rhythms (Kalsbeek et al., 2010; Kondratova and Kondratov, 2012) and numerous central functions such as synaptic transmission, control of body temperature, memory, and behavior (Barberis and Tribollet, 1996; Wersinger et al., 2002).

Knowledge of the functional anatomy, physiology, and pathophysiology of AVP in the regulation of the HPA axis is mainly based on studies carried out on rodents. There are two major vasopressinergic systems in the brain. The first system consists of hypothalamic magnocellular neurons in the PVN and supraoptic nucleus, which project to the neurohypophysis and deliver AVP and oxytocin to the peripheral circulation; it is largely responsible for the peripheral actions of AVP that maintain water homeostasis and blood pressure (Knepper, 1997; Koshimizu et al., 2006). The second system is represented by the CRH-producing parvicellular neurons of the PVN, which also synthesizes AVP. AVP produced by the latter neuron is secreted into the pituitary portal circulation from axon terminals in the external zone of the median eminence; they are involved in regulation of the HPA axis (Antoni, 1993). It has been shown in non-stressed rats that 50% of CRH neurosecretory cells coexpress AVP (Whitnall, 1987). In humans, there is evidence that all CRH neurons in the hypothalamus may contain AVP (Mouri et al., 1993; Dinan and Scott, 2005). In primates, including humans, large numbers of immunoreactive AVP neurons have been demonstrated in the limbic system, notably the bed nucleus of the stria terminalis, the hippocampus and the amygdala, and also in the pituitary intermediate lobe, the granular layers of cerebellar cortex, and the dentate gyrus. Lower levels are found in the medial habenula, adenohypophysis, area postrema, pineal body, subfornical and subcommissural organs (see review Dinan and Scott, 2005). It is thought that the AVP levels in the pituitary portal vascular system is derived from the PVN, but morphological and neurochemical studies suggest that AVP from supraoptic magnocellular AVP-secreting cells also accesses the hypophyseal portal blood (Antoni et al., 1990; Dinan and Scott, 2005). AVP neurons in the medial amygdala and the bed nucleus of the stria terminalis project to the lateral septum and ventral hippocampal sites affecting memory and behavior (Caff et al., 1987; Aguilera, 2011). Finally, AVP is expressed in the suprachiasmatic nucleus (SCN), which is involved in the regulation of circadian rhythms (Rhodes and Rubin, 1999; Arima et al., 2002; Kalsbeek et al., 2010; Kondratova and Kondratov, 2012).

#### *AVP receptors*

The actions of AVP are mediated through interaction with specific plasma membrane receptors of target cells that have been identified and cloned (Jard et al., 1987; Birnbaumer, 2000; Derick et al., 2004). AVP receptors belong to the family of GPCRs, i.e., they transmit a signal to the cell through G-protein (guanyl-nucleotide-binding protein) (Jard et al., 1987; Birnbaumer, 2000; Thibonnier et al., 2002; Derick et al., 2004). AVP receptors have been divided into three major types: V1a, V1b (or V3), and V2 according to their pharmacological and G-protein-coupled properties. The V1a and V1b subtypes are both coupled to Gq and signal via phospholipase C (Jard et al., 1987; Thibonnier et al., 2002; Roper et al., 2011). The V2 receptor subtype is coupled to Gs that signal via adenylate cyclase (Thibonnier et al., 2002; Derick et al., 2004). The V1a receptor is predominantly found in vascular smooth muscle where it is involved in control of vasoconstrictor effects and blood pressure (Koshimizu et al., 2006; Vantyghem et al., 2011). The renal V2 AVP receptor is responsible for water resorption in collecting ducts of the kidney by promoting the translocation of aquaporin-2 channels to the plasma membrane (Knepper, 1997). The V1b receptor is primarily located in corticotrophs of the anterior pituitary where it stimulates ACTH release (Antoni, 1993; Derick et al., 2004; Roper et al., 2011). A number of studies utilizing *in situ* hybridization histochemistry and reverse transcription-polymerase chain reaction in rodents have shown that V1b receptor mRNA is also expressed at a lower level in some brain regions (hippocampus, PVN, olfactory bulb, and amygdala) and a number of peripheral tissues (kidney, pancreas, heart, lung, breast, adrenal medulla, and others) (Grazzini et al., 1996; Roper et al., 2011), where its function is unknown (Roper et al., 2011).

#### *Effects of AVP on the HPA axis function and interaction with CRH*

The ability of both neuropeptides CRH and AVP to stimulate the secretion of ACTH has been demonstrated in humans (DeBold et al., 1984; Salata et al., 1988; Favrod-Coune et al., 1993) and various other species, including non-human primates (Goncharova and Lapin, 2002; Goncharova, 2009a), rats (Vale et al., 1983; Antoni, 1993), mice (Muller et al., 2000; Lolait et al., 2007), horses (Evans et al., 1993), and sheep (McFarlane et al., 1995; Hassan et al., 2003). The relative importance of each seems to vary depending on the species. For example, in humans (DeBold et al., 1984; Favrod-Coune et al., 1993), non-human primates (Goncharova, 2009a), rats (Vale et al., 1983; Antoni, 1993; Serradeil-Le Gal et al., 2005), and horses (Evans et al., 1993), CRH is a much more potent secretagogue than AVP. At the same time, some groups have reported that in the sheep AVP is the more potent secretagogue (Familari et al., 1989; Hassan et al., 2003). In all cases, a marked synergism between CRH and AVP has been observed (Antoni, 1993; Favrod-Coune et al., 1993; Aguilera et al., 1994; Aguilera, 1998; Serradeil-Le Gal et al., 2005). The impact of AVP on ACTH secretion is often regarded as ancillary to CRH as far as AVP alone is a weak ACTH secretagogue but acts synergistically with CRH to facilitate ACTH release both in humans (DeBold et al., 1984; Salata et al., 1988; Favrod-Coune et al., 1993) and rodents (Rivier and Vale, 1983; Antoni, 1993). It has been shown that the corticotroph AVP/V1b and the CRH/CRHR1 signaling pathways converge to increase ACTH secretion (Abou-Samra et al., 1986; Roper et al., 2011). In particular, it has been suggested that AVP plays a role in stimulating the primary nuclear transcripts induced by CRH in pituitary corticotrophs (Antoni, 1993). Studies in recent years suggest that the CRH–AVP synergism may also be conditioned by change in the physical state of corticotroph V1b and CRHR1 receptors (Young et al., 2007; Roper et al., 2011). The two receptors may physically heterodimerize (Young et al., 2007).

## VASOPRESSINERGIC REGULATION OF STRESS RESPONSIVENESS OF THE HPA AXIS

### AVP IN REGULATION OF HPA AXIS REACTIVITY IN RESPONSE TO ACUTE STRESS

#### *Acute stress*

Acute immobilization stress has been observed to lead to up-regulation of AVP mRNA along with up-regulation of CRH mRNA expression in parvicellular neurons of the PVN (Bartanusz et al., 1993). Moreover, compensatory increase in basal vasopressinergic system in mice lacking the CRHR1 gene was revealed (Muller et al., 2000). All this allows us to consider AVP as an important modulator of the ACTH response to stress, as a compensatory mechanism to maintain the activity of the HPA axis when the CRH/CRHR1 signaling pathway is damaged (Muller et al., 2000). The importance of AVP along with CRH as physiological modulators of ACTH secretion in response to insulin-induced hypoglycemia has been demonstrated in humans (DeBold et al., 1984; Ellis et al., 1990).

The precise role of AVP production in response to stress remains controversial because most studies have involved indirect or correlative measurements of activation of AVP-producing neurons after exposure to stress (DeBold et al., 1984; Ellis et al., 1990; Makara et al., 2004; Lolait et al., 2007). Some of the best evidence for AVP involvement in the response of the HPA axis response to stress is derived from studies that have shown that immunoneutralization of AVP diminish the increase in plasma ACTH produced by various stressors such as restraint, insulin-induced hypoglycemia, or injection of bacterial lipopolysaccharide (LPS) (Turnbull et al., 1998; see introduction in Lolait et al., 2007). In addition, studies in which AVP levels have been sampled in pituitary portal blood indicate that AVP may be secreted preferentially over CRH in response to acute stressors such as insulin-induced hypoglycemia (Plotsky et al., 1985; Engler et al., 1989).

Nevertheless, several studies do not support the conclusion of an important role for AVP in the regulation of HPA axis stress responsiveness. Animals in some studies using modern genetic and pharmacological models to create an AVP deficit have, nevertheless shown a normal response of the HPA axis in acute stress, specifically to restraint, resident-intruder, and LPS stressors (Lolait et al., 2007; Chen et al., 2008a; Zelena et al., 2011). For example, mice lacking AVP V1b receptors exhibited normal corticosterone responses to acute physical–psychological stress in the resident-intruder paradigm (Wersinger et al., 2002).

In other studies using genetic and pharmacological models of AVP deficit the pituitary–adrenal responses to acute stress were substantially reduced. Thus, recent studies with the V1b receptor knockout mice demonstrated reduced plasma levels of ACTH and corticosterone or only ACTH in response to insulin-induced hypoglycemia (Lolait et al., 2007), forced-swimming (Tanoue et al., 2004; Stewart et al., 2008), novel environment (Stewart et al., 2008), mild restraint (Stewart et al., 2008), and in response to some of the other stressors (Roper et al., 2011) compared to wild-type mice. The use of SSR149415, the first selective V1b receptor antagonist, at 2 h after treatment significantly suppressed the increase in ACTH after a 5 min forced-swimming stress and decreased the dramatic elevation in plasma corticosterone concentrations in mice (Serradeil-Le Gal et al., 2005). Acute administration of another antagonist of V1b receptor (Org) also reduced ACTH secretion following both restraint and LPS but did not antagonize the ACTH response to noise (Spiga et al., 2009). Interestingly, the Org V1b antagonist, while reducing the stress-induced increase in ACTH secretion, had no effect on plasma corticosterone levels (Spiga et al., 2009). Similar results were obtained when another V1b receptor antagonist (SSR149415) was used: the ACTH plasma level was reduced in rats in response to restraint compared to controls, but showed no inhibitory effect on the secretion of corticosterone (Serradeil-Le Gal et al., 2003).

Findings from studies of the role of AVP in responsiveness of the HPA axis in acute stress using V1b receptor antagonists in rodents are consistent with studies of naturally AVP-deficient Brattleboro rats (Zelena et al., 2009; Makara et al., 2012). The ACTH response of homozygous animals to severe stressors, such as those mentioned above, as well as to anaphylactoid stress (hypertonic saline, egg white injection), elevated plus-maze, and novelty, was sharply decreased compared to that of heterozygous littermates. The ACTH response also was decreased in response to volume load, restraint, or aggressive attack in AVP-deficient rats. At the same time, there were no significant differences in the ACTH reaction in response to such stressors as social avoidance, footshock, and ether inhalation. Differences were also observed in the corticosterone response to the three groups of stressors. It did not change in response to the first group of stressors, decreased in parallel with ACTH in AVP-deficient rats in response to the second group of stressors and, like ACTH, did not change, in response to the third group of stressors (Zelena et al., 2009; Makara et al., 2012). Herman et al. (1996) and Zelena et al. (2009) suggest that the brain categorizes stressors and utilizes neural response pathways that vary in accord with their assigned category as well as that AVP increase the ACTH response to stress in a context-specific manner (Zelena et al., 2009).

Age can also influence the importance of AVP for the HPA axis response to acute stress. Reduced ACTH and corticosterone release was observed in AVP-deficient rats in the neonatal period, while adult rats of the same strain demonstrated a normal response of the pituitary–adrenal axis to LPS injection (Zelena et al., 2011).

#### *Basal conditions*

There is a wide range of studies on the role of AVP in the HPA axis regulation not only in response to acute stressors but during basal conditions. Studies using AVP immunoneutralization have not identified a role of AVP in basal ACTH regulation (Ono et al., 1985; Tilders et al., 1985). Studies using genetic models of AVP deficit based on knocking out the corticotroph V1b receptor resulted either in reduced (Tanoue et al., 2004) or normal (Lolait et al., 2007) resting ACTH and corticosterone levels. A selective V1b receptor antagonist (Org), which decreased restraint- and LPS-induced ACTH secretion, did not affect the resting levels or stress-induced corticosterone responses (Spiga et al., 2009). The resting pituitary ACTH concentration of homozygous Brattleboro rats appeared to be normal (Lolait et al., 1986; Zelena et al., 2009), although there was a trend toward elevated corticosterone at decapitation (Zelena et al., 2009) and also there are publications of impaired basal ACTH and corticosterone plasma levels (Burgess and Balment, 1992).

### AVP REGULATION OF HPA AXIS RESPONSIVITY TO CHRONIC STRESS

Regulation of V1b receptors in the pituitary gland appears to play a major role in corticotroph responses to chronic stressors, as a good correlation has been established between the concentration of the receptor and the secretion of ACTH by the pituitary gland (Aguilera, 1994; Aguilera et al., 1994). Furthermore, increased expression of AVP mRNA in parvicellular neurons of the PVN has been demonstrated along with a positive correlation between the density of corticotroph V1b receptors and ACTH release in response to chronic stress (Aguilera, 1994).

Numerous studies performed in rats have revealed a shift of hypothalamic CRH/AVP signal in favor of AVP in some chronic stress states. This is manifested by enhanced AVP synthesis in CRH-producing cells in parvicellular neurons of the PVN after repeated restraint (Whitnall, 1989; De Goeij et al., 1992; Bartanusz et al., 1993; Aguilera, 1994), foot shock (Sawchenko et al., 1993), intraperitoneal injection of hypertonic saline (Ma and Aguilera, 1999), and AVP storage in the CRH-containing nerve terminals in the external zone of the median eminence (De Goeij et al., 1992). An increased proportion of hypothalamic neurons coexpressing AVP has also been demonstrated with such stressors (De Goeij et al., 1992). At the same time, CRH production remained unchanged or decreased (De Goeij et al., 1992). CRH expression increased only in cases of chronic stress when circulating ACTH and glucocorticoid levels increased, for example, in response to stress caused by repeated injections of intraperitoneal hypertonic saline or footshock (Imaki et al., 1991; Ma and Aguilera, 1999).

The results of direct manipulation of the HPA axis reinforce the idea that chronic stress induces a shift of the hypothalamic CRH/AVP signal in favor of AVP. Prolonged administration of CRH by osmotic minipumps led to a reduction in CRH receptor number in the pituitary corticotrophs of control rats (Tizabi and Aguilera, 1992), which was enhanced by the simultaneous infusion of AVP. At the same time adrenalectomized Brattleboro rats lacking hypothalamic AVP, showed only a minimal reduction in CRH receptor number, which was increased by AVP infusion in the period after adrenalectomy (Tizabi and Aguilera, 1992).

Repeated restraint stress or repeated hypertonic saline injections were found to produce sustained increases in the expression of V1b receptor mRNA in the pituitary (Rabadan-Diehl et al., 1995). This suggests an up-regulation of AVP receptors in situations of chronic stress, which may explain the preserved enhanced response to novel superimposed acute stress exposure (so-called heterotypic stressor) in these animal models. Thus, the study using V1b receptor knockout mice demonstrated the importance of AVP and V1b receptor for a normal response of the HPA axis to heterotypic stressor (hypoglycemia) in chronic stress induced by repeated restraint (Tanoue et al., 2004; Lolait et al., 2007). In addition, the plasma ACTH response to repeated mild restraint, forced-swimming, and novel environments in V1b receptor knockout mice was decreased in comparison with wild-type mice (Stewart et al., 2008; Roper et al., 2011).

The sensitivity of CRH and AVP transcription to glucocorticoid feedback is markedly different (Bilezijian et al., 1987). CRH mRNA and CRH receptor mRNA levels are reduced by elevated glucocorticoids, whereas V1b receptor mRNA levels and coupling of the receptor to phospholipase C are stimulated by glucocorticoids, effects which may contribute to the refractoriness of AVP-stimulated ACTH secretion to glucocorticoid feedback (Rabadan-Diehl and Aguilera, 1998; Aguilera and Rabadan-Diehl, 2000). This suggest that vasopressinergic regulation of the HPA axis is critical for sustained corticotroph responsiveness in the presence of high circulating glucocorticoid levels during chronic stress (Rabadan-Diehl and Aguilera, 1998; Aguilera and Rabadan-Diehl, 2000).

All these findings support the proposal that CRH plays a predominantly permissive role in the HPA axis regulation in conditions of chronic stress, but AVP is a dynamic modulator of ACTH release (Plotsky, 1991; Dinan and Scott, 2005).

Some recent studies of chronic stress in naturally AVP-deficient Brattleboro rats, suggest that the role of V1b and AVP in adaptation of the HPA axis to chronic stress may not be as convincing as first thought. Experiments on Brattleboro rats and control heterozygous littermates utilized three different chronic stress models: repeated restraint to produce physical–psychological stress (Zelena et al., 2004; Makara et al., 2012); repeated short periods of morphine withdrawal (Domokos et al., 2008; Makara et al., 2012); streptozotocin induced diabetes (Zelena et al., 2006; Makara et al., 2012). The changes characteristic to chronic stress, including body weight reduction, involution of the thymus, adrenal gland hypertrophy, and increases in basal POMC mRNA and plasma corticosterone, developed in all three models, but no difference was observed between the genotypes. Both male AVP-deficient Brattleboro rats and their heterozygous littermates exposed to chronic unpredictable stress, exhibited elevated levels of POMC mRNA in the anterior lobe of the pituitary and plasma ACTH along with a less significant increase in plasma corticosterone (Varga et al., 2011). In addition, the ACTH and corticosterone response to repeated shaker stress in V1b receptor knockout mice is not different from that seen in wild-type mice (Roper et al., 2011). There are also studies using pharmacological models of AVP-deficiency that have shown adequate HPA axis responses to chronic stress in the absence of AVP (Chen et al., 2008b). These data suggest that AVP is not so important for the development of the chronic stress response.

Perhaps the contradictory results can be explained in terms of age and species differences in the HPA function of rodents and primates, including humans. Some evidence suggests that AVP is the main regulator of the HPA axis during the perinatal period (Zelena et al., 2008; Makara et al., 2012). And in some key aspects of HPA function non-human primates are a more appropriate animal model for human than rodents. For example, the adrenal cortex of monkeys, in contrast to rodents, produces DHEA and DHEAS (Goncharova, 1997; Kemnitz et al., 2000; Conley et al., 2004), which are involved in stress response of the HPA axis and may regulate the release of AVP (Deuster et al., 2005). It is apparent that we need more in-depth research on the role of AVP in the HPA axis regulation in response to different types of chronic stress on various rodent models, including both wild-type and homozygous AVP-deficient Brattleboro mutant strains, as well as V1b receptor knockout rodents. It should also investigate in detail the function of the HPA axis in AVP-deficient lines in basal conditions using various functional tests to get a solid baseline data that are comprehensively characterize the artificial models. Extensive basic research is required on the effects of V1b receptors antagonists and agonists on the HPA axis function in resting and stress conditions in primates.

## DEVELOPMENTAL SPECIALTIES OF VASOPRESSINERGIC HPA AXIS REGULATION

### FETAL DEVELOPMENT

Extensive clinical and experimental data indicate variation in the importance of AVP in regulation of the HPA axis, including its stress responsiveness, at different stages of ontogeny and under different physiological conditions. The role of AVP in regulation of the HPA axis in the fetus has been described only in a few studies (Carey et al., 2007, 2009). In fetal sheep late in gestation, secretion of ACTH by the pituitary gland increases in response to stimulation with AVP. This effect is associated with an increase in the generation of inositol 1,4,5-trisphosphate, a second messenger of activated V1b receptors (Carey et al., 2007). The same study also found that hypothalamo-pituitary disconnection significantly impaired this ontogenetic development and prevents the developmental increase in fetal plasma cortisol concentrations in late gestation (Carey et al., 2007). Another study confirmed the hypothesis that cortisol is an important modulator of pituitary responsiveness to AVP in the late gestation sheep fetus (Carey et al., 2009).

### NEONATAL PERIOD

Developmental studies have shown that neonatal rodents (Yi and Baram, 1994; Dent et al., 1999; Schmidt et al., 2009; Zelena et al., 2011) and humans (Gunnar and Donzella, 2002) show a reduced adrenocortical response to stress. Thus, this period is called the stress-hyporesponsive period (Yi and Baram, 1994; Dent et al., 1999; Schmidt et al., 2009). In some studies the reduced response of the pituitary–adrenal axis to stressors was not associated with significant change in CRH gene transcription (Yi and Baram, 1994) or even mentioned its decrease in response to certain stressors, such as endotoxin (Dent et al., 1999). The use of conditional knockout mice with a deletion of the GR at the pituitary (GRPOMCCre) showed that during the neonatal period expression of CRH mRNA in parvicellular neurons of the PVN is reduced while expression of AVP mRNA is increased (Schmidt et al., 2009). Similar data were obtained in 10-day-old pups of AVP-deficient Brattleboro rats, which showed significantly lower resting CRH mRNA levels in the PVN and have revealed that AVP-deficiency abolishes the ACTH stress response in perinatal rats compared to control littermates (Zelena et al., 2008). Recent studies by this research group using the V1b antagonist, SSR149415, confirmed a primary role for AVP in ACTH stress responsiveness of control rats during the neonatal period (Zelena et al., 2011; Makara et al., 2012). Apparently, the shift in the ratio CRH/AVP in favor AVP (Whitnall, 1989; Dinan and Scott, 2005) can take place not only in adult individuals under chronic stress or acute stress induced by a severe stressor, as noted in Section "Vasopressinergic Regulation of Stress Responsiveness of the HPA Axis" above but also in the neonatal period.

### LATE PREGNANCY, LACTATION

Such important physiological conditions of the organism as pregnancy and lactation are of considerable interest in terms of vasopressinergic regulation of stress reactivity of the HPA axis. It is well known that the HPA axis response to stressors is markedly attenuated in late pregnancy and during lactation period in women (Altemus et al., 1995; de Weerth and Buitelaar, 2005) and female rodents (Fischer et al., 1995; Neumann et al., 1998; Walker et al., 2001; Ma et al., 2005; Brunton et al., 2008). The precise mechanisms of maternal HPA axis hyporesponsiveness in these two states are different (see review Brunton et al., 2008), but both states are characterized by marked changes in AVP secretion from parvicellular neurons of the PVN and subsequent change in the secretion of ACTH in response to stress. The rat's response to stress exposure late in pregnancy is associated with reduced AVP expression (Ma et al., 2005) or reduced expression of both AVP and CRH (da Costa et al., 1996; Douglas et al., 2003). On the contrary, AVP mRNA expression in parvicellular neurons of the PVN in postpartum females exposed to restraint stress during lactation was greater than that of virgin females (Fischer et al., 1995; Walker et al., 2001). At the same time, the expression of CRH mRNA in the PVN significantly decreased during lactation (Fischer et al., 1995; Shanks et al., 1999; Walker et al., 2001). It suggests that AVP may play an important role in the stimulation of ACTH secretion during lactation in rats (Walker et al., 2001). Thus, as in the fetus and neonate, AVP performs an important role in regulation of the HPA axis stress reactivity with a shift in the CRH/AVP ratio in favor of AVP in pregnant and lactating females.

Gestation and early postnatal periods, as we know, are the most vulnerable periods of ontogenesis in terms of programing disruptions of the HPA axis for adulthood (Schmidt et al., 2009; Long et al., 2010; Renard et al., 2010) and aging (Goncharova, 2009b; Solas et al., 2010). Reduced HPA axis response to stressors during late pregnancy, lactation, and the neonatal period, apparently, is an adaptive response of the body that provides protection of the fetus and newborn from an excess of toxic glucocorticoids and that can also have a programing effect on the development of the HPA axis and other physiological systems in later life.

## AVP IN REGULATION OF HPA AXIS STRESS RESPONSIVENESS DURING AGING

### ACTIVITY OF THE HPA AXIS DURING AGING

It is generally accepted that mainly hyperactivation of the HPA axis occurs during aging. In small laboratory animals hyperactivation of the HPA axis in the aging process develops at all levels of the system. Thus, aged rodents demonstrated elevated resting ACTH and corticosterone plasma levels (Sapolsky et al., 1986; Tizabi et al., 1992; Hauger et al., 1994; Sapolsky, 1999; Meijer et al., 2005; Lo et al., 2006), an increased release of resting hypothalamic CRH (Scaccianoce et al., 1990; Hauger et al., 1994; Sapolsky, 1999), a decreased sensitivity of the adrenal glands to ACTH (Tang and Phillips, 1978; Sapolsky et al., 1986), of the anterior pituitary to CRH (Hylka et al., 1984; Sapolsky et al., 1986; Hauger et al., 1994; Sapolsky, 1999), of the pituitary, hippocampus, and hypothalamus to the level of circulating glucocorticoids (Sapolsky et al., 1986; Tizabi et al., 1992; Hatzinger et al., 2000; Revskoy and Redei, 2000). In old rodents, hyperactivity of the HPA axis is likely to reflect loss of resiliency and reduced sensitivity to negative glucocorticoid feedback, which mainly reflects hippocampal receptor damage (Sapolsky et al., 1986; Seeman and Robbins, 1994; Pedersen et al., 2001; Giordano et al., 2005). As a result, older animals tend to show a more prolonged elevation of corticosterone in response to stress exposure (Sapolsky et al., 1986; Seeman and Robbins, 1994; Sapolsky, 1999). Marked disturbances have been shown in the reaction of aged rat adrenals to stress.

These have been expressed mainly as increases in the maximum peak values of plasma corticosterone rise and the prolongation of elevated corticosterone secretion (Sapolsky et al., 1986; Seeman and Robbins, 1994; Sapolsky, 1999; Lo et al., 2006). Some studies, however, have shown individual and species differences ranging from unchanged and reduced basal and stress responses in aged rats compared to young rats (Cizza et al., 1994; Hauger et al., 1994; Lightman et al., 2000).

Hyperactivation of the HPA axis during aging in humans and non-human primates is generally associated with elevated plasma levels of ACTH and cortisol in basal conditions (Sapolsky and Altman, 1991; Guazzo et al., 1996; Lupien et al., 1999, 2007). Decrease in HPA axis sensitivity to glucocorticoid regulation by a feedback mechanism with age has also been observed in humans (Born et al., 1995; Heuser et al., 2000; Giordano et al., 2005) and non-human primates (Sapolsky and Altman, 1991; Brooke et al., 1994; Goncharova et al., 2000; Gust et al., 2000; Goncharova and Lapin, 2002, 2004). However, in contrast to rodents there was an increase in response of the pituitary–adrenal axis to CRH and ACTH injection in humans (Born et al., 1995; Kudielka et al., 1999; Ferrari et al., 2001) and monkeys (Goncharova and Lapin, 2002, 2004; Goncharova et al., 2002), as was a higher responsiveness of the pituitary–adrenal axis to combined administration of CRH and AVP (Born et al., 1995). With healthy aging basal activity of CRH-producing neurons in the hypothalamic PVN slightly increased in the human (see review Swaab et al., 2005).

It should be noted that aging is associated with an increase in the variability of disturbances in the HPA axis both in primates and rodents but to a greater extent in humans and non-human primates than in rodents. Many authors have failed to observe significant age-related changes in basal plasma levels of ACTH and cortisol in humans (Ohashi et al., 1986; Waltman et al., 1991; Goncharova, 1997; Goncharova et al., 2002) and monkeys (Moore et al., 1979; Goncharova and Lapin, 2000, 2002; Goncharova et al., 2000; Kemnitz et al., 2000). Some even have observed decreased basal cortisol levels in humans (Blichert-Toft, 1978; Sherman et al., 1985) and monkeys (Gust et al., 2000). Other researchers have found no marked age-related changes in sensitivity of the HPA axis to inhibition by glucocorticoid feedback (Blichert-Toft, 1978; Waltman et al., 1991; Huizenga et al., 1998). There was no change in the reaction of the adrenal cortex to injection of CRH, ACTH, or insulin in humans (Blichert-Toft, 1978; Ohashi et al., 1986) or non-human primates (Goncharova and Lapin, 2000; Goncharova et al., 2000).

Some researchers have found higher responses to acute psycho-emotional stress in physically untrained aged individuals (Traustadóttir et al., 2005). Older men responded to psychological stress with increased cortisol levels and more intense cardiovascular responses compared to women of similar age (Traustadottir et al., 2003). Comparative analysis of cortisol response to various pharmacological stimuli including dexamethasone, CRH, naloxone, ACTH, insulin, epinephrine, metapyrone, physostigmine, and hypertonic saline, as well as to psychological stressors in healthy volunteers, young and old age through the analysis of the data published by different authors in 45 articles, allowed the authors (Otte et al., 2005) to come to a conclusion about a higher HPA axis response in older subjects compared to younger persons. The effect of age on the release of cortisol was significantly greater in women.

At the same time, no age-related differences in ACTH and cortisol levels in response to acute psychosocial stress have been reported in postmenopausal women compared to young women (Kudielka et al., 1999). The response to acute psychological stress in the elderly who were aerobically fit did not differ from that of young adults (Traustadóttir et al., 2005). Marked difference in function of the HPA axis in response to surgical stress is not seen between young persons and centenarians (Kudoh et al., 2001), even though clinical observations indicate that the mortality rate of elderly patients, undergoing surgery is much higher than that of young patients (Blichert-Toft, 1978). The higher rate may be due to reduced adaptive ability of the aging body and deterioration of HPA axis function.

Experiments on healthy non-human primates (*Macaca mulatta*) revealed that age-related dysfunctions of the HPA axis are associated with adaptive behavior of animals (Goncharova et al., 2010). Monkeys with depression-like behavior show age-related changes in the HPA axis function that are accompanied by maximal absolute and relative hypercortisolemia (high cortisol/DHEAS molar ratio) under resting conditions, as well as by a significantly greater increase in plasma cortisol levels with acute psycho-emotional stress. Young aggressive monkeys, in comparison with young monkeys of other behavior groups, demonstrated the highest plasma levels of DHEAS and the lowest molar ratios of cortisol to DHEAS. Such differences were not exhibited by old monkeys with aggressive behavior. Minimal age-related changes in the HPA axis have been observed in monkeys with average (standard) behavior.

It should be noted that a striking difference in physiology of the HPA axis between primates and rodents is the secretion of large amounts of DHEA and DHEAS by the primate adrenal cortex, which undergoes a decline with age (Orentreich et al., 1992; Goncharova, 1997; Yen and Laughlin, 1998; Ferrari et al., 2001; Goncharova and Lapin, 2002; Conley et al., 2004; Heaney et al., 2012). DHEA and DHEAS serve as precursors to androgens and estrogens (Yen and Laughlin, 1998; Labrie et al., 2001; Mellon and Vaudry, 2001). In addition, they may act as functional antagonists to the effects of glucocorticoids (Yen and Laughlin, 1998; Maninger et al., 2009). In the brain, they are neuromodulators of neuronal receptors, such as GABA-A and *N*-methyl-D-aspartate (NMDA) receptors (Baulieu, 1998; Yen and Laughlin, 1998; Mellon and Vaudry, 2001), which are part of the neurons of afferents nerves regulating – among others – the PVN activity (Arvat et al., 2002; Deuster et al., 2005).

**CIRCADIAN RHYTHMS**

Significant variability has been found with respect to age-related changes in circadian rhythms of ACTH and glucocorticoid secretion both in humans and animals. While a number of studies have failed to show marked circadian disorders of cortisol and ACTH in humans and non-human primates (Chambers et al., 1982; Waltman et al., 1991; Ceresini et al., 2000) and some strains of rats (Honma et al., 1996), an increasing number of studies have shown disruption of circadian rhythms in HPA axis activity with aging in both humans and animals. Many authors have reported age-associated increases in basal ACTH and cortisol concentrations in terms of basal evening levels and nadirs in humans (Ferrari et al., 2001; Giordano et al., 2005; Hofman and Swaab, 2006) and non-human primates (Gust et al., 2000; Khavinson et al., 2001; Goncharova et al., 2002, 2006b; Zhdanova et al., 2011), and fall of the levels of ACTH and corticosterone in the evening and increase during the circadian trough in rodents (Hauger et al., 1994; Lightman et al., 2000; Froy, 2011). A damaged daily rhythm may involve the SCN, as fetal transplants containing SCN can restore the circadian rhythm in old Sprague-Dawley rats (Cai et al., 1997).

The master circadian clock is located in the SCN of the hypothalamus. Its activity is synchronized with the natural day–night cycle, and it coordinates the circadian rhythms of the body, including the HPA axis rhythm (Reppert and Weaver, 2002; Kalsbeek et al., 2010; Walker et al., 2010; Kondratova and Kondratov, 2012). A characteristic feature of the SCN in many species, including humans and other primates is a subpopulation of AVP-containing neurons (Kalsbeek et al., 2010). The SCN regulates HPA axis activity through the PVN via AVP, which serves as a neurotransmitter in the SCN afferents to the hypothalamic PVN (Kalsbeek et al., 2010). The regulatory function of these afferents is confirmed by experiments with microinjections of AVP-cytotoxic monoclonal antibodies into the SCN, which produce a significant reduction of immunoreactive AVP and AVP mRNA expression there as well as in parvicellular neurons of the PVN (Gomez et al., 1997). Study of post-mortem human brains revealed a pronounced circadian variation in the activity of AVP-containing neurons in the SCN (Kalsbeek et al., 2010). Animal experiments have shown an important role for SCN-derived AVP in the control of neuroendocrine day/night rhythms of the HPA axis (Kalsbeek et al., 2010). The number of AVP-expressing neurons in the SCN declines with age in humans (Swaab et al., 1985), non-human primates (Cayetanot et al., 2005), and rats (Roozendaal et al., 1987). Decreased AVP-producing neurons in the SCN in aged humans and animals are accompanied by deterioration of the circadian rhythms of HPA axis function (Kalsbeek et al., 2010).

**AVP REGULATION OF STRESS RESPONSIVENESS OF THE HPA AXIS WITH AGING**

Age-related changes in AVP production vary depending on location in the brain. While secretion of AVP decreases with aging in the SCN of animals and humans (Cai et al., 1997; Cayetanot et al., 2005; Hofman and Swaab, 2006; Kalsbeek et al., 2010), its secretion in the PVN seems to increase. This is indicated by immunocytochemical studies of human post-mortem brains that have revealed increased amounts of AVP in AVP-expressing cells and in the size of AVP-containing neurons in the PVN of aged humans (Lucassen et al., 1993; Prelevic and Jacobs, 1997; Ishunina and Swaab, 1999). In addition, an age-dependent change in colocalization of CRH and AVP in favor of AVP in the human PVN has been identified (Raadsheer et al., 1993). Moreover, old rats showed signs of hyperactive AVP-expressing neurons (Terwell et al., 1992; Bazhanova et al., 2000). Other studies, however, provide indications of a modest activation of CRH neurons with aging in healthy persons (see review Swaab et al., 2005).

In the literature there are several studies that investigated the role of the AVP/V1b receptor system in the regulation of stress responsiveness of the HPA axis with aging. Most of these studies have been performed in experiments on rodents. Features of vasopressinergic regulation of stress responsiveness of the HPA axis during aging has been studied significantly less in humans and non-human primates.

***Rodents***

On the other hand, the idea that secretion of AVP in the PVN can increase with aging is evidenced by the results of studies on the role of AVP in the regulation of stress reactivity of the HPA axis, performed mainly on rodents. Thus, some reports in the literature describe work with rats of the Fischer-344/N strain, in which aging is associated with a progressive decline in hypothalamic CRH production associated with increased production of AVP (Cizza et al., 1994). In this case, basal plasma ACTH levels were similar across age groups. Injection of exogenous rat CRH elicited significantly greater ACTH and corticosterone responses in aged rats, which was consistent with the observation of hypothalamic CRH deficiency. CRH mRNA levels in the PVN, CRH content, and *in vitro* secretion of CRH by whole explanted hypothalamus showed progressive and significant reductions with age, whereas the steady state levels of AVP mRNA significantly increased with age (Cizza et al., 1994). Perhaps the importance of PVN-derived AVP for HPA axis regulation increases with advancing age, while the importance of CRH is reduced.

Subsequent studies have confirmed the important role of AVP expressed in parvicellular neurons of the PVN in the regulation of ACTH secretion in response to stimulus. Application of the combined DEX/CRH test to old male Wistar rats resulted in excessive release of ACTH and corticosterone as compared to young rats. Administration of a V1b receptor antagonist between the dexamethasone and CRH injections blocked the effect (Hatzinger et al., 2000). In DEX-pretreated aged rats the authors detected increased numbers of AVP mRNA-expressing neurons in the PVN; this was in combination with increased numbers and activity of CRH mRNA-expressing neurons. This study provided the first direct evidence of the involvement of excessive activity of AVP-expressing neurons in age-dependent hyperactivity of the HPA axis. The results of this study suggest an important role of AVP in the mechanism of increased HPA axis activity in aging rats, possibly secondary to defective function of corticosteroid receptors (Hatzinger et al., 2000).

Another study has demonstrated an increase in the content of AVP within the PVN in basal conditions. The approximately twofold increase correlated with an increase of ACTH and corticosterone basal plasma levels in old rats (Keck et al., 2000). However, in response to acute stressor, forced-swimming, the responses of AVP, ACTH, and cortisol were significantly lower than in young animals (Keck et al., 2000). Some authors report that aging in rats is likely to be associated with reduced production of AVP and hypersecretion of CRH in the hypothalamus and subsequent down-regulation of corticotroph CRH receptor (Hauger et al., 1994).

Some of the contradictory results reported in the above papers may by attributable to individual differences in HPA axis function both in resting and stress conditions. Thus, in the study of Meijer et al. (2005) young and aged rats had previously been classified as inferior and superior learners on the basis of their performance in a water maze test. The authors tested for a correlation between the production of the hypothalamic neuropeptides, CRH and AVP, and their status as inferior and superior learners. They found that AVP expression in parvicellular neurons of the PVN was virtually unchanged with aging in animals of either group. CRH expression, however, decreased significantly in old animals compared to young animals in the superior learning group, which produced a change in the ratio of CRH/AVP expression in favor of AVP. By contrast, the ratio of CRH/AVP expression in inferior learners was virtually unchanged with aging. Apparently, there are marked individual differences in rats of the same strain, as well as differences between strains in aging of the brain in general and aging of the HPA axis in particular. This conclusion is supported by the results of studies that demonstrate differences in the functioning of the HPA axis in adult rats of the same species with high and low trait anxiety (Keck et al., 2002). Using surgical microdialysis *in vivo*, the investigators showed that the content of AVP in the PVN is significantly higher in rats with increased anxiety (Keck et al., 2002).

Thus, reports on the possible role of the AVP/V1b receptor system in the increase of HPA axis hyperactivity with aging in rodents are contradictory, suggesting (a) the possible increase of the AVP production in the PVN for aged rodents, (b) the possible lack of any age changes in the AVP secretion in basal and stress conditions, and (c) the possible reduced basal AVP production along with the CRH hypersecretion.

#### *Humans and non-human primates*

Only a few studies have addressed age-related changes in vasopressinergic regulation of HPA axis stress reactivity in humans and non-human primates (Raskind et al., 1995; Deuster et al., 2005; Goncharova, 2009a). Most studies have focused on age differences in response of the pituitary–adrenal axis to stress. The cross-species findings are quite variable with regard to responsiveness of the HPA axis in old age. They depend not only on the nature, intensity and duration of exposure of the stressor, the genetic characteristics of the individual, and the environment in old age, but also on the influence of genetic and environmental factors in the early stages of development, particularly the fetal and neonatal periods. Environmental stress in early life may program the future development, including disruptions of HPA axis stress responsiveness in old age (Pivina et al., 2007; Goncharova, 2009b; Solas et al., 2010).

It has been noted that the healthy elderly exhibit a more pronounced adrenocortical response to hypertonic saline infusion than young people (Raskind et al., 1995). The increase in levels of AVP and plasma osmolarity was similar in representatives of both age groups, but no rise in the levels of ACTH was observed in either older or young subjects. The authors, therefore, suggested that the increased cortisol secretion in response to stimulation with the hypertonic solution was due to age-related changes in the adrenocortical level of the HPA axis (Raskind et al., 1995). Perhaps, stimulation of cortisol secretion was influenced by increased levels of AVP in the general circulation. This effect could be a direct AVP effect on the adrenal gland as the pituitary contains predominantly V1b receptor, but the adrenal cortex has V1a receptor (Grazzini et al., 1996; Vezzosi et al., 2007; Roper et al., 2011). Thus, there is evidence that AVP potentiates cortisol secretion *in vitro* by normal human adrenal cortex and some cortisol-producing adrenocortical tumors or hyperplasia through the activation of V1a receptors (Perraudin et al., 1993, 1995).

Interestingly, chronic administration of DHEA to healthy young men significantly increased exercise-induced release of AVP along with ACTH and cortisol secretion (Deuster et al., 2005). Perhaps, the stimulating effect of DHEA on pituitary–adrenal axis stress responsiveness is due to its action as antagonist of GABA-A receptors restrained the HPA axis and the stimulating effect of DHEA on NMDA receptors, involved in AVP release (Rossi and Chen, 2002; Deuster et al., 2005). In this regard, DHEA deficiency during aging in humans and non-human primates may play an important role in development of the age-related disturbances of the HPA axis and, in particular, of its stress responsiveness (Kudielka et al., 1998; Goncharova et al., 2000).

Recent experiments on non-human primates (Goncharova, 2006, 2009a; Goncharova et al., 2006a, 2008b), had shown that stress responsiveness of the HPA axis depends to a large extent on the time of day when stimulus is applied as well as on initial sensitivity of the HPA axis. It was shown that the circadian rhythm of ACTH and cortisol level is evident not only in basal conditions but also in response to acute psycho-emotional stress. Young (6–8 years old) female rhesus monkeys showed a much higher increase in ACTH and cortisol levels in response to a 2 h restraint stress imposed at 15:00 h than to the same stress imposed at 09:00 h. This difference attenuates with aging. Old (20–27 years old) female animals showed much lower responsiveness of the HPA axis to the afternoon stress and a tendency toward higher responsiveness to the morning stress. A similar circadian rhythm in responsiveness of the HPA axis to mild acute stress was observed in young pregnant women (De Weerth et al., 2007). The time-dependent responsiveness of the HPA axis to acute immobilization stress was observed in young male *Papio hamadryas* (Chirkov et al., 1987) and young female Wistar rats (Pivina et al., 2007). Moreover, senescent rats demonstrated flattening of circadian rhythm in stress reactivity of the HPA axis (Pivina et al., 2007).

The attempt to understand the mechanism of decreasing stress reactivity of the pituitary–adrenal axis with aging led to a series of experiments with the administration of a standard dose of CRH and AVP (1 μg/kg b.w., intravenously) to young and old female rhesus monkeys at different times of day (09:00 and 15:00 h). The response of the pituitary–adrenal axis to the injection of CRH revealed a circadian rhythm with a more pronounced response in the afternoon; this rhythm was not affected by aging (Goncharova, 2009a). Apparently, the circadian rhythm in the secretion of CRH underlies the circadian rhythm in the stress reactivity of the pituitary–adrenal axis of the HPA axis. At the same time, the rise of ACTH and cortisol levels in response to AVP injection did not show a dependence on the time of the day in either young or old animals. A significant age-related difference in the rise of ACTH and cortisol in response to AVP injection was, however, found in the response to AVP administered in the afternoon; lower values were seen in older animals (Goncharova, 2009a). It appears that age differences in response of the anterior pituitary to AVP may underlie age-related differences in stress responsiveness of the HPA axis in primates in the afternoon. Perhaps age differences in response of the anterior pituitary to AVP underlie age-related differences in stress responsiveness of the HPA axis in primates in the afternoon.

## CONCLUSION

(1) The role of CRH and AVP in the stimulation of ACTH secretion varies depending upon the species. For humans, non-human primates, and rats CRH seems to be a more important secretagogue than AVP, in humans, all parvicellular neurons of the PVN, which produce CRH in the basal conditions, produce AVP as well, whereas in rats not more than half produce AVP.

(2) AVP is an important regulator of the ACTH response to acute stress. AVP contributes to the acute ACTH secretion to stress in a context-specific manner. AVP is needed for the acute ACTH secretion for most of the known stressors.

(3) Current data on the role of AVP in the regulation of HPA axis responsiveness to chronic stress in adulthood are contradictory and require further research.

(4) The importance of the vasopressinergic regulation of stress responsiveness of the HPA axis is elevated during the fetal development, in neonatal period, and in the lactating adult.

(5) (a) Aging is associated with increased variability in several parameters of HPA axis function including basal state, responsiveness to stressors, and special testing. This increased variability in the aged compared to normal adults has been observed in some form in multiple species including rodents, non-human primates, and humans.
(b) For the most experiments on rodents, the hyperactivation of the HPA axis was observed at all levels of the HPA organization with aging under the basal and stress conditions.
(c) With healthy aging of non-human primates and humans the HPA hyperactivation is usually associated with the increase of the cortisol level in the evening time, the slight changes in the regulation of the HPA axis by glucocorticoid feedback with relative hypercortisolemia due to the decline in secretion of the adrenal antagonists of cortisol – DHEA and DHEAS.

(6) Reports on the possible role of the AVP/V1b receptor system in the increase of HPA axis hyperactivity with aging are contradictory, suggesting
(a) the possible increase of the AVP production in the PVN for aged rodents and humans,
(b) the possible lack of any age changes in the AVP secretion in basal and stress conditions,
(c) the possible reduced basal AVP production along with the CRH hypersecretion.

(7) Age-related changes in response of the HPA axis to the moderate acute restraint stress were observed in rhesus monkeys with much higher increase of ACTH and cortisol secretion in young monkeys in response to the stress imposed at 15:00 h. In addition, these age changes were associated with age-related disturbances in vasopressinergic regulation.

## REFERENCES


Abou-Samra, A. B., Catt, K. J., and Aguilera, G. (1986). Involvement of protein kinase C in the regulation of adrenocorticotropin release from rat anterior pituitary cells. *Endocrinology* 118, 212–217.

Aguilera, G. (1994). Regulation of pituitary ACTH secretion during chronic stress. *Front. Neuroendocrinol.* 15, 321–350.

Aguilera, G. (1998). Corticotropin releasing hormone, receptor regulation and the stress response. *Trends Endocrinol. Metab.* 9, 329–336.

Aguilera, G. (2011). HPA axis responsiveness to stress: implications for healthy aging. *Exp. Gerontol.* 46, 90–95.

Aguilera, G., Pham, Q., and Rabadan-Diehl, C. (1994). Regulation of pituitary vasopressin receptors during chronic stress: relationship with corticotroph responsiveness. *J. Neuroendocrinol.* 6, 299–304.

Aguilera, G., and Rabadan-Diehl, C. (2000). Vasopressinergic regulation of the hypothalamic-pituitary-adrenal axis: implications for stress adaptation. *Regul. Pept.* 96, 23–29.

Altemus, M., Deuster, P. A., Galliven, E., Carter, C. S., and Gold, P. W. (1995). Suppression of hypothalamic-pituitary-adrenal axis responses to stress in lacting women. *J. Clin. Endocrionol. Metab.* 80, 2954–2959.

Antoni, F., Fink, G., and Sheward, W. (1990). Corticotrophin-releasing peptides in rat hypophysial portal blood after paraventricular lesions: a marked reduction in the concentration of 41-residue corticotropin-releasing factor, but no change in vasopressin. *J. Endocrinol.* 125, 175–183.

Antoni, F. A. (1993). Vasopressinergic control of pituitary-adrenal secretion comes of age. *Front. Neuroendocrinol.* 14, 76–122.

Arima, H., House, S. B., Gainer, H., and Aguilera, G. (2002). Neuronal activity is required for the circadian rhythm of vasopressin gene transcription in the suprachiasmatic nucleus in vitro. *Endocrinology* 143, 4165–4171.

Arvat, E., Giordano, R., Grottoli, S., and Ghigo, E. (2002). Benzodiazepines and anterior pituitary function. *J. Endocrinol. Invest.* 25, 735–747.

Autelitano, D. J., Lundblud, J. R., Blum, M., and Roberts, J. L. (1989). Hormonal regulation of POMC gene expression. *Annu. Rev. Physiol.* 51, 715–726.

Bale, T. L., and Vale, W. W. (2004). CRF and CRF receptors: role in stress responsivity and other behaviors. *Annu. Rev. Pharmacol. Toxicol.* 44, 525–557.

Barberis, C., and Tribollet, E. (1996). Vasopressin and oxytocin receptors in the central nervous system. *Crit. Rev. Neurobiol.* 10, 119–154.

Bartanusz, V., Aubry, J. M., Jezova, D., Baffi, J., and Kiss, J. Z. (1993). Up-regulation of vasopressin mRNA in paraventricular hypophysiotropic neurons after acute immobilization stress. *Neuroendocrinology* 58, 625–629.

Baulieu, E. E. (1998). Neurosteroids: a novel function of the brain. *Psychoneuroendocrinology* 29, 963–987.

Bazhanova, E. D., Chernigovskaya, E. V., and Danilova, O. A. (2000). Different pathways of neurohormonal hypothalamic control of the adrenal cortex function in young and old rats. *Mech. Ageing Dev.* 118, 91–102.

Bilezijian, L. M., Blount, A. V., and Vale, W. W. (1987). The cellular actions of vasopressin on corticotrophs of the anterior pituitary: resistance to glucocorticoid action. *Mol. Endocrinol.* 1, 451–458.

Birnbaumer, M. (2000). Vasopressin receptors. *Trends Endocrinol. Metab.* 1, 406–410.

Blichert-Toft, M. (1978). "The adrenal glands in old age," in *Geriatric Endocrinology. Aging*, Vol. 5, ed. R. B. Greenblatt (New York: Raven Press), 81–104.

Born, J., Ditschuneit, I., Schreiber, M., Dodt, C., and Fehm, H. L. (1995). Effect of age and gender on pituitary-adrenocortical responsiveness in humans. *Eur. J. Endocrinol.* 132, 705–711.

Brooke, S. M., de Haas-Johnson, A. M., Kaplan, J. R., Manuck, S. B., and Sapolsky, R. M. (1994). Dexamethasone resistance among nonhuman primates associated with a selective decrease of glucocorticoid receptors in the hippocampus and a history of social instability. *Neuroendocrinology* 60, 134–140.

Brunton, P. J., Russell, J. A., and Douglas, A. J. (2008). Adaptive responses of the maternal hypothalamic-pituitary-adrenal axis during pregnancy and lactation. *J. Neuroendocrinol.* 20, 764–777.

Burgess, W. J., and Balment, R. J. (1992). Plasma atrial natriuretic peptide in vasopressin deficiency: the effect of acute water deprivation in rats. *J. Endocrinol.* 135, 431–438.

Caff, A. R., van Leeuwen, F. W., and Luiten, P. G. (1987). Vasopressin cells in the medial amygdala of the rat project to the lateral septum and ventral hippocampus. *J. Comp. Neurol.* 261, 237–252.

Cai, A., Scarbrough, K., Hinkle, A., and Wise, P. M. (1997). Fetal grafts containing suprachiasmatic nuclei restore the diurnal rhythm of CRH and POMC mRNA in aging rats. *Am. J. Physiol. Regul. Integr. Comp. Physiol.* 273, R1764–R1770.

Carey, L. C., Tatter, S. B., and Rose, J. C. (2007). Ontogeny and effects of hypothalamic pituitary disconnection on formation of inositol trisphosphate in fetal sheep pituitary cells. *Endocrinology* 148, 1440–1444.

Carey, L. C., Tatter, S. B., and Rose, J. C. (2009). Cortisol infusion in late-gestation hypothalamo-pituitary disconnected sheep fetus pituitary cell responsiveness to arginine vasopressin. *Am. J. Physiol. Endocrinol. Metab.* 296, E300–E304.

Cayetanot, F., Bentivoglio, M., and Aujard, E. (2005). Arginine-vasopressin and vasointestinal polypeptide rhythms in the suprachiasmatic nucleus of the mouse lemur reveal aging-related alterations of circadian pacemaker neurons in a non-human primate. *Eur. J. Neurosci.* 22, 902–910.

Ceresini, G., Morganti, S., Rebecchi, I., Freddi, M., Ceda, G. P., Banchini, A., et al. (2000). Evaluation of the circadian profiles of serum dehygroepiandrosterone (DHEA), cortisol, and cortisol/DHEA molar ratio after a single oral administration of DHEA in elderly subjects. *Metab. Clin. Exp.* 49, 548–551.

Chambers, K. S., Resko, J. A., and Phoenix, C. H. (1982). Correlation of diurnal changes in hormones with sexual behavior and age in male rhesus macaques. *Neurobiol. Aging* 3, 37–42.

Chen, J., Volpi, S., and Aguilera, G. (2008a). Anti-apoptotic actions of vasopressin in H32 neurons involve map kinase transactivation and bad phosphorylation. *Exp. Neurol.* 211, 529–538.

Chen, J., Young, S., Subburaju, S., Sheppard, J., Kiss, A., Atkinson, H., et al. (2008b). Vasopressin does not mediate hypersensitivity of the hypothalamic pituitary adrenal axis during chronic stress. *Ann. N. Y. Acad. Sci.* 1148, 349–359.

Chirkov, A. M., Chirkova, S. K., and Startsev, V. G. (1987). *Emotional Stress in Monkeys.* Leningrad: Nauka.

Chrousos, G. P. (2000). The role of stress and the hypothalamic-pituitary-adrenal axis in the pathogenesis of the metabolic syndrome: neuroendocrine and target tissue-related causes. *Int. J. Obes. Relat. Metab. Disord.* 24(Suppl. 2), S50–S55.

Cizza, G., Calogero, A. E., Brady, L. S., Bagdy, G., Bergamini, E., Blackman, M. R., et al. (1994). Male Fischer 344/N rats show a progressive central impairment of the hypothalamic-pituitary-adrenal axis with advancing age. *Endocrinology* 134, 1611–1621.

Conley, A. J., Pattison, J. C., and Bird, I. M. (2004). Variations in adrenal androgen productions among (non-human) primates. *Semin. Reprod. Med.* 22, 311–326.

da Costa, A. P. C., Wood, S., Ingram, C. D., and Lightman, S. L. (1996). Region-specific reduction in stress-induced c-foc mRNA expression during pregnancy and lactation. *Brain Res.* 742, 177–184.

Dallman, M. F., Akana, S. F., Levin, N., Walker, C.-D., Bradbury, M. J., Suemaru, S., et al. (1994). Corticosteroids and the control of function in the hypothalamo-pituitary-adrenal (HPA) axis. *Ann. N. Y. Acad. Sci.* 746, 22–28.

DeBold, C. R., Sheldon, W. R., DeCherney, G. S., Jackson, R. V., Alexander, A. N., Vale, W., et al. (1984). Arginine vasopressin potentiates adrenocorticotropin release induced by ovine corticotropin-releasing factor. *J. Clin. Invest.* 73, 533–538.

De Goeij, D., Djikstra, H., and Tilders, F. (1992). Chronic psychosocial stress enhances vasopressin but not corticotropin-releasing factor, in the external zone of the median eminence of male rats: relationship to subordinate status. *Endocrinology* 131, 847–853.

de Kloet, C. S., Vermetten, E., Geuze, E., Wiegant, V. M., and Westenberg, H. G. (2008). Elevated plasma arginine vasopressin levels in veterans with posttraumatic stress disorder. *J. Psychiatr. Res.* 42, 192–198.

de Kloet, E. R., Joels, M., and Holsboer, F. (2005). Stress and the brain: from adaptation to disease. *Nat. Rev. Neurosci.* 6, 463–475.

de Weerth, C., and Buitelaar, J. K. (2005). Physiological stress reactivity in human pregnancy: a review. *Neurosci. Biobehav. Rev.* 29, 295–312.

De Weerth, C., Wied, C. C., Jansen, L. M., and Buitelaar, J. K. (2007). Cardiovascular and cortisol responses to a psychological stressor during pregnancy. *Acta Obstet. Gynecol. Scand.* 29, 1–12.

de Winter, R. F., van Hemert, A. M., Derijk, R. H., Zwindermann, K. H., Frankhuijzen-Sierevogel, A. C., Wiegant, V. M., et al. (2003). Anxious-retarded depression: relation with plasma vasopressin and cortisol. *Neuropsychopharmacology* 28, 140–147.

Dent, G. W., Smith, M. A., and Levine, S. (1999). The ontogeny of the neuroendocrine response to endotoxin. *Brain Res. Dev. Brain Res.* 117, 21–29.

Derick, S., Pena, A., Durroux, N., Wagnon, J., Serradeil-Le Gal, C., Hibert, M., et al. (2004). Key amino acid located within the transmembrane domains 5 and 7 account for the pharmacological specificity of the human V1b vasopressin receptor. *Mol. Endocrinol.* 18, 2777–2789.

Deuster, P. A., Faraday, M. M., Chrousos, G. P., and Poth, M. A. (2005). Effects of dehydroepiandrosterone and alprazolam on hypothalamic-pituitary responses to exercise. *J. Clin. Endocrinol. Metab.* 90, 4777–4783.

Dinan, T. G., and Scott, L. V. (2005). Anatomy of melancholia: focus on hypothalamic-pituitary-adrenal axis overactivity and the role of vasopressin. *J. Anat.* 207, 259–264.

Domokos, A., Mergle, Z., Barna, I., Makara, G. B., and Zelena, D. (2008). Congenital vasopressin deficiency and acute and chronic opiate effects on hypothalamo-pituitary-adrenal axis activity in Brattleboro rats. *J. Endocrinol.* 196, 113–121.

Douglas, A. J., Brunton, P. J., Bosach, O. J., Russell, J. A., and Neumann, A. D. (2003). Neuroendicrine responses to stress in mice: hyporesponsiveness in pregnancy and parturition. *Endocrinology* 144, 5268–5276.

Ellis, M. J., Schmidli, R. S., Donald, R. A., Liversey, J. H., and Espiner, E. A. (1990). Plasma corticotrophin-releasing factor and vasopressin responses to hypoglycemia in normal man. *Clin. Endocrinol. (Oxf.)* 32, 93–100.

Engler, D., Pham, T., Fullerton, M. J., Ooi, G., Funder, J. W., and Clarke, I. J. (1989). Studies of the secretion of corticotrophin-releasing factor and arginine vasopressin into the hypophysial-portal circulation of the conscious sheep. I. Effect of an audiovisual stimulus and insulin-induced hypoglycemia. *Neuroendocrinology* 49, 367–381.

Evans, M. J., Marshall, A. G., Kitson, N. E., Summers, K., and Donald, R. A. (1993). Factors affecting ACTH release from perfused equine anterior pituitary cells. *J. Endocrinol.* 137, 391–401.

Familari, M., Smith, A. I., Smith, R., and Funder, J. W. (1989). Arginine vasopressin is a much more potent stimulus to ACTH release from ovine anterior pituitary cells than ovine corticotrophin-releasing factor. *Neuroendocrinology* 50, 152–157.

Favrod-Coune, C., Raux-Demay, M., Proeschel, M., Bertagna, X., Girard, F., and Luton, J. P. (1993). Potentiation of the classic ovine corticotropin-releasing hormone stimulation test by the combined administration of small doses of lysine vasopressin. *Clin. Endocrinol. (Oxf.)* 38, 405–410.

Fenoglio, K. A., Brunson, K. L., Vishai-Eliner, S., Chen, Y., and Baram, T. Z. (2004). Region-specific onset of handling-induced changes in corticotropin-releasing factor and glucocorticoid receptor expression. *Endocrinology* 145, 2702–2706.

Ferrari, E., Cravello, L., Muzzoni, B., Casarotti, D., Paltro, M., Solerte, S. B., et al. (2001). Age-related changes of the hypothalamic-pituitary-adrenal axis: pathophysiological correlates. *Eur. J. Endocrinol.* 144, 319–329.

Fischer, D., Patchev, V. K., Hellbach, S., Hassan, A. H., and Almeida, O. F. (1995). Lactation as a model for naturally reversible hypercortisolism plasticity in the mechanisms governing hypothalamo-pituitary-adrenocortical activity in rats. *J. Clin. Invest.* 96, 1208–1215.

Froy, O. (2011). Circadian rhythms, aging, and life span in mammals. *Physiology (Bethesda)* 26, 225–235.

Funder, J. W. (1997). Glucocorticoid and mineralocorticoid receptors: biology and clinical relevance. *Annu. Rev. Med.* 48, 231–240.

Giordano, R., Bo, M., Pellegrino, M., Vezzari, M., Baldi, M., Picu, A., et al. (2005). Hypothalamus-pituitary-adrenal hyperactivity in human aging is partially refractory to stimulation by mineralocorticoid receptor blockade. *J. Clin. Endocrinol. Metab.* 90, 5656–5662.

Gomez, F., Chapleur, M., Fernette, B., Burlet, C., Nicolas, J. P., and Burlet, A. (1997). Arginine vasopressin (AVP) depletion in neurons of the suprachiasmatic nuclei affects the AVP content of the paraventricular neurons and stimulates adrenocorticotropic hormone release. *J. Neurosci. Res.* 50, 565–574.

Goncharova, N. D. (1997). Hormonal function of the adrenal glands in men and monkeys in hemoblastoses and during aging. *Bull. Exp. Biol. Med.* 124, 804–807.

Goncharova, N. D. (2006). Hypothalamic-pituitary-adrenal axis and antioxidant enzymes: circadian rhythms, stress, and aging. *Front. Neuroendocrinol.* 27, 52–53.

Goncharova, N. D. (2009a). "The hypothalamic-pituitary-adrenal axis in nonhuman primates: circadian rhythms of stress responsiveness and aging," in *Primatology:Theories, Methods and Research*, eds E. Potocki and J. Krasinski (New York: Nova Science Publishers), 29–52.

Goncharova, N. D. (2009b). Individual life history, behavior, and biomarkers of ageing. *J. Nutr. Health Aging* 13(Suppl. 1), S215.

Goncharova, N. D., and Lapin, B. A. (2000). Changes of hormonal function of the adrenal and baboons of different age groups. *J. Med. Primatol.* 29, 26–35.

Goncharova, N. D., and Lapin, B. A. (2002). Effects of aging on hypothalamic-pituitary-adrenal system function in non-human primates. *Mech. Ageing Dev.* 123, 1191–1201.

Goncharova, N. D., and Lapin, B. A. (2004). Age-related endocrine dysfunction in nonhuman primates. *Ann. N. Y. Acad. Sci.* 1019, 321–325.

Goncharova, N. D., Lapin, B. A., and Khavinson, V. K. (2002). Age-associated endocrine dysfunctions and approaches to their correction. *Bull. Exp. Biol. Med.* 134, 417–421.

Goncharova, N. D., Marenin, V. Y., and Bogatyrenko, T. N. (2008a). Stress, aging and reliability of antioxidant enzyme defense. *Curr. Aging Sci.* 1, 22–29.

Goncharova, N. D., Shmaliy, A. V., Marenin, V. Y., Smelkova, S. A., and Lapin, B. A. (2008b). Circadian and age-related changes in stress responsiveness of the adrenal cortex and erythrocyte antioxidant enzymes in female rhesus monkeys. *J. Med. Primatol.* 37, 229–238.

Goncharova, N. D., Marenin, V. Y., and Oganyan, T. E. (2010). Aging of the hypothalamic-pituitary-adrenal axis in nonhuman primates with depression-like and aggressive behavior. *Aging* 2, 854–866.

Goncharova, N. D., Oganyan, T. E., and Smelkova, S. A. (2006a). Effect of aging on stress reactivity of the adrenal cortex in laboratory primates. Dependence on the time of day. *Bull. Exp. Biol. Med.* 141, 368–371.

Goncharova, N. D., Shmaliy, A. V., Bogatyrenko, T. N., and Koltover, V. K. (2006b). Correlation between activity of antioxidant enzymes and circadian rhythms of corticosteroids in *Macaca mulatta* monkeys of different age. *Exp. Gerontol.* 41, 778–783.

Goncharova, N. D., Oganyan, T. E., and Taranov, A. G. (2000). Functions of the hypothalamo-hypophyseal-adrenal system in aging in female monkeys. *Neurosci. Behav. Physiol.* 30, 717–721.

Grazzini, E., Lodboerer, A. M., Perez-Martin, A., Joubert, D., and Guillon, G. (1996). Molecular and functional characterization of the V1b receptor in rat adrenal medulla. *Endocrinology* 137, 3906–3914.

Guazzo, E. P., Kirkpatrick, P. J., Goodyer, I. M., Shiers, H. M., and Herbert, J. (1996). Cortisol, dehydroepiandrosterone (DHEA), and DHEA sulfate in the cerebrospinal fluid of man: relation to blood levels and the effects of age. *J. Clin. Endocrinol. Metab.* 81, 3951–3960.

Gunnar, M. R., and Donzella, B. (2002). Social regulation of the cortisol levels in early human development. *Psychoneuroendocrinology* 27, 199–220.

Gust, D. A., Wilson, M. E., Stocker, T., Conrad, S., Plotsky, P. M., and Gordon, T. P. (2000). Activity of the hypothalamic-pituitary-adrenal axis is altered by aging and exposure to social stress in female rhesus monkeys. *J. Clin. Endocrinol. Metab.* 85, 2556–2563.

Harbuz, M. S., and Lightman, S. L. (1989). Glucocorticoid inhibition of stress-induced changes in hypothalamic corticotrophin-releasing factor messenger RNA and proenkephalin A messenger RNA. *Neuropeptides* 14, 17–20.

Hassan, A., Chacko, S., and Mason, D. (2003). Desensitization of the adrenocorticotropin responses to arginine vasopressin and corticotrophin-releasing hormone in ovine anterior pituitary cells. *J. Endocrinol.* 178, 491–501.

Hatzinger, M., Wotjak, C. T., Naruo, T., Simchen, R., Kewck, M. E., Landgraf, R., et al. (2000). Endogenous vasopressin contributes to hypothalamic-pituitary-adrenocortical alterations in aged rats. *J. Endocrinol.* 164, 197–205.

Hauger, B. L., Thrivikraman, K. V., and Plotsky, P. M. (1994). Age-related alterations of hypothalamic-pituitary-adrenal axis function in male Fischer 344 rats. *Endocrinology* 134, 1528–1536.

Heaney, J. L. J., Phillips, A. C., and Carroll, D. (2012). Ageing, physical function, and the diurnal rhythms of cortisol and dehydroepiandrosterone. *Psychoneuroendocrinology* 37, 341–349.

Herman, J. P. (1995). In situ hybridization analysis of vasopressin gene transcription in the paraventricular and supraoptic nuclei of the rat: regulation by stress and glucocorticoids. *J. Comp. Neurol.* 363, 15–27.

Herman, J. P., Prewitt, C. M., and Cullinan, W. E. (1996). Neuronal circuit regulation of the hypothalamo-pituitary-adrenocortical stress axis. *Crit. Rev. Neurobiol.* 10, 371–394.

Heuser, I., Deuschle, M., Weber, A., Kniest, A., Ziegler, C., Weber, B., et al. (2000). The role of mineralocorticoid receptors in the circadian activity of the human hypothalamus-pituitary-adrenal system: effect of age. *Neurobiol. Aging* 21, 585–589.

Hofman, M. A., and Swaab, D. F. (2006). Living by the clock: the circadian pacemaker in older people. *Ageing Res. Rev.* 5, 33–51.

Honma, S., Katsuno, Y., Abe, H., and Honma, K. (1996). Aging affects development and persistence of feeding-associated circadian rhythm in rat plasma corticosterone. *Am. J. Physiol. Regul. Integr. Comp. Physiol.* 271, R1514–R1520.

Huizenga, N. A. T. M., Koper, J. W., De Lange, P., Pols, H. A. P., Stolk, R. P., Grobbee, D. E., et al. (1998). Interperson variability but interperson stability of baseline plasma cortisol concentrations, and its relation to feedback sensitivity of the hypothalamo-pituitary-adrenal axis to low dose of dexamethasone in elderly individuals. *J. Clin. Endocrinol. Metab.* 83, 47–54.

Hylka, V., Sonntag, W., and Meites, J. (1984). Reduced ability of old male rats to release ACTH and corticosterone in response to CRF administration. *Proc. Soc. Exp. Biol. Med.* 175, 1–3.

Imaki, T., Nahan, J. L., Rivier, C., Sawchenko, P. E., and Vale, W. (1991). Differential regulation of corticotropin-releasing factor mRNA in rat brain regions by glucocorticoids and stress. *J. Neurosci.* 11, 585–599.

Ishunina, T. A., and Swaab, D. F. (1999). Vasopressin and oxytocin neurons of the human supraoptic and paraventricular nucleus; size changes in relation to age and sex. *J. Clin. Endocrinol. Metab.* 84, 4637–4644.

Jacobson, L., Muglia, L. J., Weninger, S. C., Pacak, K., and Majzoub, J. A. (2000). CRH deficiency impairs but does not block pituitary-adrenal responses to diverse stressors. *Neuroendocrinology* 71, 79–87.

Jacobson, L., and Sapolsky, R. (1991). The role of hippocampus in feedback regulation of the hypothalamic-pituitary-adrenocortical axis. *Endocr. Rev.* 12, 118–134.

Jard, S., Barberis, C., Audigier, S., and Tribollet, E. (1987). Neurohypophyseal hormone receptor systems in brain and periphery. *Prog. Brain Res.* 72, 173–187.

Kalsbeek, A., Fliers, E., Hofman, M. A., Swaab, D. F., and Buijs, R. M. (2010). Vasopressin and the output of the hypothalamic biological clock. *J. Neuroendocrinol.* 22, 362–372.

Keck, M. E., Hatzinger, M., Wotjak, C. T., Landgraf, R., Holsboer, F., and Neumann, I. D. (2000). Ageing alters intrahypothalamic release patterns of vasopressin and oxytocin in rats. *Eur. J. Neurosci.* 12, 1487–1494.

Keck, M. E., Wigger, A., Welt, T., Muller, M. B., Gesing, A., Reul, J. M. H. M., et al. (2002). Vasopressin mediates the response of the combined dexamethasone/CRH test in hyper-anxious rats: implications for pathogenesis of affective disorders. *Neuropsychopharmacology* 26, 94–105.

Kemnitz, J. W., Roecker, E. B., Haffa, A. L. M., Pinheiro, J., Kurzman, I., Ramsey, J. J., et al. (2000). Serum dehydroepiandrosterone sulfate concentrations across the life span of laboratory-housed rhesus monkeys. *J. Med. Primatol.* 29, 330–337.

Khavinson, V. Kh., Goncharova, N. D., and Lapin, B. A. (2001). Synthetic tetrapeptide epitalon restores disturbed neuroendocrine regulation in senescent monkeys. *Neuroendocrinol. Lett.* 22, 251–254.

Knepper, M. A. (1997). Molecular physiology of urinary concentrating mechanism: regulation of aquaporin water channels by vasopressin. *Am. J. Physiol.* 272, F3–F12.

Kondratova, A. A., and Kondratov, R. V. (2012). The circadian clock and pathology of the ageing brain. *Nat. Rev. Neurosci.* 13, 325–335.

Koshimizu, T., Nasa, Y., Tanoue, A., Oikawa, R., Kawahara, Y., Kiyono, Y., et al. (2006). V1a vasopression receptors maintain normal blood pressure by regulation circulating blood volume and baroreflex sensitivity. *Proc. Natl. Acad. Sci. U.S.A.* 103, 7807–7812.

Kovacs, K., Kiss, J. Z., and Makara, G. B. (1986). Glucocorticoid implants around the hypothalamic paraventricular nucleus prevent the increase of corticotrophin releasing factor and arginine vasopressin immunostaining induced by adrenalectomy. *Neuroendocrinology* 44, 229–234.

Kudielka, B. M., Hellhammer, J., Hellhammer, D. H., Wolf, O. T., Pirke, K. M., Varadi, E., et al. (1998). Sex differences in endocrine and psychological responses to psychosocial stress in healthy elderly subjects and the impact of a 2-week dehydroepiandrosterone treatment. *J. Clin. Endocrinol. Metab.* 83, 1756–1761.

Kudielka, B. M., Schmidt-Reinwald, A. K., Hellhammer, D. H., and Kirschbaum, C. (1999). Psychological and endocrine responses to psychosocial stress and dexamethasone/corticotropin-releasing hormone in healthy postmenopausal women and young controls: the impact of age and a two-week estradiol treatment. *Neuroendocrinology* 70, 422–430.

Kudoh, A., Katagai, H., and Takazawa, T. (2001). Endocrine response to surgical stress in three patients over 100 yr. *Can. J. Anaesth.* 48, 340–343.

Labrie, F., Luu-The, V., Labrie, C., and Simard, J. (2001). DHEA and its transformation into androgens and estrogens in peripheral target tissues: intracrinology. *Front. Neuroendocrinol.* 22, 185–212.

Lightman, S. L., Windle, R. J., Julian, M. D., Harbuz, M. S., Shanks, N., Wood, S. A., et al. (2000). "Significance of pulsatility in the HPA axis," in *Mechanisms and Significance of Pulsatile Hormone Secretion*, ed. J. D. Veldhuis (Chichester: John Wiley), 244–260.

Liposits, Z., Uht, R. M., Harrison, R. W., Gibbs, F. P., Paull, W., and Bohn, M. C. (1987). Ultrastructural localization of glucocorticoid receptor (GR) in hypothalamic paraventricular neurons synthesizing corticotropin releasing factor (CRF). *Histochem. Cell Biol.* 87, 407–412.

Lo, M. L., Kau, M. M., and Wang, P. S. (2006). Effect of aging on corticosterone secretion in diestrous rats. *J. Cell. Biochem.* 97, 351–358.

Lolait, S. J., Markwick, A. J., McNally, M., Abraham, J., Smith, A. I., and Funder, J. W. (1986). Anterior pituitary cells from Brattleboro (di/di), Long-Evans and Sprague-Dawley rats contain immunoreactive arginine vasopressin. *Neuroendocrinology* 43, 577–583.

Lolait, S. L., Stewart, L. Q., Jessop, D. S., Young, W. S., and O'Carroll, A.-M. (2007). The hypothalamic-pituitary adrenal axis response to stress in mice lacking functional vasopressin V1b receptors. *Endocrinology* 148, 849–856.

Long, N. M., Nijland, M. J., Nathanielsz, P. W., and Ford, S. P. (2010). The effect of early to mid-gestational nutrient restriction on female offspring fertility and hypothalamic-pituitary-adrenal axis response to stress. *J. Anim. Sci.* 88, 2029–2037.

Lucassen, P. J., David, R., Gonatas, N. K., and Swaab, D. F. (1993). Activation of the human supraoptic and paraventricular nucleus neurons with aging and in Alzheimer's disease as judged from increasing size of the Golgi apparatus. *Brain Res.* 632, 105–113.

Lupien, S. J., Maheu, F., Tu, M., Fiocco, A., and Schramek, T. E. (2007). The effects of stress and stress hormones on human cognition: implications for the field of brain and cognition. *Brain Cogn.* 65, 209–237.

Lupien, S. J., McEwen, B. S., Gunnar, M. R., and Heim, C. (2009). Effects of stress throughout the lifespan on the brain, behavior and cognition. *Nat. Rev. Neurosci.* 10, 434–445.

Lupien, S. J., Nair, N. P. V., Briere, S., Maheu, F., Tu, M. T., Lemay, M., et al. (1999). Increased cortisol levels and impaired cognition in human aging: implication for depression and dementia in later life. *Rev. Neurosci.* 10, 117–139.

Lupien, S. J., Wilkinson, C. W., Briere, S., Menard, C., Kin, N. M. K. N. Y., and Nair, N. P. V. (2002). The modulatory effects of corticosteroids on cognition: studies in young human populations. *Psychoneuroendocrinology* 27, 401–416.

Ma, S., Shipston, M. J., Morilak, D., and Russel, J. A. (2005). Reduced hypothalamic vasopressin secretion underlies attenuated adrenocorticotropin stress responses in pregnant rats. *Endocrinology* 146, 1626–1637.

Ma, X. M., and Aguilera, G. (1999). Transcriptional responses of the vasopressin and corticotropin-releasing hormone genes to acute and repeated intraperitoneal hypertonic saline injection in rats. *Brain Res.* 68, 129–140.

Makara, G. B., Mergl, Z., and Zelena, D. (2004). The role of vasopressin in hypothalamo-pituitary-adrenal axis activation during stress: an assessment of the evidence. *Ann. N. Y. Acad. Sci.* 1018, 151–161.

Makara, G. B., Varga, J., Barna, I., Pinter, O., Klausz, B., and Zelena, D. (2012). The vasopressin-deficient Brattleboro rat: lessons for the hypothalamo-pituitary-adrenal axis regulation. *Cell. Mol. Neurobiol.* 32, 759–766.

Makino, S., Schulkin, J., Smith, M. A., Pacak, K., Palkovits, M., and Gold, P. W. (1995). Regulation of corticotropin-releasing hormone receptor messenger ribonucleic acid in the rat brain and pituitary by glucocorticoids and stress. *Endocrinology* 136, 4517–4525.

Maninger, N., Wolkowitz, O. M., Reus, V. I., Epel, E. S., and Mellon, S. H. (2009). Neurobiological and neuropsychiatric effects of dehydroepiandrosterone (DHEA) and DHEA sulfate (DHEAS). *Front. Neuroendocrinol.* 30, 65–91.

McEwen, B. S. (2007). Physiology and neurobiology of stress and adaptation: central role of the brain. *Physiol. Rev.* 87, 873–904.

McFarlane, A. R., Coghlan, J., Tresham, J., and Wintour, E. M. (1995). Corticotropin-releasing factor alone, but not arginine vasopressin alone, stimulates the release of adrenocorticotropin in the conscious intact sheep. *Endocrinology* 136, 1821–1827.

Meijer, J. C., Topic, D., Steenbergen, P. J., Jochan, G., Huston, J. P., and Oitzl, M. S. (2005). Correlations between hypothalamic-pituitary-adrenal axis parameters depend on age and learning capacity. *Endocrinology* 146, 1372–1381.

Mellon, S. H., and Vaudry, H. (2001). Biosynthesis of neurosteroids and regulation of their synthesis. *Int. Rev. Neurobiol.* 46, 33–78.

Moore, R. N., Shiller, H., and Bowden, D. M. (1979). "Adrenal structure and function," in *Aging in Non-human Primates*, ed. D. M. Bowden (New York: Van Nostrand Reinhold Company), 229–247.

Mouri, T., Itoi, K., Takahashi, K., Suda, T., Murakami, O., Yoshinaga, K., et al. (1993). Co-localization of corticotropin-releasing factor and vasopressin in the paraventricular nucleus of human hypothalamus. *Neuroendocrinology* 57, 34–39.

Muller, M. B., Landgraf, R., Preil, J., Sillaber, I., Kresse, A. E., Keck, M. E., et al. (2000). Selective activation of the hypothalamic vasopressinergic system in mice deficient for the corticotropin-releasing hormone receptor 1 is dependent on glucocorticoids. *Endocrinology* 141, 4262–4269.

Neumann, I. D., Johnstone, H. A., Hatzinger, M., Liebsch, G., Shipston, M., Russell, J. A., et al. (1998). Attenuated neuroendocrine responses to emotional and physical stressors in pregnant rats involve adenohypophysial changes. *J. Physiol. (Lond.)* 508, 289–300.

Ohashi, M., Fujio, N., Kato, K., Nawata, H., and Ibayashi, H. (1986). Aging is without effect on the pituitary-adrenal axis in men. *Gerontology* 32, 335–339.

Ono, N., Bedran de Castro, J., Khorram, O., and McCann, S. M. (1985). Role of arginine vasopressin in control of ACTH and LH release during stress. *Life Sci.* 36, 1779–1786.

Orentreich, N., Brind, J. L., Vogelman, J. H., Andres, R., and Baldwin, H. (1992). Long-term longitudinal measurements of plasma dehydroepiandrosterone sulfate in normal men. *J. Clin. Endocrinol. Metab.* 75, 1002–1004.

Otte, C., Hart, S., Neylan, T. C., Marmar, C. R., Yaffe, K., and Mohr, D. C. (2005). A meta-analysis of cortisol response to challenge in human aging: importance of gender. *Psychoneuroendocrinology* 30, 80–91.

Pedersen, W. A., Wan, R., and Mattson, M. P. (2001). Impact of aging on stress-responsive neuroendocrine systems. *Mech. Ageing Dev.* 122, 963–983.

Perez-Neri, I., Montes, S., Ojeda-Lopez, C., Ramirez-Bermudez, J., and Rios, C. (2008). Modulation of neurotransmitter systems by dehydroepiandrosterone and dehydroepiandrosterone sulfate: mechanism of action and relevance to psychiatric disorders. *Prog. Neuropsychopharmacol. Biol. Psychiatry* 32, 1118–1130.

Perraudin, V., Delarue, C., de Keyzer, Y., Bertagna, X., Kuhn, J. M., Contesse, V., et al. (1995). Vasopressin-responsive adrenocortical tumor in a mild Cushing's syndrome: in vivo and in vitro studies. *J. Clin. Endocrinol. Metab.* 80, 2661–2667.

Perraudin, V., Delarue, C., Lefebvre, H., Contesse, V., Kuhn, J. M., and

Vaudry, H. (1993). Vasopressin stimulates cortisol secretion from human adrenocortical tissue through activation of V1 receptors. *J. Clin. Endocrinol. Metab.* 76, 1522–1528.

Pivina, C. G., Akulova, V. K., and Ordyan, N. E. (2007). Changed activity of the hypothalamic-pituitary-adrenocortical system in prenatally stressed female rat during aging. *Bull. Exp. Biol. Med.* 143, 740–743.

Plotsky, P. (1991). Pathways to the secretion of adrenocortictropin: a view from the portal. *J. Neuroendocrinol.* 3, 1–9.

Plotsky, P. M., Bruhn, T. O., and Vale, W. (1985). Hypophysiotropic regulation of adrenocorticotropin secretion in response to insulin-induced hypoglycemia. *Endocrinology* 117, 323–329.

Prelevic, G. M., and Jacobs, H. S. (1997). Menopause and post-menopause. *Baillieres Clin. Endocrinol. Metab.* 11, 311–340.

Raadsheer, F. C., Sluiter, A. A., Ravid, R., Tilders, F. J. H., and Swaab, D. F. (1993). Localization of corticotrophin-releasing hormone (CRH) neurons in the paraventricular nucleus of the human hypothalamus; age-dependent colocalization with vasopressin. *Brain Res.* 615, 50–62.

Rabadan-Diehl, C., and Aguilera, G. (1998). Glucocorticoids increase vasopressin V1b receptor coupling to phospholipase C. *Endocrinology* 139, 3220–3226.

Rabadan-Diehl, C., Lolait, S., and Aguilera, G. (1995). Regulation of the pituitary V1b receptor mRNA during stress in the rat. *J. Neuroendocrinol.* 7, 903–910.

Raskind, M. A., Peskind, E. R., Pascualy, M., Edland, S. D., Dobie, D. J., Murray, S., et al. (1995). The effects of normal aging on cortisol and adrenocorticotropin responses to hypertonic saline infusion. *Psychoneuroendocrinology* 20, 637–644.

Ratka, A., Sutanto, W., Bloemers, M., and de Kloet, E. R. (1989). On the role of brain mineralocorticoid (type I) and glucocorticoid (type II) receptors in neuroendocrine regulation. *Neuroendocrinology* 50, 117–123.

Renard, G. M., Rivarola, M. A., and Suarez, M. M. (2010). Gender-dependent effects of early maternal separation and variable chronic stress on vasopressinergic activity and glucocorticoid receptor expression in adult rats. *Dev. Neurosci.* 32, 71–80.

Reppert, S. M., and Weaver, D. R. (2002). Coordination of circadian timing in mammals. *Nature* 418, 935–941.

Revskoy, S., and Redei, E. (2000). Decreased in vitro sensitivity to dexamethasone in corticotropes from middle-age rats. *Exp. Gerontol.* 35, 237–242.

Rhodes, M. E., and Rubin, R. (1999). Functional sex differences ("sexual diergism") of central nervous system cholinergic systems, vasopressin, and hypothalamic-pituitary-adrenal activity in mammals: a selective review. *Brain Res. Brain Res. Rev.* 30, 135–152.

Rivier, C., and Vale, W. (1983). Interaction of corticotrophin-releasing factor and arginine vasopressin on adrenocorticotropin secretion in vivo. *Endocrinology* 113, 939–942.

Roozendaal, V., Van Gool, W. A., Swaab, D. F., Hoogendijk, J. E., and Mirmiran, M. (1987). Changes in vasopressin cells of the rat suprachiasmatic nucleus with aging. *Brain Res.* 409, 259–264.

Roper, J. A., O'Carroll, A.-M., Young, W. S., and Lolait, S. J. (2011). The vasopressin Avpr1b receptor: molecular and pharmacological studies. *Stress* 14, 98–115.

Rossi, N. F., and Chen, H. (2002). Modulation of ET (B) receptor-induced arginine-vasopressin secretion by N-methyl-D-aspartate (NMDA) and γ-aminobutyric acid (GABA)-dependent mechanisms in hypothalamo-neurohypophysial explants. *Clin. Sci.* 103(Suppl. 48), 162S–166S.

Rubin, R. T., and Rhodes, M. E. (2002). Sexual diergism of hypothalamo-pituitary-adrenal cortical responses to low-dose physostigmine in elderly vs. young women and men. *Neuropsychopharmacology* 26, 672–681.

Russell, G. M., Henley, D. E., Leendertz, J., Douthwaite, J. A., Wood, S. A., Stevens, A., et al. (2010). Rapid glucocorticoid receptor-mediated inhibition of hypothalamic-pituitary-adrenal ultradian activity in healthy males. *J. Neurosci.* 30, 6106–6115.

Salata, R. A., Jarrett, D. B., Verbalis, J. G., and Robinson, A. G. (1988). Vasopressin stimulation of adrenocorticotropin hormone (ACTH) in humans. In vivo bioassay of corticotropin-releasing factor (CRF) which provides evidence for CRF mediation of the diurnal rhythm of ACTH. *J. Clin. Invest.* 81, 766–774.

Sapolsky, R., and Altman, J. (1991). Incidences of hypercortisolism and dexamethasone resistance increase with age among wild baboons. *Biol. Psychiatry* 30, 1008–1013.

Sapolsky, R. M. (1999). Glucocorticoids, stress, and their adverse neurological effects: relevance to aging. *Exp. Gerontol.* 34, 721–732.

Sapolsky, R. M., Krey, L. C., and McEwen, B. S. (1986). The neuroendocrinology of stress and aging: the glucocorticoid cascade hypothesis. *Endocr. Rev.* 7, 284–301.

Sawchenko, P. E. (1987). Evidence for a local site of action for glucocorticoids in inhibiting CRF and vasopressin expression in the paraventricular nucleus. *Brain Res.* 403, 213–224.

Sawchenko, P. E., Arias, C. A., and Mortrud, M. T. (1993). Local tetrodotoxin blocks chronic stress effects on corticotrophin-releasing factor and vasopressin messenger ribonucleic acids in hypophysiotropic neurons. *J. Neuroendocrinol.* 5, 341–348.

Scaccianoce, S., DeSciullo, A., and Angelucci, L. (1990). Age-related changes in hypothalamo-pituitary-adrenocortical axis activity in the rat. *Neuroendocrinology* 52, 150–155.

Schmidt, M. V., Sterlemann, V., Wagner, K., Niederleitner, B., Ganea, K., Liebl, C., et al. (2009). Postnatal glucocorticoid excess due to pituitary glucocorticoid receptor deficiency: differential short- and long-term consequences. *Endocrinology* 150, 2709–2716.

Seeman, T. E., and Robbins, R. J. (1994). Aging and hypothalamic-pituitary-adrenal response to challenge in humans. *Endocr. Rev.* 15, 233–260.

Serradeil-Le Gal, C., Derick, S., Brossard, G., Manning, M., Simiand, J., Gaillard, R., et al. (2003). Functional and pharmacological characterization of the first specific agonist and antagonist for the V1b receptor in mammals. *Stress* 6, 199–206.

Serradeil-Le Gal, C., Wagnon, J., Tonnerre, B., Roux, R., Garcia, G., Griebel, G., et al. (2005). An overview of SSR149415, a selective nonpeptide vasopressin V1b receptor antagonist for the treatment of stress-related disorders. *CNS Drug Rev.* 2005, 53–68.

Shanks, N., Windle, R. J., Perks, P., Wood, S., Ingram, C. D., and Lightman, S. L. (1999). The hypothalamic-pituitary-adrenal axis response to endotoxin is attenuated during lactation. *J. Neuroendocrinol.* 11, 857–865.

Sherman, B., Wysham, C., and Pfohl, B. (1985). Age-related changes in the circadian rhythm of plasma cortisol in man. *J. Clin. Endocrinol. Metab.* 61, 439–443.

Solas, M., Aisa, B., Mugueta, M. C., Del Rio, J., Tordera, R. M., and Ramirez, M. J. (2010). Interactions between age, stress and insulin on cognition: implications for Alzheimer's disease. *Neuropsychopharmacology* 35, 1–10.

Spiga, F., Harrison, L., Wood, S., Knight, D. M., MacSweeney, C. P., Thomson, F., et al. (2009). Blockade of the V1b receptor reduces ACTH, but not corticosterone secretion induced by stress without affecting basal hypothalamic-pituitary-adrenal axis activity. *J. Endocrinol.* 200, 273–283.

Stewart, L. Q., Roper, J. A., Young, W. S., O'Carroll, A.-M., and Lolait, S. J. (2008). Pituitary-adrenal response to acute and repeated mild restraint, forced swim and change in environment stress in arginine vasopressin receptor 1b knockout mice. *J. Neuroendocrinol.* 20, 597–605.

Swaab, D. F., Bao, A. M., and Lucassen, P. L. (2005). The stress system in the human brain in depression and neurodegeneration. *Ageing Res. Rev.* 4, 141–194.

Swaab, D. F., Fliers, E., and Partiman, T. S. (1985). The suprachiasmatic nucleus of the human brain in relation to sex, age and senile dementia. *Brain Res.* 342, 37–44.

Tang, G., and Phillips, R. (1978). Some age-related changes in pituitary-adrenal function in the male laboratory rat. *J. Gerontol.* 33, 377–382.

Tanoue, A., Ito, S., Honda, K., Oshikawa, S., Kitagawa, Y., Koshimuzu, T., et al. (2004). The vasopressin V1b receptor critically regulates hypothalamic-pituitary-adrenal axis activity under both stress and resting conditions. *J. Clin. Invest.* 113, 302–309.

Terwell, D., Markerink, M., and Jolles, J. (1992). Age-related changes in concentrations of vasopressin in the central nervous system and plasma of the male Wistar rat. *Mech. Ageing Dev.* 65, 127–136.

Thibonnier, M., Coles, P., Thibonnier, A., and Shoham, M. (2002). Molecular pharmacology and modeling of vasopressin receptors. *Prog. Brain Res.* 139, 179–196.

Tilders, F. J., Berkenbosch, F., Vermes, I., Linton, E. A., and Smelik, P. G. (1985). Role of epinephrine and vasopressin in the control of the pituitary–adrenal response to stress. *Fed. Proc.* 44, 155–160.

Tizabi, Y., and Aguilera, G. (1992). Desensitization of the hypothalamic–pituitary–adrenal axis following prolonged administration of corticotropin-releasing hormone and vasopressin. *Neuroendocrinology* 56, 611–618.

Tizabi, Y., Aguilera, G., and Gilad, G. M. (1992). Age-related reduction in pituitary corticotropin-releasing hormone receptors in two rat strains. *Neurobiol. Aging* 13, 227–230.

Traustadottir, T., Bosch, P. R., and Matt, K. S. (2003). Gender differences in cardiovascular and hypothalamic-pituitary-adrenal axis responses to psychological stress in healthy older adult men and women. *Stress* 6, 133–140.

Traustadóttir, T., Bosch, P. R., and Matt, K. S. (2005). The HPA axis response to stress in women: effects of aging and fitness. *Psychoneuroendocrinology* 30, 392–402.

Tuckermann, J. P., Kleiman, A., McPherson, K. G., and Reichardt, H. M. (2005). Molecular mechanisms of glucocorticoids in the control of inflammation and lymphocyte apoptosis. *Crit. Rev. Clin. Lab. Sci.* 42, 71–104.

Turnbull, A. V., Lee, S., and Rivier, C. (1998). Mechanisms of hypothalamic-pituitary-adrenal axis stimulation by immune signals in the adult rat. *Ann. N. Y. Acad. Sci.* 840, 434–443.

Vale, W., Rivier, C., Brown, M. R., Spiess, J., Koob, G., Swanson, L., et al. (1983). Chemical and biological characterization of corticotropin releasing factor. *Recent Prog. Horm. Res.* 39, 245–270.

Van Cauter, E., Polonsky, K. S., and Scheen, A. J. (1997). Roles of circadian rhythmicity and sleep in human glucose regulation. *Endocr. Rev.* 18, 716–738.

Vantyghem, M. C., Balavoine, A. S., Wemeau, J. L., and Douillard, C. (2011). Hyponatremia and antidiuresis syndrome. *Ann. Endocrinol. (Paris)* 72, 500–512.

Varga, J., Domokos, A., Barna, I., Jankord, R., Bagdy, G., and Zelena, D. (2011). Lack of vasopressin does not prevent the behavioral and endocrine changes induced by chronic unpredictable stress. *Brain Res. Bull.* 84, 45–52.

Vegiopoulos, A., and Herzig, S. (2007). Glucocorticoids, metabolism and metabolic diseases. *Mol. Cell. Endocrinol.* 275, 43–61.

Vezzosi, D., Cartier, D., Regnier, C., Otal, P., Bennet, F., Parmentier, F., et al. (2007). Familian adrenocorticotropin-independent macronodular adrenal hyperplasia with aberrant serotonin and vasopressin adrenal receptors. *Eur. J. Endocrinol.* 156, 21–31.

Volpi, S., Rabadan-Diehl, C., and Aguilera, G. (2004). Vasopressinergic regulation of the hypothalamic pituitary adrenal axis and stress adaptation. *Stress* 7, 75–83.

Walker, C. D., Tilders, F. J., and Burlet, A. (2001). Increased colocalization of corticotropin-releasing factor and arginine vasopressin in paraventricular neurons of the hypothalamus in lacting rats: evidence from immunotargeted lesions and immunohistochemistry. *J. Neuroendocrinol.* 13, 74–85.

Walker, J. J., Terry, J. R., and Lightman, S. L. (2010). Origin of ultradian pulsatility in the hypothalamic-pituitary-adrenal axis. *Proc. Biol. Sci.* 277, 1627–1633.

Waltman, C., Blackman, M. R., Chrousos, G. P., Riemann, C., and Harman, S. M. (1991). Spontaneous and glucocorticoid-inhibited adrenocorticotropic hormone and cortisol secretion are similar in healthy young and old men. *J. Clin. Endocrinol. Metab.* 73, 495–502.

Wellhoener, P., Born, J., Fehm, H. L., and Dodt, C. (2004). Elevated resting and exercise-induced cortisol levels after mineralcorticoid receptor blockade with canrenoate in healthy humans. *J. Clin. Endocrinol. Metab.* 89, 5048–5052.

Wersinger, S. R., Ginns, E. I., O'Carrol, A. M., Lolait, S. J., and Young, W. S. III. (2002). Vasopressin V1b receptor knockout reduces aggressive behavior in male mice. *Mol. Psychiatry* 7, 975–984.

Whitnall, M. (1987). Vasopressin co-exists in half of the corticotropin-releasing factor neurones in the external zone of the median eminence in normal rats. *Neuroendocrinology* 45, 420–424.

Whitnall, M. (1989). Stress selectively activates the vasopressin-containing subset of corticotrophin-releasing hormone neurons. *Neuroendocrinology* 50, 702–707.

Yen, S. S. C., and Laughlin, G. A. (1998). Aging and the adrenal cortex. *Exp. Gerontol.* 33, 897–910.

Yi, S.-J., and Baram, T. Z. (1994). Corticotropin-releasing hormone mediates the response to cold stress in the neonatal rat without compensatory enhancement of the peptide's gene expression. *Endocrinology* 135, 2364–2368.

Yoshimura, A., Masui, A., Jinde, S., Kanai, H., Kato, N., and Okawa, M. (2007). Influence of age or circadian time on bcl-2 and bax mRNA expression in the rat hippocampus after corticosterone exposure. *Brain Res. Bull.* 73, 254–258.

Young, S. F., Griffante, C., and Aguilera, G. (2007). Dimerization between vasopressin V1b and corticotrophin releasing hormone type 1 receptors. *Cell. Mol. Neurobiol.* 27, 439–461.

Zelena, D., Barna, I., Pinter, O., Klausz, B., Varga, J., and Makara, G. B. (2011). Congenital absence of vasopressin and age-related changes in ACTH and corticosterone stress responses in rats. *Stress* 14, 420–430.

Zelena, D., Domokos, A., Barna, I., Mergl, Z., Haller, J., and Makara, G. B. (2008). Control of the hypothalamo-pituitary-adrenal axis in the neonatal period: adrenocorticotropin and corticosterone stress responses dissociate in vasopressin-deficient Brattleboro rats. *Endocrinology* 149, 2576–2583.

Zelena, D., Domokos, A., Jain, S. K., Jankord, R., and Filaretova, L. (2009). The stimuli-specific role of vasopressin in the hypothalamus-pituitary-adrenal axis response to stress. *J. Endocrinol.* 202, 263–278.

Zelena, D., Filaretova, L., Mergle, Z., Barna, I., Toth, Z. E., and Makara, G. B. (2006). Hypothalamic paraventricular nucleus, but not vasopressin, participates in chronic hyperactivity of the HPA axis in diabetic rats. *Am. J. Physiol. Endocrinol. Metab.* 290, E243–E250.

Zelena, D., Foldes, A., Mergl, Z., Barna, I., Kovacs, K. J., and Makara, G. B. (2004). Effects of repeated restraint stress of hypothalamo-pituitary-adrenocortical function in vasopressin deficient Brattleboro rats. *Brain Res. Bull.* 63, 521–530.

Zhdanova, I. V., Masuda, K., Quasarano-Kourkoulis, C., Rosene, D. L., Killiany, R. J., and Wang, S. (2011). Aging of intrinsic circadian rhythms and sleep in a diurnal nonhuman primate, *Macaca mulatta*. *J. Biol. Rhythms* 26, 149–159.

Zorrilla, E. P., and Koob, G. F. (2010). Progress in corticotropin-releasing factor-1 antagonist development. *Drug Discov. Today* 15, 371–383.

3

# Regulation of gonadotropins by corticotropin-releasing factor and urocortin

***Kazunori Kageyama****

*Department of Endocrinology and Metabolism, Hirosaki University Graduate School of Medicine, Hirosaki, Aomori, Japan*

***Edited by:***
*Hubert Vaudry, University of Rouen, France*

***Reviewed by:***
*David Lovejoy, University of Toronto, Canada*
*Jae Young Seong, Korea University, South Korea*

****Correspondence:***
*Kazunori Kageyama, Department of Endocrinology and Metabolism, Hirosaki University Graduate School of Medicine, 5 Zaifu-cho, Hirosaki, Aomori 036-8562, Japan.*
*e-mail: kkageyama@hkg.odn.ne.jp*

While stress activates the hypothalamic–pituitary–adrenal (HPA) axis, it suppresses the hypothalamic–pituitary–gonadal (HPG) axis. Corticotropin-releasing factor (CRF) is a major regulatory peptide in the HPA axis during stress. Urocortin 1 (Ucn1), a member of the CRF family of peptides, has a variety of physiological functions and both CRF and Ucn1 contribute to the stress response via G protein-coupled seven transmembrane receptors. Ucn2 and Ucn3, which belong to a separate paralogous lineage from CRF, are highly selective for the CRF type 2 receptor ($CRF_2$ receptor). The HPA and HPG axes interact with each other, and gonadal function and reproduction are suppressed in response to various stressors. In this review, we focus on the regulation of gonadotropins by CRF and Ucn2 in pituitary gonadotrophs and of gonadotropin-releasing hormone (GnRH) via CRF receptors in the hypothalamus. In corticotrophs, stress-induced increases in CRF stimulate Ucn2 production, which leads to the inhibition of gonadotropin secretion via the $CRF_2$ receptor in the pituitary. GnRH in the hypothalamus is regulated by a variety of stress conditions. CRF is also involved in the suppression of the HPG axis, especially the GnRH pulse generator, via CRF receptors in the hypothalamus. Thus, complicated regulation of GnRH in the hypothalamus and gonadotropins in the pituitary via CRF receptors contributes to stress responses and adaptation of gonadal functions.

**Keywords: corticotropin-releasing factor, urocortin, stress, gonadotropin**

## INTRODUCTION

A variety of stressors have been shown to suppress gonadal function (Chand and Lovejoy, 2011). Proteins that play key roles in vertebrate reproduction include the neuropeptides gonadotropin-releasing hormone (GnRH) and kisspeptin and their receptors (Kim et al., 2012): kisspeptin stimulates GnRH release from hypothalamic GnRH neurons via Gpr54, a G protein-coupled receptor (Messager et al., 2005), while the gonadal steroid estrogen mediates its inhibitory effect on GnRH secretion by acting on kisspeptin-expressing neurons of the arcuate nucleus (Oakley et al., 2009; Ohkura et al., 2009). The expression of kisspeptin and kisspeptin receptor mRNA is downregulated by stressors including restraint, hypoglycemia, and lipopolysaccharide, which suggests that kisspeptin/kisspeptin receptor signaling plays a critical role in the transduction of stress-induced suppression of reproduction (Kinsey-Jones et al., 2009). In fact, kisspeptin–GPR54 signaling in the arcuate nucleus of the mediobasal hypothalamus is a critical neural component of the hypothalamic GnRH pulse generator (Li et al., 2009).

Gonadotropin-inhibitory hormone (GnIH), an RFamide-related peptide, can also modulate the reproduction of vertebrates (Ubuka et al., 2008). GnIH neurons interact directly with GnRH neurons, and the action of GnIH is mediated by a novel G protein-coupled receptor, Gpr147 (Ubuka et al., 2008). In mice, higher concentrations of GnIH-like substances are expressed in the hypothalamus and GnIH reduces GnRH release from the mouse hypothalamus (Bentley et al., 2010). The glucocorticoid and corticotropin-releasing factor (CRF) receptors are expressed in a large population of GnIH/RFamide-related peptide-expressing cells (Kirby et al., 2009). Glucocorticoids increase the inhibitory actions of GnIH on GnRH secretion (Kirby et al., 2009), while the regulation of GnIH via the CRF receptor remains to be determined.

Corticotropin-releasing factor activates and regulates the hypothalamic–pituitary–adrenal (HPA) axis during stress (Vale et al., 1981, 1997). Stress-induced CRF synthesis and secretion from the hypothalamic paraventricular nucleus (PVN) stimulates adrenocorticotropic hormone (ACTH) release from pituitary corticotrophs (Gillies et al., 1982; Mouri et al., 1993), which, in turn, stimulates the release of glucocorticoids from the adrenal glands (Whitnall, 1993). These glucocorticoids then moderate the stress response by inhibiting hypothalamic PVN production of CRF and pituitary production of ACTH (Whitnall, 1993). Urocortin 1 (Ucn1), a 40-amino acid peptide originally cloned from the Edinger–Westphal nucleus, is a member of the CRF family of peptides (Vaughan et al., 1995). Both CRF and Ucn1 contribute to stress responses and cardiovascular and gonadal functions via G protein-coupled seven transmembrane receptors (Vale et al., 1997; Kageyama et al., 1999a; Suda et al., 2004). CRF exhibits high affinity for CRF type 1 receptor ($CRF_1$ receptor; $IC_{50} = 1.6$ nM) but not for CRF type 2b receptor ($CRF_{2b}$ receptor; $IC_{50} = 42$ nM), while Ucn1 exhibits similar affinity for $CRF_1$ receptor ($IC_{50} = 0.16$ nM) and $CRF_{2b}$ receptor ($IC_{50} = 0.86$ nM; Jahn et al., 2004). $CRF_1$ receptor is predominately expressed in the brain and pituitary gland (Chang et al., 1993; Chen et al., 1993; Vita et al., 1993; Potter et al., 1994). In the pituitary, the $CRF_1$ receptor is mainly expressed by corticotrophs and is responsible for mediating the effects of hypothalamic CRF on ACTH secretion in response to stress (Wynn et al., 1985; Antoni, 1986).

Ucn2 and Ucn3 prohormones were identified in the human genome database and in mouse genomic DNA, respectively (Hsu and Hsueh, 2001; Lewis et al., 2001; Reyes et al., 2001), from which the identity and existence of endogenous peptides were predicted (Fekete and Zorrilla, 2007). Ucn2 and Ucn3 are more similar to each other than to CRF with regard to receptor binding (Kishimoto et al., 1995; Lovenberg et al., 1995a; Perrin et al., 1995; Stenzel et al., 1995). Ucn2 exhibits high affinity for $CRF_{2b}$ receptor ($IC_{50} = 0.25$ nM) but low affinity for $CRF_1$ receptor ($IC_{50} > 350$ nM; Jahn et al., 2004). Similarly, Ucn3 binds with moderate affinity to $CRF_{2b}$ receptor ($IC_{50} = 14$ nM), but its specific binding to $CRF_1$ receptor is not detectable ($IC_{50} > 2000$ nM; Jahn et al., 2004). It is hypothesized that an ancient gene duplication event is behind why Ucn1 belongs to the CRF lineage and why Ucn2 and Ucn3 represent a separate paralogous lineage (Fekete and Zorrilla, 2007).

The $CRF_1$ receptor is primarily involved in stress responses and depression, while the $CRF_2$ receptor is believed to mediate "stress-coping" responses in the brain, such as anxiolysis (Suda et al., 2004), because mice deficient in the $CRF_2$ receptor or treated with a $CRF_2$ receptor antagonist display increased anxiety-like behaviors and hypersensitive stress responses (Bale et al., 2000). Furthermore, both Ucn2 and Ucn3 act as anorexigenic neuropeptides via the $CRF_2$ receptor (Fekete et al., 2011; Chao et al., 2012) and Ucn3 regulates glucose-stimulated insulin secretion and energy homeostasis (Li et al., 2007). Ucn3 signaling through the $CRF_2$ receptor is also a critical molecular mediator in the ventromedial nucleus of the hypothalamus in regulating feeding and peripheral energy metabolism (Chao et al., 2012).

Corticotropin-releasing factor is involved in the suppression of the hypothalamic–pituitary–gonadal (HPG) axis (Rivier et al., 1986), especially the GnRH pulse generator in the hypothalamus (Knobil, 1992). Stress profoundly inhibits the reproductive function by suppressing the pulsatile release of GnRH and consequently luteinizing hormone (LH), at least in part via the CRF system as well as through the GABAergic system (Lin et al., 2012). Although CRF and Ucn clearly have potent effects on the HPG system, their possible roles and how they are regulated have yet to be fully determined. In this review, we focus on the regulation and the roles of Ucn2 in pituitary gonadotrophs and discuss the regulation of GnRH via CRF receptors in the hypothalamus.

## REGULATION OF GONADOTROPINS BY CRF AND Ucn2 IN THE PITUITARY

Changes in $CRF_1$ receptor expression and desensitization of the receptor in pituitary corticotrophs play a major role in modulating adaptive responses to stressors (Kageyama et al., 2006). CRF, vasopressin, lipopolysaccharides, cytokines, and glucocorticoids can negatively modulate the levels of pituitary $CRF_1$ receptor mRNA (Pozzoli et al., 1996; Sakai et al., 1996; Aubry et al., 1997). However, $CRF_2$ receptor mRNA is also found in the anterior pituitary and combined immunohistochemistry and *in situ* hybridization have demonstrated that $CRF_2$ receptor mRNA colocalizes mainly with gonadotrophs, not corticotrophs (**Figure 1**).

RNase protection assays of anterior pituitary mRNA show that the dominant receptor type is the CRF type 2a receptor ($CRF_{2a}$) receptor and not the $CRF_{2b}$ receptor (Lovenberg et al., 1995a; Kageyama et al., 2003). Rat $CRF_{2a}$ receptor, linked to various roles in the brain, is expressed primarily in several discrete brain regions, including the hypothalamus, lateral septum, and raphe nuclei (Lovenberg et al., 1995b), whereas the $CRF_{2b}$ receptor is found predominately in peripheral tissues such as the heart, gastrointestinal tract, arterioles, and muscles (Kageyama et al., 1999b). These data suggest that the $CRF_{2a}$ receptor in pituitary gonadotrophs is involved in the modulation of gonadotropin secretion and/or gonadal function.

Activation of the stress system could potentially influence reproduction at any level of the HPG axis (Tilbrook et al., 2002). The stress-induced decreases in LH/follicle-stimulating hormone (FSH) secretion influence gonadal functions such as sex steroidogenesis and sperm production (Demura et al., 1989; Tilbrook et al., 2002). Ucn2 is expressed mainly in corticotrophs of rat pituitary (Yamauchi et al., 2005), and its secretion and expression levels are increased by CRF and suppressed by glucocorticoids (Nemoto et al., 2007).

The $CRF_2$ receptor-selective ligand Ucn2 suppresses both expression and secretion of gonadotropins in rats, while a $CRF_2$ receptor antagonist increases the secretion of gonadotropins (Nemoto et al., 2009). In addition, an anti-CRF antibody blocks stress-induced increases in plasma ACTH and corticosterone, and an anti-Ucn2 antibody blocks stress-induced suppression of LH secretion without affecting stress-induced ACTH and corticosterone release (Nemoto et al., 2010). Stress-induced increases in microRNA-325-3p also suppress gonadotropin secretion (Nemoto et al., 2012). Although the presence and/or secretion of mature Ucn2 has not been determined in the pituitary or other tissues, it is possible that stress-induced increases in CRF stimulate Ucn2 in corticotrophs, which inhibits gonadotropin secretion via $CRF_2$ receptors in the pituitary.

## REGULATION OF GnRH BY CRF AND Ucn VIA CRF RECEPTORS IN THE HYPOTHALAMUS

Although peripheral administration of CRF fails to affect LH secretion (D'Agata et al., 1984; Rivier and Vale, 1984), central injection of CRF inhibits secretion of gonadotropins (Rivier et al., 1986). These effects of CRF probably reflect a central mechanism that involves modulation of the activity of GnRH neurons in the hypothalamus (Petraglia et al., 1987; Li et al., 2010). Indeed, in monkeys, a CRF antagonist attenuates suppression of the GnRH pulse generator in response to hypoglycemic stress (Chen et al., 1996). Furthermore, a recent *in vivo* rat study indicated that CRF innervation of the dorsolateral bed nucleus of the stria terminalis plays a central role in stress-induced suppression of the GnRH pulse generator (Li et al., 2011).

Corticotropin-releasing factor also suppresses GnRH gene expression levels in murine GnRH GT1-7 cells (Kinsey-Jones et al., 2006). In fact, GT1-7 GnRH-producing cells have been used extensively in studies of the basic control mechanisms involved in GnRH neuronal function. Belsham and colleagues have managed to develop cell lines that are representative of the enormous range of cell types of the hypothalamus (Dalvi et al., 2011). N39,

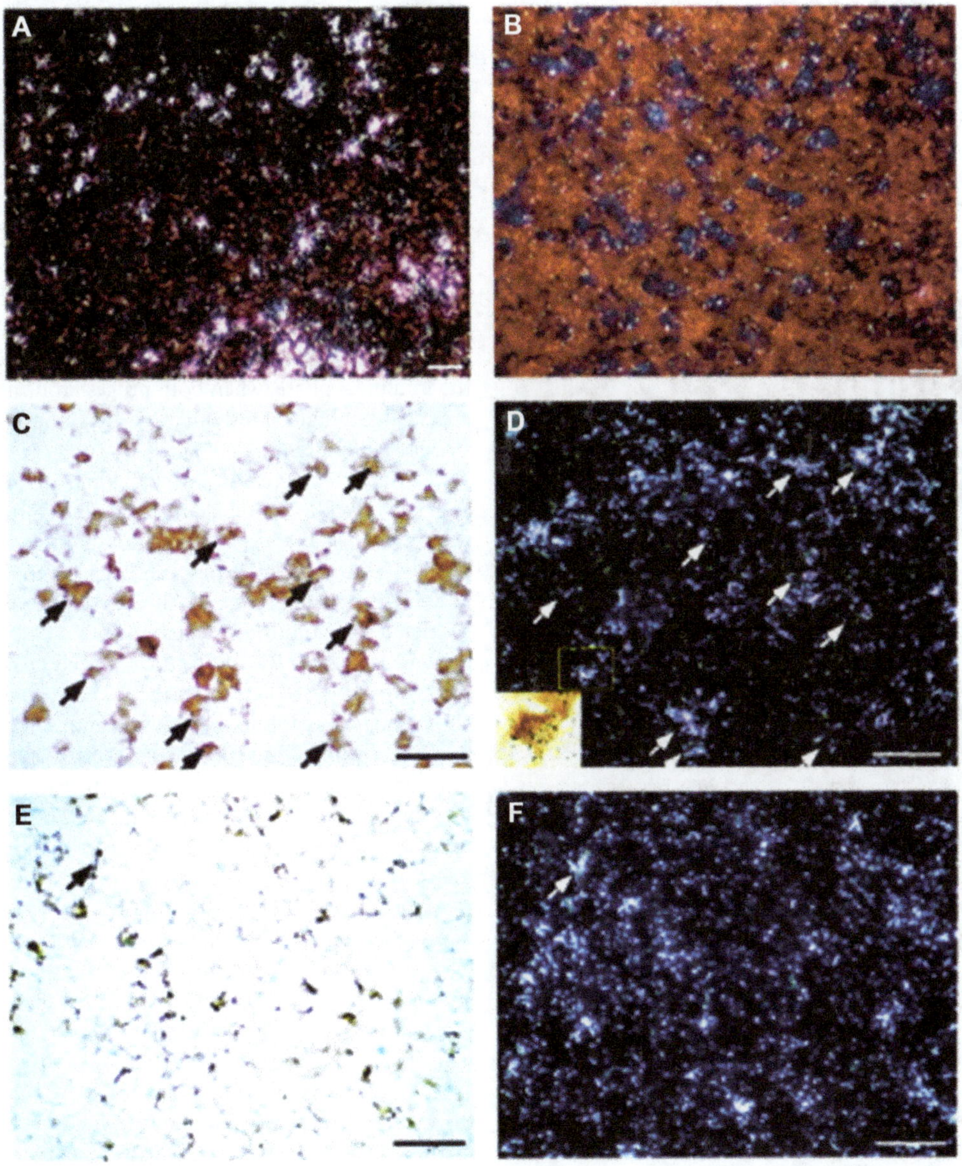


**FIGURE 1 | Localization of $CRF_2$ receptor mRNA in the rat anterior pituitary gland.** Representative dark-field photomicrographs showing anterior pituitary sections probed with either antisense **(A)** or sense **(B)** *in situ* hybridization probes for $CRF_2$ receptor mRNA. Positive signals (indicated by *silver grain clusters*) were found only in the tissues probed with antisense probes; no signals were found in the sense control. **(C)** Bright-field photomicrograph showing LH-immunoreactive cells in the rat anterior pituitary. Gonadotrophs (visualized by the *brown* DAB precipitate) represent LH-immunoreactive cells. **(D)** Dark-field image of the same area as panel **(C)** showing $CRF_2$ receptor mRNA-positive cells (*silver grain clusters*). Some of the cells that are double-labeled by immunostaining for LH and *in situ* hybridization for $CRF_2$ receptor mRNA are indicated by *arrows*. *Inset*: High-power magnification of the *boxed area* of panel **(D)** to illustrate a LH-positive cell that shows a positive signal for $CRF_2$ receptor mRNA (scattered *black silver grains*). **(E)** Representative bright-field photomicrograph of the anterior pituitary showing ACTH-immunoreactive cells (*brown* DAB precipitate). **(F)** Dark-field image of the same area as panel **(E)** showing $CRF_2$ receptor mRNA signals (*silver grain clusters*). Only a few ACTH-immunoreactive and $CRF_2$ receptor mRNA double-labeled cells (*arrow*) were observed. *Scale bar*, 50 μm. Reproduction from Kageyama et al. (2003) with permission of the publisher. Copyright 2003, The Endocrine Society.

developed from primary mouse fetal hypothalamic culture, is one of these homologous neuronal cell lines. To further understand the possible function of Ucn and the regulation of GnRH by CRF receptors in the hypothalamus, hypothalamic N39 cells have been studied because they express both $CRF_1$ and $CRF_2$ receptor mRNA and protein (Kageyama et al., 2012). It has been shown in these cells that a $CRF_1$ receptor antagonist, antalarmin, inhibits CRF-induced decreases in GnRH mRNA levels, which suggests that CRF decreases GnRH mRNA levels via the $CRF_1$ receptor (**Figure 2**).

The $CRF_2$ receptor may also be involved in the regulation of GnRH gene expression. It has been reported that CRF regulates

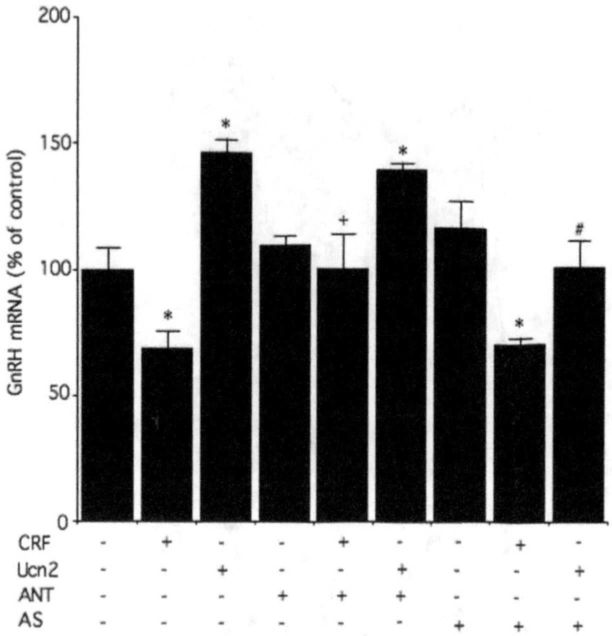


**FIGURE 2 | Effects of a CRF receptor antagonist on the effects of CRF and Ucn2 on GnRH mRNA levels in N39 cells.** Cells were pre-incubated with medium containing 1 μM antalarmin (ANT), antisauvagine-30 (AS), or vehicle for 30 min, and then incubated for 6 h with medium containing 100 nM CRF, 100 nM Ucn2, or vehicle. Reproduction from Kageyama et al. (2012) with permission of the publisher. Copyright 2012, Elsevier.

GnRH mRNA levels via, at least in part, the CRF2 receptor in GT1-7 cells (Kinsey-Jones et al., 2006). In N39 cells, Ucn2 increases GnRH mRNA levels, and these Ucn2-induced increases in GnRH mRNA levels are blocked by the $CRF_2$ receptor antagonist antisauvagine-30 (**Figure 2**). These results suggest that Ucn2 stimulates GnRH mRNA levels via the $CRF_2$ receptor in hypothalamic cells. In an *in vivo* study, hypoglycemia- and lipopolysaccharide-induced suppression of LH involves activation of $CRF_2$ receptor while restraint stress-induced inhibition of LH pulses involves both $CRF_1$ and $CRF_2$ receptors (Li et al., 2006). On the other hand, a more recent *in vivo* study showed that a $CRF_1$ receptor antagonist blocks the acute stress-induced increases in gonadotropin secretion on the morning of proestrus while a $CRF_2$ receptor antagonist weakly blocks the increase in FSH secretion (Traslaviña and Franci, 2012). Although GnRH production and secretion may be differentially modulated via CRF receptors under different stressors, further study will be required to elucidate the involvement of CRF receptors.

Glucocorticoids were recently shown to increase $CRF_{2a}$ receptor expression while simultaneously inhibiting $CRF_1$ receptor expression in pancreatic β cell-derived insulinoma MIN6 cells expressing glucocorticoid receptors (Huising et al., 2011). The differential effects of the glucocorticoids on the expression of these receptors in the endocrine pancreas represent a mechanism of shifting sensitivity from $CRF_1$ to $CRF_2$ receptor ligands (Huising et al., 2011). In the hypothalamus, glucocorticoids, released in response to stress, inhibit GnRH and gonadotropins through activation of GnIH (Kirby et al., 2009). It has yet to be determined whether glucocorticoid-induced changes in CRF and Ucn are involved in the regulation of GnRH and gonadotropins.

## RELATION BETWEEN SEXUAL DIFFERENCES AND THE CRF SYSTEM IN THE HYPOTHALAMUS

Sexual dimorphism is associated with stress sensitivity and interaction of the HPA and HPG axes (Chand and Lovejoy, 2011). Estrogens are implicated in the differing stress responses between the sexes and modulate activation of the HPA axis; females, but not males, generally have slight hypercortisolism (Magiakou et al., 1997). Estrogen replacement increases the basal levels of ACTH in ovariectomized rats (Ochedalski et al., 2007) and in postmenopausal women (Fonseca et al., 2001). Moreover, women in the midluteal phase, when both progesterone and estrogen levels are relatively high, show enhanced ACTH levels in response to a stressor (Altemus et al., 2001).

Estrogens acting centrally, including in the pituitary corticotrophs and the hypothalamus, are able to modulate the stress responses (Nakano et al., 1991), and direct estrogenic regulation of CRF gene expression has also been demonstrated in various tissues (Vamvakopoulos and Chrousos, 1993; Dibbs et al., 1997). As high levels of estrogen replacement increase the basal levels of CRF mRNA in the PVN of ovariectomized rats (Ochedalski et al., 2007), estrogen would regulate the HPA axis *in vivo* by stimulating CRF gene expression in the hypothalamus. CRF mRNA levels in the PVN are not affected by estrogen treatment in either gonadectomized estrogen receptor (ER) type β (ERβ) knockout mice or wild-type male mice (Nomura et al., 2002). Therefore, it is likely that estrogen modulates CRF gene expression in a sex-dependent manner.

Hypothalamic 4B cells show characteristics of the parvocellular neurons of the PVN because these cells express CRF, vasopressin, $CRF_1$ receptor, and glucocorticoid receptors. Estrogen directly stimulates CRF gene expression in hypothalamic 4B cells (Ogura et al., 2008), suggesting that estrogen is involved in the positive regulation of CRF gene expression in the parvocellular region of the PVN *in vitro*. Neurons expressing both CRF and ERβ are found in the medial parvocellular division (Miller et al., 2004) and project to the median eminence, and CRF in parvocellular PVN neurons exerts effects on corticotroph ACTH secretion (Gillies et al., 1982; Mouri et al., 1993). Therefore, estrogen and ERβ would contribute to the enhancement of stress responses through stimulation of CRF neurons of the hypothalamus, and may constitute the basis of sexual dimorphism in the regulation of the CRF gene (Straub, 2007). In addition, estrogen also enhances CRF- and stress-induced suppression of pulsatile LH secretion (Cates et al., 2004), and upregulation of the $CRF_2$ receptor may contribute to the sensitizing influence of estradiol on the CRF- and stress-induced suppression of the GnRH pulse generator (Kinsey-Jones et al., 2006).

Meanwhile, Ucn1 in the non-preganglionic Edinger–Westphal nucleus plays an important role in stress adaptation. Estrogens exert a differential transcriptional regulation of the Ucn1 gene through either ER type α (ERα) or ERβ receptors (Haeger et al., 2006). Ucn1 mRNA levels in the non-preganglionic Edinger–Westphal nucleus of male rats are much higher than those of females (Derks et al., 2010), and estrogens may

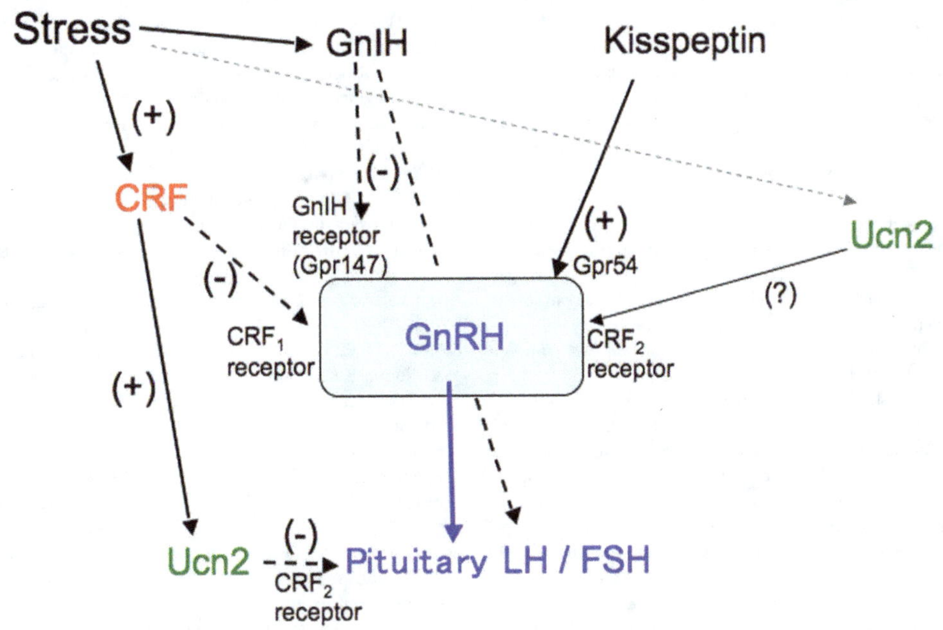


**FIGURE 3 | A schematic model of the regulation of gonadotropins by CRF and Ucn.** Stress-induced increases in CRF stimulate Ucn2 in corticotrophs, which inhibits gonadotropin secretion via the CRF$_2$ receptor in the pituitary. CRF inhibits the stress-induced suppression of the GnRH pulse generator and decreases GnRH mRNA levels via the CRF$_1$ receptor in the hypothalamus. The CRF$_2$ receptor may also be involved in the regulation of GnRH.

contribute to stress adaptation through modulation of Ucn1 production.

## CONCLUSION

In summary, Ucn2, mainly produced in corticotrophs in response to CRF, acts on gonadotrophs expressing the CRF$_2$ receptor and inhibits the production of gonadotropins in the pituitary (**Figure 3**). CRF is involved in the suppression of the HPG axis, especially the GnRH pulse generator in the hypothalamus, and also decreases GnRH mRNA levels via the CRF$_1$ receptor (**Figure 3**). The CRF$_2$ receptor may be involved in the regulation of GnRH production and secretion. GnRH production and secretion may be differentially modulated via CRF receptors in response to different stressors. Thus, complicated regulation of GnRH and gonadotropins via the CRF receptors contributes to stress responses and adaptation in gonadal functions.

## ACKNOWLEDGMENT

This work was supported in part by Health and Labour Sciences Research Grants (Research on Measures for Intractable Diseases) from the Ministry of Health, Labour, and Welfare of Japan.

## REFERENCES

Altemus, M., Roca, C., Galliven, E., Romanos, C., and Deuster, P. (2001). Increased vasopressin and adrenocorticotropin responses to stress in the midluteal phase of the menstrual cycle. *J. Clin. Endocrinol. Metab.* 86, 2525–2530.

Antoni, F. A. (1986). Hypothalamic control of adrenocorticotropin secretion: advances since the discovery of 41-residue corticotropin-releasing factor. *Endocr. Rev.* 7, 351–378.

Aubry, J.-M., Turnbull, A. V., Pozzzoli, G., Rivier, C., and Vale, W. (1997). Endotoxin decreases corticotropin-releasing factor receptor 1 messenger ribonucleic acid levels in rat pituitary. *Endocrinology* 138, 1621–1626.

Bale, T. L., Contarino, A., Smith, G. W., Chan, R., Gold, L. H., Sawchenko, P. E., et al. (2000). Mice deficient for corticotropin-releasing hormone receptor-2 display anxiety-like behaviour and are hypersensitive to stress. *Nat. Genet.* 24, 410–414.

Bentley, G. E., Tsutsui, K., and Kriegsfeld, L. J. (2010). Recent studies of gonadotropin-inhibitory hormone (GnIH) in the mammalian hypothalamus, pituitary and gonads. *Brain Res.* 1364, 62–71.

Cates, P. S., Li, X. F., and O'Byrne, K. T. (2004). The influence of 17beta-oestradiol on corticotrophin-releasing hormone induced suppression of luteinising hormone pulses and the role of CRH in hypoglycaemic stress-induced suppression of pulsatile LH secretion in the female rat. *Stress* 7, 113–118.

Chand, D., and Lovejoy, D. A. (2011). Stress and reproduction: controversies and challenges. *Gen. Comp. Endocrinol.* 171, 253–257.

Chang, C. P., Pearse, R. I., O'Connell, S., and Rosenfeld, M. G. (1993). Identification of a seven transmembrane helix receptor for corticotropin-releasing factor and sauvagine in mammalian brain. *Neuron* 11, 1187–1195.

Chao, H., Digruccio, M., Chen, P., and Li, C. (2012). Type 2 corticotropin-releasing factor receptor in the ventromedial nucleus of hypothalamus is critical in regulating feeding and lipid metabolism in white adipose tissue. *Endocrinology* 153, 166–176.

Chen, M. D., Ordög, T., O'Byrne, K. T., Goldsmith, J. R., Connaughton, M. A., and Knobil, E. (1996). The insulin hypoglycemia-induced inhibition of gonadotropin-releasing hormone pulse generator activity in the rhesus monkey: roles of vasopressin and corticotropin-releasing factor. *Endocrinology* 137, 2012–2021.

Chen, R., Lewis, K. A., Perrin, M. H., and Vale, W. W. (1993). Expression cloning of a human corticotropin-releasing-factor receptor. *Proc. Natl. Acad. Sci. U.S.A.* 90, 8967–8971.

D'Agata, R., Cavagnini, F., Invitti, C., Mongioi, A., Fossati, R., Scapagnini, U., et al. (1984). Effect of CRF on the release of anterior pituitary hormones in normal subjects and patients with Cushing's disease. *Pharmacol. Res. Commun.* 16, 303–311.

Dalvi, P. S., Nazarians-Armavil, A., Tung, S., and Belsham, D. D. (2011). Immortalized neurons for the study of hypothalamic function. *Am. J. Physiol. Regul. Integr. Comp. Physiol.* 300, R1030–R1052.

Demura, R., Suzuki, T., Nakamura, S., Komatsu, H., Odagiri, E., and Demura, H. (1989). Effect of immobilization stress on testosterone and inhibin in male rats. *J. Androl.* 10, 210–213.

Derks, N. M., Gaszner, B., Roubos, E. W., and Kozicz, L. T. (2010). Sex differences in urocortin 1 dynamics in the non-preganglionic Edinger–Westphal nucleus of the rat. *Neurosci. Res.* 66, 117–123.

Dibbs, K. I., Anteby, E., Mallon, M. A., Sadovsky, Y., and Adler, S. (1997). Transcriptional regulation of human placental corticotropin-releasing factor by prostaglandins and estradiol. *Biol. Reprod.* 57, 1285–1292.

Fekete, E. M., Zhao, Y., Szücs, A., Sabino, V., Cottone, P., Rivier, J., et al. (2011). Systemic urocortin 2, but not urocortin 1 or stressin 1-A, suppresses feeding via CRF2 receptors without malaise and stress. *Br. J. Pharmacol.* 164, 1959–1975.

Fekete, E. M., and Zorrilla, E. P. (2007). Physiology, pharmacology, and therapeutic relevance of urocortins in mammals: ancient CRF paralogs. *Front. Neuroendocrinol.* 28, 1–27.

Fonseca, E., Basurto, L., Velazquez, S., and Zarate, A. (2001). Hormone replacement therapy increases ACTH/dehydroepiandrosterone sulfate in menopause. *Maturitas* 39, 57–62.

Gillies, G. E., Linton, E. A., and Lowry, P. J. (1982). Corticotropin releasing activity of the new CRF is potentiated several times by vasopressin. *Nature* 299, 355–357.

Haeger, P., Andrés, M. E., Forray, M. I., Daza, C., Araneda, S., and Gysling, K. (2006). Estrogen receptors alpha and beta differentially regulate the transcriptional activity of the urocortin gene. *J. Neurosci.* 26, 4908–4916.

Hsu, S. Y., and Hsueh, A. J. (2001). Human stresscopin and stresscopin-related peptide are selective ligands for the type 2 corticotropin-releasing hormone receptor. *Nat. Med.* 7, 605–611.

Huising, M. O., Pilbrow, A. P., Matsumoto, M., van der Meulen, T., Park, H., Vaughan, J. M., et al. (2011). Glucocorticoids differentially regulate the expression of CRFR1 and CRFR2α in MIN6 insulinoma cells and rodent islets. *Endocrinology* 152, 138–150.

Jahn, O., Tezval, H., van Werven, L., Eckart, K., and Spiess, J. (2004). Three-amino acid motifs of urocortin II and III determine their CRF receptor subtype selectivity. *Neuropharmacology* 47, 233–242.

Kageyama, K., Bradbury, M. J., Zhao, L., Blount, A. L., and Vale, W. W. (1999a). Urocortin messenger ribonucleic acid: tissue distribution in the rat and regulation in thymus by lipopolysaccharide and glucocorticoids. *Endocrinology* 140, 5651–5658.

Kageyama, K., Gaudriault, G. E., Bradbury, M. J., and Vale, W. W. (1999b). Regulation of corticotropin-releasing factor receptor type 2 β messenger ribonucleic acid in the rat cardiovascular system by urocortin, glucocorticoids, and cytokines. *Endocrinology* 141, 2285–2293.

Kageyama, K., Hanada, K., Moriyama, T., Nigawara, T., Sakihara, S., and Suda, T. (2006). G protein-coupled receptor kinase 2 involvement in desensitization of corticotropin-releasing factor (CRF) receptor type 1 by CRF in murine corticotrophs. *Endocrinology* 147, 441–450.

Kageyama, K., Hasegawa, G., Akimoto, K., Yamagata, S., Tamasawa, N., and Suda, T. (2012). Differential regulation of gonadotropin-releasing hormone by corticotropin-releasing factor family peptides in hypothalamic N39 cells. *Peptides* 33, 149–155.

Kageyama, K., Li, C., and Vale, W. W. (2003). Corticotropin-releasing factor receptor type 2 messenger ribonucleic acid in rat pituitary: localization and regulation by immune challenge, restraint stress, and glucocorticoids. *Endocrinology* 144, 1524–1532.

Kim, D. K., Cho, E. B., Moon, M. J., Park, S., Hwang, J. I., Do Rego, J. L., et al. (2012). Molecular coevolution of neuropeptides gonadotropin-releasing hormone and kisspeptin with their cognate G protein-coupled receptors. *Front. Neurosci.* 6:3. doi: 10.3389/fnins.2012.00003

Kinsey-Jones, J. S., Li, X. F., Bowe, J. E., Lightman, S. L., and O'Byrne, K. T. (2006). Corticotrophin-releasing factor type 2 receptor-mediated suppression of gonadotrophin-releasing hormone mRNA expression in GT1-7 cells. *Stress* 9, 215–222.

Kinsey-Jones, J. S., Li, X. F., Knox, A. M., Wilkinson, E. S., Zhu, X. L., Chaudhary, A. A., et al. (2009). Down-regulation of hypothalamic kisspeptin and its receptor, Kiss1r, mRNA expression is associated with stress-induced suppression of luteinising hormone secretion in the female rat. *J. Neuroendocrinol.* 21, 20–29.

Kirby, E. D., Geraghty, A. C., Ubuka, T., Bentley, G. E., and Kaufer, D. (2009). Stress increases putative gonadotropin inhibitory hormone and decreases luteinizing hormone in male rats. *Proc. Natl. Acad. Sci. U.S.A.* 106, 11324–11329.

Kishimoto, T., Pearse, R. V. II, Lin, C. R., and Rosenfield, M. G. (1995). A sauvagine/corticotropin-releasing factor receptor expressed in heart and skeletal muscle. *Proc. Natl. Acad. Sci. U.S.A.* 92, 1108–1112.

Knobil, E. (1992). Remembrance: the discovery of the hypothalamic gonadotropin-releasing hormone pulse generator and of its physiological significance. *Endocrinology* 131, 1005–1006.

Lewis, K., Li, C., Perrin, M. H., Blount, A., Kunitake, K., Donaldson, C., et al. (2001). Identification of urocortin III, an additional member of the corticotropin-releasing factor (CRF) family with high affinity for the CRF2 receptor. *Proc. Natl. Acad. Sci. U.S.A.* 98, 7570–7575.

Li, C., Chen, P., Vaughan, J., Lee, K. F., and Vale, W. (2007). Urocortin 3 regulates glucose-stimulated insulin secretion and energy homeostasis. *Proc. Natl. Acad. Sci. U.S.A.* 104, 4206–4211.

Li, X. F., Bowe, J. E., Kinsey-Jones, J. S., Brain, S. D., Lightman, S. L., and O'Byrne, K. T. (2006). Differential role of corticotrophin-releasing factor receptor types 1 and 2 in stress-induced suppression of pulsatile luteinising hormone secretion in the female rat. *J. Neuroendocrinol.* 18, 602–610.

Li, X. F., Kinsey-Jones, J. S., Cheng, Y., Knox, A. M., Lin, Y., Petrou, N. A., et al. (2009). Kisspeptin signalling in the hypothalamic arcuate nucleus regulates GnRH pulse generator frequency in the rat. *PLoS ONE* 4:e8334. doi: 10.1371/journal.pone.0008334

Li, X. F., Knox, A. M., and O'Byrne, K. T. (2010). Corticotrophin-releasing factor and stress-induced inhibition of the gonadotrophin-releasing hormone pulse generator in the female. *Brain Res.* 1364, 153–163.

Li, X. F., Lin, Y. S., Kinsey-Jones, J. S., Milligan, S. R., Lightman, S. L., and O'Byrne, K. T. (2011). The role of the bed nucleus of the stria terminalis in stress-induced inhibition of pulsatile luteinising hormone secretion in the female rat. *J. Neuroendocrinol.* 23, 3–11.

Lin, Y. S., Li, X. F., Shao, B., Hu, M. H., Goundry, A. L., Jeyaram, A., et al. (2012). The role of GABAergic signalling in stress-induced suppression of gonadotrophin-releasing hormone pulse generator frequency in female rats. *J. Neuroendocrinol.* 24, 477–488.

Lovenberg, T. W., Chalmers, D. T., Liu, C., and De Souza, E. B. (1995a). CRF 2 α and CRF2 β receptor mRNAs are differentially distributed between the rat central nervous system and peripheral tissues. *Endocrinology* 136, 4139–4142.

Lovenberg, T. W., Liaw, C. W., Grigoriadis, D. E., Clevenger, W., Chalmers, D. T., De Souza, E. B., et al. (1995b). Cloning and characterization of a functionally distinct corticotropin-releasing factor receptor subtype from rat brain. *Proc. Natl. Acad. Sci. U.S.A.* 92, 836–840.

Magiakou, M. A., Mastorakos, G., Webster, E., and Chrousos, G. P. (1997). The hypothalamic–pituitary–adrenal axis and the female reproductive system. *Ann. N. Y. Acad. Sci.* 816, 42–56.

Messager, S., Chatzidaki, E. E., Ma, D., Hendrick, A. G., Zahn, D., Dixon, J., et al. (2005). Kisspeptin directly stimulates gonadotropin-releasing hormone release via G protein-coupled receptor 54. *Proc. Natl. Acad. Sci. U.S.A.* 102, 1761–1766.

Miller, W. J., Suzuki, S., Miller, L. K., Handa, R., and Uht, R. M. (2004). Estrogen receptor (ER) beta isoforms rather than ERalpha regulate corticotropin-releasing hormone promoter activity through an alternate pathway. *J. Neurosci.* 24, 10628–10635.

Mouri, T., Itoi, K., Takahashi, K., Suda, T., Murakami, O., Yoshinaga, K., et al. (1993). Colocalization of corticotropin-releasing factor and vasopressin in the paraventricular nucleus of the human hypothalamus. *Neuroendocrinology* 57, 34–39.

Nakano, Y., Suda, T., Sumitomo, T., Tozawa, F., and Demura, H. (1991). Effects of sex steroids on beta-endorphin release from rat hypothalamus in vitro. *Brain Res.* 553, 1–3.

Nemoto, T., Iwasaki-Sekino, A., Yamauchi, N., and Shibasaki, T. (2007). Regulation of the expression and secretion of urocortin 2 in rat pituitary. *J. Endocrinol.* 192, 443–452.

Nemoto, T., Iwasaki-Sekino, A., Yamauchi, N., and Shibasaki, T. (2010). Role of urocortin 2 secreted by the pituitary in the stress-induced suppression of luteinizing hormone secretion in rats. *Am. J. Physiol. Endocrinol. Metab.* 299, E567–E575.

Nemoto, T., Mano, A., and Shibasaki, T. (2012). Increased expression of miR-325-3p by urocortin 2 and its involvement in stress-induced suppression of LH secretion in rat pituitary. *Am. J. Physiol. Endocrinol. Metab.* 302, E781–E787.

Nemoto, T., Yamauchi, N., and Shibasaki, T. (2009). Novel action of pituitary urocortin 2 in the regulation of expression and secretion of gonadotropins. *J. Endocrinol.* 201, 105–114.

Nomura, M., McKenna, E., Korach, K. S., Pfaff, D. W., and Ogawa, S. (2002). Estrogen receptor-beta regulates transcript levels for oxytocin and arginine vasopressin in the hypothalamic paraventricular nucleus of male mice. *Brain Res. Mol. Brain Res.* 109, 84–94.

Oakley, A. E., Clifton, D. K., and Steiner, R. A. (2009). Kisspeptin signaling in the brain. *Endocr. Rev.* 30, 713–743.

Ochedalski, T., Subburaju, S., Wynn, P. C., and Aguilera, G. (2007). Interaction between oestrogen and oxytocin on hypothalamic–pituitary–adrenal axis activity. *J. Neuroendocrinol.* 19, 189–197.

Ogura, E., Kageyama, K., Hanada, K., Kasckow, J., and Suda, T. (2008). Effects of estradiol on regulation of corticotropin-releasing factor gene and interleukin-6 production via estrogen receptor type beta in hypothalamic 4B cells. *Peptides* 29, 456–464.

Ohkura, S., Uenoyama, Y., Yamada, S., Homma, T., Takase, K., Inoue, N., et al. (2009). Physiological role of metastin/kisspeptin in regulating gonadotropin-releasing hormone (GnRH) secretion in female rats. *Peptides* 30, 49–56.

Perrin, M., Donaldson, C., Chen, R., Blount, A., Berggren, T., Bilezikjian, L., et al. (1995). Identification of a second CRF receptor gene and characterization of a cDNA expressed in heart. *Proc. Natl. Acad. Sci. U.S.A.* 92, 2969–2973.

Petraglia, F., Sutton, S., Vale, W., and Plotsky, P. (1987). Corticotropin-releasing factor decreases plasma luteinizing hormone levels in female rats by inhibiting gonadotropin-releasing hormone release into hypophysial-portal circulation. *Endocrinology* 120, 1083–1088.

Potter, E., Sutton, S., Donaldson, C., Chen, R., Perrin, M., Lewis, K., et al. (1994). Distribution of corticotropin-releasing factor receptor mRNA expression in the rat brain and pituitary. *Proc. Natl. Acad. Sci. U.S.A.* 91, 8777–8781.

Pozzoli, G., Bilezikjian, L. M., Perrin, M. H., Blount, A. L., and Vale, W. W. (1996). Corticotropin-releasing factor (CRF) and glucocorticoids modulate the expression of type 1 CRF receptor messenger ribonucleic acid in rat anterior pituitary cell cultures. *Endocrinology* 137, 65–71.

Reyes, T. M., Lewis, K., Perrin, M. H., Kunitake, K. S., Vaughan, J., Arias, C. A., et al. (2001). Urocortin II: a member of the corticotropin-releasing factor (CRF) neuropeptide family that is selectively bound by type 2 CRF receptors. *Proc. Natl. Acad. Sci. U.S.A.* 98, 2843–2848.

Rivier, C., Rivier, J., and Vale, W. (1986). Stress-induced inhibition of reproductive functions: role of endogenous corticotropin-releasing factor. *Science* 231, 607–609.

Rivier, C., and Vale, W. (1984). Influence of corticotropin-releasing factor on reproductive functions in the rat. *Endocrinology* 114, 914–921.

Sakai, K., Horiba, N., Sakai, Y., Tozawa, F., Demura, H., and Suda, T. (1996). Regulation of corticotropin-releasing factor receptor messenger ribonucleic acid in rat anterior pituitary. *Endocrinology* 137, 1758–1763.

Stenzel, P., Kesterson, R., Yeung, W., Cone, R. D., Rittenberg, M. B., and Stenzel-Poore, M. P. (1995). Identification of a novel murine receptor for corticotropin-releasing hormone expressed in the heart. *Mol. Endocrinol.* 9, 637–645.

Straub, R. H. (2007). The complex role of estrogens in inflammation. *Endocr. Rev.* 28, 521–574.

Suda, T., Kageyama, K., Sakihara, S., and Nigawara, T. (2004). Physiological roles of urocortins, human homologues of fish urotensin 1, and their receptors. *Peptides* 25, 1689–1701.

Tilbrook, A. J., Turner, A. I., and Clarke, I. J. (2002). Stress and reproduction: central mechanisms and sex differences in non-rodent species. *Stress* 5, 83–100.

Traslaviña, G. A., and Franci, C. R. (2012). Divergent roles of the CRH receptors in the control of gonadotropin secretion induced by acute restraint stress at proestrus. *Endocrinology* 153, 4838–4848.

Ubuka, T., Kim, S., Huang, Y. C., Reid, J., Jiang, J., Osugi, T., et al. (2008). Gonadotropin-inhibitory hormone neurons interact directly with gonadotropin-releasing hormone-I and -II neurons in European starling brain. *Endocrinology* 149, 268–278.

Vale, W., Spiess, J., Rivier, C., and Rivier, J. (1981). Characterization of a 41-residue ovine hypothalamic peptide that stimulates secretion of corticotropin and beta-endorphin. *Science* 213, 1394–1397.

Vale, W., Vaughan, J., and Perrin, M. H. (1997). Corticotropin-releasing factor (CRF) family ligands and their receptors. *Endocrinologist* 7, 3S–9S.

Vamvakopoulos, N. C., and Chrousos, G. P. (1993). Evidence of direct estrogenic regulation of human corticotropin-releasing hormone gene expression. Potential implications for the sexual dimorphism of the stress response and immune/inflammatory reaction. *J. Clin. Invest.* 92, 1896–1902.

Vaughan, J., Donaldson, C., Bittencourt, J., Perrin, M. H., Lewis, K., Sutton, S., et al. (1995). Urocortin, a mammalian neuropeptide related to fish urotensin I and to corticotropin-releasing factor. *Nature* 378, 287–292.

Vita, N., Laurent, P., Lefort, S., Chalon, P., Lelias, J. M., Kaghad, M., et al. (1993). Primary structure and functional expression of mouse pituitary and human brain corticotrophin releasing factor receptors. *FEBS Lett.* 335, 1–5.

Whitnall, M. H. (1993). Regulation of the hypothalamic corticotropin-releasing hormone neurosecretory system. *Prog. Neurobiol.* 40, 573–629.

Wynn, P. C., Harwood, J. P., Catt, K. J., and Aguilera, G. (1985). Regulation of corticotropin-releasing factor (CRF) receptors in the rat pituitary gland: effects of adrenalectomy on CRF receptors and corticotroph responses. *Endocrinology* 116, 1653–1659.

Yamauchi, N., Otagiri, A., Nemoto, T., Sekino, A., Oono, H., Kato, I., et al. (2005). Distribution of urocortin 2 in various tissues of the rat. *J. Neuroendocrinol.* 17, 656–663.

# 4

# Neuromedins U and S involvement in the regulation of the hypothalamo–pituitary–adrenal axis

***Ludwik K. Malendowicz*, Agnieszka Ziolkowska and Marcin Rucinski***

*Department of Histology and Embryology, Poznan University of Medical Sciences, Poznan, Poland*

***Edited by:***
*Hubert Vaudry, University of Rouen, France*

***Reviewed by:***
*James A. Carr, Texas Tech University, USA*
*Gábor B. Makara, Hungarian Academy of Sciences, Hungary*

****Correspondence:***
*Ludwik K. Malendowicz, Department of Histology and Embryology, Poznan University of Medical Sciences, 6 Swięcicki St., 60-781 Poznan, Poland.*
*e-mail: lkm@amp.edu.pl*

We reviewed neuromedin U (NMU) and neuromedin S (NMS) involvement in the regulation of the hypothalamo–pituitary–adrenal (HPA) axis function. NMU and NMS are structurally related and highly conserved neuropeptides. They exert biological effects via two GPCR receptors designated as NMUR1 and NMUR2 which show differential expression. NMUR1 is expressed predominantly at the periphery, while NMUR2 in the central nervous system. Elements of the NMU/NMS and their receptors network are also expressed in the HPA axis and progress in molecular biology techniques provided new information on their actions within this system. Several lines of evidence suggest that within the HPA axis NMU and NMS act at both hypothalamic and adrenal levels. Moreover, new data suggest that NMU and NMS are involved in central and peripheral control of the stress response.

**Keywords: neuromedin U, neuromedin S, hypothalamus, pituitary, adrenal**

## INTRODUCTION

In search for new biologically active peptides, the group of Minamino, Kangawa, and Matsuo in the 1980s isolated numerous small neuropeptides from porcine spinal cord. All of them exerted potent smooth-muscle stimulating activity. These short peptides have been named neuromedins (Minamino et al., 1985). Their sequences and biological activities are similar to some known neuropeptides and therefore they are commonly divided into four groups (classes):

Bombesin-like neuromedins—neuromedin B (NMB) and neuromedin C (NMC) (Minamino et al., 1983, 1984b).
Kassinin-like neuromedins—neuromedin K (NMK) and neuromedin L (NML) (Kangawa et al., 1983; Minamino et al., 1984a).
Neurotensin-like neuromedins—neuromedin N (NMN) (Minamino et al., 1984c).
Neuromedins U (NMU), for which no substantial homology with other known neuropeptides was found (Minamino et al., 1985). This group, however, was expanded in 2005, when Mori et al. (2005, 2008) isolated neuromedin S (NMS) from rat brain. NMS is composed of 36 amino acid residues and both peptides share the same amidated C-terminal heptapeptide. Furthermore, both NMU and NMS appeared to be endogenous ligands for the orphan G protein-coupled receptors FM-3/GPR66 and FM-4/TGR-1, identified earlier as type-1 and type-2 NMU receptors (NMUR1 and NMUR2), respectively (Tan et al., 1998; Howard et al., 2000; Raddatz et al., 2000; Mori et al., 2005).

**Abbreviations:** CRH, corticotropin releasing hormone; GPCR, G protein coupled receptor; HPA, hypothalamo–pituitary–adrenal; icv, intracerebroventrical; iPVN, intraparaventricular nucleus; KO, knock out; NMS, neuromedin S; NMU, neuromedin U; NMUR1, neuromedin U receptor 1; NMUR2, neuromedin U receptor 2; PCR, polymerase chain reaction; PVN, paraventricular nucleus; QPCR, quantitative real time polymerase chain reaction; RT-PCR, reverse transcription PCR; sc, subcutaneously; WT, wild type.

Identification of specific NMU receptors (NMUR1 and NMUR2) and its anorexigenic action have enhanced interest in physiological role of NMU and NMS (Howard et al., 2000; Ida et al., 2005). Advances in these studies were recently reviewed (Brighton et al., 2004; Mori et al., 2008; Mitchell et al., 2009a; Budhiraja and Chugh, 2009). Present review, on the other hand, will focus on expression and of role of NMU/NMS system in hypothalamo–pituitary–adrenal (HPA) axis functioning, updating thus our earlier reviews (Malendowicz and Markowska, 1994; Malendowicz, 1998; Malendowicz et al., 2013).

## ISOLATION, STRUCTURE, AND SYNTHESIS OF NMU AND NMS

Originally NMU was isolated from porcine spinal cord in two molecular forms, one containing 25 (NMU25) and the other 8 (NMU8) amino acid residues (Minamino et al., 1985). Subsequently NMU was isolated from other vertebrates, among them humans (Austin et al., 1995), rat (Conlon et al., 1988), guinea pig (Murphy et al., 1990), dog (O'Harte et al., 1991a), rabbit (Kage et al., 1991), chicken (O'Harte et al., 1991b; Domin et al., 1992), frogs—*Rana temporaria*, *Litoria caerulea*, and *Bombina maxima* (Domin et al., 1989b; Salmon et al., 2000; Lee et al., 2005), and goldfish (Maruyama et al., 2008). Amino acid sequences of NMU from different species are shown in **Figure 1**.

In the mammalian NMUs a common C-terminal sequence—Phe-Leu-Phe-Arg-Pro-Arg-Asn-$NH_2$—contains the active site of the neuropeptide, which is formed by the amino acid residues between positions 2 and 8 (Hashimoto et al., 1991; Sakura et al., 1991). Recent data indicate that in most species studied, the five amino acids at the C-terminus of the NMUs are totally conserved, suggesting that this region is of major importance for biological activity (Lo et al., 1992; Brighton et al., 2004; Mitchell et al., 2009b). Amidation of the C-terminus of NMU is required for receptor activation (for review see Brighton et al., 2004).

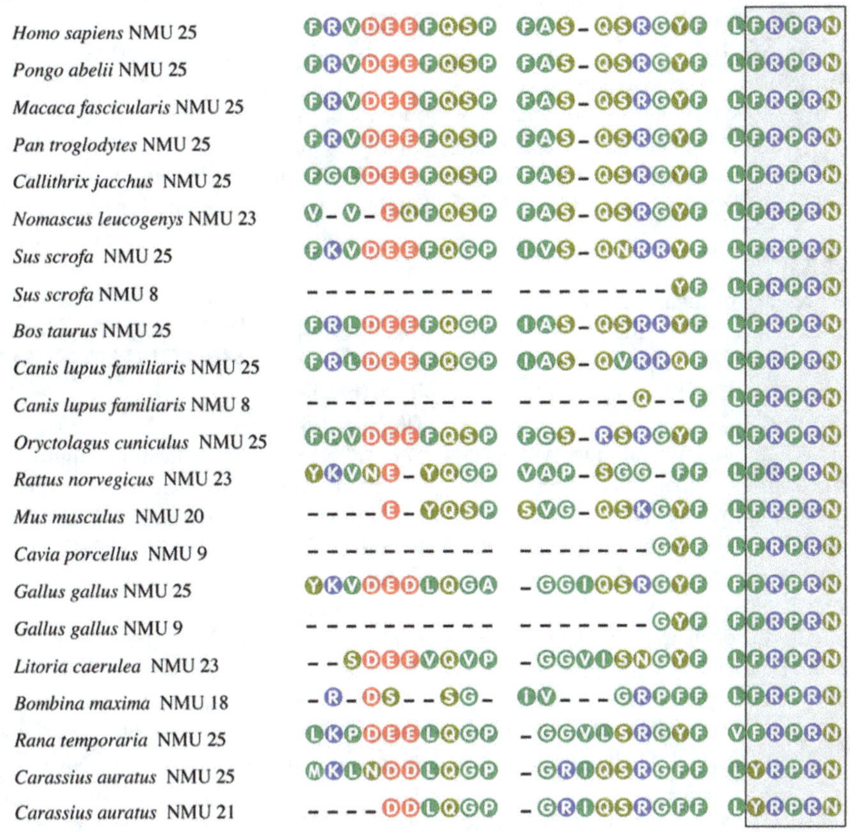


**FIGURE 1 | Amino acid sequences of neuromedin U from some mammalian, avian, piscine, and amphibian species.** The box, highlighting the C-terminal pentapeptide, shows conservation of this sequence in vertebrates, except of goldfish. From Mitchell et al. (2009a), modified. Amino acid sequences were acquired from NCBI. Numbers after NMU denote peptide length.

Unexpectedly, in 2005, Mori et al. (2005) isolated from the rat brain a new 36 amino acid peptide related to NMU, which appeared to be another endogenous ligand of FM-4/TGR-1 receptor. This neuropeptide is highly expressed in the suprachiasmiatic nucleus of the hypothalamus and therefore was designed as NMS. Human NMS, on the other hand, is composed of 33 amino acid residues. All NMS share a C-terminal core structure with NMU. NMU and NMS share the same amidated C-terminal heptapeptide and bind to the same receptors NMUR1 and NMUR2. Amino acid sequences of NMS from different species are shown in **Figure 2**.

It should be emphasized that NMU and NMS genes are located on different chromosomes (NMU on 4q12 and NMS on 2q11.2) (Mori et al., 2005). Moreover, evidences indicate that during the

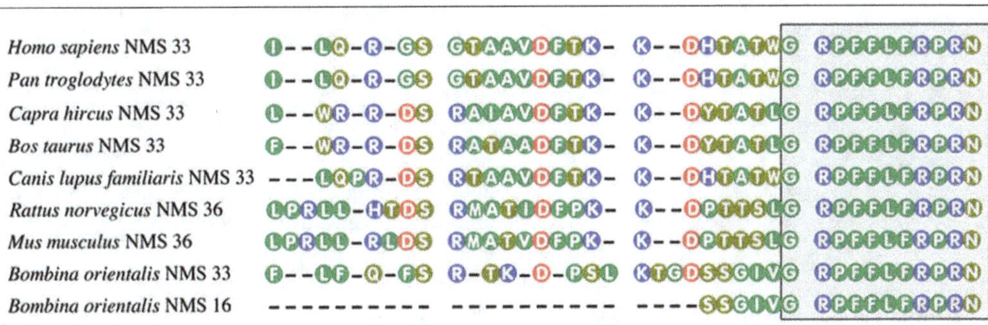


**FIGURE 2 | Amino acid sequences of neuromedin S from some mammalian and amphibian species.** The box, highlighting the C-terminal decapeptide, shows conservation of this sequence in vertebrates. NMU and NMS share the same amidated C-terminal heptapeptide. Amino acid sequences were acquired from NCBI. Numbers after NMS denote peptide length.

process of evolution NMU and NMS genes had already diverged at the level of the Amphibia (Chen et al., 2006).

In humans both NMU and NMS genes are composed of 10 exons and 9 introns. The mRNA lengths encoded by these genes are 816 and 485 bp, respectively. The exon–intron boundaries in the NMU and NMS prepro-proteins are comparably conserved (Mori et al., 2008). General structures of encoded prepro-NMU and prepro-NMS are shown in **Figure 3**.

## NMU AND NMS RECEPTORS

Early studies revealed the presence of highly specific $^{125}$I-NMU binding sites on membranes prepared from the rat uterus. The binding was saturable and specific and Scatchard analysis suggested a single class of binding site with a $K_d$ of 0.35 nM (Nandha et al., 1993).

By means of modern molecular biology techniques two receptors for NMU were identified. In 1998, Tan et al. (1998) cloned a GPCR (FM-3) from human and murine cDNA libraries. This DNA segment has homology to the growth hormone secretagogue receptor and the neurotensin receptor. Subsequently, by means of a "reverse pharmacological" method NMU was identified as an endogenous ligand for the orphan human GPCR, FM-3 (or GPR66) (Fujii et al., 2000; Hedrick et al., 2000; Hosoya et al., 2000; Howard et al., 2000; Kojima et al., 2000; Raddatz et al., 2000; Shan et al., 2000; Szekeres et al., 2000). After identification of the second NMU receptor, the first one had been named NMUR1.

The NMUR2 (FM-4, TGR1) gene, on the other hand, was identified based on its sequence similarity with NMUR1 (Hosoya et al., 2000; Howard et al., 2000; Raddatz et al., 2000; Shan et al., 2000). NMUR1 gene is located on human chromosome 2—position q37.1 and NMUR2 gene on chromosome 5—position q33.1 (Mitchell et al., 2009a).

In humans NMUR1 gene consists of 3 exons and 2 introns, the size of encoded mRNA is 3274 bp and the receptor is composed of 426 aa residues. NMUR2 gene, on the other hand, consists of 4 exons and 3 introns. The size of its mRNA is 2067 bp and the receptor is composed of 415 aa residues (**Figure 4**).

NMS has also been identified as an endogenous ligand of NMUR1 and NMUR2 receptors and some data indicate that NMUR2 has greater affinity to NMS than NMU (Mori et al., 2005).

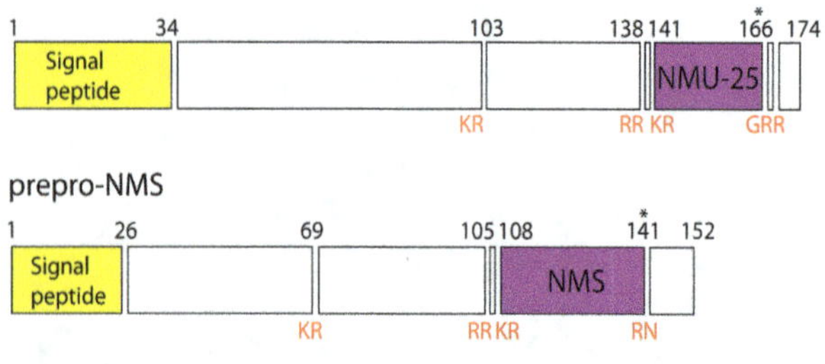


**FIGURE 3 | Schematic structure of prepro-NMU and prepro-NMS in humans.** Data from Protein Knowledgebase (UniProtKB) P48645 and Q5H8A3, respectively. Schematic structure of prepro-NMU is modified from Austin et al. (1995). Numbers refer to residues and cleavage sites are given in red. Asterisk marks amidated asparagine.

Interaction of NMU and NMS with their receptors results in intracellular calcium mobilization and subsequent stimulation of inositol phosphates. These effects are mediated by both $G_{q/11}$ and $G_{i/0}$ proteins (Raddatz et al., 2000; Shan et al., 2000; Szekeres et al., 2000; Funes et al., 2002; Mori et al., 2005; Maruyama et al., 2011). Moreover, both neuromedins are also able to activate the mitogen activated protein kinase ERK1 and ERK2 (Brighton et al., 2004).

## EXPRESSION OF NMU AND NMS AND THEIR RECEPTORS IN THE HYPOTHALAMO–PITUITARY–ADRENAL AXIS

### HYPOTHALAMUS

#### *NMU and NMS*

Soon after NMU identification, high concentrations of NMU-like immunoreactivity were found in extracts of the rat, mouse, and human hypothalamus (Domin et al., 1986, 1988). In rat hypothalamus concentration of NMU-like immunoreactivity was reported as 31.2 ± 5.6 pmol/g (nearly 6 times higher than in the anterior pituitary lobe). Subsequent immunohistochemical studies demonstrated the presence of NMU-like substances in the hypothalamic paraventricular (PVN) and arcuate nucleus of the rat (Honzawa et al., 1987; Ballesta et al., 1988; Steel et al., 1988). On the other hand, molecular biology techniques demonstrated low to moderate levels of NMU mRNA in rat (RT-PCR) and human (QPCR) hypothalamus (Fujii et al., 2000; Szekeres et al., 2000). Single-cell reverse transcription-multiplex polymerase chain reaction (single-cell RT-mPCR) technique revealed that 14.7% parvocellular neurons of the rat PVN expressed NMU mRNA (Chu et al., 2012).

NMU mRNA is present in hypothalamus of WT mice and, in contrast, NMU mRNA could not be detected in NMU KO mice (Fukue et al., 2006).

In the frog (*Rana esculenta*) NMU-like immunoreactivity was observed in perikaria of the dorsal nucleus of the hypothalamus and the caudal part of the infundibulum (Maderdrut et al., 1996). Although authors emphasize that this pattern of immunoreactivity distribution differs notably from that seen in mammals, it is necessary to emphasize that the ventral infundibular nucleus of the frog is homologous to the mammalian arcuate nucleus (Neary and Northcutt, 1983; Ten Donkelaar, 1998).

The highest expression of NMS mRNA was found by RT-PCR in rat hypothalamus (Mori et al., 2005). Subsequently, *in situ* hybridization demonstrated that this neuropeptide was specifically expressed in the hypothalamic suprachiasmatic nuclei (SCN). In the rat hypothalamus expression of NMS gene was nearly 3-fold higher than that of NMU gene (Rucinski et al., 2007). During postnatal development levels of NMS mRNA attained maximum at prepubertal stage and adulthood (Vigo et al., 2007).

#### *NMU receptors*

Earliest studies revealed that NMUR1 is expressed predominantly in periphery while NMUR2 in the central nervous system (for review see Brighton et al., 2004; Mitchell et al., 2009a). In agreement with this principle in the rat hypothalamus, by means

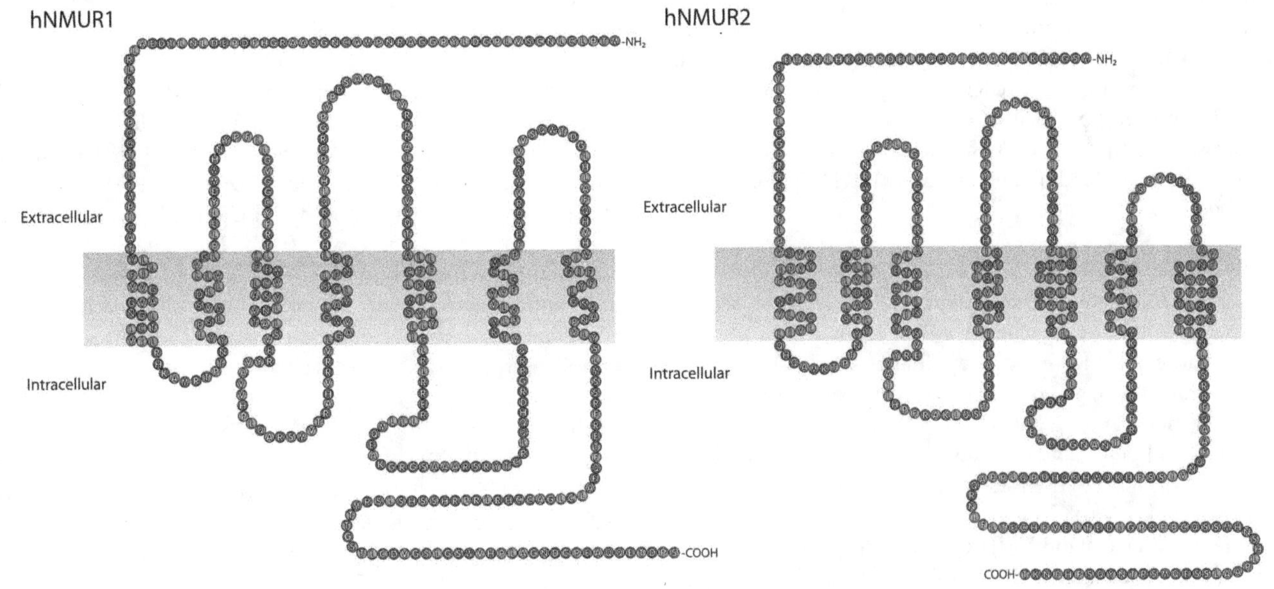


**FIGURE 4 | Schematic representation of human NMUR1 and NMUR2 receptors.** NMUR1 receptor is composed of 426 amino acid residues while NMUR2 of 415. Amino acid sequences were acquired from NCBI, accession numbers AAG24793.1 and EAW61653.1, respectively.

of QPCR Raddatz et al. (2000) demonstrated high expression of NMUR2 and a notably lower one of NMUR1. This finding was confirmed by numerous groups (Fujii et al., 2000; Howard et al., 2000; Qiu et al., 2005; Rucinski et al., 2007; Vigo et al., 2007). NMUR2 gene is also expressed in the PVN. By means of the single-cell RT-mPCR analysis (multiplex) Qiu et al. (2005) demonstrated that NMU-sensitive PVN neurons abundantly expressed NMUR2 mRNA but expressed NMUR1 mRNA to a lesser extent or not at all.

Detailed mapping of NMUR2 mRNA expression in the rat brain by *in situ* hybridization revealed the most intense signal in ependymal cells of the third ventricle and moderate signal in the PVN (Guan et al., 2001; Graham et al., 2003). Presence of NMUR2 receptors in these regions of the brain had also been confirmed by receptor autoradiography (Mangold et al., 2008).

Similar pattern of NMU receptor expressions is observed in human hypothalamus, with high expression of NMUR2 and a negligible one of NMUR1 (Szekeres et al., 2000; Gartlon et al., 2004).

## PITUITARY GLAND

### *NMU and NMS*

High concentrations of NMU-like immunoreactivity were found in the pituitary gland of the rat as early as in 1987 (Domin et al., 1987, 1988, 1989a). In rat anterior lobe concentration of NMU-like immunoreactive substances was 6.3 pmol/gland (mean) while in posterior lobe 0.3 pmol/gland only. Furthermore, Northern blot analysis using total RNA extracted from rat anterior pituitary demonstrated high levels of NMU mRNA in the gland (Lo et al., 1992).

High concentrations of NMU protein in rat pituitary gland are accompanied by high expression of NMU gene (Fujii et al., 2000). High expression of this gene in anterior pituitary lobe of the rat was confirmed by QPCR (Rucinski et al., 2007; Shimizu et al., 2008). It should be emphasized that NMU mRNA is also expressed in cultured pituitary cells of the rat. Using quantitative *in situ* hybridization, high concentration of NMU transcripts was also found in part tuberalis of the rat pituitary (Ivanov et al., 2002; Nogueiras et al., 2006).

Immunohistochemistry demonstrated the presence of NMU-immunoreactive substances in the intermediate and the anterior pituitary gland lobes of mouse, rat, and human (Ballesta et al., 1988; Steel et al., 1988). Electron microscopy studies revealed NMU-like immunoreactivity in some thyrotropes and most corticotropes of the rat pituitary gland. NMU is colocalized with galanin and ACTH in the same secretory granules (Cimini et al., 1993; for review see Malendowicz, 1998; Cimini, 2003).

In developing rat NMU-immunopositive cells appear in anterior pituitary at day E15 (Cimini, 2003). Their number increases at day E20 and then decreases. More than 60% of NMU-immunoreactive cells contain ACTH at E15, and, after falling to about 40% at E16, this value is more or less constant until E21.

NMU mRNA is expressed in pituitary gland of WT mice, but in contrast, NMU mRNA could not be detected in NMU KO mice (Fukue et al., 2006).

Expression of NMS gene in rat pituitary gland was found by Mori et al. (2005). In rat anterior pituitary expression level of NMS gene however, was notably lower than that of NMU gene (Rucinski et al., 2007).

### *NMU receptors*

Conflicting data were reported on expression of NMUR1 and NMUR2 in pituitary gland. By means of QPCR low expression of both receptors in human pituitary gland was reported by Raddatz et al. (2000). These data were confirmed by other groups (Shan et al., 2000; Gartlon et al., 2004).

The earliest studies did not reveal NMUR1 gene expression in the rat pituitary gland while that of NMUR2 was very low (Fujii et al., 2000; Gartlon et al., 2004). On the other hand, in rat adenohypophysis expression of NMUR1 gene, but not of NMUR2 was observed by our group (Rucinski et al., 2007).

Expression of both NMUR1 and NMUR2 genes was observed in mouse pituitary gland of both WT and NMU KO mice (Fukue et al., 2006).

#### ADRENAL GLAND

Only scanty data are available on expression of NMU–NMS and their receptors in adrenal glands. Very low levels of NMU mRNA in the rat adrenal were reported by Fujii et al. (2000). Detailed studies on rat adrenal gland revealed very low expression of NMU and NMS genes at mRNA levels (Rucinski et al., 2007).

In human adrenal gland both NMUR2 mRNA (PCR) and protein (dot blot method) were identified in 2000 (Raddatz et al., 2000; Shan et al., 2000).

In the rat adrenal gland NMUR2 mRNA could not be demonstrated (Hosoya et al., 2000; Fujii et al., 2000). In immature rat adrenal NMUR1 was expressed at both mRNA and protein (immunohistochemistry) levels while the signal from NMUR2 was absent. NMUR1 mRNA was detected in all adrenocortical zones and in medulla of the gland (Ziolkowska et al., 2008). Moreover, the presence of NMUR1 mRNA in isolated zona glomerulosa and fasciculata/reticularis cells rules out the possibility that the expression was due to the presence in the specimens assayed of the non-parenchymal components of the gland. Expression of NMUR1 as mRNA and protein was demonstrated in adrenal gland of intact rat, in enucleation-induced regenerating gland, in hemiadrenalectomized animals (compensatory adrenal growth) as well as in ACTH-stimulated one (Trejter et al., 2008, 2009; Malendowicz et al., 2009).

### NMU AND NMS IN THE HYPOTHALAMO–PITUITARY–ADRENAL AXIS FUNCTIONING

#### HYPOTHALAMUS

The above described localization of elements of NMU/NMS and NMUR2 system in hypothalamus forms a base of regulation by NMU and NMS of HPA axis functioning.

The earliest experiments with intracerebroventricular (icv) injection of NMU demonstrated a strong increase in Fos-immunoreactive nuclei in the PVN and supraoptic nucleus (SON) of the rat hypothalamus (Niimi et al., 2001; Ozaki et al., 2002). Almost all CRH-containing neurons in the parvocellular divisions of the PVN expressed Fos-like immunoreactivity 90 min after icv administration of NMU (Yokota et al., 2004).

Subsequent studies demonstrated direct NMU effects on CRH and arginine vasopressin (AVP) release by rat hypothalamic explants *in vitro* (Wren et al., 2002). At the 100 nM NMU concentration CRH and AVP release was nearly doubled when compared to controls. Moreover, results of whole cell patch-clamp recordings revealed that NMU directly depolarized the subpopulation of PVN parvocellular, but not magnocellular neurons via enhancement of the hyperpolarization-activated inward current (Qiu et al., 2003). Direct effects of both neuromedins on PVN was also suggested by *in vitro* electrophysiological studies which showed that NMU and NMS increased the neuronal firing rates in both arcuate and PVN nuclei slices (Nakahara et al., 2010).

NMU also regulates HPA axis in birds. Icv administration of NMU in chicks significantly upregulated mRNA expression of CRH in the hypothalamus (Kamisoyama et al., 2007).

NMS likewise affects CRH neurons in PVN. In the rat icv administration of this neuromedin increased POMC mRNA expression in the arcuate nucleus and CRH mRNA in the PVN (Ida et al., 2005; Nakahara et al., 2010). NMS notably stimulated Fos-immunoreactive cells in both hypothalamic nuclei. NMS also significantly increased firing rate of PVN cells. Stimulating effects of NMS on Fos-immunoreactive cells of the PVN was confirmed by another group (Sakamoto et al., 2007, 2008).

#### PITUITARY

Expression of NMUR1 in pituitary gland and colocalization of NMU and ACTH in pituitary corticotropes suggest NMU and NMS involvement in regulation of ACTH secretion. Regarding this, there is a growing body of evidence that in the rat NMU administered icv, into PVN or subcutaneously increases blood ACTH concentrations, via stimulation of CRH release.

First reports demonstrated that a single sc injection of NMU8 resulted in a transient increase in ACTH blood concentration while after 2–6-day treatment (low NMU8 dose) blood ACTH level remained unchanged (Malendowicz et al., 1993, 1994b; Trejter et al., 2009). Only the higher dose of NMU8 (6 μg/100 g/day for 6 days) increased the level of circulating ACTH.

In the rat unilateral adrenalectomy notably increased plasma ACTH concentrations and NMU administration (sc) into hemiadrenalectomized rats did not significantly change corticotropin levels (Malendowicz et al., 2009).

In the rat icv administration of NMU (0.1, 1, and 3 nmol/rat) resulted in a dose-dependent increase of plasma ACTH concentrations, an effect significantly reduced by pretreatment with anti-NMU IgG (Ozaki et al., 2002). Similar dose-dependent effects of NMU on plasma ACTH concentrations were found after iPVN neuropeptide administration (Wren et al., 2002). Again, chronic iPVN NMU administration (twice-daily of 0.3 nmol NMU for 7 days) did not change plasma ACTH concentrations (Thompson et al., 2004). Only one group was unable to demonstrate stimulating effect of icv administered NMU on plasma ACTH concentrations in the rat (Rokkaku et al., 2003).

Unfortunately, no studies have as yet investigated direct effects of NMU and NMS on pituitary ACTH secretion. Our preliminary data indicate that neither NMU nor NMS affect ACTH release by quarters of the rat adenohypophysis, while the response to CRH was normal. This observation may suggest that observed *in vivo* stimulating effect of NMU/NMS on ACTH secretion is mediated via hypothalamus.

#### ADRENAL

Potent stimulating effects of exogenous NMU on adrenocortical steroid secretion in the rat have been described as early as in 1993. A single sc injection of NMU resulted in a transient increase in ACTH blood concentration (between 3 and 12 h) and a sustained (24 h) elevation of plasma corticosterone concentration (Malendowicz et al., 1993, 1994b). These data demonstrated stimulating effect of neuropeptide on adrenal cortex, possibly partially due to the direct effect of NMU on the gland.

In subsequent searches for mode of NMU action on corticosteroid secretion our group found that NMU had no effect on basal and ACTH-stimulated corticosterone secretion by freshly isolated or cultured inner zone adrenocortical cells, nor did it change their cytosolic $Ca^{2+}$ concentration (Malendowicz et al., 1994b; confirmed by Ziolkowska et al., 2008). However, this neuropeptide stimulated corticosterone output by adrenal slices, but not by fragments of adrenocortical autotransplants lacking medullary chromaffin cells (Malendowicz et al., 1994a). Detailed analysis revealed that at all concentrations tested NMU increased basal pregnenolone and total post-pregnenolone steroid output by gland slices containing both cortex and medulla. The increase in total post-pregnenolone steroid output induced by low concentrations of NMU8 was due to similar rises in the production of non-18-hydroxylated steroids; conversely, that provoked by higher concentrations of the peptide was almost exclusively caused by the rise in the yield of 18-hydroxylated steroids. The stimulating effect of NMU8 on pregnenolone output was blocked by both alpha-helical-CRH and corticotropin-inhibiting peptide, which are competitive inhibitors of CRH and ACTH, respectively. These data suggest that NMU affects corticosteroid secretion indirectly by acting on the medullary chromaffin cells, which in turn may paracrinally stimulate cortex of the gland. We also suggested that the medullary mediator of NMU action on adrenal cortex may activate 18-hydroxylation and aldosterone synthase activity. On the other hand, we cannot rule out the possibility of NMU action on adrenal cortex via stimulation of adrenaline secretion by adrenal medulla. Recently it has been demonstrated that centrally administered NMU evokes secretion of adrenaline from the adrenal medulla (Sasaki et al., 2008). Medullary adrenaline may in turn modulate secretion of corticosteroids (for review see Nussdorfer, 1996; Bornstein et al., 1997; Ehrhart-Bornstein et al., 1998).

Stimulating effects of NMU on corticosteroid secretion also were observed after icv or iPVN neuropeptide administration. In the rat acute iPVN administration of NMU dose-dependently increased plasma corticosterone concentrations (Wren et al., 2002). Similar effect was observed after icv NMU administration (Ozaki et al., 2002). In contrast, another group reported lack of icv NMU administration effects on plasma corticosterone levels (Gartlon et al., 2004).

Stimulating effects of icv administered NMU on plasma corticosterone levels were confirmed by experiments with anti-NMU IgG (Jethwa et al., 2006). In rats administration of anti-NMU IgG significantly attenuated the dark phase rise in plasma corticosterone concentrations.

In contrast to acute administration, chronic iPVN administration of NMU produced an elevation of plasma corticosterone levels while plasma ACTH concentrations remained unchanged (Thompson et al., 2004). Thus, in chronically NMU administered rats elevated plasma corticosterone levels, not accompanied by increased ACTH concentrations, were independent of the mode of NMU administration (sc vs iPVN) (Malendowicz et al., 1993, 1994b; Thompson et al., 2004).

The stimulating effect of sc administered NMU on plasma corticosterone concentrations also was found in rats during enucleation-induced regeneration, as well as in rats treated with low ACTH doses (Trejter et al., 2008, 2009). On the other hand, NMU8 administration to immature rats was found to raise aldosterone, but not corticosterone concentrations (Ziolkowska et al., 2008).

NMS, like NMU also stimulates corticosteroid secretion. In rats icv NMS administration resulted in nearly 5-fold increase in plasma corticosterone concentrations and the effect was dependent on neuropeptide dose (Jászberényi et al., 2007). Likewise, in castrated Holstein steers both NMS and NMU evoked a dose-related increase in plasma cortisol concentrations (Yayou et al., 2009). Of interest is that also in chicks icv NMS administration stimulated corticosterone release (Tachibana et al., 2010).

In contrast to the above described NMS effects on corticosterone/cortisol secretion, an opposite effect was seen in Rhesus monkeys (Jahan et al., 2011). In their experiments NMS was infused through a teflon cannula implanted into saphenous vein. Blood samples were collected 45 min before and 120 min after NMS administration at 15 min intervals. Under these conditions NMS resulted in a significant decrease in plasma cortisol levels at 40 and 60 nmol doses while a non-significant difference was observed at 20 nmol. This unexpected finding may suggest that in non-human primates NMS exerts inhibitory effect on HPA axis functioning. However this finding remains to be confirmed.

Recent data also demonstrated direct stimulating effect of NMU on proliferative activity of immature rat inner adrenocortical cells in primary culture (Ziolkowska et al., 2008). Moreover, in enucleation-induced adrenal regeneration NMU notably enhanced proliferative activity of adrenocortical cells (Trejter et al., 2008). A similar stimulating effect of sc administered NMU on proliferative activity (metaphase index) was seen in ACTH treated rats (Trejter et al., 2009). In contrast, in hemiadrenalectomized rats NMU notably inhibited adrenocortical cell proliferation in both zona glomerulosa and zona fasciculata, as assessed by the metaphase index (Malendowicz et al., 2009). Since these effects were independent of changes in blood ACTH, they could reflect an interaction of NMU with the neural system innervating the adrenal gland, which is responsible for compensatory adrenal growth.

## INVOLVEMENT OF NMU AND NMS IN THE STRESS RESPONSE

As it follows from the above presented data, NMU and NMS are linked to the HPA axis functioning. Independently of mode of administration (icv, iPVN, or sc) NMU activates CRH containing neurons and stimulates CRH secretion, which in turn triggers pituitary ACTH and adrenal corticosterone/cortisol secretion. In this regard it is not astonishing that NMU and NMS are involved in central and peripheral control of the stress response. These studies were initiated by Hanada et al. (2001) who observed stress-related behavior (gross locomotor activity, face washing and grooming) in icv NMU administered rats. This response was attenuated by pretreatment with alpha-helical CRH (antagonist of CRH) or anti-CRH IgG. Furthermore, NMU-induced increases in oxygen consumption and body temperature were attenuated in CRH KO mice. Subsequent studies demonstrated that blood corticosterone levels were significantly increased after 10 min of immobilization stress in wild-type mice, but not in NMU KO mice (Nakahara et al., 2004). Excessive grooming induced by icv NMU administration were abolished in the NMUR2 KO mice, an observation suggesting that NMUR2 plays a decisive role in stress/anxiety induction (Zeng et al., 2006).

Stress related behavior induced by icv NMU or NMS administration was also observed in cattle (Yayou et al., 2009). Administration of both neuropeptides tended to shorten the duration of lying and increase the number of head shaking in studied cattle. These behavioral changes were accompanied by increased levels of plasma cortisol.

## CONCLUDING REMARKS

The above reviewed data clearly demonstrate NMU and NMS involvement in regulation of HPA axis growth and functions. However, their mechanism of action is far from being completely understood. The available experimental data suggest that within the HPA axis these neuromedins may exert both endocrine and/or paracrine/autocrine effects on target cells.

Endocrine effects of discussed neuropeptides require their release into the bloodstream. Only scanty data are available on NMU and NMS presence in general circulation. Manufacturers' manuals for various kits contain data on NMU and NMS concentration in plasma and comparable figures are shown in clinical studies (Ketterer et al., 2009). However, experimental data suggest that neither endogenous NMU nor NMS are circulating, at least in the rat (Peier et al., 2009). Furthermore, in general circulation the biological half-life of NMU is shorter than 5 min.

At the hypothalamus level the actions of NMU and NMS are rather well documented. Stimulation of CRH, arginine-vasopresssin and oxytocin release both *in vivo* and *in vitro* activates HPA axis and apart from elevation of ACTH and corticosterone/cortisol secretion, triggers behavioral parameters typical for stress reaction.

More puzzling is the effect of NMU on pituitary gland. As discussed earlier, in pituitary gland high levels of NMU are present, and the gland contains high concentration of NMU-like immunoreactive substances and is provided with NMUR1 receptor. NMU is colocalized with ACTH and numerous NMU-like immunoreactive cells are present in human extrapituitary corticotropinomas (Steel et al., 1988). Denef (2008) suggests that in the pituitary NMU may paracrinally regulate function of adjacent cells and a similar mode of action may be present in extrapituitary corticotropinomas. So far, direct effects of NMU/NMS on pituitary ACTH secretion have not been reported. Our preliminary data indicate that neither NMU nor NMS affect ACTH release by quarters of the rat adenohypophysis. It remains to be established whether inability of NMU and NMS to directly stimulate ACTH release from pituitary gland may be caused by possible high receptor occupancy by endogenous NMU.

In view of these findings, questions arise concerning the possible role of NMU in pituitary tumor formation. In their review on pituitary tumorogenesis Korbonits et al. (2004) mention NMU only as a potential messenger in the anterior pituitary. Thus, the possible role of NMU in development of pituitary and extrapituitary corticotropinomas requires further investigation. As far as endocrine system is concerned, an elevated expression of NMU gene was found in human ovarian cancer cell lines (Euer et al., 2005).

The available experimental data suggest that at the adrenal level NMU affects the steroid secretion indirectly by acting on the medullary chromaffin cells. On the other hand some data suggest direct effect of neuromedin on proliferation and growth of rat adrenocortical cells.

Thus, although great progress has been made in understanding NMU and NMS action within the HPA axis during the past years, much remains to be learned about their mechanisms of action within this system. Recent development of a metabolically stable analog of NMU, based on derivatization of the native peptide with high molecular weight poly(ethylene) glycol (PEG) ("PEGylation") may be helpful in these attempts (Ingallinella et al., 2012).

## ACKNOWLEDGMENTS

Review was prepared using funds from the grant no N N401 227839 from the Ministry of Science and Education in Poland.

## REFERENCES

Austin, C., Lo, G., Nandha, K. A., Meleagros, L., and Bloom, S. R. (1995). Cloning and characterization of the cDNA encoding the human neuromedin U (NmU) precursor: NmU expression in the human gastrointestinal tract. *J. Mol. Endocrinol.* 14, 157–169.

Ballesta, J., Carlei, F., Bishop, A. E., Steel, J. H., Gibson, S. J., Fahey, M., et al. (1988). Occurrence and developmental pattern of neuromedin U-immunoreactive nerves in the gastrointestinal tract and brain of the rat. *Neuroscience* 25, 797–816.

Bornstein, S. R., Ehrhart-Bornstein, M., and Scherbaum, W. A. (1997). Morphological and functional studies of the paracrine interaction between cortex and medulla in the adrenal gland. *Microsc. Res. Tech.* 36, 520–533.

Brighton, P. J., Szekeres, P. G., and Willars, G. B. (2004). Neuromedin U and its receptors: structure, function, and physiological roles. *Pharmacol. Rev.* 56, 231–248.

Budhiraja, S., and Chugh, A. (2009). Neuromedin U: physiology, pharmacology and therapeutic potential. *Fundam. Clin. Pharmacol.* 23, 149–157.

Chen, T. B., Zhou, M., Walker, B., Harriot, P., Mori, K., Miyazato, M., et al. (2006). Structural and functional analogs of the novel mammalian neuropeptide, neuromedin S (NmS), in the dermal venoms of Eurasian bombinid toads. *Biochem. Biophys. Res. Commun.* 345, 377–384.

Chu, C.-P., Xu, C.-J., Kannan, H., and Qui, D.-L. (2012). Corticotrophin-releasing factor inhibits neuromedin U mRNA expressing neuron in the rat hypothalamic paraventricular nucleus *in vitro*. *Neurosci. Lett.* 511, 79–83.

Cimini, V. (2003). Neuropeptides in anterior pituitary development. *Int. J. Dev. Neurosci.* 21, 291–301.

Cimini, V., Van Noorden, S., Timson, C. M., and Polak, J. M. (1993). Modulation of galanin and neuromedin U-like immunoreactivity in rat corticotropes after alteration of endocrine status. *Cell Tissue Res.* 272, 137–146.

Conlon, J. M., Domin, J., Thim, L., DiMarzo, V., Morris, H. R., and Bloom, S. R. (1988). Primary structure of neuromedin U from the rat. *J. Neurochem.* 51, 988–991.

Denef, C. (2008). Paracrinicity: The story of 30 years of cellular pituitary crosstalk. *J. Neuroendocrinol.* 20, 1–70.

Domin, J., Benito-Orfila, M. A., Nandha, K. A., Aitken, A., and Bloom, S. R. (1992). The purification and sequence analysis of an avian neuromedin U. *Regul. Pept.* 41, 1–8.

Domin, J., Ghatei, M. A., Chochan, P., and Bloom, S. R. (1986). Characterization of neuromedin U-like immunoreactivity in rat, porcine, guinea pig and human tissue extracts using a specific radioimmunoassay. *Biochem. Biophys. Res. Commun.* 140, 1127–1134.

Domin, J., Ghatei, M. A., Chohan, P., and Bloom, S. R. (1987). Neuromedin U: a study of its distribution in the rat. *Peptides* 8, 779–784.

Domin, J., Polak, J. M., and Bloom, S. R. (1988). The distribution and biological effects of neuromedins B and U. *Ann. N.Y. Acad. Sci.* 547, 391–403.

Domin, J., Steel, J. H., Adolphus, N., Burrin, J. M., Leonhardt, U., Polak, J. M., et al. (1989a). The anterior pituitary content of neuromedin U-like immunoreactivity is altered by thyrotrophin-releasing hormone and thyroid hormone status in the rat. *J. Endocrinol.* 122, 471–476.

Domin, J., Yiangou, Y. G., Spokes, R. A., Aitken, A., Parmar, K. B., Chrysanthou, B. J., et al. (1989b). The distribution, purification, and pharmacological action of an amphibian neuromedin U. *J. Biol. Chem.* 264, 20881–20885.

Ehrhart-Bornstein, M., Hinson, J. P., Bornstein, S. R., Scherbaum, W. A., and Vinson, G. P. (1998). Intraadrenal interactions in the regulation of adrenocortical steroidogenesis. *Endocr. Rev.* 19, 101–143.

Euer, N. I., Kaul, S., Deissler, H., Möbus, V. J., Zeilunger, R., and Weidle, U. H. (2005). Identification of L1CAM, Jagged2 and Neuromedin U as ovarian cancer-associated antigens. *Oncol. Rep.* 13, 375–387.

Fujii, R., Hosoya, M., Fukusumi, S., Kawamata, Y., Habata, Y., Hinuma, S., et al. (2000). Identification of neuromedin U as the cognate ligand of the orphan G-protein-coupled receptor FM-3. *J. Biol. Chem.* 275, 21068–21074.

Fukue, Y., Sato, T., Teranishi, H., Hanada, R., Takahashi, T., Nakashima, Y., et al. (2006). Regulation of gonadotropin secretion and puberty onset by neuromedin U. *FEBS Lett.* 580, 3485–3488.

Funes, S., Hedrick, J. A., Yang, S. J., Shan, L. X., Bayne, M., Monsma, F. J. Jr., et al. (2002). Cloning and characterization of murine neuromedin U receptors. *Peptides* 23, 1607–1615.

Gartlon, J., Szekeres, P., Pullen, M., Sarau, H. M., Aiyar, N., Shabon, U., et al. (2004). Localisation of NMU1R and NMU2R in human and rat central nervous system and effects of neuromedin-U following central administration in rats. *Psychopharmacology (Berl.)* 177, 1–14.

Graham, E. S., Turnbull, Y., Fotheringham, P., Nilaweera, K., Mercer, J. G., Morgan, P. J., et al. (2003). Neuromedin U and Neuromedin U receptor-2 expression in the mouse and rat hypothalamus: effects of nutritional status. *J. Neurochem.* 87, 1165–1173.

Guan, X. M., Yu, H., Jiang, Q., Van Der Ploeg, L. H., and Liu, Q. (2001). Distribution of neuromedin U receptor subtype 2 mRNA in the rat brain. *Brain Res. Gene Expr. Patterns* 1, 1–4.

Hanada, R., Nakazato, M., Murakami, N., Sakihara, S., Yoshimatsu, H., Toshinai, K., et al. (2001). A role for neuromedin U in stress response. *Biochem. Biophys. Res. Commun.* 289, 225–228.

Hashimoto, T., Masui, H., Uchida, Y., Sakura, N., and Okimura, K. (1991). Agonistic and antagonistic activities of neuromedin U-8 analogs substituted with glycine or D-amino acid on contractile activity of chicken crop smooth muscle preparations. *Chem. Pharm. Bull.* 39, 2319–2322.

Hedrick, J. A., Morse, K., Shan, L. X., Qiao, X. D., Pang, L., Wang, S., et al. (2000). Identification of a human gastrointestinal tract and immune system receptor for the peptide neuromedin U. *Mol. Pharmacol.* 58, 870–875.

Honzawa, M., Sudok, T., Minamino, N., Tokyama, M., and Matsuo, H. (1987). Topographic localization of neuromedin U-like structures in the rat brain: an immunohistochemical study. *Neuroscience* 23, 1103–1122.

Hosoya, M., Moriya, T., Kawamata, Y., Ohkubo, S., Fujii, R., Matsui, H., et al. (2000). Identification and functional characterization of a novel subtype of neuromedin U receptor. *J. Biol. Chem.* 275, 29528–29532.

Howard, A. D., Wang, R. P., Pong, S. S., Mellin, T. N., Strack, A., Guan, X. M., et al. (2000). Identification of receptors for neuromedin U and its role in feeding. *Nature (Lond.)* 406, 70–74.

Ida, T., Mori, K., Miyazato, M., Egi, Y., Abe, S., Nakahara, K., et al. (2005). Neuromedin s is a novel anorexigenic hormone. *Endocrinology* 146, 4217–4223.

Ingallinella, P., Peier, A. M., Pocai, A., Di Marco, A., Desai, K., Zytko, K., et al. (2012). PEGylation of Neuromedin U yields a promising candidate for the treatment of obesity and diabetes. *Bioorg. Med. Chem.* 20, 4751–4759.

Ivanov, T. R., Lawrence, C. B., Stanley, P. J., and Luckman, S. M. (2002). Evaluation of neuromedin U actions in energy homeostasis and pituitary function. *Endocrinology* 143, 3813–3821.

Jahan, S., Ahmed, S., and Shah, N. A. (2011). Role of neuromedin S in plasma testosterone and cortisol concentrations in male adult rhesus monkey (*Macaca mulatta*). *Pak. J. Zool.* 43, 147–153.

Jászberényi, M., Bagosi, Z., Thurzó, B., Földesi, I., and Telegdy, G. (2007). Endocrine and behavioral effects of neuromedin S. *Horm. Behav.* 52, 631–639.

Jethwa, P. H., Smith, K. L., Small, C. J., Abbott, C. R., Darch, S. J., Murphy, K. G., et al. (2006). Neuromedin U partially mediates leptin-induced hypothalamo-pituitary adrenal (HPA) stimulation and has a physiological role in the regulation of the HPA axis in the rat. *Endocrinology* 147, 2886–2892.

Kage, R., O'Harte, F., Thim, L., and Conlon, J. M. (1991). Rabbit neuromedin U-25: lack of conservation of a posttranslational processing site. *Regul. Pept.* 33, 191–198.

Kamisoyama, H., Honda, K., Saneyasu, T., Sugahara, K., and Hasegawa, S. (2007). Central administration of neuromedin U suppresses food intake in chicks. *Neurosci Lett.* 420, 1–5.

Kangawa, K., Minamino, N., Fukuda, A., and Matsuo, H. (1983). Neuromedin K: a novel mammalian tachykinin identified in porcine spinal cord. *Biochem. Biophys. Res. Commun.* 114, 533–540.

Ketterer, K., Kong, B., Frank, D., Giese, N. A., Bauer, A., Hoheisel, J., et al. (2009). Neuromedin U is overexpressed in pancreatic cancer and increases invasiveness via the hepatocyte growth factor c-Met pathway. *Cancer Lett.* 277, 72–81.

Kojima, M., Haruno, R., Nakazato, M., Date, Y., Murakami, N., Hanada, R., et al. (2000). Purification and identification of neuromedin U as an endogenous ligand for an orphan receptor GPR66 (FM3). *Biochem. Biophys. Res. Commun.* 276, 435–438.

Korbonits, M., Morris, D. G., Nanzer, A., Kola, B., and Grossman, A. B. (2004). Role of regulatory factors in pituitary tumour formation. *Front. Horm. Res.* 32, 63–95.

Lee, W. H., Liu, S. B., Shen, J. H., Jin, Y., Lai, R., and Zhang, Y. (2005). Identification and molecular cloning of a novel neuromedin U analog from the skin secretions of toad *Bombina maxima*. *Regul. Pept.* 129, 43–47.

Lo, G., Legon, S., Austin, C., Wallis, S., Wang, Z., and Bloom, S. R. (1992). Characterization of complementary DNA encoding the rat neuromedin U precursor. *Mol. Endocrinol.* 6, 1538–1544.

Maderdrut, J. L., Lázár, G., Kozicz, T., and Merchenthaler, I. (1996). Distribution of neuromedin U-like immunoreactivity in the central nervous system of *Rana esculenta*. *J. Comp. Neurol.* 369, 438–450.

Malendowicz, L. K. (1998). Role of neuromedins in the regulation of adrenocortical function. *Horm. Metab. Res.* 30, 374–383.

Malendowicz, L. K., Andreis, P. G., Markowska, A., Nowak, M., Warchol, J. B., Neri, G., et al. (1994a). Effects of neuromedin U-8 on the secretory activity of the rat adrenal cortex: evidence for an indirect action requiring the presence of the zona medullaris. *Res. Exp. Med. (Berl.)* 194, 69–79.

Malendowicz, L. K., Nussdorfer, G. G., Markowska, A., Tortorella, C., Nowak, M., and Warchol, J. B. (1994b). Effects of neuromedin U (NMU)-8 on the rat hypothalamo-pituitary-adrenal axis. Evidence of a direct effect of NMU-8 on the adrenal gland. *Neuropeptides* 26, 47–53.

Malendowicz, L. K., Guidolin, D., Trejter, M., Rucinski, M., Porzionato, A., de Caro, R., et al. (2009). Neuromedin-U inhibits unilateral adrenalectomy-induced compensatory adrenal growth in the rat. *Peptides* 30, 935–939.

Malendowicz, L. K., and Markowska, A. (1994). Neuromedins and their involvement in the regulation of growth, structure and function of the adrenal cortex. *Histol. Histopathol.* 9, 591–601.

Malendowicz, L. K., Nussdorfer, G. G., Nowak, K. W., and Mazzocchi, G. (1993). Effects of neuromedin U-8 on the rat pituitary-adrenocortical axis. *In Vivo* 7, 419–422.

Malendowicz, L. K., Rucinski, M., and Ziolkowska, A. (2013). "Neuromedins U/S," in *Handbook of Biologically Active Peptides: Section XI Endocrine Peptides*, ed A. Kastin (Amsterdam: Elsevier Inc.).

Mangold, C., Ksiazek, I., Yun, S. W., Berger, E., and Binkert, C. (2008). Distribution of neuromedin U binding sites in the rat CNS revealed by *in vitro* receptor autoradiography. *Neuropeptides* 42, 377–386.

Maruyama, K., Kaiya, H., Miyazato, M., Konno, N., Wakasugi, T., Uchiyama, M., et al. (2011). Isolation and characterisation of two cDNAs encoding the neuromedin U receptor from goldfish brain. *J. Neuroendocrinol.* 23, 282–291.

Maruyama, K., Konno, N., Ishiguro, K., Wakasugi, T., Uchiyama, M., Shioda, S., et al. (2008). Isolation and characterisation of four cDNAs encoding neuromedin U (NMU) from the brain and gut of goldfish, and the inhibitory effect of a deduced NMU on food intake and locomotor activity. *J. Neuroendocrinol.* 20, 71–78.

Minamino, N., Kangawa, K., Fukuda, A., and Matsuo, H. (1984a). Neuromedin L: a novel mammalian tachykinin identified in porcine spinal cord. *Neuropeptides* 4, 157–166.

Minamino, N., Kangawa, K., and Matsuo, H. (1984b). Neuromedin C: a bombesin-like peptide identified in porcine spinal cord. *Biochem. Biophys. Res. Commun.* 119, 14–20.

Minamino, N., Kangawa, K., and Matsuo, H. (1984c). Neuromedin N: a novel neurotensin-like peptide identified in porcine spinal cord. *Biochem. Biophys. Res. Commun.* 122, 542–549.

Minamino, N., Kangawa, K., and Matsuo, H. (1983). Neuromedin B: a novel bombesin-like peptide identified in porcine spinal cord. *Biochem. Biophys. Res. Commun.* 114, 541–548.

Minamino, N., Sudoh, T., Kangawa, K., and Matsuo, H. (1985). Neuromedins: novel smooth-muscle stimulating peptides identified in porcine spinal cord. *Peptides* 6, 245–248.

Mitchell, J. D., Maguire, J. J., and Davenport, A. P. (2009a). Emerging pharmacology and physiology of neuromedin U and the structurally related peptide neuromedin S. *Br. J. Pharmacol.* 158, 87–103.

Mitchell, J. D., Maguire, J. J., Kuc, R. E., and Davenport, A. P. (2009b). Expression and vasoconstrictor function of anorexigenic peptides neuromedin U-25 and S in the human cardiovascular system. *Cardiovasc. Res.* 81, 353–361.

Mori, K., Miyazato, M., Ida, T., Murakami, N., Serino, R., Ueta, Y., et al. (2005). Identification of neuromedin S and its possible role in the mammalian circadian oscillator system. *EMBO J.* 24, 325–335.

Mori, K., Miyazato, M., and Kangawa, K. (2008). Neuromedin S: discovery and functions. *Results Probl. Cell Differ.* 46, 201–212.

Murphy, R., Turner, C. A., Furness, J. B., Parker, L., and Giraud, A. (1990). Isolation and microsequence analysis of a novel form of neuromedin-U from guinea-pig small-intestine. *Peptides* 11, 613–617.

Nakahara, K., Katayama, T., Maruyama, K., Ida, T., Mori, K., Miyazato, M., et al. (2010). Comparison of feeding suppression by the anorexigenic hormones neuromedin U and neuromedin S in rats. *J. Endocrinol.* 207, 185–193.

Nakahara, K., Kojima, M., Hanada, R., Egi, Y., Ida, T., Miyazato, M., et al. (2004). Neuromedin U is involved in nociceptive reflexes and adaptation to environmental stimuli in mice. *Biochem. Biophys. Res. Commun.* 323, 615–620.

Nandha, K. A., Benito-Orfila, M. A., Smith, D. M., and Bloom, S. R. (1993). Characterization of the rat uterine neuromedin-U receptor. *Endocrinology* 133, 482–486.

Neary, T., and Northcutt, R. G. (1983). Nuclear organization of the bullfrog diencephalon. *J. Comp. Neurol.* 213, 262–278.

Niimi, M., Murao, K., and Taminato, T. (2001). Central administration of neuromedin U activates neurons in ventrobasal hypothalamus and brainstem. *Endocrine* 16, 201–206.

Nogueiras, R., Tovar, S., Mitchell, S. E., Barrett, P., Rayner, D. V., Dieguez, C., et al. (2006). Negative energy balance and leptin regulate neuromedin-U expression in the rat pars tuberalis. *J. Endocrinol.* 190, 545–553.

Nussdorfer, G. G. (1996). Paracrine control of adrenal cortical function by medullary chromaffin cells. *Pharmacol. Rev.* 48, 495–530.

O'Harte, F., Bockman, C. S., Abel, P. W., and Conlon, J. M. (1991a). Isolation, structural characterization and pharmacological activity of dog neuromedin U. *Peptides* 12, 11–15.

O'Harte, F., Bockman, C. S., Zeng, W., Abel, P. W., Harvey, S., and Conlon, J. M. (1991b). Primary structure and pharmacological activity of a nonapeptide related to neuromedin U isolated from chicken intestine. *Peptides* 12, 809–812.

Ozaki, Y., Onaka, T., Nakazato, M., Saito, J., Kanemoto, K., Matsumoto, T., et al. (2002). Centrally administered neuromedin U activates neurosecretion and induction of c-fos messenger ribonucleic acid in the paraventricular and supraoptic nuclei of rat. *Endocrinology* 143, 4320–4329.

Peier, A., Kosinski, J., Cox-York, K., Qian, Y., Desai, K., Feng, Y., et al. (2009). The antiobesity effects of centrally administered Neuromedin U and Neuromedin S are mediated predominantly by the Neuromedin U receptor 2 (NMUR2). *Endocrinology* 150, 3101–3109.

Qiu, D. L., Chu, C. P., Shirasaka, T., Nabekura, T., Kunitake, T., Kato, K., et al. (2003). Neuromedin U depolarizes rat hypothalamic paraventricular nucleus neurons *in vitro* by enhancing IH channel activity. *J. Neurophysiol.* 90, 843–850.

Qiu, D.-L., Chu, C.-P., Tsukino, H., Shirasaka, T., Nakao, H., Kato, K., et al. (2005). Neuromedin U receptor-2 mRNA and HCN channels mRNA expression in NMU-sensitive neurons in rat hypothalamic paraventricular nucleus. *Neurosci. Lett.* 374, 69–72.

Raddatz, R., Wilson, A. E., Artymyshyn, R., Bonini, J. A., Borowsky, B., Boteju, L. W., et al. (2000). Identification and characterization of two neuromedin U receptors differentially expressed in peripheral tissues and the central nervous system. *J. Biol. Chem.* 275, 32452–32459.

Rokkaku, K., Onaka, T., Okada, N., Ideno, J., Kawakami, A., Honda, K., et al. (2003). Neuromedin U facilitates oxytocin release from the pituitary via beta adrenoceptors. *Neuroreport* 14, 1997–2000.

Rucinski, M., Ziolkowska, A., Neri, G., Trejter, M., Zemleduch, T., Tyczewska, M., et al. (2007). Expression of neuromedins S and U and their receptors in the hypothalamus and endocrine glands of the rat. *Int. J. Mol. Med.* 20, 255–259.

Sakamoto, T., Mori, K., Miyazato, M., Kangawa, K., Sameshima, H., Nakahara, K., et al. (2008). Involvement of neuromedin S in the oxytocin release response to suckling stimulus. *Biochem. Biophys. Res. Commun.* 375, 49–53.

Sakamoto, T., Mori, K., Nakahara, K., Miyazato, M., Kangawa, K., Sameshima, H., et al. (2007). Neuromedin S exerts an antidiuretic action in rats. *Biochem. Biophys. Res. Commun.* 361, 457–461.

Sakura, N., Ohta, S., Uchida, Y., Kurosawa, K., Okimura, K., and Hashimoto, T. (1991). Structure-activity relationships of rat neuromedin U for smooth muscle contraction. *Chem. Pharm. Bull.* 39, 2016–2020.

Salmon, A. L., Johnsen, A. H., Bienert, M., McMurray, G., Nandha, K. A., Bloom, S. R., et al. (2000). Isolation, structural characterization, and bioactivity of a novel neuromedin U analog from the defensive skin secretion of the Australasian tree frog, *Litoria caerulea. J. Biol. Chem.* 275, 4549–4554.

Sasaki, T., Shimizu, T., Wakiguchi, H., and Yokotani, K. (2008). Centrally administered neuromedin U elevates plasma adrenaline by brain prostanoid TP receptor-mediated mechanisms in rats. *Eur. J. Pharmacol.* 592, 81–86.

Shan, L. X., Qiao, X. D., Crona, J. H., Behan, J., Wang, S., Laz, T., et al. (2000). Identification of a novel neuromedin U receptor subtype expressed in the central nervous system. *J. Biol. Chem.* 275, 39482–39486.

Shimizu, F., Matsuzaki, T., Iwasa, T., Minakuchi, M., Kuwahara, A., Yasui, T., et al. (2008). Estradiol suppresses NMU mRNA expression during sexual maturation in the female rat pituitary. *Int. J. Dev. Neurosci.* 26, 381–384.

Steel, J. H., Van Noorden, S., Ballesta, J., Gibson, S. J., Ghatei, M. A., Burrin, J., et al. (1988). Localization of 7B2, neuromedin B, and neuromedin U in specific cell types of rat, mouse, and human pituitary, in rat hypothalamus, and in 30 human pituitary and extrapituitary tumors. *Endocrinology* 122, 270–282.

Szekeres, P. G., Muir, A. I., Spinage, L. D., Miller, J. E., Butler, S. I., Smith, A., et al. (2000). Neuromedin U is a potent agonist at the orphan G protein-coupled receptor FM3. *J. Biol. Chem.* 275, 20247–20250.

Tachibana, T., Matsuda, K., Khan, M. S., Ueda, H., and Cline, M. A. (2010). Feeding and drinking response following central administration of neuromedin S in chicks. *Comp. Biochem. Physiol. A Mol. Integr. Physiol.* 157, 63–67.

Tan, C. P., McKee, K. K., Liu, Q. Y., Palyha, O. C., Feighner, S. D., Hreniuk, D. L., et al. (1998). Cloning and characterization of a human and murine T-cell orphan G-protein-coupled receptor similar to the growth hormone secretagogue and neurotensin receptors. *Genomics* 52, 223–229.

Ten Donkelaar, H. J. (1998). "Urodeles," in *The Central Nervous System of Vertebrates, Vol. 1*, eds R. Nieuwenhuys, H. J. Donkelaar, and C. Nicholson (Berlin: Springer Verlag), 1045–1149.

Thompson, E. L., Murphy, K. G., Todd, J. F., Martin, N. M., Small, C. J., Ghatei, M. A., et al. (2004). Chronic administration of NMU into the paraventricular nucleus stimulates the HPA axis but does not influence food intake or body weight.

*Biochem. Biophys. Res. Commun.* 323, 65–71.

Trejter, M., Guidolin, D., Nowak, M., Macchi, V., Majchrzak, M., De Caro, R., et al. (2009). Neuromedin U enhances proliferation of ACTH-stimulated adrenocortical cells in the rat. *Int. J. Mol. Med.* 23, 99–104.

Trejter, M., Neri, G., Rucinski, M., Majchrzak, M., Nussdorfer, G. G., and Malendowicz, L. K. (2008). Neuromedin-U stimulates enucleation-induced adrenocortical regeneration in the rat. *Int. J. Mol. Med.* 21, 683–687.

Vigo, E., Roa, J., López, M., Castellano, J. M., Fernandez-Fernandez, R., Navarro, V. M., et al. (2007). Neuromedin s as novel putative regulator of luteinizing hormone secretion. *Endocrinology* 148, 813–823.

Wren, A. M., Small, C. J., Abbott, C. R., Jethwa, P. H., Kennedy, A. R., Murphy, K. G., et al. (2002). Hypothalamic actions of neuromedin U. *Endocrinology* 143, 4227–4234.

Yayou, K., Kitagawa, S., Ito, S., Kasuya, E., and Sutoh, M. (2009). Effects of intracerebroventricular administration of neuromedin U or neuromedin S in steers. *Gen. Comp. Endocrinol.* 163, 324–328.

Yokota, M., Ozaki, Y., Sakamoto, F., Yamada, S., Saito, J., Fujihara, H., et al. (2004). Fos expression in CRF-containing neurons in the rat paraventricular nucleus after central administration of neuromedin U. *Stress* 7, 109–112.

Zeng, H., Gragerov, A., Hohmann, J. G., Pavlova, M. N., Schimpf, B. A., Xu, H., et al. (2006). Neuromedin U receptor 2-deficient mice display differential responses in sensory perception, stress, and feeding. *Mol. Cell. Biol.* 26, 9352–9363.

Ziolkowska, A., Macchi, C., Trejter, M., Rucinski, M., Nowak, M., Nussdorfer, G. G., et al. (2008). Effects of neuromedin-U on immature rat adrenocortical cells: *in vitro* and *in vivo* studies. *Int. J. Mol. Med.* 21, 303–307.

# How does angiotensin $AT_2$ receptor activation help neuronal differentiation and improve neuronal pathological situations?

***Marie-Odile Guimond and Nicole Gallo-Payet****

*Division of Endocrinology, Department of Medicine, Faculté de Médecine et des Sciences de la Santé, Université de Sherbrooke, Sherbrooke, QC, Canada*

***Edited by:***
*Hubert Vaudry, University of Rouen, France*

***Reviewed by:***
*Lie Gao, University of Nebraska Medical Center, USA*
*Thomas Unger, Maastricht University, Netherlands*

****Correspondence:***
*Nicole Gallo-Payet, Service d'Endocrinologie, Département de Médecine, Faculté de Médecine et des Sciences de la Santé, Université de Sherbrooke, 3001, 12e Avenue Nord, Sherbrooke, QC, Canada J1H 5N4.*
*e-mail: nicole.gallo-payet@usherbrooke.ca*

The angiotensin type 2 ($AT_2$) receptor of angiotensin II has long been thought to be limited to few tissues, with the primary effect of counteracting the angiotensin type 1 ($AT_1$) receptor. Functional studies in neuronal cells have demonstrated $AT_2$ receptor capability to modulate neuronal excitability, neurite elongation, and neuronal migration, suggesting that it may be an important regulator of brain functions. The observation that the $AT_2$ receptor was expressed in brain areas implicated in learning and memory led to the hypothesis that it may also be implicated in cognitive functions. However, linking signaling pathways to physiological effects has always proven challenging since information relative to its physiological functions has mainly emerged from indirect observations, either from the blockade of the $AT_1$ receptor or through the use of transgenic animals. From a mechanistic standpoint, the main intracellular pathways linked to $AT_2$ receptor stimulation include modulation of phosphorylation by activation of kinases and phosphatases or the production of nitric oxide and cGMP, some of which are associated with the Gi-coupling protein. The receptor can also interact with other receptors, either G protein-coupled such as bradykinin, or growth factor receptors such as nerve growth factor or platelet-derived growth factor receptors. More recently, new advances have also led to identification of various partner proteins, thus providing new insights into this receptor's mechanism of action. This review summarizes the recent advances regarding the signaling pathways induced by the $AT_2$ receptor in neuronal cells, and discussed the potential therapeutic relevance of central actions of this enigmatic receptor. In particular, we highlight the possibility that selective $AT_2$ receptor activation by non-peptide and selective agonists could represent new pharmacological tools that may help to improve impaired cognitive performance in Alzheimer's disease and other neurological cognitive disorders.

**Keywords: $AT_2$ receptor, angiotensin, brain, differentiation, regeneration, neurodegenerative disorders, signaling, cognitive functions**

## INTRODUCTION

It is now well accepted that the effects of the various components of the renin-angiotensin system (RAS) range in various aspects of peripheral and brain functions well beyond those of regulating blood pressure and hydro-mineral balance. In particular, the existence of a complete RAS in the brain is fully acknowledged. Its activation leads to angiotensin II (Ang II) production, which is usually viewed as the end-product of this system (de Gasparo et al., 2000). Ang II binds two receptors from the G protein-coupled receptor family (GPCR), namely the angiotensin type 1 ($AT_1$) and angiotensin type 2 ($AT_2$) receptor. Although physiological functions of the $AT_1$ receptor are relatively well-established, ranging from vasoconstriction and aldosterone release to cell growth, the effects associated with the $AT_2$ receptor are surrounded by controversy. Both $AT_1$ and $AT_2$ receptors are expressed in various brain areas involved in the regulation of fluid and electrolyte balance and in the regulation of arterial pressure, as well as in structures involved in cognition, behavior, and locomotion (Phillips and de Oliveira, 2008; Horiuchi et al., 2010; Horiuchi and Mogi, 2011; Wright and Harding, 2011, 2012; Mogi and Horiuchi, 2012).

One of the biggest challenges in studying the $AT_2$ receptor is to apply what has been observed using cell lines to *in vivo* models. Indeed, studies using cell lines expressing the $AT_2$ receptor either endogenously or by transfection, have provided paramount information regarding its intracellular mechanisms of action, although associating these mechanisms with biological functions has proven to be much more difficult. Indeed, most of the relevant information regarding $AT_2$ receptor functions in the brain has emerged from indirect observations, either by use of $AT_1$ receptor blockers (ARB) or *via* transgenic "knock-down" animals for $AT_2$ receptor expression. The present review summarizes recent advances in $AT_2$ receptor signaling pathways, and discusses how they could be related to the neuroprotective functions of the receptor.

## BRAIN EXPRESSION AND ROLE OF THE $AT_2$ RECEPTOR

As summarized in several reviews (de Gasparo et al., 2000; Porrello et al., 2009; Gallo-Payet et al., 2011; Wright and Harding,

2011; Mogi and Horiuchi, 2012), the $AT_2$ receptor is widely expressed during fetal life, which decreases rapidly after birth (Grady et al., 1991; Breault et al., 1996; Schutz et al., 1996; Nuyt et al., 1999), although a recent study has reported opposite results (Yu et al., 2010). This study is indeed in sharp contrast with previous reports using more specific methods, like autoradiography or *in situ* hybridization. In the adult, $AT_2$ receptor expression is limited to a few tissues and cell types, such as vascular endothelial cells, adrenal gland, kidney, heart, myometrial cells, and ovaries (review in Porrello et al., 2009; Gallo-Payet et al., 2011, 2012; Verdonk et al., 2012). In the adult central nervous system (CNS), the $AT_2$ receptor is observed in certain specific brain areas involved in the control and learning of motor activity, control of autonomous functions, sensory areas, and selected limbic system structures (Lenkei et al., 1996, 1997). In particular, it is the major Ang II receptor in the medulla oblongata (control of autonomous functions), septum and amygdala (associated with anxiety-like behavior), thalamus (sensory perception), superior colliculus (control of eye movements in response to visual information) as well as subthalamic nucleus and cerebellum (areas associated with learning of motor functions). On the other hand, certain areas involved in cardiovascular functions, learning, behavior, and stress reactions (cingulate cortex, molecular layer of the cerebellar cortex, superior colliculus, and paraventricular nuclei) contain both $AT_1$ and $AT_2$ receptors (Millan et al., 1991; Tsutsumi and Saavedra, 1991; Lenkei et al., 1996, 1997). More recently, expression of the $AT_2$ receptor was also detected in the substantia nigra pars compacta, an area involved in dopaminergic signals and associated with Parkinson's disease (Grammatopoulos et al., 2007), and in the hippocampus (Arganaraz et al., 2008; AbdAlla et al., 2009). At the cellular level, the $AT_2$ receptor is expressed in neurons, but not in astrocytes (Bottari et al., 1992a; Lenkei et al., 1996; Gendron et al., 2003). Evidence also suggests that the $AT_2$ receptor is expressed in the vasculature wall, where it acts on cerebral blood flow (review in Horiuchi and Mogi, 2011; Horiuchi et al., 2012). It should also be noted that existence of a non-$AT_1$/non-$AT_2$ receptor in the CNS has been suggested, which displays high affinity for Ang I, II, and III (Karamyan and Speth, 2007).

## ROLE OF THE $AT_2$ RECEPTOR IN NEURONAL EXCITABILITY

One of the first roles of the $AT_2$ receptor to be identified was the modulation of neuronal excitability, which plays a crucial role not only in neuronal differentiation, but also in neuronal functions (review in Gendron et al., 2003; Gao et al., 2011). In particular, in cells of neuronal origin, activation of the $AT_2$ receptor decreases activity of T-type calcium channels (Buisson et al., 1992, 1995). On the other hand, in rat brain neuronal culture, Kang et al. (1994) showed that the $AT_2$ receptor stimulates a delayed rectifier $K^+$ current ($I_K$) and a transient $K^+$ current ($I_A$), an effect dependent on the G-protein Gi and the serine/threonine phosphatase PP2A. Consistent with these observations, a recent study showed that $AT_2$ receptor induces a hyperpolarization and a decrease in firing rate in rostral ventrolateral medulla (RVLM) neurons suggesting that central activation of the $AT_2$ receptor in this region decreases excitability (Matsuura et al., 2005). More recently, another study using C21/M024 demonstrated that selective stimulation of $AT_2$ receptor in the neuronal cell line (called CATH.a neurons) increases the potassium current activity ($I_{Kv}$) in a nitric oxide (NO)-dependant pathway (Gao et al., 2011). Moreover, intracerebroventricular infusion of C21/M024 was associated with a decrease in norepinephrine excretion and in blood pressure. Indeed, the modulation of the receptor on neuronal excitability in this region could be one of the mechanism associated with its effect on blood pressure, since RVLM is often considered as the main regulator of vascular tone (review in Dupont and Brouwers, 2010). An inhibitory effect of the $AT_2$ receptor on neuronal excitability has also been observed in the locus coeruleus from brain slice preparations (Xiong and Marshall, 1994) and in the superior colliculus (Merabet et al., 1997). Finally, using the selective agonist C21/M024, Jing et al. (2012) recently demonstrated that direct stimulation of cerebral $AT_2$ receptor increases postsynaptic potential, thus corroborating previous *in vitro* observations. Interestingly, $AT_2$ receptor-induced neuronal activation of delayed rectifier potassium channels has also been demonstrated to have a neuroprotective effect (Grammatopoulos et al., 2004a). In fact, these $AT_2$ receptor effects on ionic channel activity suggest that it may be implicated in synaptic plasticity, an important process involved in learning and memory.

## ROLE OF THE $AT_2$ RECEPTOR IN NEURONAL DIFFERENTIATION

One of the best recognized effects of $AT_2$ receptor stimulation in neuronal cells is the induction of neurite outgrowth (review in Gallo-Payet et al., 2011). In the early 1990s, our group observed that stimulation of the $AT_2$ receptor with its selective agonist CGP42112A induces neurite outgrowth in the neuronal NG108-15 cell line (Laflamme et al., 1996), results that were further confirmed using the recently developed non-peptide selective $AT_2$ receptor agonist C21/M024 (Wan et al., 2004). This effect was associated with an increase in mature neural cell markers, such as βIII-tubulin, and microtubule-associated proteins (MAPs) such as MAP2c (Laflamme et al., 1996), both known to stabilize tubulin in a polymerized state, thus participating actively in differentiation (Sanchez et al., 2000). Similar results have also been reported in the pheochromocytoma-derived cell line PC12W, where Ang II was found to promoted neuronal differentiation characterized by an increase in neurite elongation (Meffert et al., 1996) and enhanced levels of polymerized βIII-tubulin and MAP2 associated with microtubules (Stroth et al., 1998). However, neurite outgrowth in PC12W cells has also been associated with a reduced expression of MAP1B (Stroth et al., 1998) and neurofilament M (Gallinat et al., 1997), two proteins specifically associated with axon elongation (Gordon-Weeks, 1991). These results were further confirmed in primary neuronal cultures, including retinal explants (Lucius et al., 1998), microexplant cultures of the cerebellum (Coté et al., 1999), in neurospheres from mouse fetal brain (Mogi et al., 2006) as well as primary cultures of newborn brain cortex neurons (Li et al., 2007) and hippocampal neurons (Jing et al., 2012). Some studies also showed that this neurite elongation was associated with an increase in the repair of damaged DNA by induction of methyl methanesulfonate sensitive-2 (MMS2), a neural-differentiating factor (Mogi et al., 2006; Jing et al., 2012). Altogether, these results suggest that activation of the $AT_2$ receptor is associated with important rearrangements of the cytoskeleton necessary for induction of neurite elongation.

### ROLE OF THE AT$_2$ RECEPTOR IN NEURONAL MIGRATION

In cerebellar microexplants, where both neuronal and glial cells are present, AT$_2$ receptor activation induces not only neurite outgrowth, but cell migration as well (Coté et al., 1999). Indeed, application of Ang II in this model induced cell migration of neurons from the center toward the periphery of the microexplant (Coté et al., 1999). These effects were more pronounced in cells treated with Ang II and DUP 753 (known as the ARB losartan) or in cells treated with 10 nM of CGP42112A an AT$_2$ receptor agonist, and conversely blocked with the AT$_2$ receptor antagonist PD123,319. Similar cell migration has also been observed during AT$_2$ receptor-induced regeneration of post-natal retinal microexplants (Lucius et al., 1998). During migration and neurite outgrowth, cells are characterized by a myriad of advancing, retracting, turning, and branching behavioral patterns. Such dynamics and plasticity are driven by the reorganization of actin and the microtubular cytoskeleton. In particular, during the process of migration, actin filaments play a major role and are putatively considered as the primary target of guidance cues, due to their localization at the cell periphery, and in filopodium in the growth cone, where they are considered to be the driving force for the forward extension of the cell membrane (Gallo and Letourneau, 2004; Kalil and Dent, 2005). Our results on NG108-15 cells have shown that the underlying mechanism involves an Ang II-induced decrease in the amount of F-actin in filopodium and an increase in the pool of unpolymerized actin, through a pertussis toxin (PTX)-sensitive increase in ADF/cofilin activity. These latter effects were found to be AT$_2$ receptor-dependent, since the increase in the rate of migration was abolished by the selective antagonist PD123,319, but not by the selective AT$_1$ receptor antagonist losartan. Interestingly, some co-localization of F-actin with microtubules was also observed in control conditions, but which disappeared during Ang II-induced migration (Kilian et al., 2008). Among the candidate molecules that possibly cross-link actin filaments and microtubules are MAP2c and MAP1B (Dehmelt et al., 2003; Dehmelt and Halpain, 2004), proteins previously shown by our group to be affected during the process of AT$_2$ receptor-stimulated neurite outgrowth, both in NG108-15 cells and in cerebellar granule cells (Laflamme et al., 1996; Coté et al., 1999).

## MAIN SIGNALING PATHWAYS OF THE AT$_2$ RECEPTOR

Although the AT$_2$ receptor displays most of the classical features of a GPCR, it is usually considered as an atypical member of this family, since it fails to induce all of the classical signaling pathways such as cAMP, production of inositol triphosphate (IP3) or intracellular calcium release. Signaling pathways associated with the AT$_2$ receptor mainly involve a balance between phosphatase and kinase activities and according to whether the cell is undifferentiated or differentiated and whether it expresses angiotensin AT$_1$ receptors or not. Thus, there is still much controversy surrounding this receptor, and its effects, either protective or deleterious, remain a subject of debate (Widdop et al., 2003; Steckelings et al., 2005, 2010; Porrello et al., 2009; Horiuchi et al., 2012; Verdonk et al., 2012). In our endeavor to elucidate the mechanisms associated with AT$_2$ receptor-induced neurite outgrowth, we and others have investigated signaling pathways activated by this receptor, including G-protein coupling, regulation of kinase activity, interaction with growth factor receptors, and production of NO. Moreover, recent observations have also delineated new partners for the AT$_2$ receptor which play key functions in its regulation (**Figure 1**).

### G-PROTEIN COUPLING

While coupling of G-protein to AT$_1$ receptors is well described (de Gasparo et al., 2000; Hunyady and Catt, 2006), such coupling is not the rule for the AT$_2$ receptor. Former studies have described a coupling to subunit G$\alpha_{i2}$ and G$\alpha_{i3}$ in rat fetus (Zhang and Pratt, 1996). In some models (rat hippocampal neurons and other selected cell types), blocking G$\alpha_i$ with PTX or antibodies directed against G$\alpha_i$ inhibited the AT$_2$ receptor effects on actin depolymerization, activation of endothelial NO synthase (NOS), stimulation of neuronal $K^+$ current and on anti-proliferative activity (Kang et al., 1994; Ozawa et al., 1996; Li et al., 2004; Olson et al., 2004; Kilian et al., 2008), indicating that coupling of the AT$_2$receptor to G$\alpha_i$ is at least implicated in these pathways. However, aside from a few exceptions (Kang et al., 1994), PTX failed to inhibit either p42/p44$^{mapk}$ activation in the neuronal cell line NG108-15 (Gendron et al., 2002) or phosphatase activity in several models (for review see Nouet and Nahmias, 2000; Gendron et al., 2003).

### REGULATION OF KINASE ACTIVITY

#### *AT$_2$ Receptor-induced phosphatase activation*

Phosphatase activation has been one of the first signals associated with AT$_2$ receptor activation. After the earlier studies in PC12W cells (Bottari et al., 1992b; Brechler et al., 1994), results have been confirmed in other cell lines, including N1E-115 cells (Nahmias et al., 1995), NG108-15 cells (Buisson et al., 1995), and R3T3 fibroblasts (Tsuzuki et al., 1996a,b). This phosphatase activation by the AT$_2$ receptor is essential for its anti-proliferative and pro-apoptotic effects (for reviews, see Nouet and Nahmias, 2000; Steckelings et al., 2005; Porrello et al., 2009; Verdonk et al., 2012). Currently, three main phosphatases have been implicated in AT$_2$ receptor signaling, namely SH2-domain-containing phosphatase 1 (SHP-1), mitogen-activated protein kinase phosphatase 1 (MKP-1), and the serine–threonine phosphatase PP2A.

SHP-1 is a cytosolic phosphatase rapidly activated by the AT$_2$ receptor following Ang II binding. Activation of SHP-1 is associated with AT$_2$-induced growth inhibition in various cells, including neuronal cells (Bedecs et al., 1997; Elbaz et al., 2000; Feng et al., 2002; Li et al., 2007), vascular smooth muscle cells (Cui et al., 2001; Matsubara et al., 2001), CHO, and COS-7 cells transfected with the AT$_2$ receptor (Elbaz et al., 2000; Feng et al., 2002). Activation of SHP-1 is associated with inhibitory effects of the AT$_2$ receptor on the AT$_1$ receptor, including transactivation of the epidermal growth factor (EGF) receptor and activation of c-Jun N-terminal kinase (JNK) (Matsubara et al., 2001; Shibasaki et al., 2001), but also on insulin-induced activation of the phosphatidylinositol 3-kinase (PI3K), its association with the insulin receptor substrate IRS-2 and phosphorylation of Akt (Cui et al., 2001). This inhibition of insulin signaling by AT$_2$ receptor-induced SHP-1 activation has also been associated with an increase in PC12W

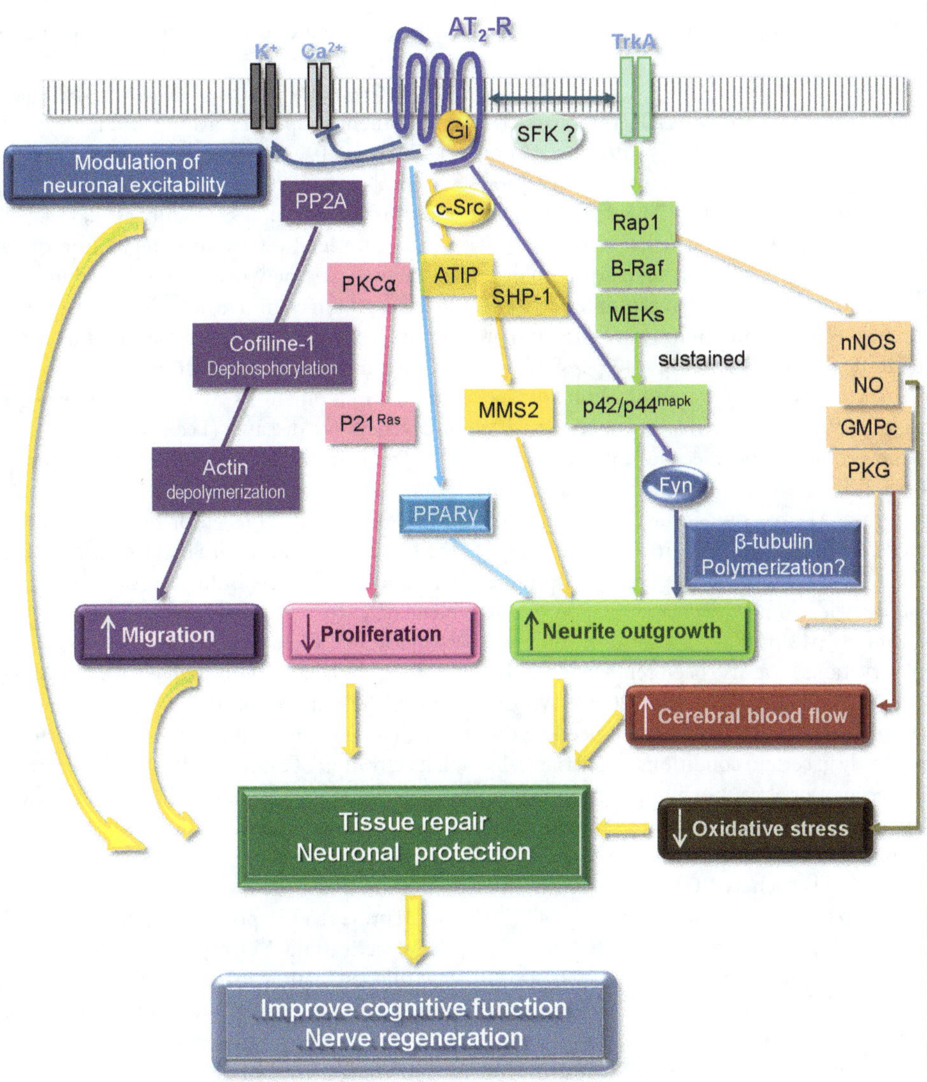


**FIGURE 1 | Main signaling pathways associated with $AT_2$ receptor activation leading to neuroprotective effects (see text for details).** Adapted from Gallo-Payet et al. (2011).

cell apoptosis (Cui et al., 2002). More recently, Li et al. (2007) have shown that induction of neurite outgrowth in fetal rat neurons by $AT_2$ receptor involves the association of SHP-1 with the newly identified $AT_2$-receptor interacting protein (ATIP; see section $AT_2$ Receptor Interacting Proteins) and an increase in MMS2 protein (Li et al., 2007). Finally, although the mechanisms associated with $AT_2$ receptor-induced activation of SHP-1 have yet to be fully elucidated, implication of G-protein coupling (Bedecs et al., 1997; Feng et al., 2002) as well as activation of Src kinase (Alvarez et al., 2008) have been reported; other studies have also implicated a constitutive association between $AT_2$ receptor and SHP-1 in overexpressing models (Feng et al., 2002; Miura et al., 2005). Another phosphatase associated with $AT_2$ receptor activation is MKP-1, which is a key regulator of $p42/p44^{mapk}$ activity. $AT_2$ receptor-activated MKP-1 has been observed in various cell types, including PC12W cells (Yamada et al., 1996), fibroblasts (Horiuchi et al., 1997; Calo et al., 2010), and cardiac myocytes (Fischer et al., 1998; Hiroi et al., 2001). Activation of MKP-1 by $AT_2$ leads to a decrease in $p42/p44^{mapk}$ activity, and is associated to growth inhibition induced by the $AT_2$ receptor. Moreover, Horiuchi et al. (1997) demonstrated that $AT_2$ receptor-induced MKP-1 activation is implicated in apoptotic effects of the $AT_2$ receptor, leading to Bcl-2 dephosphorylation and an increase in Bax, resulting in cell death. Finally, the serine–threonine phosphatase PP2A is also activated by the $AT_2$ receptor following Ang II binding and may be associated with $AT_2$ receptor regulation of $p42/p44^{mapk}$. Indeed, in primary neuronal cultures, $AT_2$ receptor-induced activation of PP2A is associated with inhibition of $AT_1$ receptor-induced $p42/p44^{mapk}$ phosphorylation (Huang et al., 1995, 1996a,b) and is implicated in $AT_2$-induced modulation of potassium currents (Huang et al., 1995, 1996a; Caballero et al., 2004). More recently, we have also shown an implication of PP2A activation in actin depolymerization and an increase in neuronal migration (Kilian et al., 2008; **Figure 1**).

### *Mitogen-activated protein kinase p42/p44*

Among all signaling pathways associated with $AT_2$ receptor activation, regulation of p42/p44$^{mapk}$ is probably the one where variability is the most important. The effect of $AT_2$ receptor stimulation on activation or inhibition of p42/p44$^{mapk}$ activity is dependent on the models studied, on whether they express $AT_1$ receptors or not and whether cells are under physiological or pathological conditions. Thus, $AT_2$ receptor effects on p42/p44$^{mapk}$ remain controversial. Many studies have shown that the $AT_2$ receptor leads to dephosphorylation of p42/p44$^{mapk}$ *via* one the phosphatases associated with $AT_2$ receptor signaling (see above). This decrease in p42/p44$^{mapk}$ activity is associated with inhibition of growth and pro-apoptotic effects of the $AT_2$ receptor (review in Nouet et al., 2004; Porrello et al., 2009). In addition to activation of phosphatase, $AT_2$ receptor-induced inhibition of p42/p44$^{mapk}$ can be mediated by inhibition of growth factor receptors. Indeed, in vascular smooth muscle cells overexpressing the $AT_2$ receptor, stimulation with Ang II decreases EGF receptor phosphorylation and inhibits p42/p44$^{mapk}$ activation (Shibasaki et al., 2001). Similar observations have also been reported in CHO cells overexpressing the $AT_2$ receptor (Elbaz et al., 2000). Worthy of note is the fact that inhibition of p42/p44$^{mapk}$ induced by the $AT_2$ receptor is observed only in certain conditions, such as in cells overexpressing the $AT_2$ receptor or already exhibiting pathological conditions such as serum-starving (Bedecs et al., 1997; Horiuchi et al., 1997; Elbaz et al., 2000; Cui et al., 2001; Shibasaki et al., 2001).

By contrast, in neuronal cells such as NG108-15 and PC12W cells, the $AT_2$ receptor leads to sustained activation of p42/p44$^{mapk}$. In these cells, activation of p42/p44$^{mapk}$ is essential to $AT_2$ receptor-induced neurite elongation (Gendron et al., 1999; Stroth et al., 2000). In NG108-15 cells, we observed that this increase in p42/p44$^{mapk}$ activity was associated with the Rap1/B-Raf pathway. However, this Rap1 activation appears to be dependent of nerve growth factor receptor TrkA activation (see latter; Plouffe et al., 2006) rather than through cAMP and protein kinase A (PKA), as usually observed with other GPCR (**Figure 1**). This activation of p42/p44$^{mapk}$ by the $AT_2$ receptor has also been observed in non-neuronal COS-7 and NIH3T3 cells overexpressing the $AT_2$ receptor (Hansen et al., 2000; De Paolis et al., 2002).

### *Src family kinase*

There are few studies showing an implication of Src family members in $AT_2$ receptor signaling. However, Src family kinases (SFKs) are key regulators in cell growth and differentiation and are implicated in most growth factor signaling pathways. In the CNS, five members of SFK are expressed, namely Src, Fyn, Lyn, Lck, and Yes, where they act as modulators of neurotransmitter receptors as well as in the regulation of excitatory transmission (review in Kalia et al., 2004; Theus et al., 2006; Ohnishi et al., 2011). Recently, we have shown that stimulation of the $AT_2$ receptor in NG108-15 cells leads to rapid but transient activation of SFK and that expression of inactive Fyn abolished $AT_2$ receptor-induced neurite outgrowth in these cells (Guimond et al., 2010). However, inhibition of Fyn had no effect on other signaling pathways induced by the $AT_2$ receptor, including p42/p44$^{mapk}$ and Rap1 activation, suggesting that it may be involved either downstream of these proteins, or in a parallel pathway. Of note, among the five SFKs expressed in the brain, only a deficiency in Fyn-induced neurological deficits, including impairment in spatial learning and in hippocampal development (Grant et al., 1992; Kojima et al., 1997). Interestingly, similar physiological perturbations were also observed in mice lacking the $AT_2$ receptor (Hein et al., 1995; Ichiki et al., 1995; Okuyama et al., 1999; Maul et al., 2008). Therefore, regulation of Fyn activity could be considered as a new player implicated in the protective effect of this receptor in cognitive disorders. Indeed, Fyn has been shown to be involved in tau phosphorylation, thus regulating its affinity for tubulin and stability of microtubules, two parameters implicated in the development of Alzheimer's disease (AD) and other neurodegenerative diseases (Lee et al., 1998, 2004). Thus, it appears that Fyn is involved in the final steps of induction of elongation, but not in the initial events of $AT_2$ receptor activation. This implication of Fyn in $AT_2$ receptor signaling is further strengthened by the fact that activation of SFKs, as the $AT_2$ receptor, was shown to be important for the induction of long-term potentiation, a key element in learning and memory, in CA1 pyramidal neurons of hippocampal slices (Yu et al., 1997).

To the best of our knowledge, only one other group has demonstrated the implication of a Src family member in $AT_2$ receptor signaling (Alvarez et al., 2008). In this latter study, it was shown that activation of c-Src was present in an immunocomplex including the tyrosine phosphatase SHP-1 and the $AT_2$ receptor following Ang II stimulation in rat fetal membranes. Pre-incubation of membranes with the non-selective inhibitor PP2 inhibited SHP-1 activation and c-Src association. These results indicate that c-Src may represent an important step leading to $AT_2$ receptor-induced SHP-1 activation. More recently, the same group demonstrated that this association also occurred in hindbrain membranes from post-natal day 15 rats, and was associated with focal adhesion kinase (p85FAK) (Seguin et al., 2012). These observations strongly suggest that c-Src may also be implicated in cytoskeleton remodeling associated with neurite elongation and neuronal migration induced by the $AT_2$ receptor.

## LINKING THE $AT_2$ RECEPTOR WITH THE GROWTH FACTOR RECEPTORS

Recently, we demonstrated that activation of Rap1/B-Raf/p42/p44$^{mapk}$ pathway by the $AT_2$ receptor was dependent on the nerve growth factor receptor TrkA, although the mechanism involved remains unknown (Plouffe et al., 2006). In addition, we further showed that a SFK member was essential for the initial activation of TrkA by the $AT_2$ receptor, since pre-incubation of NG108-15 cells with the non-selective inhibitor PP1 disrupted this effect (Guimond et al., 2010). However, although Fyn was essential for neurite outgrowth induced by the $AT_2$ receptor, it did not appear to be implicated in TrkA activation, since expression of a dominant negative form did not impede $AT_2$-induced TrkA activation (Guimond et al., 2010). In light of recent data obtained by Ciuffo's group regarding the involvement of c-Src and other SFK members with $AT_2$ receptors (Alvarez et al., 2008; Seguin et al., 2012), it would be of interest to see whether the association of the $AT_2$ receptor with SHP-1 and c-Src is implicated in this transactivation, and whether TrkA could be involved in

FAK activation. Interestingly, transactivation of the TrkA receptor in neurons has also been observed for the pituitary adenylyl cyclase-activating polypeptide receptor (PACAP; Rajagopal et al., 2004), which is also associated with neuronal development in the cerebellum (Basille et al., 2006).

Curiously, although the expression of inactive Fyn is known to disrupt $AT_2$ receptor-induced neurite elongation, non-selective inhibition of SFK in NG108-15 cells with the inhibitor PP1 is sufficient to increase neurite elongation to levels similar to those observed with $AT_2$ receptor stimulation (Guimond et al., 2010), which could be a consequence of a decrease in proliferative signal. Indeed, our group showed that induction of neurite outgrowth was associated with a decrease in cell proliferation through inhibition of PKC$\alpha$ and $p21^{Ras}$ (Gendron et al., 1999; Beaudry et al., 2006). Moreover, as in the case of SFK, inhibition of the platelet-derived growth factor (PDGF) receptor was sufficient to induce neurite outgrowth and to increase microtubule polymerization more extensively than Ang II alone (Plouffe et al., 2006). These findings are in agreement with a previous report demonstrating that expression of an inactive form of the PDGF receptor in PC12 cells was sufficient to increase neurite elongation (Vetter and Bishop, 1995). However, whether $AT_2$ receptor directly inhibits PDGF receptor or inhibits its signaling pathway is still unknown.

## NITRIC OXIDE AND cGMP PRODUCTION – A ROLE FOR BRADYKININ

Nitric oxide has been shown to regulate several types of $K^+$ channels, including ATP-dependent $K^+$ channels and $Ca^{2+}$-activated $K^+$ channels (review in Prast and Philippu, 2001). Indeed, in neuronal cell lines, observations with the selective $AT_2$ receptor agonist C21/M024 revealed that this production of NO induced by $AT_2$ was necessary for $AT_2$-induced hyperpolarization of potassium channel function (Gao and Zucker, 2011). Production of NO following $AT_2$ receptor stimulation has been observed in various cell types, such as neuronal cells (Chaki and Inagami, 1993; Coté et al., 1998; Gendron et al., 2002; Zhao et al., 2003; Muller et al., 2010), vascular endothelial cells (Wiemer et al., 1993; Seyedi et al., 1995; Saito et al., 1996; Thorup et al., 1998; Baranov and Armstead, 2005) as well as in smooth muscle cells (de Godoy et al., 2004). It is already well accepted that $AT_2$ receptor activation plays an important role in the control of renal function particularly in chronic kidney diseases. The $AT_2$ receptor is believed to counterbalance the effects of the $AT_1$ receptor at least by influencing vasodilation through NO production and natriuresis (Carey and Padia, 2008; Siragy, 2010; Siragy and Carey, 2010). This promoter effect of $AT_2$ on natriuresis in pathological conditions (obese Zucker rats) was also recently confirmed using C21/M024 (Ali and Hussain, 2012). Activation of NOS by the $AT_2$ receptor can occur by direct signaling such as in neuronal cells, or indirectly *via* stimulation of bradykinin production and subsequent activation of its receptor B2. Indeed, heterodimerization between the $AT_2$ receptor and bradykinin has also been described in PC12W cells (Abadir et al., 2006). Moreover, it is already known that bradykinin can modulate $AT_2$ receptor-induced NO production (Siragy and Carey, 1996; Gohlke et al., 1998; Searles and Harrison, 1999). Such involvement of B2 receptors in $AT_2$ receptor-induced production of NO is of prime importance in the modulation of cerebral blood flow. Indeed, an $AT_2$-induced increase in spatial learning was recently observed to be associated with an increase in cerebral blood flow, an effect reduced by co-administration of the B2 receptor antagonist icatibant. This observation strongly suggests that the beneficial effect of the $AT_2$ receptor in cognitive function is partly dependent on bradykinin (Jing et al., 2012). In addition, Abadir et al. (2003) demonstrated in conscious bradykinin B2-null and wild-type mice that the $AT_2$ receptor can induce production of NO in both null and wild-type models, indicating that the B2 receptor may participate in this process, although is not the only means for the $AT_2$ receptor to induce NO production.

## $AT_2$ RECEPTOR ASSOCIATED PROTEINS

### *ATIP*

Recently, using a yeast two-hybrid system, the ATIP was cloned and identified as a protein interacting with the C-terminal tail of the $AT_2$ receptor (Nouet et al., 2004). This protein is expressed as five different transcripts, namely ATIP1, ATIP2, ATIP3a, ATIP3b, and ATIP4 (review in Rodrigues-Ferreira and Nahmias, 2010; Horiuchi et al., 2012). While ATIP3 appears to be the major transcript in tissues, ATIP1 and ATIP4 are mainly expressed in the brain, indicating that they may play biological roles in brain functions. ATIP2, on the other hand, is almost undetectable by real-time PCR (Di Benedetto et al., 2006). In CHO cells expressing the $AT_2$ receptor, ATIP is known to decrease growth factor-induced $p42/p44^{mapk}$ activation and DNA synthesis, therefore decreasing cell proliferation, as well as decrease insulin receptor autophosphorylation, similarly to the $AT_2$ receptor. Of particular interest is the fact that, although expression of the $AT_2$ receptor was essential in this instance, stimulation by Ang II was not necessary, and that ATIP was able to exert its effect by its sole expression. Implication of ATIP in $AT_2$ receptor-induced neurite outgrowth has also been reported. In this context, Ang II stimulation of the $AT_2$ receptor induces translocation of ATIP with SHP-1 into the nucleus, resulting in the transactivation of MMS2 (Li et al., 2007). Moreover, ATIP, also known as ATBP50 ($AT_2$ receptor binding protein of 50 kDa), has been reported as a membrane-associated Golgi protein implicated in intracellular localization of the $AT_2$ receptor and necessary for its membrane expression (Wruck et al., 2005). ATIP3, which is also expressed in the CNS, has been shown to strongly interact with stabilized microtubules in a model of breast cancer, suggesting an implication on cell division, where it induces a delayed metaphase, thus decreasing tumor progression (Rodrigues-Ferreira et al., 2009). The brain-specific isoform ATIP4 is highly expressed in the cerebellum and fetal brain, two sites where the $AT_2$ receptor is also highly expressed. Therefore considering (i) the previously described function of the $AT_2$ receptor in preservation of cognitive function, (ii) the role of ATIP protein in $AT_2$ receptor function, and (iii) the link between ATIP protein and microtubule cytoskeleton, it could be suggested that regulation of ATIP expression and regulation of its association with the $AT_2$ receptor could be an important element to consider with regard to the development of neurological disorders, such as AD.

### *PLZF*

Association between the $AT_2$ receptor and the promyelocytic leukemia zinc finger (PLZF) protein has been observed using a yeast two-hybrid system (Senbonmatsu et al., 2003). In CHO cells expressing both PLZF and $AT_2$ receptors, Ang II stimulation induces co-localization of PLZF with the $AT_2$ receptor, followed by internalization of the complex. This observation is in contrast with other studies observing no internalization of the $AT_2$ receptor following Ang II stimulation (Hunyady et al., 1994; Hein et al., 1997). Since internalization of the receptor was observed only in cells expressing PLZF, this could represent a new regulatory pathway of $AT_2$ receptor function, specific only to selected cell types. However, beside internalization of $AT_2$ receptor, a recent study showed that PLZF was implicated in neuroprotection in a stroke model (Seidel et al., 2011). In this study, the authors showed that PLZF exerts neuroprotective effect in a model of *in vitro* glutamate toxicity. They also showed that overexpression of PLZF in neuronal cells in culture induced a significant increase in $AT_2$ receptor expression, suggesting that PLZF could also be implicated in the regulation of $AT_2$ receptor expression.

#### *PPARγ*

A new partner for the $AT_2$ receptor has recently emerged from the study of Zhao et al. (2005) who observed that neurite outgrowth induced by $AT_2$ receptor stimulation in PC12W cells was dependent on the activation of peroxisome proliferator-activated receptor gamma (PPARγ). This observation is in keeping with the implication of PPARγ in NGF-induced neurite outgrowth in the same cell type (Fuenzalida et al., 2005), clearly suggesting a possible crosstalk between the $AT_2$ receptor and NGF pathways. This hypothesis is further reinforced by the observation that inhibition of the NGF receptor TrkA significantly decreases $AT_2$ receptor-induced neurite outgrowth (Plouffe et al., 2006). Moreover, Iwai et al. (2009), using atherosclerotic ApoE-KO mice with an $AT_2$ receptor deficiency (AT2R/ApoE double knockout mice), observed that the lack of $AT_2$ receptor expression decreased the expression of PPARγ in adipocytes cells. These observations strongly suggest a link between the $AT_2$ receptor and PPARγ functions. PPARγ is a transcriptional factor regulating the expression of multiple genes, hence promoting the differentiation and development of various tissues, specifically in adipose tissue, brain, placenta, and skin. Interestingly, neuroprotective effects of PPARγ agonist have also been observed (review in Gillespie et al., 2011). However, a major component of the hypothesis regarding the possible implication of PPARγ in $AT_2$ receptor function is the PPARγ-like activity associated with certain ARBs, including telmisartan, irbesartan, and candesartan (Benson et al., 2004; Schupp et al., 2004; review in Horiuchi et al., 2012). Indeed, there is some evidence suggesting that this PPARγ activation following blockade of the $AT_1$ receptor could be part of its anti-inflammatory and anti-oxidative effects, leading to neuroprotection against ischemia and amyloid β (Aβ) accumulation (Tsukuda et al., 2009; Iwanami et al., 2010; Washida et al., 2010). PPARγ has also been implicated in neural cell differentiation and death, as well as inflammatory and neurodegenerative conditions (review in Gillespie et al., 2011).

## LESSONS FROM NEURONAL DIFFERENTIATION: HOW CAN THE $AT_2$ RECEPTOR IMPROVE BRAIN FUNCTION?

### ROLE OF THE $AT_2$ RECEPTOR IN NEURONAL REGENERATION

The capacity for nerve regeneration in lower vertebrates has been mostly lost in higher vertebrates and regeneration within the CNS in mammals is essentially inexistent. However, after injury in the peripheral nervous system, regeneration can be achieved successfully. Observations that $AT_2$ receptor stimulation induces neurite elongation associated with modulation of MAP expression strongly suggested that this effect could also be observed following nerve injury. In 1998, two studies demonstrated that the $AT_2$ receptor improved nerve recovery in both optic (Lucius et al., 1998) and sciatic (Gallinat et al., 1998) nerve following nerve crush or in perivascular nerves implicated in vasodilation (Hobara et al., 2007). This effect was accompanied by an increase in $AT_2$ receptor expression, the activation of NFκB and induction of growth-associated protein (GAP-43) leading to a reduction in lesion size. Moreover, Reinecke et al. (2003) demonstrated that activation of NFκB by the $AT_2$ receptor was an essential step to recovery following sciatic nerve crush. This implication of $AT_2$ receptor in neuronal regeneration has even led to the suggestion that Ang II, *via* the $AT_2$ receptor, could act as a neurotrophic factor.

### $AT_2$ RECEPTOR IN COGNITIVE FUNCTION

There is increasing evidence suggesting that the $AT_2$ receptor could be associated with improvement of cognitive function following cerebral ischemia-induced neuronal injury (Iwai et al., 2004; Li et al., 2005; Mogi et al., 2006; McCarthy et al., 2009). Indeed, it has been shown that central administration of CGP42112A increases neuronal survival and minimizes experimental post-stroke injury (McCarthy et al., 2009), indicating that activation of brain $AT_2$ receptors exhibits a neuroprotective effect. More recently, stimulation of the $AT_2$ receptor with the selective agonist C21/M024 was observed to prevent cognitive decline in an AD mouse model with intracerebroventricular injection of Aβ(1-40) (Jing et al., 2012). Indeed, some of the signaling pathways described above may be linked to improvement in impaired signaling functions as observed in AD. One of the major hallmarks of AD is Aβ deposition in senile plaques and the presence of neurofibrillary tangles (NFTs). Formation of NFTs is a consequence of protein tau accumulation, due to its hyperphosphorylation, and the dissociation of microtubules. Thus, regulation of tau phosphorylation is of paramount importance with regard to AD progression. On the other hand, several studies have reported that the $AT_2$ receptor activates PP2A phosphatase (Huang et al., 1995, 1996a; Kilian et al., 2008), which is markedly deficient in AD (Gong et al., 1993, 2000; Wang et al., 2007) and implicated in glycogen synthase kinase-3 (GSK-3) inactivation *via* a sustained increase in $p42/p44^{mapk}$. Since tau is a substrate for PP2A phosphatase, GSK-3 and Fyn, the latter of which is also implicated in the $AT_2$ receptor effect on neurite outgrowth (Guimond et al., 2010), $AT_2$ receptor activation could participate in controlling the equilibrium between tau phosphorylation and dephosphorylation (Hernandez and Avila, 2008; Hanger et al., 2009; Hernandez et al., 2009). In addition to acting on tau regulation, the $AT_2$ receptor may also improve neurite architecture, through effects on MAPs, as observed in neuronal cell lines (Laflamme et al., 1996; Meffert et al., 1996; Coté et al., 1999; Li et al., 2007). The observation that central $AT_2$ receptor activation using its selective agonist C21/M024 decreases cognitive loss induced by Aβ intracerebroventricular injection lends further support to this hypothesis (Jing et al., 2012). Although the mechanisms underlying these neuroprotective effects of the $AT_2$

receptor remain to be fully elucidated, they may include PPARγ and the protein MMS2 (Mogi et al., 2006, 2008; for recent reviews see Gallo-Payet et al., 2011, 2012).

Moreover, as indicated earlier, another important feature of $AT_2$ receptor signaling is induction of NO and cGMP production. Recently, Jing et al. (2012) observed that direct stimulation of central $AT_2$ receptors increases NO *via* a bradykinin-dependent pathway, an effect which leads to an increase in cerebral blood flow and enhanced spatial memory. A further study also showed that administration of C21/M024 reduced early renal inflammatory response with production of NO and cGMP (Matavelli et al., 2011). This increase in NO-cGMP production has also been shown to lead to a decrease in nicotinamide adenine dinucleotide phosphate-oxidase (NADPH) superoxide production (Volpe et al., 2003; Widdop et al., 2003; de la Torre, 2004; Steckelings et al., 2005; Iadecola et al., 2009), thus reducing oxidative stress and potentially associated neuronal apoptosis. This hypothesis is coherent with the observation that the $AT_2$ receptor attenuates chemical hypoxia-induced caspase-3 activation in primary cortical neuronal cultures (Grammatopoulos et al., 2004b). Finally, inflammation is also a common feature of neurodegenerative diseases. In this regard, a recent study conducted in primary cultures of human and murine dermal fibroblasts, has shown that C21/M024 has anti-inflammatory effects, inhibiting tumor necrosis factor (TNF)-α-induced interleukin-6 levels and NFκB activity. This effect was notably initiated through increased activation of protein phosphatases and increased synthesis of epoxyeicosatrienoic acid (Rompe et al., 2010).

## CONCLUSION

Since its identification in the early 90s, the $AT_2$ receptor has been and still is shrouded by controversy, its low expression in the adult and its atypical signaling pathways adding to the challenge of studying this receptor. Thanks to the major advances achieved in the past few years, several studies have confirmed that stimulation of the $AT_2$ receptor activates multiple signaling pathways which are linked to beneficial effects on neuronal functions (including excitability, differentiation, and regeneration), inflammation, oxidative stress, and cerebral blood flow (**Figure 1**). Several neurodegenerative diseases (including cognitive deficits and dementia) are closely associated with these neuronal and synaptic dysfunctions (Iadecola, 2004; Zlokovic, 2005; LaFerla et al., 2007; Boissonneault et al., 2009; Mucke, 2009; Nelson et al., 2009). Moreover, an increasing number of studies suggest that the protective effects of ARBs on brain damage and cognition may result not only from the inhibition of $AT_1$ receptor effects, but also from the beneficial effect due to unopposed activation of the $AT_2$ receptor. Thus, if further research confirms the promising early results obtained with the recently developed selective non-peptide $AT_2$ receptor agonist C21/M024, the latter may represent a new pharmacological tool in the fight against neurological cognitive disorders. In addition, unraveling the underlying effects of the $AT_2$ receptor on neuronal plasticity may lead to the development of even more potent and selective therapies.

## ACKNOWLEDGMENTS

The authors are grateful to Pierre Pothier for critical reading of the manuscript and editorial assistance (Les Services PM-SYS Enr., Sherbrooke). This work presented in this review was supported by grants from the Canadian Institutes of Health Research (MOP-82819 to Nicole Gallo-Payet) and from the Alzheimer's Society of Canada to Nicole Gallo-Payet with Louis Gendron (Université de Sherbrooke) and Thomas Stroh (McGill University) and by the Canada Research Chair program to Nicole Gallo-Payet. Nicole Gallo-Payet is a past holder of the Canada Research Chair in Endocrinology of the Adrenal Gland. Marie-Odile Guimond is a postdoctoral fellowship in the laboratory of Nicole Gallo-Payet. Nicole Gallo-Payet and Marie-Odile Guimond are both members of the FRSQ-funded Centre de recherche clinique Étienne-Le Bel.

## REFERENCES

Abadir, P. M., Carey, R. M., and Siragy, H. M. (2003). Angiotensin AT2 receptors directly stimulate renal nitric oxide in bradykinin B2-receptor-null mice. *Hypertension* 42, 600–604.

Abadir, P. M., Periasamy, A., Carey, R. M., and Siragy, H. M. (2006). Angiotensin II type 2 receptor-bradykinin B2 receptor functional heterodimerization. *Hypertension* 48, 316–322.

AbdAlla, S., Lother, H., el Missiry, A., Langer, A., Sergeev, P., el Faramawy, Y., et al. (2009). Angiotensin II AT2 receptor oligomers mediate G-protein dysfunction in an animal model of Alzheimer disease. *J. Biol. Chem.* 284, 6554–6565.

Ali, Q., and Hussain, T. (2012). AT(2) receptor non-peptide agonist C21 promotes natriuresis in obese Zucker rats. *Hypertens. Res.* 35, 654–660.

Alvarez, S. E., Seguin, L. R., Villarreal, R. S., Nahmias, C., and Ciuffo, G. M. (2008). Involvement of c-Src tyrosine kinase in SHP-1 phosphatase activation by Ang II AT2 receptors in rat fetal tissues. *J. Cell. Biochem.* 105, 703–711.

Arganaraz, G. A., Konno, A. C., Perosa, S. R., Santiago, J. F., Boim, M. A., Vidotti, D. B., et al. (2008). The renin-angiotensin system is upregulated in the cortex and hippocampus of patients with temporal lobe epilepsy related to mesial temporal sclerosis. *Epilepsia* 49, 1348–1357.

Baranov, D., and Armstead, W. M. (2005). Nitric oxide contributes to AT2 but not AT1 angiotensin II receptor-mediated vasodilatation of porcine pial arteries and arterioles. *Eur. J. Pharmacol.* 525, 112–116.

Basille, M., Cartier, D., Vaudry, D., Lihrmann, I., Fournier, A., Freger, P., et al. (2006). Localization and characterization of pituitary adenylate cyclase-activating polypeptide receptors in the human cerebellum during development. *J. Comp. Neurol.* 496, 468–478.

Beaudry, H.,Gendron, L., Guimond, M. O., Payet, M. D., and Gallo-Payet, N. (2006). Involvement of protein kinase C alpha (PKC alpha) in the early action of angiotensin II type 2 (AT2) effects on neurite outgrowth in NG108-15 cells: AT2-receptor inhibits PKC alpha and p21ras activity. *Endocrinology* 147, 4263–4272.

Bedecs, K., Elbaz, N., Sutren, M., Masson, M., Susini, C., Strosberg, A. D., et al. (1997). Angiotensin II type 2 receptors mediate inhibition of mitogen-activated protein kinase cascade and functional activation of SHP-1 tyrosine phosphatase. *Biochem. J.* 325, 449–454.

Benson, S. C., Pershadsingh, H. A., Ho, C. I., Chittiboyina, A., Desai, P., Pravenec, M., et al. (2004). Identification of telmisartan as a unique angiotensin II receptor antagonist with selective PPARgamma-modulating activity. *Hypertension* 43, 993–1002.

Boissonneault, V., Filali, M., Lessard, M., Relton, J., Wong, G., and Rivest, S. (2009). Powerful beneficial effects of macrophage colony-stimulating factor on beta-amyloid deposition and cognitive impairment in Alzheimer's disease. *Brain* 132, 1078–1092.

Bottari, S. P., King, I. N., Reichlin, S., Dahlstroem, I., Lydon, N., and de Gasparo, M. (1992a). The angiotensin AT2 receptor stimulates protein tyrosine phosphatase activity and mediates inhibition of particulate guanylate cyclase. *Biochem. Biophys. Res. Commun.* 183, 206–211.

Bottari, S. P., Obermuller, N., Bogdal, Y., Zahs, K. R., and Deschepper, C. F. (1992b). Characterization and distribution of angiotensin II binding sites in fetal and neonatal astrocytes from different rat brain regions. *Brain Res.* 585, 372–376.

Breault, L., Lehoux, J. G., and Gallo-Payet, N. (1996). The angiotensin AT2 receptor is present in the human fetal adrenal gland throughout the second trimester of gestation. *J. Clin. Endocrinol. Metab.* 81, 3914–3922.

Brechler, V., Reichlin, S., De Gasparo, M., and Bottari, S. P. (1994). Angiotensin II stimulates protein tyrosine phosphatase activity through a G-protein independent mechanism. *Recept. Channels* 2, 89–98.

Buisson, B., Bottari, S. P., de Gasparo, M., Gallo-Payet, N., and Payet, M. D. (1992). The angiotensin AT2 receptor modulates T-type calcium current in non-differentiated NG108-15 cells. *FEBS Lett.* 309, 161–164.

Buisson, B., Laflamme, L., Bottari, S. P., de Gasparo, M., Gallo-Payet, N., and Payet, M. D. (1995). A G protein is involved in the angiotensin AT2 receptor inhibition of the T-type calcium current in non-differentiated NG108-15 cells. *J. Biol. Chem.* 270, 1670–1674.

Caballero, R., Gomez, R., Moreno, I., Nunez, L., Gonzalez, T., Arias, C., et al. (2004). Interaction of angiotensin II with the angiotensin type 2 receptor inhibits the cardiac transient outward potassium current. *Cardiovasc. Res.* 62, 86–95.

Calo, L. A., Schiavo, S., Davis, P. A., Pagnin, E., Mormino, P., D'Angelo, A., et al. (2010). Angiotensin II signaling via type 2 receptors in a human model of vascular hyporeactivity: implications for hypertension. *J. Hypertens.* 28, 111–118.

Carey, R. M., and Padia, S. H. (2008). Angiotensin AT2 receptors: control of renal sodium excretion and blood pressure. *Trends Endocrinol. Metab.* 19, 84–87.

Chaki, S., and Inagami, T. (1993). New signaling mechanism of angiotensin II in neuroblastoma neuro-2A cells: activation of soluble guanylyl cyclase via nitric oxide synthesis. *Mol. Pharmacol.* 43, 603–608.

Coté, F., Do, T. H., Laflamme, L., Gallo, J. M., and Gallo-Payet, N. (1999). Activation of the AT(2) receptor of angiotensin II induces neurite outgrowth and cell migration in microexplant cultures of the cerebellum. *J. Biol. Chem.* 274, 31686–31692.

Coté, F., Laflamme, L., Payet, M. D., and Gallo-Payet, N. (1998). Nitric oxide, a new second messenger involved in the action of angiotensin II on neuronal differentiation of NG108-15 cells. *Endocr. Res.* 24, 403–407.

Cui, T., Nakagami, H., Iwai, M., Takeda, Y., Shiuchi, T., Daviet, L., et al. (2001). Pivotal role of tyrosine phosphatase SHP-1 in AT2 receptor-mediated apoptosis in rat fetal vascular smooth muscle cell. *Cardiovasc. Res.* 49, 863–871.

Cui, T. X., Nakagami, H., Nahmias, C., Shiuchi, T., Takeda-Matsubara, Y., Li, J. M., et al. (2002). Angiotensin II subtype 2 receptor activation inhibits insulin-induced phosphoinositide 3-kinase and Akt and induces apoptosis in PC12W cells. *Mol. Endocrinol.* 16, 2113–2123.

de Gasparo, M., Catt, K. J., Inagami, T., Wright, J. W., and Unger, T. (2000). International union of pharmacology. XXIII. The angiotensin II receptors. *Pharmacol. Rev.* 52, 415–472.

de Godoy, M. A., de Oliveira, A. M., and Rattan, S. (2004). Angiotensin II-induced relaxation of anococcygeus smooth muscle via desensitization of AT1 receptor, and activation of AT2 receptor associated with nitric-oxide synthase pathway. *J. Pharmacol. Exp. Ther.* 311, 394–401.

de la Torre, J. C. (2004). Is Alzheimer's disease a neurodegenerative or a vascular disorder? Data, dogma, and dialectics. *Lancet Neurol.* 3, 184–190.

De Paolis, P., Porcellini, A., Savoia, C., Lombardi, A., Gigante, B., Frati, G., et al. (2002). Functional cross-talk between angiotensin II and epidermal growth factor receptors in NIH3T3 fibroblasts. *J. Hypertens.* 20, 693–699.

Dehmelt, L., and Halpain, S. (2004). Actin and microtubules in neurite initiation: are MAPs the missing link? *J. Neurobiol.* 58, 18–33.

Dehmelt, L., Smart, F. M., Ozer, R. S., and Halpain, S. (2003). The role of microtubule-associated protein 2c in the reorganization of microtubules and lamellipodia during neurite initiation. *J. Neurosci.* 23, 9479–94790.

Di Benedetto, M., Bieche, I., Deshayes, F., Vacher, S., Nouet, S., Collura, V., et al. (2006). Structural organization and expression of human MTUS1, a candidate 8p22 tumor suppressor gene encoding a family of angiotensin II AT2 receptor-interacting proteins, ATIP. *Gene* 380, 127–136.

Dupont, A. G., and Brouwers, S. (2010). Brain angiotensin peptides regulate sympathetic tone and blood pressure. *J. Hypertens.* 28, 1599–1610.

Elbaz, N., Bedecs, K., Masson, M., Sutren, M., Strosberg, A. D., and Nahmias, C. (2000). Functional trans-inactivation of insulin receptor kinase by growth-inhibitory angiotensin II AT2 receptor. *Mol. Endocrinol.* 14, 795–804.

Feng, Y. H., Sun, Y., and Douglas, J. G. (2002). Gbeta gamma -independent constitutive association of Galpha s with SHP-1 and angiotensin II receptor AT2 is essential in AT2-mediated ITIM-independent activation of SHP-1. *Proc. Natl. Acad. Sci. U.S.A.* 99, 12049–12054.

Fischer, T. A., Singh, K., O'Hara, D. S., Kaye, D. M., and Kelly, R. A. (1998). Role of AT1 and AT2 receptors in regulation of MAPKs and MKP-1 by ANG II in adult cardiac myocytes. *Am. J. Physiol.* 275, H906–H916.

Fuenzalida, K. M., Aguilera, M. C., Piderit, D. G., Ramos, P. C., Contador, D., Quinones, V., et al. (2005). Peroxisome proliferator-activated receptor gamma is a novel target of the nerve growth factor signaling pathway in PC12 cells. *J. Biol. Chem.* 280, 9604–9609.

Gallinat, S., Csikos, T., Meffert, S., Herdegen, T., Stoll, M., and Unger, T. (1997). The angiotensin AT2 receptor down-regulates neurofilament M in PC12W cells. *Neurosci. Lett.* 227, 29–32.

Gallinat, S., Yu, M., Dorst, A., Unger, T., and Herdegen, T. (1998). Sciatic nerve transection evokes lasting up-regulation of angiotensin AT2 and AT1 receptor mRNA in adult rat dorsal root ganglia and sciatic nerves. *Brain Res. Mol. Brain Res.* 57, 111–122.

Gallo, G., and Letourneau, P. C. (2004). Regulation of growth cone actin filaments by guidance cues. *J. Neurobiol.* 58, 92–102.

Gallo-Payet, N., Guimond, M.-O., Bilodeau, L., Wallinder, C., Alterman, M., and Hallberg, A. (2011). Angiotensin II, a neuropeptide at the frontier between endocrinology and neuroscience: is there a link between the angiotensin II type 2 receptor (AT2R) and Alzheimer's disease? *Front. Endocrinol.* 2:17. doi: 10.3389/fendo.2011.00017

Gallo-Payet, N., Shum, M., Baillargeon, J.-P., Langlois, M.-F., Alterman, M., Hallberg, A., et al. (2012). AT2 receptor agonists: exploiting the beneficial arm of Ang II signaling. *Curr. Hypertens. Rev.* 8, 47–59.

Gao, J., Zhang, H., Le, K. D., Chao, J., and Gao, L. (2011). Activation of central angiotensin type 2 receptors suppresses norepinephrine excretion and blood pressure in conscious rats. *Am. J. Hypertens.* 24, 724–730.

Gao, L., and Zucker, I. H. (2011). AT2 receptor signaling and sympathetic regulation. *Curr. Opin. Pharmacol.* 11, 124–130.

Gendron, L., Coté, F., Payet, M. D., and Gallo-Payet, N. (2002). Nitric oxide and cyclic GMP are involved in angiotensin II AT(2) receptor effects on neurite outgrowth in NG108-15 cells. *Neuroendocrinology* 75, 70–81.

Gendron, L., Laflamme, L., Rivard, N., Asselin, C., Payet, M. D., and Gallo-Payet, N. (1999). Signals from the AT2 (angiotensin type 2) receptor of angiotensin II inhibit p21ras and activate MAPK (mitogen-activated protein kinase) to induce morphological neuronal differentiation in NG108-15 cells. *Mol. Endocrinol.* 13, 1615–1626.

Gendron, L., Payet, M. D., and Gallo-Payet, N. (2003). The angiotensin type 2 receptor of angiotensin II and neuronal differentiation: from observations to mechanisms. *J. Mol. Endocrinol.* 31, 359–372.

Gillespie, W., Tyagi, N., and Tyagi, S. C. (2011). Role of PPARgamma, a nuclear hormone receptor in neuroprotection. *Indian J. Biochem. Biophys.* 48, 73–81.

Gohlke, P., Pees, C., and Unger, T. (1998). AT2 receptor stimulation increases aortic cyclic GMP in SHRSP by a kinin-dependent mechanism. *Hypertension* 31, 349–355.

Gong, C. X., Lidsky, T., Wegiel, J., Zuck, L., Grundke-Iqbal, I., and Iqbal, K. (2000). Phosphorylation of microtubule-associated protein tau is regulated by protein phosphatase 2A in mammalian brain. Implications for neurofibrillary degeneration in Alzheimer's disease. *J. Biol. Chem.* 275, 5535–5544.

Gong, C. X., Singh, T. J., Grundke-Iqbal, I., and Iqbal, K. (1993). Phosphoprotein phosphatase activities in Alzheimer disease brain. *J. Neurochem.* 61, 921–927.

Gordon-Weeks, P. R. (1991). Control of microtubule assembly in growth cones. *J. Cell Sci. Suppl.* 15, 45–49.

Grady, E. F., Sechi, L. A., Griffin, C. A., Schambelan, M., and Kalinyak, J. E. (1991). Expression of AT2 receptors in the developing rat fetus. *J. Clin. Invest.* 88, 921–933.

Grammatopoulos, T. N., Johnson, V., Moore, S. A., Andres, R., and Weyhenmeyer, J. A. (2004a). Angiotensin type 2 receptor neuroprotection against chemical hypoxia is dependent on the delayed rectifier K+ channel, Na+/Ca2+ exchanger and Na+/K+ ATPase in primary cortical cultures. *Neurosci. Res.* 50, 299–306.

Grammatopoulos, T. N., Morris, K., Bachar, C., Moore, S., Andres, R., and Weyhenmeyer, J. A. (2004b). Angiotensin II attenuates chemical hypoxia-induced caspase-3 activation in primary cortical neuronal cultures. *Brain Res. Bull.* 62, 297–303.

Grammatopoulos, T. N., Jones, S. M., Ahmadi, F. A., Hoover, B. R., Snell, L. D., Skoch, J., et al. (2007). Angiotensin type 1 receptor antagonist losartan, reduces MPTP-induced degeneration of dopaminergic neurons in substantia nigra. *Mol. Neurodegener.* 2, 1–17.

Grant, S. G., O'Dell, T. J., Karl, K. A., Stein, P. L., Soriano, P., and Kandel, E. R. (1992). Impaired long-term potentiation, spatial learning, and hippocampal development in fyn mutant mice. *Science* 258, 1903–1910.

Guimond, M. O., Roberge, C., and Gallo-Payet, N. (2010). Fyn is involved in angiotensin II type 2 receptor-induced neurite outgrowth, but not in p42/p44mapk in NG108-15 cells. *Mol. Cell. Neurosci.* 45, 201–212.

Hanger, D. P., Anderton, B. H., and Noble, W. (2009). Tau phosphorylation: the therapeutic challenge for neurodegenerative disease. *Trends Mol. Med.* 15, 112–119.

Hansen, J., Servant, G., Baranski, T., Fujita, T., Iiri, T., and Sheikh, S. (2000). Functional reconstitution of the angiotensin II type 2 receptor and G(i) activation. *Circ. Res.* 87, 753–759.

Hein, L., Barsh, G. S., Pratt, R. E., Dzau, V. J., and Kobilka, B. K. (1995). Behavioural and cardiovascular effects of disrupting the angiotensin II type-2 receptor in mice. *Nature* 377, 744–747.

Hein, L., Meinel, L., Pratt, R. E., Dzau, V. J., and Kobilka, B. K. (1997). Intracellular trafficking of angiotensin II and its AT1 and AT2 receptors: evidence for selective sorting of receptor and ligand. *Mol. Endocrinol.* 11, 1266–1277.

Hernandez, F., and Avila, J. (2008). The role of glycogen synthase kinase 3 in the early stages of Alzheimers' disease. *FEBS Lett.* 582, 3848–3854.

Hernandez, F., Gomez de Barreda, E., Fuster-Matanzo, A., Lucas, J. J., and Avila, J. (2009). GSK3: a possible link between beta amyloid peptide and tau protein. *Exp. Neurol.* 223, 322–325.

Hiroi, Y., Hiroi, J., Kudoh, S., Yazaki, Y., Nagai, R., and Komuro, I. (2001). Two distinct mechanisms of angiotensin II-induced negative regulation of the mitogen-activated protein kinases in cultured cardiac myocytes. *Hypertens. Res.* 24, 385–394.

Hobara, N., Goda, M., Yoshida, N., Takatori, S., Kitamura, Y., Mio, M., and Kawasaki, H. (2007). Angiotensin II type 2 receptors facilitate reinnervation of phenol-lesioned vascular calcitonin gene-related peptide-containing nerves in rat mesenteric arteries. *Neuroscience* 150, 730–741.

Horiuchi, M., Hayashida, W., Kambe, T., Yamada, T., and Dzau, V. J. (1997). Angiotensin type 2 receptor dephosphorylates Bcl-2 by activating mitogen-activated protein kinase phosphatase-1 and induces apoptosis. *J. Biol. Chem.* 272, 19022–19026.

Horiuchi, M., Iwanami, J., and Mogi, M. (2012). Regulation of angiotensin II receptors beyond the classical pathway. *Clin. Sci. (Lond)* 123, 193–203.

Horiuchi, M., and Mogi, M. (2011). Role of angiotensin II receptor subtype activation in cognitive function and ischaemic brain damage. *Br. J. Pharmacol.* 163, 1122–1130.

Horiuchi, M., Mogi, M., and Iwai, M. (2010). The angiotensin II type 2 receptor in the brain. *J. Renin Angiotensin Aldosterone Syst.* 11, 1–6.

Huang, X. C., Richards, E. M., and Sumners, C. (1995). Angiotensin II type 2 receptor-mediated stimulation of protein phosphatase 2A in rat hypothalamic/brainstem neuronal cocultures. *J. Neurochem.* 65, 2131–2137.

Huang, X. C., Richards, E. M., and Sumners, C. (1996a). Mitogen-activated protein kinases in rat brain neuronal cultures are activated by angiotensin II type 1 receptors and inhibited by angiotensin II type 2 receptors. *J. Biol. Chem.* 271, 15635–15641.

Huang, X. C., Sumners, C., and Richards, E. M. (1996b). Angiotensin II stimulates protein phosphatase 2A activity in cultured neuronal cells via type 2 receptors in a pertussis toxin sensitive fashion. *Adv. Exp. Med. Biol.* 396, 209–215.

Hunyady, L., Bor, M., Balla, T., and Catt, K. J. (1994). Identification of a cytoplasmic Ser-Thr-Leu motif that determines agonist-induced internalization of the AT1 angiotensin receptor. *J. Biol. Chem.* 269, 31378–37382.

Hunyady, L., and Catt, K. J. (2006). Pleiotropic AT1 receptor signaling pathways mediating physiological and pathogenic actions of angiotensin II. *Mol. Endocrinol.* 20, 953–970.

Iadecola, C. (2004). Neurovascular regulation in the normal brain and in Alzheimer's disease. *Nat. Rev. Neurosci.* 5, 347–360.

Iadecola, C., Park, L., and Capone, C. (2009). Threats to the mind: aging, amyloid, and hypertension. *Stroke* 40, S40–S44.

Ichiki, T., Labosky, P. A., Shiota, C., Okuyama, S., Imagawa, Y., Fogo, A., et al. (1995). Effects on blood pressure and exploratory behaviour of mice lacking angiotensin II type-2 receptor. *Nature* 377, 748–750.

Iwai, M., Liu, H. W., Chen, R., Ide, A., Okamoto, S., Hata, R., et al. (2004). Possible inhibition of focal cerebral ischemia by angiotensin II type 2 receptor stimulation. *Circulation* 110, 843–848.

Iwai, M., Tomono, Y., Inaba, S., Kanno, H., Senba, I., Mogi, M., and Horiuchi, M. (2009). AT2 receptor deficiency attenuates adipocyte differentiation and decreases adipocyte number in atherosclerotic mice. *Am. J. Hypertens.* 22, 784–791.

Iwanami, J., Mogi, M., Tsukuda, K., Min, L. J., Sakata, A., Jing, F., et al. (2010). Low dose of telmisartan prevents ischemic brain damage with peroxisome proliferator-activated receptor-gamma activation in diabetic mice. *J. Hypertens.* 28, 1730–1737.

Jing, F., Mogi, M., Sakata, A., Iwanami, J., Tsukuda, K., Ohshima, K., et al. (2012). Direct stimulation of angiotensin II type 2 receptor enhances spatial memory. *J. Cereb. Blood Flow Metab.* 32, 248–255.

Kalia, L. V., Gingrich, J. R., and Salter, M. W. (2004). Src in synaptic transmission and plasticity. *Oncogene* 23, 8007–8016.

Kalil, K., and Dent, E. W. (2005). Touch and go: guidance cues signal to the growth cone cytoskeleton. *Curr. Opin. Neurobiol.* 15, 521–526.

Kang, J., Posner, P., and Sumners, C. (1994). Angiotensin II type 2 receptor stimulation of neuronal K+ currents involves an inhibitory GTP binding protein. *Am. J. Physiol.* 267, C1389–C1397.

Karamyan, V. T., and Speth, R. C. (2007). Identification of a novel non-AT1, non-AT2 angiotensin binding site in the rat brain. *Brain Res.* 1143, 83–91.

Kilian, P., Campbell, S., Bilodeau, L., Guimond, M. O., Roberge, C., Gallo-Payet, N., et al. (2008). Angiotensin II type 2 receptor stimulation increases the rate of NG108-15 cell migration via actin depolymerization. *Endocrinology* 149, 2923–2933.

Kojima, N., Wang, J., Mansuy, I. M., Grant, S. G., Mayford, M., and Kandel, E. R. (1997). Rescuing impairment of long-term potentiation in fyn-deficient mice by introducing Fyn transgene. *Proc. Natl. Acad. Sci. U.S.A.* 94, 4761–4765.

LaFerla, F. M., Green, K. N., and Oddo, S. (2007). Intracellular amyloid-beta in Alzheimer's disease. *Nat. Rev. Neurosci.* 8, 499–509.

Laflamme, L., Gasparo, M., Gallo, J. M., Payet, M. D., and Gallo-Payet, N. (1996). Angiotensin II induction of neurite outgrowth by AT2 receptors in NG108-15 cells. Effect counteracted by the AT1 receptors. *J. Biol. Chem.* 271, 22729–22735.

Lee, G., Newman, S. T., Gard, D. L., Band, H., and Panchamoorthy, G. (1998). Tau interacts with src-family non-receptor tyrosine kinases. *J. Cell Sci.* 111(Pt. 21), 3167–3177.

Lee, G., Thangavel, R., Sharma, V. M., Litersky, J. M., Bhaskar, K. Fang, S. M., et al. (2004). Phosphorylation of tau by fyn: implications for Alzheimer's disease. *J. Neurosci.* 24, 2304–2312.

Lenkei, Z., Palkovits, M., Corvol, P., and Llorens-Cortes, C. (1996). Distribution of angiotensin II type-2 receptor (AT2) mRNA expression in the adult rat brain. *J Comp. Neurol.* 373, 322–339.

Lenkei, Z., Palkovits, M., Corvol, P., and Llorens-Cortes, C. (1997). Expression of angiotensin type-1 (AT1) and type-2 (AT2) receptor mRNAs in the adult rat brain: a functional neuroanatomical review. *Front. Neuroendocrinol.* 18:383–439. doi: 10.1006/frne.1997.0155

Li, J., Culman, J., Hortnagl, H., Zhao, Y., Gerova, N., Timm, M., et al. (2005). Angiotensin AT2 receptor protects against cerebral ischemia-induced neuronal injury. *FASEB J.* 19, 617–619.

Li, J. M., Mogi, M., Tsukuda, K., Tomochika, H., Iwanami, J., Min, L. J., et al. (2007). Angiotensin II-induced neural differentiation via angiotensin II type 2 (AT2) receptor-MMS2 cascade involving interaction between AT2 receptor-interacting protein and Src homology 2 domain-containing protein-tyrosine phosphatase 1. *Mol. Endocrinol.* 21, 499–511.

Li, X., Lerea, K. M., Li, J., and Olson, S. C. (2004). Src kinase mediates angiotensin II-dependent increase in pulmonary endothelial nitric oxide synthase. *Am. J. Respir. Cell Mol. Biol.* 31, 365–372.

Lucius, R., Gallinat, S., Rosenstiel, P., Herdegen, T., Sievers, J., and Unger, T. (1998). The angiotensin II type 2 (AT2) receptor promotes axonal regeneration in the optic nerve of adult rats. *J. Exp. Med.* 188, 661–670.

Matavelli, L. C., Huang, J., and Siragy, H. M. (2011). Angiotensin AT receptor stimulation inhibits early renal inflammation in renovascular hypertension. *Hypertension* 57, 308–313.

Matsubara, H., Shibasaki, Y., Okigaki, M., Mori, Y., Masaki, H., Kosaki, A. et al. (2001). Effect of angiotensin II type 2 receptor on tyrosine kinase Pyk2 and c-Jun NH2-terminal kinase via SHP-1 tyrosine phosphatase activity: evidence from vascular-targeted transgenic mice of AT2 receptor. *Biochem. Biophys. Res. Commun.* 282, 1085–1091.

Matsuura, T., Kumagai, H., Onimaru, H., Kawai, A., Iigaya, K., Onami, T., et al. (2005). Electrophysiological properties of rostral ventrolateral medulla neurons in angiotensin II 1a receptor knockout mice. *Hypertension* 46, 349–354.

Maul, B., von Bohlen und Halbach, O., Becker, A., Sterner-Kock, A., Voigt, J. P., Siems, W. E., et al. (2008). Impaired spatial memory and altered dendritic spine morphology in angiotensin II type 2 receptor-deficient mice. *J. Mol. Med.* 86, 563–571.

McCarthy, C. A., Vinh, A., Callaway, J. K., and Widdop, R. E. (2009). Angiotensin AT2 Receptor Stimulation Causes Neuroprotection in a Conscious Rat Model of Stroke. *Stroke* 40, 1482–1489.

Meffert, S., Stoll, M., Steckelings, U. M., Bottari, S. P., and Unger, T. (1996). The angiotensin II AT2 receptor inhibits proliferation and promotes differentiation in PC12W cells. *Mol. Cell. Endocrinol.* 122, 59–67.

Merabet, L., de Gasparo, M., and Casanova, C. (1997). Dose-dependent inhibitory effects of angiotensin II on visual responses of the rat superior colliculus: AT1 and AT2 receptor contributions. *Neuropeptides* 31, 469–481.

Millan, M. A., Jacobowitz, D. M., Aguilera, G., and Catt, K. J. (1991). Differential distribution of AT1 and AT2 angiotensin II receptor subtypes in the rat brain during development. *Proc. Natl. Acad. Sci. U.S.A.*88, 11440–11444.

Miura, S., Karnik, S. S., and Saku, K. (2005). Constitutively active homo-oligomeric angiotensin II type 2 receptor induces cell signaling independent of receptor conformation and ligand stimulation. *J. Biol. Chem.* 280, 18237–18244.

Mogi, M., and Horiuchi, M., (2012). Effect of angiotensin II type 2 receptor on stroke, cognitive impairment and neurodegenerative diseases. *Geriatr. Gerontol. Int.* doi: 10.1111/j.1447 [Epub ahead of print].

Mogi, M.,Li, J. M., Iwanami, J., Min, L. J., Tsukuda, K., Iwai, M., et al. (2006). Angiotensin II type-2 receptor stimulation prevents neural damage by transcriptional activation of methyl methanesulfonate sensitive 2. *Hypertension* 48, 141–148.

Mogi, M., Li, J. M., Tsukuda, K., Iwanami, J., Min, L. J., Sakata, A., et al. (2008). Telmisartan prevented cognitive decline partly due to PPAR-gamma activation. *Biochem. Biophys. Res. Commun.* 375, 446–449.

Mucke, L. (2009). Neuroscience: Alzheimer's disease. *Nature* 461, 895–897.

Muller, D., Greenland, K. J., Speth, R. C., and Middendorff, R. (2010). Neuronal differentiation of NG108-15 cells has impact on nitric oxide- and membrane (natriuretic peptide receptor-A) cyclic GMP-generating proteins. *Mol. Cell. Endocrinol.* 320, 118–127.

Nahmias, C., Cazaubon, S. M., Briend-Sutren, M. M., Lazard, D., Villageois, P., and Strosberg, A. D. (1995). Angiotensin II AT2 receptors are functionally coupled to protein tyrosine dephosphorylation in N1E-115 neuroblastoma cells. *Biochem. J.* 306(Pt. 1), 87–92.

Nelson, P. T., Braak, H., and Markesbery, W. R. (2009). Neuropathology and cognitive impairment in Alzheimer disease: a complex but coherent relationship. *J. Neuropathol. Exp. Neurol.* 68, 1–14.

Nouet, S., Amzallag, N., Li, J. M., Louis, S., Seitz, I., Cui, T. X., et al. (2004). Trans-inactivation of receptor tyrosine kinases by novel angiotensin II AT2 receptor-interacting protein, ATIP. *J. Biol. Chem.* 279, 28989–28997.

Nouet, S., and Nahmias, C. (2000). Signal transduction from the angiotensin II AT2 receptor. *Trends Endocrinol. Metab.* 11, 1–6.

Nuyt, A. M., Lenkei, Z., Palkovits, M., Corvol, P., and Llorens-Cortes, C., (1999). Ontogeny of angiotensin II type 2 receptor mRNA expression in fetal and neonatal rat brain. *J. Comp. Neurol.* 407, 193–206.

Ohnishi, H., Murata, Y., Okazawa, H., and Matozaki, T. (2011). Src family kinases: modulators of neurotransmitter receptor function and behavior. *Trends Neurosci.* 34, 629–637.

Okuyama, S., Sakagawa, T., Chaki, S., Imagawa, Y., Ichiki, T., and Inagami, T. (1999). Anxiety-like behavior in mice lacking the angiotensin II type-2 receptor. *Brain Res.* 821, 150–159.

Olson, S., Oeckler, R., Li, X., Du, L., Traganos, F., Zhao, X., et al. (2004). Angiotensin II stimulates nitric oxide production in pulmonary artery endothelium via the type 2 receptor. *Am. J. Physiol. Lung Cell. Mol. Physiol.* 287, L559–L568.

Ozawa, Y., Suzuki, Y., Murakami, K., and Miyazaki, H. (1996). The angiotensin II type 2 receptor primarily inhibits cell growth via pertussis toxin-sensitive G proteins. *Biochem. Biophys. Res. Commun.* 228, 328–333.

Phillips, M. I. and de Oliveira, E. M. (2008). Brain renin angiotensin in disease. *J. Mol. Med.* 86, 715–722.

Plouffe, B., Guimond, M. O., Beaudry, H., and Gallo-Payet, N. (2006). Role of tyrosine kinase receptors in angiotensin II AT2 receptor signaling: involvement in neurite outgrowth and in p42/p44mapk activation in NG108-15 cells. *Endocrinology* 147, 4646–4654.

Porrello, E. R., Delbridge, L. M., and Thomas, W. G. (2009). The angiotensin II type 2 (AT2) receptor: an enigmatic seven transmembrane receptor. *Front. Biosci.* 14:958–972. doi: 10.2741/3289

Prast, H., and Philippu, A. (2001). Nitric oxide as modulator of neuronal function. *Prog. Neurobiol.* 64, 51–68.

Rajagopal, R., Chen, Z. Y., Lee, F. S., and Chao, M. V. (2004). Transactivation of Trk neurotrophin receptors by G-protein-coupled receptor ligands occurs on intracellular membranes. *J. Neurosci.* 24, 6650–6658.

Reinecke, K., Lucius, R., Reinecke, A., Rickert, U., Herdegen, T., and Unger, T. (2003). Angiotensin II accelerates functional recovery in the rat sciatic nerve in vivo: role of the AT2 receptor and the transcription factor NF-kappaB. *FASEB J.* 17, 2094–2096.

Rodrigues-Ferreira, S., Di Tommaso, A., Dimitrov, A., Cazaubon, S., Gruel, N., Colasson, H., et al. (2009). 8p22 MTUS1 gene product ATIP3 is a novel anti-mitotic protein underexpressed in invasive breast carcinoma of poor prognosis. *PLoS ONE* 4:e7239. doi: 10.1371/journal.pone.0007239

Rodrigues-Ferreira, S., and Nahmias, C. (2010). An ATIPical family of angiotensin II AT2 receptor-interacting proteins. *Trends Endocrinol. Metab.* 21, 684–690.

Rompe, F., Artuc, M., Hallberg, A., Alterman, M., Stroder, K., Thone-Reineke, C., et al. (2010). Direct angiotensin II type 2 receptor stimulation acts anti-inflammatory through epoxyeicosatrienoic acid and inhibition of nuclear factor kappaB. *Hypertension* 55, 924–931.

Saito, S., Hirata, Y., Emori, T., Imai, T., and Marumo, F. (1996). Angiotensin II activates endothelial constitutive nitric oxide synthase via AT1 receptors. *Hypertens. Res.* 19, 201–206.

Sanchez, C., Diaz-Nido, J., and Avila, J. (2000). Phosphorylation of microtubule-associated protein 2 (MAP2) and its relevance for the regulation of the neuronal cytoskeleton function. *Prog. Neurobiol.* 61, 133–168.

Schupp, M., Janke, J., Clasen, R., Unger, T., and Kintscher, U. (2004). Angiotensin type 1 receptor blockers induce peroxisome proliferator-activated receptor-gamma activity. *Circulation* 109, 2054–2057.

Schutz, S., Le Moullec, J. M., Corvol, P., and Gasc, J. M. (1996). Early expression of all the components of the renin-angiotensin-system in human development. *Am. J. Pathol.* 149, 2067–2079.

Searles, C. D., and Harrison, D. G. (1999). The interaction of nitric oxide, bradykinin, and the angiotensin II type 2 receptor: lessons learned from transgenic mice. *J. Clin. Invest.* 104, 1013–1014.

Seguin, L. R., Villarreal, R. S., and Ciuffo, G. M. (2012). AT2 receptors recruit c-Src, SHP-1 and FAK upon activation by Ang II in PND15 rat hindbrain. *Neurochem. Int.* 60, 199–207.

Seidel, K., Kirsch, S., Lucht, K., Zaade, D., Reinemund, J., Schmitz, J., et al. (2011). The promyelocytic leukemia zinc finger (PLZF) protein exerts neuroprotective effects in neuronal cells and is dysregulated in experimental stroke. *Brain Pathol.* 21, 31–43.

Senbonmatsu, T., Saito, T., Landon, E. J., Watanabe, O., Price, E. Jr., Roberts, R. L., et al. (2003). A novel angiotensin II type 2 receptor signaling pathway: possible role in cardiac hypertrophy. *EMBO J.* 22, 6471–6482.

Seyedi, N., Xu, X., Nasjletti, A., and Hintze, T. H. (1995). Coronary kinin generation mediates nitric oxide release after angiotensin receptor stimulation. *Hypertension* 26, 164–170.

Shibasaki, Y., Matsubara, H., Nozawa, Y., Mori, Y., Masaki, H., Kosaki, A., Tsutsumi, Y., et al. (2001). Angiotensin II type 2 receptor inhibits epidermal growth factor receptor transactivation by increasing association of SHP-1 tyrosine phosphatase. *Hypertension* 38, 367–372.

Siragy, H. M. (2010). The angiotensin II type 2 receptor and the kidney. *J. Renin Angiotensin Aldosterone Syst.* 11, 33–36.

Siragy, H. M., and Carey, R. M. (1996). The subtype-2 (AT2) angiotensin receptor regulates renal cyclic guanosine 3', 5'-monophosphate and AT1 receptor-mediated prostaglandin E2 production in conscious rats. *J. Clin. Invest.* 97, 1978–1982.

Siragy, H. M., and Carey, R. M. (2010). Role of the intrarenal renin-angiotensin-aldosterone system in chronic kidney disease. *Am. J. Nephrol.* 31, 541–550.

Steckelings, U. M., Kaschina, E., and Unger, T. (2005). The AT2 receptor-a matter of love and hate. *Peptides* 26, 1401–1409.

Steckelings, U. M., Rompe, F., Kaschina, E., Namsolleck, P., Grzesiak, A., Funke-Kaiser, H., et al. (2010). The past, present and future of angiotensin II type 2 receptor stimulation. *J. Renin. Angiotensin. Aldosterone. Syst.* 11, 67–73.

Stroth, U., Blume, A., Mielke, K., and Unger T. (2000). Angiotensin AT(2) receptor stimulates ERK1 and ERK2 in quiescent but inhibits ERK in NGF-stimulated PC12W cells. *Brain Res. Mol. Brain Res.* 78, 175–180.

Stroth, U., Meffert, S., Gallinat, S., and Unger, T. (1998). Angiotensin II and NGF differentially influence microtubule proteins in PC12W cells: role of the AT2 receptor. *Brain Res. Mol. Brain Res.* 53, 187–195.

Theus, M., Wei, L., Francis, K., and Ping Yu, S. (2006). Critical roles of Src family tyrosine kinases in excitatory neuronal differentiation of cultured embryonic stem cells. *Exp. Cell Res.* 312, 3096–3107.

Thorup, C., Kornfeld, M., Winaver, J. M., Goligorsky, M. S., and Moore, L. C. (1998). Angiotensin-II stimulates nitric oxide release in isolated perfused renal resistance arteries. *Pflugers Arch.* 435, 432–434.

Tsukuda, K., Mogi, M., Iwanami, J., Min, L. J., Sakata, A., Jing, F., et al. (2009). Cognitive deficit in amyloid-beta-injected mice was improved by pretreatment with a low dose of telmisartan partly because of peroxisome proliferator-activated receptor-gamma activation. *Hypertension* 54, 782–787.

Tsutsumi, K., and Saavedra, J. M. (1991). Characterization and development of angiotensin II receptor subtypes (AT1 and AT2) in rat brain. *Am. J. Physiol.* 261, R209–R216.

Tsuzuki, S., Eguchi, S., and Inagami, T. (1996a). Inhibition of cell proliferation and activation of protein tyrosine phosphatase mediated by angiotensin II type 2 (AT2) receptor in R3T3 cells. *Biochem. Biophys. Res. Commun.* 228, 825–830.

Tsuzuki, S., Matoba, T., Eguchi, S., and Inagami, T. (1996b). Angiotensin II type 2 receptor inhibits cell proliferation and activates tyrosine phosphatase. *Hypertension* 28, 916–918.

Verdonk, K., Danser, A. H., and van Esch, J. H. (2012). Angiotensin II type 2 receptor agonists: where should they be applied? *Expert Opin. Investig. Drugs* 21, 501–513.

Vetter, M. L., and Bishop, J. M. (1995). Beta PDGF receptor mutants defective for mitogenesis promote neurite outgrowth in PC12 cells. *Curr. Biol.* 5, 168–178.

Volpe, M., Musumeci, B., De Paolis, P., Savoia, C., and Morganti, A. (2003). Angiotensin II AT2 receptor subtype: an uprising frontier in cardiovascular disease? *J. Hypertens.* 21, 1429–1443.

Wan, Y., Wallinder, C., Plouffe, B., Beaudry, H., Mahalingam, A. K., Wu, X., et al. (2004). Design, synthesis, and biological evaluation of the first selective nonpeptide AT2 receptor agonist. *J. Med. Chem.* 47, 5995–6008.

Wang, J. Z., Grundke-Iqbal, I., and Iqbal, K. (2007). Kinases and phosphatases and tau sites involved in Alzheimer neurofibrillary degeneration. *Eur. J. Neurosci.* 25, 59–68.

Washida, K., Ihara, M., Nishio, K., Fujita, Y., Maki, T., Yamada, M., et al. (2010). Nonhypotensive dose of telmisartan attenuates cognitive impairment partially due to peroxisome proliferator-activated receptor-gamma activation in mice with chronic cerebral hypoperfusion. *Stroke* 41, 1798–1806.

Widdop, R. E., Jones, E. S., Hannan, R. E., and Gaspari, T. A. (2003). Angiotensin AT2 receptors: cardiovascular hope or hype? *Br. J. Pharmacol.* 140, 809–924.

Wiemer, G., Scholkens, B. A., Wagner, A., Heitsch, H., and Linz, W. (1993). The possible role of angiotensin II subtype AT2 receptors in endothelial cells and isolated ischemic rat hearts. *J. Hypertens. Suppl.* 11, S234–S235.

Wright, J. W., and Harding, J. W. (2011). Brain renin-angiotensin–a new look at an old system. *Prog. Neurobiol.* 95, 49–67.

Wright, J. W., and Harding, J. W. (2012). The brain renin-angiotensin system: a diversity of functions and implications for CNS diseases. *Pflugers Arch.* doi: 10.1234/12345678 [Epub ahead of print].

Wruck, C. J., Funke-Kaiser, H., Pufe, T., Kusserow, H., Menk, M., Schefe, J. H., et al. (2005). Regulation of transport of the angiotensin AT2 receptor by a novel membrane-associated Golgi protein. *Arterioscler. Thromb. Vasc. Biol.* 25, 57–64.

Xiong, H., and Marshall, K. C. (1994). Angiotensin II depresses glutamate depolarizations and excitatory postsynaptic potentials in locus coeruleus through angiotensin II subtype 2 receptors. *Neuroscience* 62, 163–175.

Yamada, T., Horiuchi, M., and Dzau, V. J. (1996). Angiotensin II type 2 receptor mediates programmed cell death. *Proc. Natl. Acad. Sci. U.S.A.* 93, 156–160.

Yu, L., Zheng, M., Wang, W., Rozanski, G. J., Zucker, I. H., and Gao, L. (2010). Developmental changes in AT1 and AT2 receptor-protein expression in rats. *J. Renin Angiotensin Aldosterone Syst.* 11, 214–221.

Yu, X. M., Askalan, R., Keil, G. J. II, and Salter, M. W. (1997). NMDA channel regulation by channel-associated protein tyrosine kinase Src. *Science* 275, 674–678.

Zhang, J., and Pratt, R. E. (1996). The AT2 receptor selectively associates with Gialpha2 and Gialpha3 in the rat fetus. *J. Biol. Chem.* 271, 15026–15033.

Zhao, Y., Biermann, T., Luther, C., Unger, T., Culman, J., and Gohlke, P. (2003). Contribution of bradykinin and nitric oxide to AT2 receptor-mediated differentiation in PC12 W cells. *J. Neurochem.* 85, 759–767.

Zhao, Y., Foryst-Ludwig, A., Bruemmer, D., Culman, J., Bader, M., Unger, T., et al. (2005). Angiotensin II induces peroxisome proliferator-activated receptor gamma in PC12W cells via angiotensin type 2 receptor activation. *J. Neurochem.* 94, 1395–1401.

Zlokovic, B. V. (2005). Neurovascular mechanisms of Alzheimer's neurodegeneration. *Trends Neurosci.* 28, 202–208.

6

# Brain neuropeptides in central ventilatory and cardiovascular regulation in trout

**_Jean-Claude Le Mével[1]*, Frédéric Lancien[1], Nagi Mimassi[1] and J. Michael Conlon[2]_**

[1] *INSERM UMR 1101, Laboratoire de Traitement de l'Information Médicale, Laboratoire de Neurophysiologie, SFR ScInBioS, Faculté de Médecine et des Sciences de la Santé, Université Européenne de Bretagne, Université de Brest, CHU de Brest, Brest, France*

[2] *Department of Biochemistry, Faculty of Medicine and Health Sciences, United Arab Emirates University, Al Ain, United Arab Emirates*

**_Edited by:_**
*Hubert Vaudry, University of Rouen, France*

**_Reviewed by:_**
*Tobias Wang, University of Aarhus, Denmark*
*Pei-San Tsai, University of Colorado, USA*

**_*Correspondence:_**
*Jean-Claude Le Mével, INSERM UMR 1101, Laboratoire de Traitement de l'Information Médicale, Laboratoire de Neurophysiologie, SFR ScInBioS, Faculté de Médecine et des Sciences de la Santé, Université Européenne de Bretagne, Université de Brest, CHU de Brest, 22 avenue Camille Desmoulins, CS 93837, 29238 Brest Cedex 3, France.*
*e-mail: jean-claude.lemevel@univ-brest.fr*

Many neuropeptides and their G-protein coupled receptors (GPCRs) are present within the brain area involved in ventilatory and cardiovascular regulation but only a few mammalian studies have focused on the integrative physiological actions of neuropeptides on these vital cardio-respiratory regulations. Because both the central neuroanatomical substrates that govern motor ventilatory and cardiovascular output and the primary sequence of regulatory peptides and their receptors have been mostly conserved through evolution, we have developed a trout model to study the central action of native neuropeptides on cardio-ventilatory regulation. In the present review, we summarize the most recent results obtained using this non-mammalian model with a focus on PACAP, VIP, tachykinins, CRF, urotensin-1, CGRP, angiotensin-related peptides, urotensin-II, NPY, and PYY. We propose hypotheses regarding the physiological relevance of the results obtained.

**Keywords: neuropeptides, brain, ventilatory variables, heart rate, blood pressure, evolution, fish**

## INTRODUCTION

In addition to classical neurotransmitters, numerous brain neuropeptides and their G-protein coupled receptors (GPCRs) have been identified in several cardiovascular and ventilatory nuclei (Fuxe et al., 1986). Considerable data have accumulated in the literature concerning the central cardiovascular actions of these neuropeptides in mammals but much less is known about the roles of central neuropeptides on ventilatory regulation (Niewoehner et al., 1983; Doi and Ramirez, 2008; Pilowsky et al., 2009). Since the central ventilatory system and the cardiovascular system share some nuclei and mutually interact (Niewoehner et al., 1983; Taylor et al., 1999, 2009; Mandel and Schreihofer, 2006; Dampney et al., 2008), it is crucial to determine the integrative role of neuropeptides on these two vital regulatory mechanisms. Fish are aquatic vertebrates that use their gills to breathe, and mammals are vertebrates that breathe using their lungs. Nevertheless, there are important similarities between fish and mammals in the neuroanatomical networks and nervous mechanisms that control the ventilatory and cardiovascular systems (Taylor et al., 1999, 2010a,b; Bolis et al., 2001). In addition, neuropeptides appeared very early during evolution and the primary structures of these peptides and their receptors have been generally well conserved from fish to mammals (Holmgren and Jensen, 2001). Furthermore, in fish as in mammals, the neuropeptidergic systems are frequently present within brain areas involved in cardiovascular and ventilatory functions, including the hypothalamus and the brainstem autonomic nuclei (Batten et al., 1990; Dampney et al., 2005). Consequently, we have developed a trout model to gain insight into the effects of exogenously administered synthetic replicates of endogenous neuropeptides on ventilatory and cardiovascular functions in trout.

In this review, we summarize the neuroanatomical and functional pathways involved in cardio-respiratory control in fish. We describe the trout model and report methods to study the ventilatory and cardiovascular responses to centrally administered neuropeptides. We briefly summarize the available information regarding the primary structures of the fish neuropeptides and the similarities with their mammalian counterparts, the neuroanatomical location of the neuropeptides and their receptors in the fish brains. The neuropeptides investigated in this programme are those whose primary structures are known in the trout and whose neuroananatomical distribution is well characterized. We describe the ventilatory and cardiovascular actions of these neuropeptides following their intracerebroventricular (ICV) injection and we briefly contrast these central effects with their actions following intra-arterial (IA) injection. Finally, we propose hypotheses relating to the potential mechanisms of actions and physiological significance of central neuropeptides in the brain of the trout.

**Abbreviations:** BRS, baroreflex sensitivity; CNS, central nervous system; CPG, central pattern generator; DVN, dorsal motor nucleus of the vagus; HR, heart rate; HRV, heart rate variability; IA, intra-arterial; ICV, intracerebroventricular; NPO, preoptic nucleus; $P_{DA}$, dorsal aortic blood pressure; VF, ventilation frequency; VA, ventilation amplitude; VTOT, total ventilation.

## NEURAL PATHWAYS REGULATING CARDIO-RESPIRATORY FUNCTIONS IN FISH

The central control of cardiorespiratory functions in fish has been previously described (Taylor et al., 1999). In fish, the visceral sensory area in the medulla oblongata to which the chemoreceptor and baroreceptor afferent fibers project is homologous to the nucleus tractus solitarius (NTS) of higher vertebrates (Nieuwenhuys and Powels, 1983; Sundin et al., 2003a). The NTS is the site where the first synapse on the chemo- and baroreflexes takes place. Rhythmic ventilatory movements in fish are generated by a diffuse central pattern generator (CPG) whose activity is modulated by inputs from the peripheral chemoreceptors and also from higher brain centers, including the mesencephalon and the forebrain (Taylor et al., 1999). The CPG controls the activity of trigeminal Vth, facial VIIth, glossopharyngeal IXth, and vagal Xth motor nuclei all of which drive the breathing muscles (Taylor et al., 1999). There is a close association between the neural mechanisms controlling the ventilatory and the cardiovascular systems at the level of the medulla oblongata (Taylor et al., 1999). Furthermore, anatomical and functional links between the hypothalamus and the medullary cardio-respiratory centers in teleosts have been described (Ariëns-Kappers et al., 1936; Hornby and Demski, 1988). Electrical stimulation of hypothalamic sites in the goldfish *Carassius auratus* induces concomitant changes in ventilatory variables and heart rate (HR) (Hornby and Demski, 1988). Within the brainstem, the cardiac vagal pre-ganglionic neurons are located within the dorsal motor nucleus of the vagus (DVN). Some cardiac vagal pre-ganglionic neurons are also present in a more lateral position, probably constituting a primitive nucleus ambiguus. However, little is known regarding the neurotransmitters and/or neuropeptides and their receptors that permit integration of the various inputs at the level of the brainstem to control the final output motor impulses that ultimately govern the ventilatory and cardiovascular variables (Gilmour and Perry, 2007). In the brainstem of the dogfish *Squalus acanthias*, catecholamines regulate the electrical activity of respiratory neurons (Randall and Taylor, 1991). In the channel catfish, *Ictalurus punctatus*, glutamatergic pathways within the caudal part of the NTS are essential for the control of ventilation and studies in the shorthorn sculpin *Myoxocephalus scorpius* reveal that *N*-methyl-D-aspartate (NMDA) receptors mediate ventilatory frequency (VF), while kainate receptors mediate ventilatory amplitude (VA) (Sundin et al., 2003b; Turesson and Sundin, 2003; Turesson et al., 2010). In addition, it was shown that α-amino-3-OH-5-methyl-4-isooxazole-propionic-acid (AMPA) receptors located within the NTS control the parasympathetic activity to the heart and that NMDA and non-NMDA receptors are involved in the hypoxia activated sympathetic hypertension (Turesson et al., 2010). The hearts of teleost fish receive both a cholinergic vagal innervation and an adrenergic sympathetic supply (Taylor et al., 1999). Although humoral catecholamines increase HR after binding to β-adrenoreceptors (Wood and Shelton, 1980), the functional role of the nervous sympathetic system in teleost cardiac control is not clearly recognized (Burnstock, 1969; Taylor et al., 1999). At rest, the teleost heart is under strong inhibitory control mediated by the vagus nerve acting on muscarinic cholinergic receptors on the pacemaker cells (Laurent et al., 1983; Taylor, 1992; Taylor et al., 1999).

## THE TROUT MODEL

For the *in vivo* experiments, we use rainbow trout *Oncorhynchus mykiss* (body wt 240–270 g) of both sexes. The experiments were made on unanesthetized trout under controlled and constant levels of oxygen partial pressure in water (*P*wO2), pH and temperature, maintained at constant levels ($P$wO2 = 20 kPa; pH = 7.4 − 7.6; T = 10 − 11°C). Experimental protocols were approved by the Regional Ethics Committee in Animal Experiments of Brittany, France (registration number: 07).

An overview of trout equipped with arterial and buccal catheters, electrocardiographic (ECG) leads, and the ICV guide is presented **Figure 1**. Examples of the recorded signals are also plotted on the figure. The ventilatory and cardiovascular signals are processed off-line with custom-made programs written in LabView 6.1 (Laboratory Virtual Instrument Engineering Workbench, National Instruments).

### THE VENTILATORY SIGNAL (FIGURE 1A)

A flared cannula is inserted into a hole drilled between the nares such that its flared end is resting against the roof of the mouth. This cannula is used to record any changes in buccal ventilatory pressure (Holeton and Randall, 1967). Segments free of any movement artifacts on the ventilatory signal are selected and the VF and VA are determined. VF is calculated from the first harmonic of the power spectrum of the ventilatory signal using the fast Fourier transform (FFT) algorithm. VA is calculated from the difference between the maximal abduction phase and the maximal adduction phase for each of the ventilatory movements. The net effect of the changes in VF and VA on ventilation is determined according to the formula VTOT = VF × VA where VTOT is total ventilation. Thus, the overall ventilatory response is determined by the combined output of the VF and ventilatory stroke volume (by approximation VA).

### THE BLOOD PRESSURE SIGNAL (FIGURE 1B)

Catheterization of the dorsal aorta (Soivio et al., 1972) permits the recording of the dorsal aortic blood pressure ($P_{DA}$) and injection of various compounds, including the neuropeptides. Blood is collected via this catheter for routine hematocrit determination and for measurement of the concentration of hormones in plasma. The pulsatile $P_{DA}$ enables the measurement of systolic blood pressure (SBP) and diastolic blood pressure (DBP). Mean $P_{DA}$ is calculated as the arithmetic mean between the SBP and the DBP. The detection of the SBP along the recordings together with the R-R tachogram permits the determination of the cardiac baroreflex response. The baroreflex has been evolutionary conserved from Agnatha (lamprey) to humans (Bagshaw, 1985). The baroreflex in fish, as in humans, is working spontaneously under baseline conditions and also responds to adverse blood pressure changes (Lancien and Le Mével, 2007; Karemaker and Wesseling, 2008). In fish, the baroreflex response is probably used as a mechanism to protect the delicate vasculature of the fish gill against high blood pressure (Sundin and Nilsson, 2002). We evaluate the cardiac baroreflex sensitivity (BRS) using both a time domain

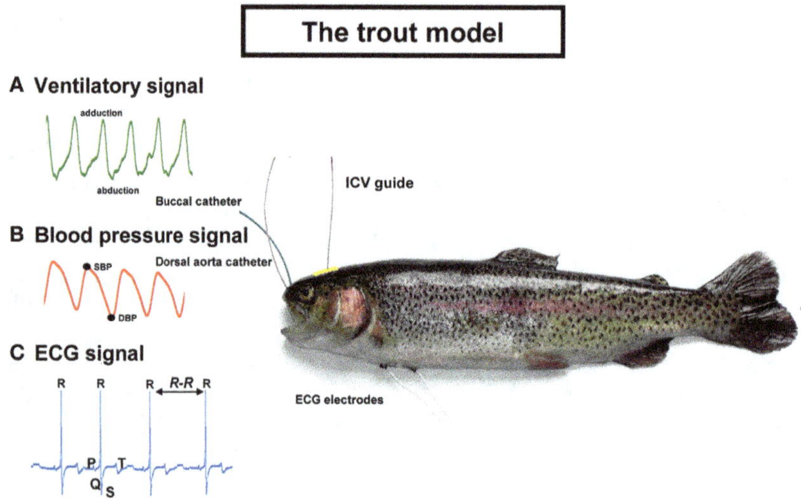


**FIGURE 1 | The trout model used for testing the intracerebroventricular and intra-arterial effects of neuropeptides on (A) ventilatory signal; (B) blood pressure signal; and (C) ECG signal.** SBP, systolic blood pressure; DBP, diastolic blood pressure; ECG, electrocardiographic; ICV, intracerebroventricular. See text for explanations.

method, the sequence method (Bertinieri et al., 1988; Lancien and Le Mével, 2007) and a frequency domain method, the cross spectral analysis technique (Parati et al., 2000; Lancien et al., 2011). In teleost fish (Lancien and Le Mével, 2007; Sandblom and Axelsson, 2011), as in mammals (Bertinieri et al., 1988), the parasympathetic nervous system plays a crucial role in the short term cardiac baroreflex response.

### THE ELECTROCARDIOGRAPHIC (ECG) SIGNAL (FIGURE 1C)

Two ECG AgCl electrodes are subcutaneously implanted ventrally and longitudinally at the level of the pectoral fins. After amplification, the ECG signal, which is very similar to the human ECG, displays its different waves (P, Q, R, S, T) (Satchell, 1991). The QRS complex is the largest deflection and the R waves are routinely measured to determine HR. The R-R interval of the ECG can be used to plot the tachogram and to quantify the heart rate variability (HRV) using either the FFT algorithm (for review see Task Force of the European Society of Cardiology, and the North American Society of Pacing and Electrophysiology, 1996) or the Poincaré plot (Brennan et al., 2001). HRV reflects modulation on a beat to beat basis of the cardiac sinus node activity by both limbs of the autonomic nervous system. The high frequency component of the HRV in humans reflects respiratory sinus arrhythmia and provides information primarily on the degree of vagal tone on the heart (Médigue et al., 2001). Interestingly, studies of HRV in teleost fish demonstrate that the parasympathetic nervous system is the main, or even the only, contributor to HRV (Altimiras et al., 1995; Le Mével et al., 2002; Grossman and Taylor, 2007). Nevertheless, the physiological significance of HRV in teleost fishes is poorly understood.

### THE ICV GUIDE

Fish do not possess large and expanded cerebral hemispheres with a developed neocortex (Nieuwenhuys et al., 1998). Consequently, these animals offer the opportunity to insert directly, under stereomicroscopic guidance, a 25-gauge needle fitted with a PE-10 polyethylene catheter between the two habenular ganglia toward the third ventricle until its tip lies between the two preoptic nuclei (NPO) (Le Mével et al., 2009a). The method is rapid and accurate since no stereotaxic placement is needed. In addition, no post-injection confirmation of the injected site is required. The rationale for this ICV implantation between the two NPO is that neuropeptides, directly or after diffusion through the cerebrospinal fluid, can access sites which are known to be critical to ventilatory and cardiovascular control. In teleost fish, as in mammals, these are the hypothalamus and the brainstem (Hornby and Demski, 1988; Taylor et al., 1999; Dampney et al., 2008).

## EFFECTS OF INTRACEREBROVENTRICULAR INJECTIONS OF NEUROPEPTIDES

### PITUITARY ADENYLATE CYCLASE-ACTIVATING POLYPEPTIDE (PACAP) AND VASOACTIVE INTESTINAL PEPTIDE (VIP)

PACAP and VIP belong to the secretin-glucagon superfamily of peptides (Sherwood et al., 2000). PACAP is found in two forms, a 38 amino-acid peptide (PACAP-38) and the C-terminally truncated 27 amino-acid peptide (PACAP-27). PACAP and VIP share sequence similarity and, in mammals, these peptides exert their actions by binding to three receptors, PAC1, VPAC1, and VPAC2 (Laburthe et al., 2007). Within the brains of mammals, PACAP and VIP are known to control multiple physiological functions including some cardiovascular and ventilatory processes (Wilson and Cumming, 2008; Vaudry et al., 2009).

PACAP and VIP appeared very early during evolution and the primary structure of these peptides and their receptors have been remarkably well conserved from fish to mammals (Wong et al., 1998; Sherwood et al., 2000; Montpetit et al., 2003). Within the central nervous system (CNS) of teleosts, PACAP- and VIP-like immunoreactivities are localized mainly in neuronal perikarya of the diencephalon at the level of the NPO.

Their fibers project not only into the adenohypophysis (Matsuda et al., 1997; Montero et al., 1998; Wong et al., 1998) but also toward many extra hypothalamo-hypophysial areas such as the mesencephalon and the medulla oblongata (Montero et al., 1998). These observations suggest that PACAP and VIP act not only as hypophysiotropic hormones (Montero et al., 1998; Wong et al., 1998) but also as neurotransmitters, and/or neuromodulators. In the goldfish, peripheral PACAP reduces food intake (Matsuda et al., 2006). We also demonstrated that trout PACAP-27 and trout VIP act on the CNS to increase ventilation (Le Mével et al., 2009b) and to reduce the cardiac BRS (Lancien et al., 2011).

After ICV injection, PACAP (25–100 pmol) evokes a dose- and time-dependent elevation of VF and VA. Consequently, the net effect of the peptide is a hyperventilatory response involving a gradual and significant dose-dependent increase in VTOT. The threshold dose for an effect of PACAP on VF is 100 pmol, but a significant effect on VA and VTOT is seen at 50 pmol and this latter effect is observed 15 min after the injection of the peptide. The actions of PACAP on the ventilatory variables are long-lasting since values have not returned to baseline levels by the end of the post-injection period of 25 min. The most pronounced action of PACAP is evoking hyperventilation through an increase in VA rather than VF. For instance, after 50 and 100 pmol PACAP this maximal change in VA, expressed as a percentage of the pre-injection value, reaches about 100 and 200%, respectively, while the elevation of VF is only about 10 and 35% (Le Mével et al., 2009b).

Upon ICV injection, the effects of trout VIP on the ventilatory variables are quite different from those following ICV injection of PACAP. VIP does not produce a significant increase in VF and VA but nonetheless the resultant action of this peptide is a small, transient but significant elevation of VTOT at the highest dose tested. Moreover, statistical analysis of the results obtained following ICV injection indicates that the maximum increase in VF, VA, and VTOT after ICV injection of 100 pmol PACAP relative to the pre-injection values is about 2.5-fold higher than the maximum ventilatory effects of the same dose of VIP.

After ICV injection, only the highest dose of PACAP produces a weak, but significant, sustained increase in $P_{DA}$. However, there is no significant change in HR. ICV injections of VIP do not cause any change in either $P_{DA}$ or HR. The greater action of PACAP on ventilation and blood pressure compared with VIP suggests that PACAP may bind preferentially to PAC1 receptors rather than to VPAC receptors. The lack of HR response to elevation of blood pressure suggests that the cardiac BRS is depressed following central PACAP. Compared with vehicle, ICV injections of PACAP and VIP (25–100 pmol) dose-dependently reduce the cardiac BRS to the same extent with a threshold dose of 50 pmol for a significant effect (Lancien et al., 2011).

In contrast to their ICV effects, IA injections of PACAP and VIP at doses of 25–100 pmol produce no change in the ventilatory variables. Peripherally injected PACAP does not cause any significant change either in $P_{DA}$ or in HR, but bolus peripheral injection of VIP produces a robust dose-dependent and sustained hypertensive response without any change in HR.

## NEUROPEPTIDE GAMMA (NPγ), NEUROKININ A (NKA) AND SUBSTANCE P (SP)

The tachykinins are a family of biologically active peptides that are characterized structurally by the common carboxy-terminal pentapeptide sequence Phe-Xaa-Gly-Leu-Met-$NH_2$. This C-terminally amidated sequence is of primary importance for the interaction with the tachykinin receptors (Conlon, 2004). In mammals, SP, NKA, NPγ, and neuropeptide K (NPK) are encoded by the single copy preprotachykinin A gene. Neurokinin B is derived from the preprotachykinin B gene while the preprotachykinin C gene encodes three peptides (hemokinin 1, endokinin C, and endokinin D) with limited structural similarity with SP (for references, see Conlon, 2004). The tachykinins exert their actions by binding to GPCRs that are widely distributed within vascular, endocrine and nervous tissues. SP is the preferential agonist of the NK-1 receptor, NKA along with NPγ and NPK are regarded as endogenous ligands of the NK-2 receptor, and NKB is the preferred agonist of the NK-3 receptor (Patacchini and Maggi, 2004). In mammals, there is strong evidence for the importance of CNS tachykinins in the control of respiration (Gray et al., 1999). In addition, central tachykinins are involved in cardiovascular regulation, neuroendocrine secretion, pain transmission, and in certain behavioral responses (Satake and Kawada, 2006).

Orthologs of the mammalian tachykinins have been isolated and structurally characterized in a wide range of tetrapod and non-tetrapod species (for references, see Conlon, 2004). In particular, SP (Jensen and Conlon, 1992), NKA (Jensen and Conlon, 1992), and NPγ (Jensen et al., 1993) have been purified from tissues of the rainbow trout *O. mykiss.* Neuroanatomical studies have revealed the presence of tachykinin-like immunoreactivity in neuronal cell bodies and fibers throughout the brains of several teleost fish, including the trout (Vecino et al., 1989; Batten et al., 1990; Holmqvist and Ekstrom, 1991; Moons et al., 1992) together with high density of tachykinin binding sites from the hypothalamus to the medulla oblongata (Moons et al., 1992). We recently demonstrated that, after ICV injection, exogenously administered trout tachykinins are differentially implicated in the neuroregulatory control of ventilation in trout (Le Mével et al., 2007).

Compared with ICV injection of vehicle, NPγ (25–100 pmol) evokes a gradual elevation of VF but a progressive dose-dependent reduction of VA. Therefore, the net effect of the peptide is a hypoventilatory response involving a significant decrease in VTOT. The threshold dose for an effect of NPγ on VF, VA, and VTOT is 50 pmol and this is observed 15 min after the injection of the peptide (**Figure 2A**). Interestingly, in some trout, the ICV injection of 100 pmol NPγ was followed by a dramatic reduction in VA to near the noise level of the recording system for periods of 10–20 s, giving the appearance of an apneic response. All actions of NPγ on the ventilatory variables are of long duration, since parameters do not return to baseline values by the end of the recording period.

In contrast to the action of NPγ, the effects of SP(50–250 pmol) on ventilation are not dose dependent and only the highest dose of SP (250 pmol) produces a significant elevation of VF, a significant reduction of VA, and a resultant

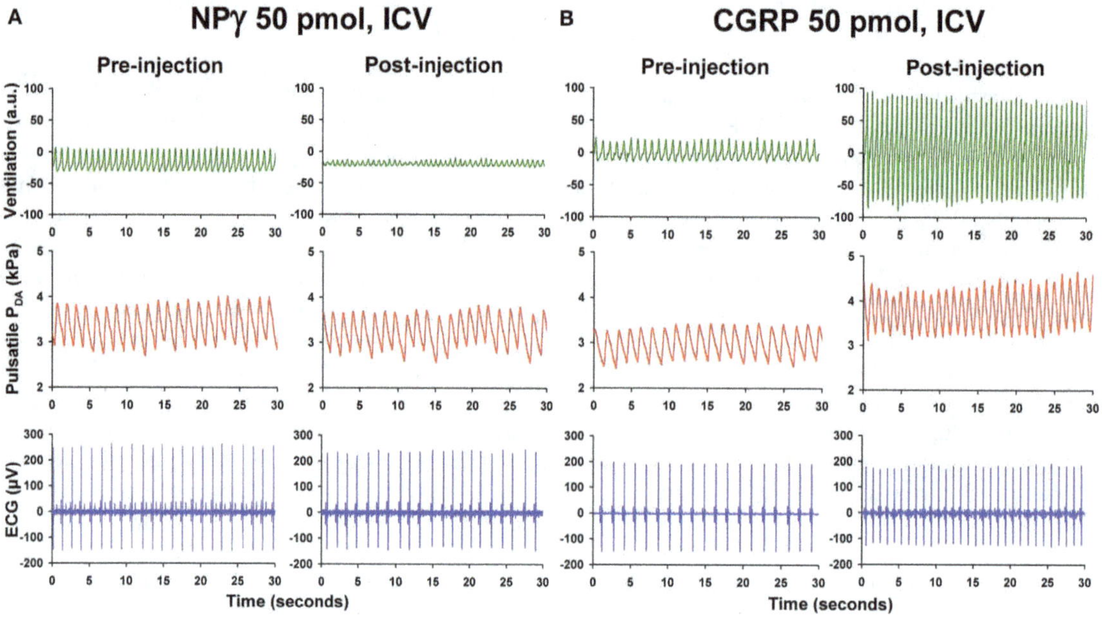


**FIGURE 2 | Recording traces of 30 s duration from two unanesthetized trout illustrating the changes observed in ventilatory movements (ventilation), pulsatile dorsal aortic blood pressure ($P_{DA}$), and electrocardiographic (ECG) signals between the pre-injection period (0–5 min) and the post-injection period (20–25 min) after intracerebroventricular (ICV) injection of (A) 50 pmol trout neuropeptide gamma (NPγ) or (B) 50 pmol trout calcitonin gene-related peptide (CGRP).** Note that ICV injection of NPγ produces an impressive reduction in the ventilatory amplitude but a slight increase in the ventilatory frequency. In contrast, ICV CGRP evokes a potent increase of the ventilation rate and amplitude. Only the ICV injection of CGRP causes a substantial elevation of blood pressure and heart rate.

significant decrease of VTOT. The changes in these parameters reach significance 10–15 min after ICV injection.

As with SP, the effect of NKA (50–250 pmol) on the ventilatory variables are relatively minor, with only the highest dose (250 pmol) producing a significant decrease in VA and an overall significant fall in VTOT. This action of NKA is of short duration with VA returning rapidly to baseline values.

None of the three tachykinin peptides produce significant changes in mean $P_{DA}$ or HR following ICV injection. Further studies are required to determine whether the central action of NPγ on ventilatory variables in trout involves interaction with a receptor that resembles the mammalian NK-2 receptor more closely than the NK1-receptor.

Because centrally controlled cardiorespiratory coupling contributes to HRV in teleost fish (Grossman and Taylor, 2007), we made the assumption that changes in the VF after central injection of NPγ and SP, but not NKA, also produce changes in HRV (Lancien et al., 2009). Compared to vehicle-injected trout, Poincaré plot analysis of HRV demonstrates that ICV injection of NPγ dose-dependently increases HRV. SP evokes a significant elevation of HRV but only at the highest dose (250 pmol). In contrast, NKA is without any effect on HRV. The physiological significance of HRV in teleost fish is poorly understood. Recent studies favor the hypothesis that HRV may be an important component of the mechanisms optimizing the efficiency of respiratory gas exchange over the counter-current at the gill lamellae (Grossman and Taylor, 2007). Taken together, our data are consistent with a possible selective central action of NPγ on neuronal networks implicated in the control of cardiorespiratory coupling in teleost fish.

IA injections of NPγ, SP or NKA at doses of 50–250 pmol produce no change in any of the ventilatory variables. However, all three tachykinins at their highest dose of 250 pmol cause a significant increase in mean $P_{DA}$ and, except for NPγ, a concomitant and significant fall in HR.

### CORTICOTROPIN-RELEASING FACTOR (CRF) AND UROTENSIN-I (U-I)

CRF, a 41-amino acid peptide originally isolated from ovine hypothalamus (Vale et al., 1981), plays a key role in regulating the release of adrenocorticotropic hormone from the pituitary during stress. In mammals, CRF and the CRF-related peptide urocortin 1, an ortholog of the fish U-I (Vaughan et al., 1995; Barsyte et al., 1999), are also known to play a crucial neurotropic role in the CNS in coordinating the autonomic and behavioral responses to stressful situations (Koob and Heinrichs, 1999). In mammals, the actions of the CRF-family peptides are mediated by two types of G-protein-coupled receptors: CRF type 1 receptor (CRF-R1) and CRF type 2 receptor (CRF-R2) (Bale and Vale, 2004). CRF, urocortin-1, and the non-mammalian CRF-related peptides U-I, and sauvagine (SVG) bind with similar affinity to CRF-R1 while CRF has only a low affinity for CRF-R2. U-I, SVG, and the urocortins bind with high affinity to CRF-R2. In mammals including humans, CRF immunoreactivity (Swanson et al., 1983) and CRF receptors (Bale and Vale, 2004) are widely distributed in brain areas involved in the control of cardiovascular regulation and breathing movements. After ICV administration,

CRF and urocortin 1 induce marked changes in cardiovascular variables (Parkes et al., 2001) and CRF acts centrally to produce a strong stimulatory effect on ventilatory movements (Bennet et al., 1990).

The CRF family of peptides and their receptors are of ancient origin (Chang and Hsu, 2004). In teleost fish, CRF, U-I, CRF receptors, and CRF binding protein are present not only in neurons of the preoptic region and hypothalamus (Olivereau and Olivereau, 1990) but also in extra-hypothalamic brain regions including the telencephalon and the posterior brain (Batten et al., 1990; Bernier et al., 1999a; Lovejoy and Balment, 1999; Alderman et al., 2008). Taken together, these neuroanatomical findings raise the possibility that CRF and U-I in teleosts also exert extra-hypothalamo-hypophyseal actions and mediate some autonomic and/or behavioral effects within the brain. In fact, physiological data have indicated that, after ICV injection, CRF and U-I are implicated in the autonomic regulation of the cardiovascular system (for review see Le Mével et al., 2006), the control of locomotor activity (Clements et al., 2002) and in the regulation of food intake (for review see Bernier, 2006). Our results demonstrate that CRF and U-I also produce a potent hyperventilatory response when injected centrally in trout (Le Mével et al., 2009a).

After ICV injection, trout CRF (1–10 pmol) evokes both gradual and dose-dependent elevations of VF and VA. The net effect of the peptide is, therefore, a hyperventilatory response involving a significant dose-dependent elevation in VTOT. The minimum dose to elicit a statistically significant response in both ventilatory variables is 5 pmol and this is observed 15 min after the injection of the peptide. In contrast to the sustained action of ICV injection of CRF on VF and VA, a significant stimulatory action of trout U-I (1–10 pmol) on these two variables appears only after ICV injection of the highest dose of peptide tested. VTOT also indicates that the significant hyperventilatory action of U-I is delayed by 10 min (U-I, 5 pmol) and 5 min (U-I, 10 pmol) compared to corresponding doses of CRF. Moreover, the maximum increase in VTOT after ICV injection of CRF relative to the pre-injection value is 2-fold higher than the hyperventilatory effect of U-I during the 25–30 min post-injection period.

At the dose of 5 pmol, only CRF transiently increases $P_{DA}$, but a clear sustained hypertension is observed for the highest dose of 10 pmol of CRF and U-I. ICV injection of either CRF or U-I has no significant effect on HR for all doses tested.

ICV administration of alpha helical $CRF_{9-41}$ ($ahCRF_{9-41}$) alone (50 pmol) does not affect the baseline ventilatory and cardiovascular variables. However, pre-treatment of the trout with this CRF antagonist at a dose ratio of $ahCRF_{9-41}$: CRF of 10:1 delays and significantly reduces (by at least 3-fold) the CRF-induced increase in VF, VA, and VTOT and inhibits CRF-induced elevation in $P_{DA}$. In fish, the pharmacological characteristics of the CRF receptors are quite different from their mammalian counterparts (see above). In catfish, where a third CRF receptor (CRF-R3) has been identified (Arai et al., 2001), CRF-R1 binds CRF, U-I, and SVG with similar affinity, while CRF-R2 preferentially binds SVG. CRF-R3 binds CRF with a 5-fold higher affinity than U-I and SVG (Arai et al., 2001). Pohl et al. (2001) concluded that, in Chum salmon, neither CRF-R1 nor CRF-R2 could discriminate between CRF and U-I. The lack of an intrinsic effect of $ahCRF_{9-41}$ when injected centrally suggests that endogenous CRF and U-I are not involved in the regulation of VA and VF in baseline situations. The fact that this antagonist significantly reduces the central hyperventilatory effects of exogenous CRF is indicative of a selective receptor-mediated hyperventilatory action of CRF in the brain of the trout. However, the type of CRF receptor involved cannot be determined at this time.

After IA injection, CRF and U-I are devoid of any ventilatory or cardiovascular activities except a transient increase in blood pressure at the highest dose of U-I (50 pmol).

### CALCITONIN GENE-RELATED PEPTIDE (CGRP)

The 37-amino- acid peptide CGRP is derived from the tissue-specific splicing of the primary transcript of the calcitonin gene (Amara et al., 1982). CGRP is thus a member of the calcitonin/CGRP peptide family that includes adrenomedullin (AM), adrenomedullin-2 (or intermedin), amylin, and calcitonin receptor-stimulating peptide (Ogoshi et al., 2006; Sawada et al., 2006). CGRP binds to a seven transmembrane G-protein-coupled calcitonin receptor-like receptor that is complexed with one of three receptor activity-modifying proteins (Tam and Brain, 2006). In mammals, CGRP and its receptors are widely distributed throughout the peripheral and central CNS. In the CNS, CGRP acts as a neurotransmitter and/or neuromodulator involved in multiple physiological and behavioral processes including the hypothalamic regulation of feeding (Krahn et al., 1984). In addition, CGRP regulates the local vasodilation of cerebral vessels contributing to the pathophysiology of migraine headache and the peptide modulates pain responses at the level of the spinal cord (Tam and Brain, 2006). Central CGRP also plays a role in the autonomic regulation of the cardiovascular system. In contrast to its hypotensive effect in the periphery, ICV injection of CGRP produces a hypertensive response by activating the sympathetic nerves in rats (Fisher et al., 1983) and CGRP augments the baroreflex controls of renal sympathetic nerve activity and HR in the unanesthetized rabbit (Matsumura et al., 1999).

CGRP has an ancient evolutionary history. In fish, cDNAs encoding for CGRP have been isolated from a number of species (Jansz and Zandberg, 1992; Clark et al., 2002; Ogoshi et al., 2006; Martinez-Alvarez et al., 2008) and CGRP mRNA is expressed in peripheral and central tissues (Clark et al., 2002; Martinez-Alvarez et al., 2008). Moreover, the primary sequence of the peptide has been highly conserved from fish to humans (Shahbazi et al., 1998). As in many cerebral regions, the hypothalamus expresses CGRP mRNA (Martinez-Alvarez et al., 2008) and some CGRP-like immunoreactive fibers represent ascending projections from brainstem areas involved in autonomic functions (Batten and Cambre, 1989; Batten et al., 1990). Interestingly, in the goldfish *Carassius auratus* and in the puffer fish *Fugu rubripes* (Clark et al., 2002) the strongest expression of calcitonin/CGRP transcripts was observed in the posterior brain at the level of autonomic nuclei and spinal cord. In addition, CGRP receptors are present within the brain and heart of the flounder *Paralichthys olivaceus* (Suzuki and Kurokawa, 2000). Collectively these neuroanatomical data support a role for CGRP not only in neuroendocrine function and behavior but also in autonomic and cardiovascular regulation in fish. The anorexigenic action of centrally administered CGRP in the goldfish *Carassius auratus* has been previously described (Martinez-Alvarez et al., 2009). The cardio-ventilatory actions of centrally administered trout CGRP in trout has been recently described (Le Mével et al., 2012).

ICV administration of CGRP (1–50 pmol) evokes a dose- and time-dependent elevation of VF and VA. As a result, the net effect of the peptide is a hyperventilatory response involving a gradual and significant dose-dependent increase in VTOT. The threshold dose for an effect of CGRP on VF is 50 pmol but only 5 pmol for VA (**Figure 2B**). As for many neuropeptides, the actions of CGRP on these ventilatory variables are long-lasting since values had not returned to baseline levels by the end of the post-injection period of 25 min. This observation suggests that CGRP may act as a long-term hyperventilatory peptide *in vivo*. The most pronounced action of CGRP is evoking hyperventilation through an increase in VA instead of VF. For instance at a dose of 50 pmol, during the 15–20 min post-injection period when VTOT is maximal and increased by 300% from baseline value, the change in VA, expressed as a percentage of pre-injection value, is more than 200% while the elevation of VF is only about 30%.

After ICV injection, CGRP produces a significant dose-dependent and sustained increase in $P_{DA}$ but the increase in HR does not reach the level of statistical significance. The receptor(s) mediating the ventilatory and cardiovascular action of CGRP in trout have not been determined. In eel, the paralogs AM2 and AM5 exhibit different central cardiovascular responses suggesting that they may act through different receptors (Ogoshi et al., 2008).

In contrast to its ICV effects, IA injections of CGRP at doses of 5–50 pmol produce no change in VF, VA, or VTOT. Nonetheless, peripherally injected CGRP causes an overall robust, dose-dependent and sustained hypertensive response without any change in HR. IA injection of the highest dose of CGRP causes at first a rapid but transient decrease in $P_{DA}$ followed by a hypertensive phase that does not return to the pre-injection level until 60 min.

#### ANGIOTENSIN PEPTIDES

Data from mammalian studies have demonstrated that angiotensin II (Ang II) and angiotensin III (Ang III) are the two main effector peptides of the brain renin-angiotensin system (RAS). However, angiotensin IV (Ang IV) and to a lesser extend angiotensin 1–7 (Ang 1–7) are also implicated in various physiological functions, particularly body fluid homeostasis and cardiovascular regulation (Paul et al., 2006; Fyhrquist and Saijonmaa, 2008). Ang II and Ang III bind to angiotensin receptor type 1 (AT1) and type 2 (AT2). Ang IV binds exclusively to angiotensin receptor type 4 (AT4). The type of receptor that mediates the actions of Ang 1–7 is somewhat controversial. Studies on the effects of the RAS on ventilation are limited and only the action of Ang II has been explored in mammals. In both anaesthetized and unanaesthetized dogs (Potter and McCloskey, 1979; Ohtake and Jennings, 1993) and in unanaesthetized rabbits (Potter and McCloskey, 1979) but not in unanaesthetized Sprague-Dawley rats (Walker and Jennings, 1996), Ang II stimulates ventilation through a central mechanism that is independent of baroreceptor or chemoreceptor stimulation (Potter and McCloskey, 1979). In spontaneous hypertensive rats (SHR), but not in normotensive control Wistar-Kyoto rats, intravenous injection of the Ang II receptor antagonist, saralasin, has a depressant action upon ventilation (O'Connor and Jennings, 2001). Because SHR rats exhibit high brain RAS activity compared with normotensive control Wistar-Kyoto rats, the authors speculated that central Ang II is involved in the control of respiration only in SHR rats. However, in anaesthetized Sprague-Dawley rats, intracisternal ANG II provokes a decrease that becomes less when the doses of Ang II are increased (Aguirre et al., 1991) and ICV injection of saralasin reduces respiratory rate and respiratory rate variability in Wistar rats (Olsson et al., 2004). These data indicate that the brain RAS plays a role in the control of ventilation in mammalian species. In humans, Ang II may be implicated in the regulation of the respiratory sensitivity during pregnancy but the mechanism involved in this effect has not been elucidated (Wolfe et al., 1998).

The RAS has an ancient evolutionary history and most of its components are present in lampreys, elasmobranchs, and teleosts (Olson, 1992; Takei et al., 1993; Nishimura, 2001; Rankin et al., 2004; Wong and Takei, 2011). In contrast to the well known peripheral cardiovascular and osmoregulatory hormonal actions of Ang II (Olson, 1992; Le Mével et al., 1993; Bernier et al., 1999b; Takei and Balment, 2009), studies in fish on the central action of Ang II are sparse. Furthermore, two Ang II isoforms [$Asn^1$]- and [$Asp^1$]-Ang are present in plasma and tissues (Conlon et al., 1996; Wong and Takei, 2012) but the physiological roles of the latter form have only been recently explored (Lancien et al., 2012). Central administration of [$Asn^1$]-Ang II into the third or fourth ventricle of the eel *Anguilla japonica* induces drinking (Kozaka et al., 2003) and increases HR and blood pressure (Nobata et al., 2011). This procedure elevates HR and blood pressure but reduces both HRV and the cardiac BRS sensitivity in the trout (Le Mével et al., 1994, 2002, 2008b; Lancien et al., 2004b; Lancien and Le Mével, 2007) In addition, local injection of [$Asn^1$]-Ang II within the DVN of the trout potently enhances HR but only weakly increases blood pressure (Pamantung et al., 1997). Taken together, these results demonstrate that in the brains of teleosts, as in mammals, Ang II may act as a neuromodulator or a neurotransmitter involved in key osmoregulatory and cardiovascular regulations. Recently, the cardio-ventilatory actions of exogenously administered [$Asn^1$]-Ang II, [$Asp^1$]-Ang II, Ang III, Ang IV, and Ang 1–7 within the third ventricle of the trout brain have been described (Lancien et al., 2012). In addition, the angiotensin peptides produced in the brain and circulating in plasma of trout were characterized using a high performance liquid chromatography (HPLC) system that can separate these peptides (Lancien et al., 2012; Wong and Takei, 2012).

After ICV injection (5–50 pmol), [$Asn^1$]-Ang II and [$Asp^1$]-Ang II gradually elevate VTOT through a selective stimulatory action on VA. However, the hyperventilatory effect of [$Asn^1$]-Ang II is 3-fold higher than the effect of [$Asp^1$]-Ang II at the 50 pmol dose. Ang III, Ang IV, and Ang 1–7 (25–100 pmol) are without effect on the ventilatory variables. In addition, both Ang II peptides and Ang III dose-dependently increase $P_{DA}$ and HR. These results suggest that the N- and C-terminal amino acid residues of Ang II are important for full effect on the central receptor(s) that mediate(s) hyperventilation and cardiovascular actions. It was previously proposed that in trout, [Asn$^1$]-Ang II was the product of angiotensinogen cleavage in plasma but that this peptide is converted to [Asp$^1$]-Ang II by plasma asparaginase (Conlon et al., 1996). In eel plasma, asparaginase activity is low and the conversion seems to occur in the tissues such as liver and kidney with angiotensinogen, not Ang II, as substrate (Wong and Takei, 2012). In brain tissue, comparable amounts of [Asn$^1$]-Ang II and [Asp$^1$]-Ang II were detected (ca. 40 fmol/mg brain tissue) but Ang III was not present, and the amount of Ang IV was about 8-fold lower than the content of the Ang II peptides. In plasma, Ang II peptides were also the major angiotensins (ca. 110 fmol/ml plasma), while significant but lower amounts of Ang III and Ang IV were present. These results demonstrate that the two Ang II peptides are present in trout plasma and brain tissue and suggest that the conversion Asn$^1$ $\rightarrow$ Asp$^1$occurs not only in plasma but also in brain. It has been proposed that the teleost AT receptor is an AT1-like receptor (Russell et al., 2001). The demonstration that both Ang II peptides and Ang III elevate $P_{DA}$ and HR while the other angiotensins were without action supports the idea that an AT1-like receptor might also be involved in the central cardiovascular actions of Ang II and Ang III. A novel receptor that binds specifically or with a higher affinity to the Ang II peptides, but not the truncated forms, might mediate the ventilatory effect of the brain RAS in trout.

Within the brain of the trout, [Asn$^1$]-Ang II affects not only the mean HR but also the beat to beat change in R-R intervals of the ECG since ICV injection of the peptide reduces HRV (Le Mével et al., 2002) and the cardiac BRS (Lancien and Le Mével, 2007).

None of the angiotensin peptides injected peripherally alter any of the ventilatory variables but the two Ang II isoforms and to a lesser extent Ang III provoke a pressor response. The concomitant decrease in HR following the IA injections of these angiotensins is not significant. In addition, Ang IV and Ang 1–7 are without effect on the cardiovascular variables. Collectively, these results support the view that the N- and C-terminal residues of the Ang II peptides play a role in optimal interaction with the putative cardiovascular angiotensin receptor in trout vascular tissue (Nishimura, 2001).

## UROTENSIN II (U-II)

U-II is a cyclic neuropeptide that was originally isolated from the caudal neurosecretory system of the teleost fish *Gillichthys mirabilis* on the basis of its smooth muscle-stimulating activity (Pearson et al., 1980; Bern et al., 1985). U-II is widely expressed in peripheral and nervous structures of species from lampreys to mammals including humans (Vaudry et al., 2010). It has now been demonstrated that U-II belongs to a family of structurally related peptides that include U-II and the UII-related peptides (URPs), URP, URP-1, and URP-2. In the teleost lineage, four U-II/URP paralogs are present but only two of these ancestral genes, U-II and URP, are found in tetrapods (Quan et al., 2012). U-II, URP, and URP isoforms exhibit the same cyclic hexapeptide core sequence (Cys-Phe-Trp-Lys-Tyr-Cys) while the N- and C-terminal regions are highly variable (Lihrmann et al., 2006; Conlon, 2008). Studies on UII/URP/URP-2 gene expression in teleosts and tetrapods suggest that U-II, URP, and URP-2 exert different functions (Parmentier et al., 2011). In teleost fish URP, URP-1, and URP-2 mRNA occur both in brain and spinal cord (Parmentier et al., 2008; Nobata et al., 2011) but in the eel, *Anguilla japonica* the U-II gene is exclusively expressed in the urophysis (Nobata et al., 2011). In tetrapods, the U-II gene is expressed primarily in motoneurons of the brainstem and spinal cord (Vaudry et al., 2010). U-II has been identified as a specific natural ligand of the orphan, G-protein-coupled receptor GPR14 (now renamed the UT receptor) in mammals (Vaudry et al., 2010) and in teleost fish (Lu et al., 2006). U-II and URP both activate the UT receptor with the same potency. The cardiovascular effects of centrally administered U-II and URP in trout and eel have been analyzed. In trout and eel, only a relatively high dose of U-II (500 pmol) evokes an increase in $P_{DA}$ with variable action on HR (Le Mével et al., 1996; Nobata et al., 2011). In addition, the central vasopressor action of URP in the eel is equally efficacious but less potent than the action of U-II (Nobata et al., 2011). The brain structures controlling the ventilatory system in trout seem to be more sensitive to the central action of U-II as only a 50 pmol dose of the peptide produces an hyperventilatory response through a significant increase in VF and VA (Lancien et al., 2004a). At this dose, U-II produces a long-lasting increase in locomotor activity (Lancien et al., 2004a). The effects of central URP and URP isoforms on the ventilatory and cardiovascular systems in trout have not yet been determined.

IA injection of U-II and URP in trout and eel evokes an elevation in $P_{DA}$. In both species, the hypertensive effect of U-II is longer-lasting than that of URP (Le Mével et al., 2008a; Nobata et al., 2011). In trout, U-II only provokes a dose-dependent bradycardia (Le Mével et al., 1996, 2008a), while in the eel, U-II and URP significantly increase HR (Nobata et al., 2011). U-II is devoid of ventilatory actions following systemic injection in trout (unpublished observations).

## NEUROPEPTIDE TYROSINE (NPY) AND PEPTIDE TYROSINE TYROSINE (PYY)

NPY and PYY are two members of the pancreatic polypeptide family of regulatory peptides. These two 36-amino acid peptides contain a tyrosine residue at their N- and C-termini. NPY is the most abundant peptide within the CNS of mammals. The peptide and its GPCRs, designated $Y_1$, $Y_2$, $Y_4$, $Y_5$, and $Y_6$, are widely distributed in nerve terminals throughout the brain (Dumont and Quirion, 2006). NPY-like immunoreactivity has been demonstrated in many noradrenergic and adrenergic neurons of the medulla oblongata (Fuxe et al., 1986). NPY-containing cell bodies are found in the lateral hypothalamus and NPY innervation of the paraventricular nucleus (PVN) of the hypothalamus arises from the medulla oblongata (Dumont and Quirion, 2006). In mammals, including rat, mouse, sheep, pig, rabbit, and pigeon, NPY has many neuroendocrine regulatory effects within the brain including an orexigenic action and regulation of food intake, anxiety, circadian rhythms, and memory. The central actions of NPY on cardiorespiratory functions remain unclear due to the fact that activation of different NPY receptors have opposite effects on cardiorespiratory variables (Fuxe et al., 1983; Scott et al., 1989; Morton et al., 1999). NPY is also present in peripheral organs, notably in blood vessels and heart. PYY is primarily located in endocrine cells of the lower intestine. In mammals, these two peptides are also involved in peripheral vasoregulation (Zukowska-Grojec et al., 1987; Playford et al., 1992).

NPY and PYY are present in both peripheral and brain tissues in fish (Jensen and Conlon, 1992; Danger et al., 1991). Seven NPY receptors subtypes ($Y_1$, $Y_2$, $Y_4$–$Y_8$) bind both NPY and PYY in fish (Salaneck et al., 2008). ICV injection of NPY in goldfish increases feeding (Volkoff et al., 2009). In trout, ICV administration of trout NPY and PYY at doses up to 100 pmol does not have any effect on ventilatory and cardiovascular variables (unpublished data). These cardiovascular results are consistent with a previous study demonstrating that ICV injection of human NPY (0.6–0.8 nmol) in trout exerts only a weak hypertensive action without any change in HR (Le Mével et al., 1991). These results obtained in trout suggest that, contrary to the actions of the other peptides mentioned in this review, NPY and PYY do not appear to have an important role in the central cardiorespiratory regulation in trout. In contrast, cod NPY causes vasodilation in the cod celiac artery (Shahbazi et al., 2002). In the elasmobranchs, the unanesthetized *Scyliorinus canicula* (Conlon et al., 1991) and the anesthetized *Heterodontus portjacksoni* (Preston et al., 1998), IA or intravenous injection of relatively high doses of dogfish NPY or PYY significantly increase blood pressure. However in trout, IA injection of trout NPY and PYY at a 100 pmol dose is devoid of significant cardiovascular effects (unpublished data). These differences between the effects of NPY and PYY in elasmobranchs and teleosts can possibly be explained by the different experimental protocols used or that the location of NPY/PYY cardiovascular receptors in the cardiovascular systems of elasmobranchs differs from that in teleost fishes.

## POSSIBLE MECHANISMS OF ACTION AND PHYSIOLOGICAL SIGNIFICANCE

In order to produce changes in ventilatory and cardiovascular variables, ICV injections of neuropeptides must access receptors critical for the control of cardio-ventilatory motor neurons. However, the receptor site(s) initiating cellular transduction mechanisms cannot be deduced from the experiments in which the peptides are injected into the third cerebral ventricle. Nevertheless, neuroanatomical prerequisites and some neurophysiological data exist that might explain the ventilatory and cardiovascular responses to ICV neuropeptides. Since the neuropeptides are injected in close proximity to a major neuroendocrine hypothalamic nucleus, the NPO, it is reasonable to assume that these exogenous neuropeptides may mimic the action of the endogenous peptides after release from neurons belonging to this nucleus. These neuropeptides can then activate arginine vasotocin (AVT) and isotocin (IT) preoptic neurons. AVT and IT preoptic neurons project to the neurohypophysis where the two nonapeptides are released into the general circulation. AVT is well known to increase vascular tone and elevate blood pressure *in vivo* (Le Mével et al., 1996; Conklin et al., 1997). In addition to this neuroendocrine pathway, projection from the preoptic neurons could influence brainstem respiratory and cardiovascular neurons including the NTS and the DVN through the neurogenic route by the release of AVT, IT or other neuropeptides or classical neurotransmitters (Batten et al., 1990; Saito et al., 2004). In the goldfish, functional-anatomical studies have demonstrated the existence of a neural pathway from the preoptic area to the DNV controlling concomitantly ventilation and HR (Hornby and Demski, 1988). In mammals, stimulation of the

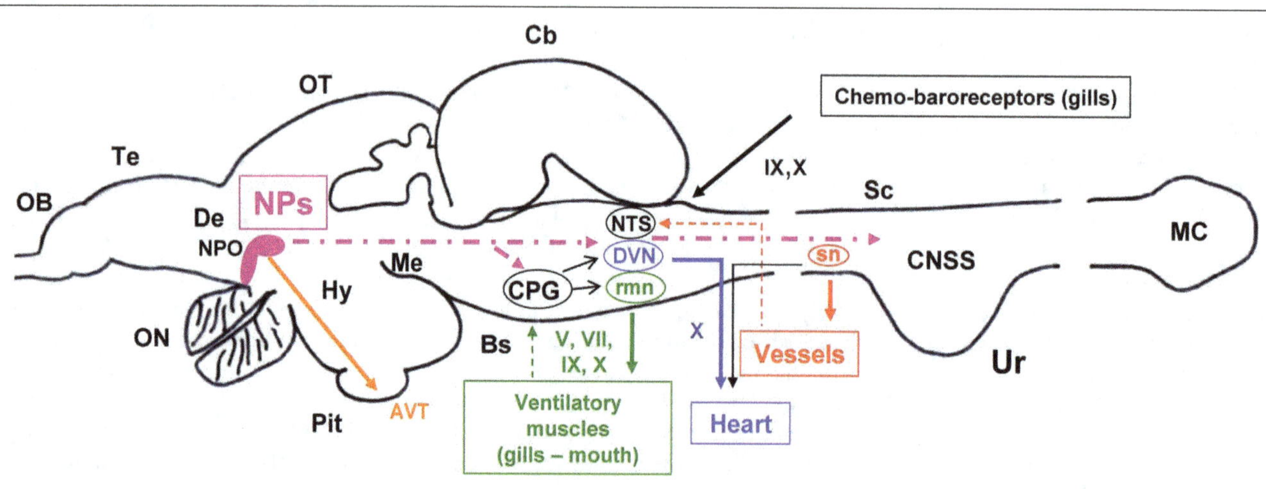


**FIGURE 3 | A model based on a parasagital view of the CNS of the trout depicting the potential central sites and pathways for the effects of intracerebroventricular administered neuropeptides (NPs) on central ventilatory and cardiovascular functions.** Target ventilatory and cardiovascular tissues are also shown. Projecting fibers from preoptic nucleus (NPO) neurons to brainstem ventilatory and cardiovascular nuclei and to spinal sympathetic neurons (sn) are shown with a bold hatched line. Motor outputs from ventilatory and cardiovascular central nuclei to peripheral effectors are shown in continuous line. Feedback information from peripheral tissues to CNS nuclei is shown using thin hatched lines. The sites and pathways described are highly schematic and speculative (see also text in section 2 and 5 for further explanations). Other abbreviations: AVT, arginine-vasotocin; Cb, cerebellum; CPG, central pattern generator; CNSS, caudal neurosecretory system; De, diencephalon; DVN, dorsal motor nucleus of the vagus; Hy, hypothalamus; MC, massa caudalis; Me, mesencephalon; NTS, nucleus tractus solitarius; OB, olfactory bulb; ON, optic nerve; OT, optic tectum; Pit, pituitary gland (hypophysis); rmn, respiratory motor nuclei; Te, telencephalon; Ur, urophysis; VC, valvula cerebelli. V, trigeminal; VII, facial; IX, glossopharyngeal; X, vagal cranial nerves.

PVN, a nucleus homologous to the teleostean NPO, can influence brainstem and spinal cord respiratory related mechanisms. Vasopressin and oxytocin parvocellular neurons of the PVN project to important respiratory-related regions of the medulla and spinal cord, including the pre-Bõtzinger complex and the phrenic motor nuclei (Mack et al., 2002). The PVN is also part of the central cardiovascular network that controls the rostral ventrolateral medulla (RVLM) (Nunn et al., 2011). Neurons of the RVLM send excitatory projections to the sympathetic preganglionic neurons in the intermediolateral cell column of the spinal cord to increase HR and blood pressure (Dampney et al., 2005; Pilowsky et al., 2009; Nunn et al., 2011). Although in fish the locations of sympathetic pre-vasomotor nuclei within the medulla are unknown, neuropeptides may also act at the medulla oblongata to influence sympathetic outflow to vascular tissue and chromaffin cells increasing blood pressure. In addition, we can speculate about a possible diffusion of the injected neuropeptides within the cerebrospinal fluid toward critical ventilatory and cardiovascular brainstem nuclei. Consistent with this, receptors for some of the aforementioned neuropeptides are also expressed within the hindbrain (Cobb and Brown, 1992; Moons et al., 1992; Lovejoy and Balment, 1999; Lu et al., 2006). However, the pharmacological characterization of these receptors using specific antagonists/agonists is difficult in fish due to the fact that only drugs designed for mammalian receptors are available. We have noted consistently that the effects exerted by the neuropeptides are usually long lasting, a characteristic that is probably related to their slow rate of metabolism. Alternatively, this long lasting effect of neuropeptides may be due to complex intracellular signalling pathways after binding to their metabotropic GPCRs.

We cannot excluded that some neuropeptides when injected at high doses within the periphery may act at central target sites to increase $P_{DA}$, through leakage of the blood brain barrier. However, a direct action of neuropeptides on vasculature is probably the physiological mechanism involved after peripheral injection.

**Figure 3** gives a summary of the proposed mechanisms for central neuropeptidergic cardio-respiratory regulation in trout.

**Table 1** provides a summary of the central ventilatory and cardiovascular actions of neuropeptides in our trout model. However, it remains to be determined whether the observed actions of exogenously administered neuropeptides can be translated into evidence for endogenous regulation of physiological functions. It is probable that a cocktail of neuropeptides within the trout brain is involved in fine control of ventilation, each peptide having a selective action either on VA or VF or on both ventilatory variables. Neuropeptides may be part of the neurochemical systems that are involved in the hypoxic ventilatory response in fish (Porteus et al., 2011). However, as previously stated, their precise implication in the CNS pathways that control the VA and VF during intermittent, repeated or chronic hypoxia is unknown. A balance between the action of hyperventilatory and hypoventilatory peptides may permit the fine control of ventilation so as to maintain homeostasis. In addition, endogenous neuropeptides may regulate cardiovascular function.

**Table 1 | Summary of the effects of intracerebroventricular injection of neuropeptides on ventilatory and cardiovascular variables in the unanesthetized trout.**

| Neuropeptides (pmol) | | Ventilatory effects | | | Cardiovascular effects | |
|---|---|---|---|---|---|---|
| | | VF | VA | VTOT | $P_{DA}$ | HR |
| PACAP | (50) | – | ↑ | ↑ | – | – |
| | (100) | ↑ | **↑** | **↑** | ↑ | – |
| VIP | (50) | – | – | – | – | – |
| | (100) | – | – | ↑ | – | – |
| NPγ | (50) | ↑ | ↓ | ↓ | – | – |
| | (100) | **↑** | **↓** | **↓** | – | – |
| SP | (100) | – | – | – | – | – |
| | (250) | ↑ | ↓ | ↓ | – | – |
| NKA | (100) | – | – | – | – | – |
| | (250) | – | ↓ | ↓ | – | – |
| CRF | (5) | ↑ | ↑ | ↑ | ↑ | – |
| | (10) | **↑** | **↑** | **↑** | **↑** | – |
| U-I | (5) | – | – | – | – | – |
| | (10) | ↑ | ↑ | ↑ | ↑ | – |
| CGRP | (5) | – | ↑ | ↑ | ↑ | – |
| | (50) | ↑ | **↑** | **↑** | **↑** | – |
| [Asn[1]]-Ang II | (5) | – | – | – | – | ↑ |
| | (50) | – | ↑ | ↑ | ↑ | **↑** |
| [Asp[1]]-Ang II | (5) | – | – | – | – | – |
| | (50) | – | ↑ | ↑ | ↑ | ↑ |
| Ang III | (50) | – | – | – | ↑ | ↑ |
| | (100) | – | – | – | **↑** | **↑** |
| Ang IV | (100) | – | – | – | – | – |
| Ang 1–7 | (100) | – | – | – | – | – |
| U II | (5) | – | – | – | – | – |
| | (50) | ↑ | ↑ | ↑ | – | ↑ |
| NPY | (100) | – | – | – | – | – |
| PYY | (100) | – | – | – | – | – |

*PACAP, pituitary adenylate cyclase-activating polypeptide; VIP, vasoactive intestinal peptide; NPγ, neuropeptide gamma; SP, substance P; NKA, neurokinin A; CRF, corticotropin-releasing factor; U-I, urotensin-I; CGRP, calcitonin gene-related peptide; [Asn[1]]-Ang II, [Asn[1]]-angiotensin II; [Asp[1]]-Ang II, [Asp[1]]-angiotensin II; Ang III, angiotensin III; Ang IV, angiotensin IV; Ang 1–7, angiotensin 1–7; U-II, urotensin-II; NPY, neuropeptide Y; PYY, peptide YY. –, no effect; ↑, increase; ↓, decrease; symbol in bold reflects a higher effect.*

The circumstances leading to the release of endogenous neuropeptides into the synaptic cleft to control the ventilatory and cardiovascular autonomic nuclei during adverse metabolic or environmental situations remain to be delineated. It may be hypothesized that the central neuropeptidergic regulation of cardio-respiratory functions may be critical for proper uptake of oxygen from the aquatic environment and distribution of oxygen to tissues during hypoxic stress for example. Hypoxic stress is known to induce an hyperventilatory response in the rainbow trout through a selective action on VA (Gilmour and Perry, 2007) and environmental hypoxia increases the expression of CRF, UI, and CRF-binding protein genes within the NPO (Bernier and Craig, 2005).

## CONCLUSION AND PERSPECTIVES

Besides conservation of the amino acid sequence of neuropeptides during evolution, our physiological results obtained with unanesthetized trout also give support for a strong conservation of cardiovascular and ventilatory functions throughout the vertebrate classes. Determination of the central ventilatory and cardiovascular actions of these neuropeptides in our trout model suggests that these neuropeptides act as neuromodulators and/or neurotransmitters. In addition, neuropeptides acting as local peptides or hormones may be involved in peripheral cardiovascular regulation. We hope that our comparative physiological studies provide new insights into evolution of the basic neuroregulatory mechanisms that operate in the CNS of vertebrates, including humans, to control these vital cardio-respiratory functions.

## REFERENCES


Aguirre, J. A., Fuxe, K., Hedlund, P., Narvaez, J. A., Cintra, A., Rosen, L., et al. (1991). Neuropeptide Y/angiotensin II interactions in central cardiovascular regulation of the rat. *Brain Res.* 566, 61–69.

Alderman, S. L., Raine, J. C., and Bernier, N. J. (2008). Distribution and regional stressor-induced regulation of corticotrophin-releasing factor binding protein in rainbow trout (*Oncorhynchus mykiss*). *J. Neuroendocrinol.* 20, 347–358.

Altimiras, J., Aissaoui, A., and Tort, L. (1995). Is the short-term modulation of heart rate in teleost fish physiologically significant? Assessment by spectral analysis techniques. *Braz. J. Med. Biol. Res.* 28, 1197–1206.

Amara, S. G., Jonas, V., Rosenfeld, M. G., Ong, E. S., and Evans, R. M. (1982). Alternative RNA processing in calcitonin gene expression generates mRNAs encoding different polypeptide products. *Nature* 298, 240–244.

Arai, M., Assil, I. Q., and Abou-Samra, A. B. (2001). Characterization of three corticotropin-releasing factor receptors in catfish: a novel third receptor is predominantly expressed in pituitary and urophysis. *Endocrinology* 142, 446–454.

Ariëns-Kappers, C. U., Huber, G. C., and Crosby, E. C. (1936). *The Comparative Anatomy of the Nervous System of Vertebrates, Including Man.* New York, NY: Macmillan.

Bagshaw, R. J. (1985). Evolution of cardiovascular baroreceptor control. *Biol. Rev. Camb. Philos. Soc.* 60, 121–162.

Bale, T. L., and Vale, W. W. (2004). CRF and CRF receptors: role in stress responsivity and other behaviors. *Annu. Rev. Pharmacol. Toxicol.* 44, 525–557.

Barsyte, D., Tipping, D. R., Smart, D., Conlon, J. M., Baker, B. I., and Lovejoy, D. A. (1999). Rainbow trout (*Oncorhynchus mykiss*) urotensin-I: structural differences between urotensins-I and urocortins. *Gen. Comp. Endocrinol.* 115, 169–177.

Batten, T. F., and Cambre, M. L. (1989). Calcitonin gene-related peptide-like immunoreactive fibres innervating the hypothalamic inferior lobes of teleost fishes. *Neurosci. Lett.* 98, 1–7.

Batten, T. F., Cambre, M. L., Moons, L., and Vandesande, F. (1990). Comparative distribution of neuropeptide-immunoreactive systems in the brain of the green molly, *Poecilia latipinna*. *J. Comp. Neurol.* 302, 893–919.

Bennet, L., Johnston, B. M., Vale, W. W., and Gluckman, P. D. (1990). The effects of corticotrophin-releasing factor and two antagonists on breathing movements in fetal sheep. *J. Physiol.* 421, 1–11.

Bern, H. A., Pearson, D., Larson, B. A., and Nishioka, R. S. (1985). Neurohormones from fish tails: the caudal neurosecretory system. I. "Urophysiology" and the caudal neurosecretory system of fishes. *Recent Prog. Horm. Res.* 41, 533–552.

Bernier, N. J. (2006). The corticotropin-releasing factor sys-tem as a mediator of the appetite-suppressing effects of stress in fish. *Gen. Comp. Endocrinol.* 146, 45–55.

Bernier, N. J., and Craig, P. M. (2005). CRF-related peptides contribute to stress response and regulation of appetite in hypoxic rainbow trout. *Am. J. Physiol.* 289, R982–R990.

Bernier, N. J., Lin, X., and Peter, R. E. (1999a). Differential expression of corticotropin-releasing factor (CRF) and urotensin I precursor genes, and evidence of CRF gene expression regulated by cortisol in goldfish brain. *Gen. Comp. Endocrinol.* 116, 461–477.

Bernier, N. J., McKendry, J. E., and Perry, S. F. (1999b). Blood pressure regulation during hypotension in two teleost species: differential involvement of the renin-angiotensin and adrenergic systems. *J. Exp. Biol.* 202, 1677–1690.

Bertinieri, G., Di Rienzo, M., Cavallazzi, A., Ferrari, A. U., Pedotti, A., and Mancia, G. (1988). Evaluation of baroreceptor reflex by blood pressure monitoring in unanesthetized cats. *Am. J. Physiol.* 254, H377–H383.

Bolis, C. L., Piccolella, M., Dalla Valle, A. Z., and Rankin, J. C. (2001). Fish as model in pharmacological and biological research. *Pharmacol. Res.* 44, 265–280.

Brennan, M., Palaniswami, M., and Kamen, P. (2001). Do existing measures of Poincare plot geometry reflect nonlinear features of heart rate variability? *IEEE Trans. Biomed. Eng.* 48, 1342–1347.

Burnstock, G. (1969). Evolution of the autonomic innervation of visceral and cardiovascular systems in vertebrates. *Pharmacol. Rev.* 21, 247–324.

Chang, C. L., and Hsu, S. Y. (2004). Ancient evolution of stress-regulating peptides in vertebrates. *Peptides* 25, 1681–1688.

Clark, M. S., Bendell, L., Power, D. M., Warner, S., Elgar, G., and Ingleton, P. M. (2002). Calcitonin: characterisation and expression in a teleost fish, *Fugu rubripes*. *J. Mol. Endocrinol.* 28, 111–123.

Clements, S., Schreck, C. B., Larsen, D. A., and Dickhoff, W. W. (2002). Central administration of corticotropin-releasing hormone stimulates locomotor activity in juvenile chinook salmon (*Oncorhynchus tshawytscha*). *Gen. Comp. Endocrinol.* 125, 319–327.

Cobb, C. S., and Brown, J. A. (1992). Angiotensin II binding to tissues of the rainbow trout, *Oncorhynchus mykiss*, studied by autoradiography. *J. Comp. Physiol. B* 162, 197–202.

Conklin, D., Chavas, A., Duff, W. D., Leroy Weaver, Jr., Zang., Y., and Olson, K. (1997). Cardiovascular effects of arginine vasotocin in the rainbow trout *Oncorhynchus mykiss*. *J. Exp. Biol.* 200, 2821–2832.

Conlon, J. M. (2004). The tachykinins peptide family, with particular emphasis on mammalian tachykinins and tachykinin receptor agonists. *Handb. Exp. Pharmacol.* 164, 25–62.

Conlon, J. M. (2008). Liberation of urotensin II from the teleost urophysis: an historical overview. *Peptides* 29, 651–657.

Conlon, J. M., Balasubramaniam, A., and Hazon, N. (1991). Structural characterization and biological activity of a neuropeptide Y-related peptide from the dogfish, *Scyliorhinus canicula*. *Endocrinology* 128, 2273–2279.

Conlon, J. M., Yano, K., and Olson, K. R. (1996). Production of [Asn1, Val5] angiotensin II and [Asp1, Val5] angiotensin II in kallikrein-treated trout plasma (T60K). *Peptides* 17, 527–530.

Dampney, R. A., Horiuchi, J., Killinger, S., Sheriff, M. J., Tan, P. S., and McDowall, L. M. (2005). Long-term regulation of arterial blood pressure by hypothalamic nuclei: some critical questions. *Clin. Exp. Pharmacol. Physiol.* 32, 419–425.

Dampney, R. A., Horiuchi, J., and McDowall, L. M. (2008). Hypothalamic mechanisms coordinating cardiorespiratory function during exercise and defensive behaviour. *Auton. Neurosci.* 142, 3–10.

Danger, J. M., Breton, B., Vallarino, M., Fournier, A., Pelletier, G., and Vaudry, H. (1991). Neuropeptide-Y in the trout brain and pituitary: localization, characterization, and action on gonadotropin release. *Endocrinology* 128, 2360–2368.

Doi, A., and Ramirez, J. M. (2008). Neuromodulation and the orchestration of the respiratory rhythm. *Respir. Physiol. Neurobiol.* 164, 96–104.

Dumont, J., and Quirion, R. (2006). "Neuropeptide, Y," in *Handbook of Biologically Active Peptides*, ed A. J. Kastin (San Diego, CA: Academic Press), 683–688.

Fisher, L. A., Kikkawa, D. O., Rivier, J. E., Amara, S. G., Evans, R. M., Rosenfeld, M. G., et al. (1983). Stimulation of noradrenergic sympathetic outflow by calcitonin gene-related peptide. *Nature* 305, 534–536.

Fuxe, K., Agnati, L. F., Harfstrand, A., Janson, A. M., Neumeyer, A., Andersson, K., et al. (1986). Morphofunctional studies on the neuropeptide Y/adrenaline costoring terminal systems in the dorsal cardiovascular region of the medulla oblongata. Focus on receptor-receptor interactions in cotransmission. *Prog. Brain Res.* 68, 303–320.

Fuxe, K., Agnati, L. F., Harfstrand, A., Zini, I., Tatemoto, K., Pich, E. M., et al. (1983). Central administration of neuropeptide Y induces hypotension bradypnea and EEG synchronization in the rat. *Acta Physiol. Scand.* 118, 189–192.

Fyhrquist, F., and Saijonmaa, O. (2008). Renin-angiotensin system revisited. *J. Intern. Med.* 264, 224–236.

Gilmour, K. M., and Perry, S. P. (2007). "Branchial chemoreceptor regulation of cardiorespiratory function," in *Fish Physiology, Sensory Systems Neuroscience, Vol. 25*, eds T. J. Hara and B. S. Zielinski (San Diego, CA: Academic Press), 97–151.

Gray, P. A., Rekling, J. C., Bocchiaro, C. M., and Feldman, J. L. (1999). Modulation of respiratory frequency by peptidergic input to rhythmogenic neurons in the preBotzinger complex. *Science* 286, 1566–1568.

Grossman, P., and Taylor, E. W. (2007). Toward understanding respiratory sinus arrhythmia: relations to cardiac vagal tone, evolution and biobehavioral functions. *Biol. Psychol.* 74, 263–285.

Holeton, G. F., and Randall, D. J. (1967). Changes in blood pressure in the rainbow trout during hypoxia. *J. Exp. Biol.* 46, 297–305.

Holmgren, S., and Jensen, J. (2001). Evolution of vertebrate neuropeptides. *Brain Res. Bull.* 55, 723–735.

Holmqvist, B. I., and Ekstrom, P. (1991). Galanin-like immunoreactivity in the brain of teleosts: distribution and relation to substance P, vasotocin, and isotocin in the Atlantic salmon (*Salmo salar*). *J. Comp. Neurol.* 306, 361–381.

Hornby, P. J., and Demski, L. S. (1988). Functional-anatomical studies of neural control of heart rate in goldfish. *Brain Behav. Evol.* 31, 181–192.

Jansz, H. S., and Zandberg, J. (1992). Identification and partial characterization of the salmon calcitonin/CGRP gene by polymerase chain reaction. *Ann. N.Y. Acad. Sci.* 657, 63–69.

Jensen, J., and Conlon, J. M. (1992). Characterization of peptides related to neuropeptide tyrosine and peptide tyrosine-tyrosine from the brain and gastrointestinal tract of teleost fish. *Eur. J. Biochem.* 210, 405–410.

Jensen, J., Olson, K. R., and Conlon, J. M. (1993). Primary structures and effects on gastrointestinal motility of tachykinins from the rainbow trout. *Am. J. Physiol.* 265, R804–R810.

Karemaker, J. M., and Wesseling, K. H. (2008). Variability in cardiovascular control: the baroreflex reconsidered. *Cardiovasc. Eng.* 8, 23–29.

Koob, G. F., and Heinrichs, S. C. (1999). A role for corticotropin releasing factor and urocortin in behavioral responses to stressors. *Brain Res.* 848, 141–152.

Kozaka, T., Fujii, Y., and Ando, M. (2003). Central effects of various ligands on drinking behavior in eels acclimated to seawater. *J. Exp. Biol.* 206, 687–692.

Krahn, D. D., Gosnell, B. A., Levine, A. S., and Morley, J. E. (1984). Effects of calcitonin gene-related peptide on food intake. *Peptides* 5, 861–864.

Laburthe, M., Couvineau, A., and Tan, V. (2007). Class II G protein-coupled receptors for VIP and PACAP: structure, models of activation and pharmacology. *Peptides* 28, 1631–1639.

Lancien, F., and Le Mével, J. C. (2007). Central actions of angiotensin II on spontaneous baroreflex sensitivity in the trout *Oncorhynchus mykiss*. *Regul. Pept.* 138, 94–102.

Lancien, F., Leprince, J., Mimassi, N., Mabin, D., Vaudry, H., and Le Mével, J. C. (2004a). Central effects of native urotensin II on motor activity, ventilatory movements, and heart rate in the trout *Oncorhynchus mykiss*. *Brain Res.* 1023, 167–174.

Lancien, F., Mimassi, N., Mabin, D., and Le Mével, J. C. (2004b). Captopril blocks the cardiac actions of centrally administered angiotensin I in the trout *Oncorhynchus mykiss*. *Brain Res.* 1007, 116–123.

Lancien, F., Mimassi, N., Conlon, J. M., and Le Mével, J. C. (2009). Central effects of trout tachykinins on heart rate variability in trout. *Ann. N.Y. Acad. Sci.* 1163, 379–382.

Lancien, F., Mimassi, N., Conlon, J. M., and Le Mével, J. C. (2011). Central pituitary adenylate cyclase-activating polypeptide (PACAP) and vasoactive intestinal peptide (VIP) decrease the baroreflex sensitivity in trout. *Gen. Comp. Endocrinol.* 171, 245–251.

Lancien, F., Wong, M., Arab, A. A., Mimassi, N., Takei, Y., and Le Mével, J. C. (2012). Central ventilator and cardiovascular actions of angiotensin peptides in trout. *Am. J. Physiol.* 303, R311–R320.

Laurent, P., Homgren, S., and Nilsson, S. (1983). Nervous and humoral control of the fish heart: structure and function. *Comp. Biochem. Physiol.* 76A, 525–542.

Le Mével, J. C., Lancien, F., Mimassi, N., Leprince, J., Conlon, J. M., and Vaudry, H. (2008a). Central and peripheral cardiovascular, ventilatory, and motor effects of trout urotensin-II in the trout. *Peptides* 29, 830–837.

Le Mével, J. C., Lancien, F., and Mimassi, N. (2008b). Central cardiovascular actions of angiotensin II in trout. *Gen. Comp. Endocrinol.* 157, 27–34.

Le Mével, J. C., Lancien, F., Mimassi, N., and Conlon, J. M. (2007). Ventilatory and cardiovascular actions of centrally administered trout tachykinins in the unanesthetized trout. *J. Exp. Biol.* 210, 3301–3310.

Le Mével, J. C., Lancien, F., Mimassi, N., and Conlon, J. M. (2009a). Central hyperventilatory action of the stress-related neurohormonal peptides, corticotropin-releasing factor and urotensin-I in the trout *Oncorhynchus mykiss*. *Gen. Comp. Endocrinol.* 164, 51–60.

Le Mével, J. C., Lancien, F., Mimassi, N., and Conlon, J. M. (2009b). Ventilatory and cardiovascular actions of centrally and peripherally administered trout pituitary adenylate cyclase-activating polypeptide (PACAP) and vasoactive intestinal peptide (VIP) in the unanaesthetized trout. *J. Exp. Biol.* 212, 3919–3927.

Le Mével, J. C., Lancien, F., Mimassi, N., Kermorgant, M., and Conlon, J. M. (2012). Central ventilatory and cardiovascular actions of calcitonin gene-related peptide in unanesthetized trout. *J. Exp. Biol.* 215, 1930–1937.

Le Mével, J. C., Mabin, D., and Vaudry, H. (1991). Intracerebroventricular injection of arginine vasotocin induces elevation of blood pressure in anesthetized trout. *Peptides* 12, 477–481.

Le Mével, J. C., Mimassi, N., Lancien, F., Mabin, D., Boucher, J. M., and Blanc, J. J. (2002). Heart rate variability, a target for the effects of angiotensin II in the brain of the trout *Oncorhynchus mykiss*. *Brain Res.* 947, 34–40.

Le Mével, J. C., Mimassi, N., Lancien, F., Mabin, D., and Conlon, J. M. (2006). Cardiovascular actions of the stress-related neurohormonal peptides, corticotropin-releasing factor and urotensin-I in the trout *Oncorhynchus mykiss*. *Gen. Comp. Endocrinol.* 146, 56–61.

Le Mével, J. C., Pamantung, T. F., Mabin, D., and Vaudry, H. (1993). Effects of central and peripheral administration of arginine vasotocin and related neuropeptides on blood pressure and heart rate in the conscious trout. *Brain Res.* 610, 82–89.

Le Mével, J. C., Pamantung, T. F., Mabin, D., and Vaudry, H. (1994). Intracerebroventricular administration of angiotensin II increases heart rate in the conscious trout. *Brain Res.* 654, 216–222.

Le Mével, J. C., Olson, K. R., Conklin, D., Waugh, D., Smith, D. D., Vaudry, H., et al. (1996). Cardiovascular actions of trout urotensin II in the conscious trout, *Oncorhynchus mykiss. Am. J. Physiol.* 271, R1335–R1343.

Lihrmann, I., Bern, H. A., and Vaudry, H. (2006). "Urotensin II and Urotensin II-related peptide," in *Handbook of Biologically Active Peptides*, ed A. J. Kastin (San Diego, CA: Academic Press), 795–803.

Lovejoy, D. A., and Balment, R. J. (1999). Evolution and physiology of the corticotropin-releasing factor (CRF) family of neuropeptides in vertebrates. *Gen. Comp. Endocrinol.* 115, 1–22.

Lu, W., Greenwood, M., Dow, L., Yuill, J., Worthington, J., Brierley, M. J., et al. (2006). Molecular characterization and expression of urotensin II and its receptor in the flounder (*Platichthys flesus*): a hormone system supporting body fluid homeostasis in euryhaline fish. *Endocrinology* 147, 3692–3708.

Mack, S. O., Kc, P., Wu, M., Coleman, B. R., Tolentino-Silva, F. P., and Haxhiu, M. A. (2002). Paraventricular oxytocin neurons are involved in neural modulation of breathing. *J. Appl. Physiol.* 92, 826–834.

Mandel, D. A., and Schreihofer, A. M. (2006). Central respiratory modulation of barosensitive neurones in rat caudal ventrolateral medulla. *J. Physiol.* 572, 881–896.

Martinez-Alvarez, R. M., Volkoff, H., Cueto, J. A., and Delgado, M. J. (2008). Molecular characterization of calcitonin gene-related peptide (CGRP) related peptides (CGRP, amylin, adrenomedullin and adrenomedullin-2/intermedin) in goldfish (*Carassius auratus*): cloning and distribution. *Peptides* 29, 1534–1543.

Martinez-Alvarez, R. M., Volkoff, H., Munoz-Cueto, J. A., and Delgado, M. J. (2009). Effect of calcitonin gene-related peptide (CGRP), adrenomedullin and adrenomedullin-2/intermedin on food intake in goldfish (*Carassius auratus*). *Peptides* 30, 803–807.

Matsuda, K., Maruyama, K., Nakamachi, T., Miura, T., and Shioda, S. (2006). Effects of pituitary adenylate cyclase-activating polypeptide and vasoactive intestinal polypeptide on food intake and locomotor activity in the goldfish, *Carassius auratus. Ann. N.Y. Acad. Sci.* 1070, 417–421.

Matsuda, K., Takei, Y., Katoh, J., Shioda, S., Arimura, A., and Uchiyama, M. (1997). Isolation and structural characterization of pituitary adenylate cyclase activating polypeptide (PACAP)-like peptide from the brain of a teleost, stargazer, *Uranoscopus japonicus. Peptides* 18, 723–727.

Matsumura, K., Abe, I., Tsuchihashi, T., and Fujishima, M. (1999). Central adrenomedullin augments the baroreceptor reflex in conscious rabbits. *Hypertension* 33, 992–997.

Médigue, C., Girard, A., Laude, D., Monti, A., Wargon, M., and Elghozi, J. L. (2001). Relationship between pulse interval and respiratory sinus arrhythmia: a time- and frequency-domain analysis of the effects of atropine. *Pflugers Arch.* 441, 650–655.

Montero, M., Yon, L., Rousseau, K., Arimura, A., Fournier, A., Dufour, S., et al. (1998). Distribution, characterization, and growth hormone-releasing activity of pituitary adenylate cyclase-activating polypeptide in the European eel, *Anguilla anguilla. Endocrinology* 139, 4300–4310.

Montpetit, C. J., Shahsavarani, A., and Perry, S. F. (2003). Localisation of VIP-binding sites exhibiting properties of VPAC receptors in chromaffin cells of rainbow trout (*Oncorhynchus mykiss*). *J. Exp. Biol.* 206, 1917–1927.

Moons, L., Batten, T. F., and Vandesande, F. (1992). Comparative distribution of substance P (SP) and cholecystokinin (CCK) binding sites and immunoreactivity in the brain of the sea bass (*Dicentrarchus labrax*). *Peptides* 13, 37–46.

Morton, K. D., McCloskey, M. J., and Potter, E. K. (1999). Cardiorespiratory responses to intracerebroventricular injection of neuropeptide Y in anaesthetised dogs. *Regul. Pept.* 81, 81–88.

Nieuwenhuys, R., and Powels, E. (1983). "The brainstem of actinopterygian fishes," in *Fish Neurobiology, 1. Brain Stem and Sense Organs*, eds R. G. Northcutt and R. E. Davies (Ann Arbor, MI: University of Michigan Press), 25–87.

Nieuwenhuys, R., Ten Donkelaar, H. J., and Nicholson, C. (1998). *The Central Nervous System of Vertebrates, Vol. 2.* Berlin: Springer.

Niewoehner, D. E., Levine, A. S., and Morley, J. E. (1983). Central effects of neuropeptides on ventilation in the rat. *Peptides* 4, 277–281.

Nishimura, H. (2001). Angiotensin receptors–evolutionary overview and perspectives. *Comp. Biochem. Physiol. A Mol. Integr. Physiol.* 128, 11–30.

Nobata, S., Donald, J. A., Balment, R. J., and Takei, Y. (2011). Potent cardiovascular effects of homologous urotensin II (UII)-related peptide and UII in unanesthetized eels after peripheral and central injections. *Am. J. Physiol.* 300, R437–R446.

Nunn, N., Womack, M., Dart, C., and Barrett-Jolley, R. (2011). Function and pharmacology of spinally-projecting sympathetic pre-autonomic neurones in the paraventricular nucleus of the hypothalamus. *Curr. Neuropharmacol.* 9, 262–277.

O'Connor, M. D., and Jennings, D. B. (2001). Respiratory and metabolic effects of decreased osmolality in conscious rats. *Can. J. Physiol. Pharmacol.* 79, 768–778.

Ogoshi, M., Inoue, K., Naruse, K., and Takei, Y. (2006). Evolutionary history of the calcitonin gene-related peptide family in vertebrates revealed by comparative genomic analyses. *Peptides* 27, 3154–3164.

Ogoshi, M., Nobata, S., and Takei, Y. (2008). Potent osmoregulatory actions of homologous adrenomedullins administered peripherally and centrally in eels. *Am. J. Physiol.* 295, R2075–R2083.

Ohtake, P. J., and Jennings, D. B. (1993). Angiotensin II stimulates respiration in awake dogs and antagonizes baroreceptor inhibition. *Respir. Physiol.* 91, 335–351.

Olivereau, M., and Olivereau, J. M. (1990). Corticotropin-like immunoreactivity in the brain and pituitary of three teleost species (goldfish, trout and eel). *Cell Tissue Res.* 262, 115–123.

Olson, K. R. (1992). "Blood and extracellular fluid volume regulation: role of the renin-angiotensin system, kallikrein-kinin system, and atrial natriuretic peptides," in *Fish Physiology: The Cardiovascular System*, eds W. S. Hoar, D. J. Randall, and A. P. Farrell (San Diego, CA: Academic Press), 135–254.

Olsson, M., Annerbrink, K., Hedner, J., and Eriksson, E. (2004). Intracerebroventricular administration of the angiotensin II receptor antagonist saralasin reduces respiratory rate and tidal volume variability in freely moving Wistar rats. *Psychoneuroendocrinology* 29, 107–112.

Pamantung, T. F., Leroy, J. P., Mabin, D., and Le Mével, J. C. (1997). Role of dorsal vagal motor nucleus in angiotensin II-mediated tachycardia in the conscious trout *Oncorhynchus mykiss. Brain Res.* 772, 167–175.

Parati, G., Di Rienzo, M., and Mancia, G. (2000). How to measure baroreflex sensitivity: from the cardiovascular laboratory to daily life. *J. Hypertens.* 18, 7–19.

Parkes, D. G., Weisinger, R. S., and May, C. N. (2001). Cardiovascular actions of CRH and urocortin: an update. *Peptides* 22, 821–827.

Parmentier, C., Hameury, E., Dubessy, C., Quan, F. B., Habert, D., Calas, A., et al. (2011). Occurrence of two distinct urotensin II-related peptides in zebrafish provides new insight into the evolutionary history of the urotensin II gene family. *Endocrinology* 152, 2330–2341.

Parmentier, C., Hameury, E., Lihrmann, I., Taxi, J., Hardin-Pouzet, H., Vaudry, H., et al. (2008). Comparative distribution of the mRNAs encoding urotensin I and urotensin II in zebrafish. *Peptides* 29, 820–829.

Patacchini, R., and Maggi, C. A. (2004). The nomenclature of tachykinins receptors. *Handb. Exp. Pharmacol.* 164, 121–139.

Paul, M., Poyan Mehr, A., and Kreutz, R. (2006). Physiology of local renin-angiotensin systems. *Physiol. Rev.* 86, 747–803.

Pearson, D., Shively, J. E., Clark, B. R., Geschwind, I. I., Barkley, M., Nishioka, R. S., et al. (1980). Urotensin II: a somatostatin-like peptide in the caudal neurosecretory system of fishes. *Proc. Natl. Acad. Sci. U.S.A.* 77, 5021–5024.

Pilowsky, P. M., Lung, M. S., Spirovski, D., and McMullan, S. (2009). Differential regulation of the central neural cardiorespiratory system by metabotropic neurotransmitters. *Philos. Trans. R. Soc. Lond. B Biol. Sci.* 364, 2537–2552.

Playford, R. J., Benito-Orfila, M. A., Nihoyannopoulos, P., Nandha, K. A., Cockcroft, J., Todd, S., et al. (1992). Effects of peptide YY on the human cardiovascular system: reversal of responses to vasoactive intestinal peptide. *Am. J. Physiol.* 263, E740–E747.

Pohl, S., Darlison, M. G., Clarke, W. C., Lederis, K., and Richter, D. (2001). Cloning and functional pharmacology of two corticotropin-releasing factor receptors from a teleost fish. *Eur. J. Pharmacol.* 430, 193–202.

Porteus, C., Hedrick, M. S., Hicks, J. W., Wang, T., and Milsom, W. K. (2011). Time domains of the hypoxic ventilatory response in ectothermic vertebrates. *J. Comp. Physiol. B* 181, 311–333.

Potter, E. K., and McCloskey, D. I. (1979). Respiratory stimulation by angiotensin II. *Respir. Physiol.* 36, 367–373.

Preston, E., Jonsson, A. C., McManus, C. D., Conlon, J. M., and Courtice, G. P. (1998). Comparative vascular responses in elasmobranchs to different structures of neuropeptide Y and peptide YY. *Regul. Pept.* 78, 57–67.

Quan, F. B., Bougerol, M., Rigour, F., Kenigfest, N. B., and Tostivint, H. (2012). Characterization of the true ortholog of the urotensin II-related peptide (URP) gene in teleosts. *Gen. Comp. Endocrinol.* 177, 205–212.

Randall, D. J., and Taylor, E. W. (1991). Evidence of a role for catecholamines in the control of breathing in fish. *Rev. Fish Biol. Fish.* 1, 139–157.

Rankin, J. C., Watanabe, T. X., Nakajima, K., Broadhead, C., and Takei, Y. (2004). Identification of angiotensin I in a cyclostome, *Lampetra fluviatilis. Zoolog. Sci.* 21, 173–179.

Russell, M. J., Klemmer, A. M., and Olson, K. R. (2001). Angiotensin signaling and receptor types in teleost fish. *Comp. Biochem. Physiol. A Mol. Integr. Physiol.* 128, 41–51.

Saito, D., Komatsuda, M., and Urano, A. (2004). Functional organization of preoptic vasotocin and isotocin neurons in the brain of rainbow trout: central and neurohypophysial projections of single neurons. *Neuroscience* 124, 973–984.

Sandblom, E., and Axelsson, M. (2011). Autonomic control of circulation in fish: a comparative view. *Auton. Neurosci.* 165, 127–139.

Salaneck, E., Larsson, T. A., Larson, E. T., and Larhammar, D. (2008). Birth and death of neuropeptide Y receptor genes in relation to the teleost fish tetraploidization. *Gene* 409, 61–71.

Satake, H., and Kawada, T. (2006). Overview of the primary structure, distribution, and functions of tachykinins and their receptors. *Curr. Drug Targets* 7, 963–974.

Satchell, G. H. (1991). *Physiology and Form of Fish Circulation.* Cambridge, MA: Cambridge University Press.

Sawada, H., Yamaguchi, H., Shimbara, T., Toshinai, K., Mondal, M. S., Date, Y., et al. (2006). Central effects of calcitonin receptor-stimulating peptide-1 on energy homeostasis in rats. *Endocrinology* 147, 2043–2050.

Scott, N. A., Webb, V., Boublik, J. H., Rivier, J., and Brown, M. R. (1989). The cardiovascular actions of centrally administered neuropeptide Y. *Regul. Pept.* 25, 247–258.

Shahbazi, F., Holmgren, S., Larhammar, D., and Jensen, J. (2002). Neuropeptide Y effects on vasorelaxation and intestinal contraction in the Atlantic cod *Gadus morhua. Am. J. Physiol.* 282, R1414–R1421.

Shahbazi, F., Karila, P., Olsson, C., Holmgren, S., Conlon, J. M., and Jensen, J. (1998). Primary structure, distribution, and effects on motility of CGRP in the intestine of the cod Gadus morhua. *Am. J. Physiol.* 275, R19–R28.

Sherwood, N. M., Krueckl, S. L., and McRory, J. E. (2000). The origin and function of the pituitary adenylate cyclase-activating polypeptide (PACAP)/glucagon superfamily. *Endocr. Rev.* 21, 619–670.

Soivio, A., Westman, K., and Nyholm, K. (1972). Improved method of dorsal aorta catheterization: haematological effects followed for three weeks in rainbow trout (*Salmo gairdneri*). *Finn. Fish. Res.* 1, 11–21.

Sundin, L., and Nilsson, S. (2002). Branchial innervation. *J. Exp. Zool.* 293, 232–248.

Sundin, L., Turesson, J., and Burleson, M. (2003a). Identification of central mechanisms vital for breathing in the channel catfish, *Ictalurus punctatus. Respir. Physiol. Neurobiol.* 138, 77–86.

Sundin, L., Turesson, J., and Taylor, E. W. (2003b). Evidence for glutamatergic mechanisms in the vagal sensory pathway initiating cardiorespiratory reflexes in the shorthorn sculpin *Myoxocephalus scorpius. J. Exp. Biol.* 206, 867–876.

Suzuki, N. T., and Kurokawa, T. (2000). Cloning of a calcitonin gene-related peptide receptor and a novel calcitonin receptor-like receptor from the gill of flounder, *Paralichthys olivaceus. Gene* 244, 81–88.

Swanson, L. W., Sawchenko, P. E., Rivier, J., and Vale, W. W. (1983). Organization of ovine corticotropin-releasing factor immunoreactive cells and fibers in the rat brain: an immunohistochemical study. *Neuroendocrinology* 36, 165–186.

Tam, C. W. L., and Brain, S. D. (2006). "Calcitonin gene-related peptides," in *Handbook of Biologically Active Peptides,* ed A. J. Kastin (San Diego, CA: Academic Press), 1181–1186.

Takei, Y., and Balment, R. (2009). "The neuroendocrine regulation of fluid intake and fluid balance," in *Fish Physiology: Fish Neuroendocrinology*, eds N. J. Bernier, G. Van Der Kraak, A. P. Farrell, and C. J. Brauner (San Diego, CA: Academic Press), 365–419.

Takei, Y., Hasegawa, Y., Watanabe, T. X., Nakajima, K., and Hazon, N. (1993). A novel angiotensin I isolated from an elasmobranch fish. *J. Endocrinol.* 139, 281–285.

Task Force of the European Society of Cardiology, and the North American Society of Pacing and Electrophysiology. (1996). Heart Rate variability: standards of measurement, physiological interpretation, and clinical use. *Circulation* 93, 1043–1065.

Taylor, E. W. (1992). "Nervous control of the heart and cardiorespiratory interactions," in *The Cardiovascular System*, eds W. S. Hoar, D. J. Randall, and A. P. Farrell (San Diego, CA: Academic Press), 343–387.

Taylor, E. W., Jordan, D., and Coote, J. H. (1999). Central control of the cardiovascular and respiratory systems and their interactions in vertebrates. *Physiol. Rev.* 79, 855–916.

Taylor, E. W., Leite, C. A., and Levings, J. J. (2009). Central control of cardiorespiratory interactions in fish. *Acta Histochem.* 111, 257–267.

Taylor, E. W., Leite, C. A., McKenzie, D. J., and Wang, T. (2010a). Control of respiration in fish, amphibians and reptiles. *Braz. J. Med. Biol. Res.* 43, 409–424.

Taylor, E. W., Leite, C. A., and Skovgaard, N. (2010b). Autonomic control of cardiorespiratory interactions in fish, amphibians and reptiles. *Braz. J. Med. Biol. Res.* 43, 600–610.

Turesson, J., Johansson, M., and Sundin, L. (2010). Involvement of non-NMDA receptors in central mediation of chemoreflexes in the shorthorn sculpin, *Myoxocephalus scorpius. Respir. Physiol. Neurobiol.* 172, 83–93.

Turesson, J., and Sundin, L. (2003). N-methyl-D-aspartate receptors mediate chemoreflexes in the shorthorn sculpin *Myoxocephalus scorpius. J. Exp. Biol.* 206, 1251–1259.

Vale, W., Spiess, J., Rivier, C., and Rivier, J. (1981). Characterization of a 41-residue ovine hypothalamic peptide that stimulates secretion of corticotropin and beta-endorphin. *Science* 213, 1394–1397.

Vaudry, H., Do Rego, J. C., Le Mével, J. C., Chatenet, D., Tostivint, H., Fournier, A., et al. (2010). Urotensin, II, from fish to human. *Ann. N.Y. Acad. Sci.* 1200, 53–66.

Vaudry, D., Falluel-Morel, A., Bourgault, S., Basille, M., Burel, D., Wurtz, O., et al. (2009). Pituitary adenylate cyclase-activating polypeptide and its receptors: 20 years after the discovery. *Pharmacol. Rev.* 61, 283–357.

Vaughan, J., Donaldson, C., Bittencourt, J., Perrin, M. H., Lewis, K., Sutton, S., et al. (1995). Urocortin, a mammalian neuropeptide related to fish urotensin I and to corticotropin-releasing factor. *Nature* 378, 287–292.

Vecino, E., Covenas, R., Alonso, J. R., Lara, J., and Aijon, J. (1989). Immunocytochemical study of substance P-like cell bodies and fibres in the brain of the rainbow trout, *Salmo gairdneri. J. Anat.* 165, 191–200.

Volkoff, E., Unniappan, S., and Scott, P. K. (2009). "The endocrine regulation of food intake," in *Fish Physiology: Fish Neuroendocrinology*, eds N. J. Bernier, G. Van Der Kraak, A. P. Farrell, and C. J. Braune (San Diego, CA: Academic Press), 421–465.

Walker, J. K., and Jennings, D. B. (1996). Ventilatory effects of angiotensin and vasopressin in conscious rats. *Can. J. Physiol. Pharmacol.* 74, 1258–1264.

Wilson, R. J., and Cumming, K. J. (2008). Pituitary adenylate cyclase-activating polypeptide is vital for neonatal survival and the neuronal control of breathing. *Respir. Physiol. Neurobiol.* 164, 168–178.

Wolfe, L. A., Kemp, J. G., Heenan, A. P., Preston, R. J., and Ohtake, P. J. (1998). Acid-base regulation and control of ventilation in human pregnancy. *Can. J. Physiol. Pharmacol.* 76, 815–827.

Wong, A. O., Leung, M. Y., Shea, W. L., Tse, L. Y., Chang, J. P., and Chow, B. K. (1998). Hypophysiotropic action of pituitary adenylate cyclase-activating polypeptide (PACAP) in the goldfish: immunohistochemical demonstration of PACAP in the pituitary, PACAP stimulation of growth hormone release from pituitary cells, and molecular cloning of pituitary type I PACAP receptor. *Endocrinology* 139, 3465–3479.

Wong, M. K., and Takei, Y. (2011). Characterization of a native angiotensin from an anciently diverged serine protease inhibitor in lamprey. *J. Endocrinol.* 209, 127–137.

Wong, M. K., and Takei, Y. (2012). Changes in plasma angiotensin subtypes in Japenese eel acclimated to various salinities from deionized water to double-stength seawater. *Gen. Comp. Endocrinol.* 178, 250–258.

Wood, C. M., and Shelton, G. (1980). Cardiovascular dynamics and adrenergic responses of the rainbow trout *in vivo*. *J. Exp. Biol.* 87, 247–270.

Zukowska-Grojec, Z., Marks, E. S., and Haass, M. (1987). Neuropeptide Y is a potent vasoconstrictor and a cardiodepressant in rat. *Am. J. Physiol.* 253, H1234–H1239.

# 7

# The stimulatory effect of the octadecaneuropeptide (ODN) on astroglial antioxidant enzyme systems is mediated through a GPCR

**Yosra Hamdi[1], Hadhemi Kaddour[1], David Vaudry[2,3,4], Salma Douiri[1], Seyma Bahdoudi[1], Jérôme Leprince[2,3,4], Hélène Castel[2,4], Hubert Vaudry[2,3,4]*, Mohamed Amri[1]*, Marie-Christine Tonon[2,4] and Olfa Masmoudi-Kouki[1]**

[1] Laboratory of Functional Neurophysiology and Pathology, Research Unit UR/11ES09, Department of Biological Sciences, Faculty of Science of Tunis, University Tunis El Manar, Tunis, Tunisia
[2] Inserm U982, Laboratory of Neuronal and Neuroendocrine Communication and Differentiation, University of Rouen, Mont-Saint-Aignan, France
[3] International Associated Laboratory Samuel de Champlain, Mont-Saint-Aignan, France
[4] Regional Platform for Cell Imaging of Haute-Normandie, Institute for Medical Research and Innovation, University of Rouen, Mont-Saint-Aignan, France

**Edited by:**
Jae Young Seong, Korea University, South Korea

**Reviewed by:**
María M. Malagón, University of Cordoba, Spain
Kouhei Matsuda, University of Toyama, Japan

***Correspondence:**
Mohamed Amri, Laboratory of Functional Neurophysiology and Pathology, Research Unit UR/11ES09, Department of Biological Sciences, Faculty of Science of Tunis, University Tunis El Manar, 2092 Tunis, Tunisia.
e-mail: mohamed.amri@fst.rnu.tn;
Hubert Vaudry, Inserm U982, Laboratory of Neuronal and Neuroendocrine Communication and Differentiation, International Associated Laboratory Samuel de Champlain, Regional Platform for Cell Imaging of Haute-Normandie, Institute for Medical Research and Innovation, University of Rouen, 76821 Mont-Saint-Aignan, France.
e-mail: hubert.vaudry@univ-rouen.fr

Astroglial cells possess an array of cellular defense systems, including superoxide dismutase (SOD) and catalase antioxidant enzymes, to prevent damage caused by oxidative stress on the central nervous system. Astrocytes specifically synthesize and release endozepines, a family of regulatory peptides including the octadecaneuropeptide (ODN). ODN is the ligand of both central-type benzodiazepine receptors (CBR), and an adenylyl cyclase- and phospholipase C-coupled receptor. We have recently shown that ODN is a potent protective agent that prevents hydrogen peroxide ($H_2O_2$)-induced inhibition of SOD and catalase activities and stimulation of cell apoptosis in astrocytes. The purpose of the present study was to investigate the type of receptor involved in ODN-induced inhibition of SOD and catalase in cultured rat astrocytes. We found that ODN induced a rapid stimulation of SOD and catalase gene transcription in a concentration-dependent manner. In addition, 0.1 nM ODN blocked $H_2O_2$-evoked reduction of both mRNA levels and activities of SOD and catalase. Furthermore, the inhibitory actions of ODN on the deleterious effects of $H_2O_2$ on SOD and catalase were abrogated by the metabotropic ODN receptor antagonist cyclo$_{1-8}$[Dleu$^5$]OP, but not by the CBR antagonist flumazenil. Finally, the protective action of ODN against $H_2O_2$-evoked inhibition of endogenous antioxidant systems in astrocytes was protein kinase A (PKA)-dependent, but protein kinase C-independent. Taken together, these data demonstrate for the first time that ODN, acting through its metabotropic receptor coupled to the PKA pathway, prevents oxidative stress-induced alteration of antioxidant enzyme expression and activities. The peptide ODN is thus a potential candidate for the development of specific agonists that would selectively mimic its protective activity.

**Keywords: astrocyte, catalase, ODN, ODN metabotropic receptor, oxidative stress, SOD, protein kinase A**

## INTRODUCTION

The octadecaneuropeptide (ODN) is a peptide generated through the proteolytic cleavage of the 86-amino acid precursor diazepam-binding inhibitor (DBI; Guidotti et al., 1983) which is exclusively expressed in astroglial cells in the central nervous system (CNS) of mammals (Malagon et al., 1993; Burgi et al., 1999; Tonon et al., 2006). DBI and its derived peptides are collectively designated by the term endozepines (Tonon et al., 2006). It was initially reported that ODN acts as an inverse agonist of central-type benzodiazepine receptors (CBR) that are intrinsic components of the $GABA_A$ receptor-chloride channel complex (Ferrero et al., 1986). It has been subsequently shown that ODN can also activate a $G_{i/0}$ protein-coupled receptor leading to the activation of phospholipase C (PLC) in astrocytes (Patte et al., 1995; Leprince et al., 2001). In addition, recent data indicate that the ODN G protein-coupled receptor can also activate adenylyl cyclase (AC; Hamdi et al., 2012). ODN exerts a wide range of biological activities which are mediated either through CBR, i.e., increase of aggressiveness and anxiety (Kavaliers and Hirst, 1986; De Mateos-Verchere et al., 1998), reduction of pentobarbital-induced sleeping time and drinking (Dong et al., 1999; Manabe et al., 2001), or through a metabotropic receptor, i.e., inhibition of food intake (Do Rego et al., 2007). Similarly, at the cellular level, the diverse effects of ODN are mediated either through CBR, i.e., stimulation of glial cell and neuroblast proliferation (Gandolfo et al., 1999; Alfonso et al., 2012) and activation of neurosteroid biosynthesis (Do Rego et al., 2001), or through a metabotropic receptor, i.e., increase of intracellular calcium concentration in astrocytes

**Abbreviations:** AC, adenylyl cyclase; CBR, central-type benzodiazepine receptors; CREB, cAMP-responsive element-binding protein; DBI, diazepam-binding inhibitor; GADPH, glyceraldehyde-3-phosphate dehydrogenase; $H_2O_2$, hydrogen peroxide; ODN, octadecaneuropeptide; PBS, phosphate buffered saline; PKA, protein kinase A; PKC, protein kinase C; PLC, phospholipase C; ROS, reactive oxygen species; SOD, superoxide dismutase.

(Leprince et al., 2001) and modulation of neuropeptide expression in neurons (Compère et al., 2003, 2004).

Oxidative stress, resulting from excessive production of reactive oxygen species (ROS), such as hydrogen peroxide ($H_2O_2$), is implicated in the pathology of several neurological disorders including cerebral ischemia and neurodegenerative diseases (Garcia et al., 2012; Hayashi et al., 2012). An excess of $H_2O_2$ induces imbalance in ROS generation, impairs cellular antioxidant defences and finally triggers cell death by apoptosis (Emerit et al., 2004; Shibata and Kobayashi, 2008). It is well known that astroglial cells contain high levels of ROS scavenger molecules such as glutathione (Dringen et al., 1999) and the antioxidant enzymes Mn- and Cu,Zn-superoxide dismutases (Mn- and Cu,Zn-SOD), catalase and glutathione peroxidase (Lindenau et al., 2000; Sokolova et al., 2001; Saha and Pahan, 2007). Nonetheless, astroglial cells can be affected, in terms of viability and functionality, by an insurmountable oxidative stress (Ferrero-Gutierrez et al., 2008; Park et al., 2009). In particular, it has been shown that inhibition of SOD and/or catalase activities in cultured astrocytes is associated with an exacerbation of oxidative damages induced by $H_2O_2$ or hypoxia (Desagher et al., 1996; Bi et al., 2008; Li et al., 2008). Reciprocally, cultured astrocytes derived from Cu,Zn-SOD-overexpressing transgenic mice exhibit increased resistance to oxidative stress (Chen et al., 2001; Wang et al., 2005). However, little is known regarding the endogenous factors that modulate glial antioxidant systems. In this context, we have previously reported that, in cultured astrocytes, ODN exerts a potent protective effect against oxidative stress-induced apoptosis, and attenuates $H_2O_2$-evoked inhibition of SOD and catalase activities (Hamdi et al., 2011). More recently, we have shown that the anti-apoptotic activity of ODN is mediated through the metabotropic endozepine receptor (Hamdi et al., 2012). In contrast, regarding the effects of ODN on endogenous antioxidant systems, the receptor and the signaling mechanism are currently unknown. The purpose of the present study was thus to examine the effects of ODN on SOD and catalase gene expression and to determine the type of receptor involved in the antioxidant action of ODN on astroglial cells.

## MATERIALS AND METHODS

### ANIMALS

All experiments were performed in accordance with American Veterinary Medical Association. Approval for these experiments was obtained from the Medical Ethical Committee for the Care and Use of Laboratory Animals of Pasteur Institute of Tunis (approval number: FST/LNFP/Pro 152012).

### REAGENTS

Dulbecco's modified Eagle's medium (DMEM), F12 culture medium, D(+)-glucose, L-glutamine, *N*-2-hydroxyethylpiperazine-*N*-2-ethane sulfonic acid (HEPES), fetal bovine serum (FBS), the antibiotic-antimycotic solution, and trypsin-EDTA were obtained from Gibco (Invitrogen, Grand Island NY, USA). Bovine liver catalase, chelerythrine, DL-epinephrine, H89, Triton X-100, and insulin were purchased from Sigma Aldrich (St. Louis, MO, USA). Flumazenil was a generous gift from Hoffmann-La Roche (Basel, Switzerland). Rat ODN and the G protein-coupled receptor antagonist cyclo$_{1-8}$[DLeu$^5$]OP were synthesized by using the standard Fmoc procedure, as previously described (Leprince et al., 2001). All other reagents were of A grade purity.

### SECONDARY CULTURES OF RAT CORTICAL ASTROCYTES

Secondary cultures of rat cortical astrocytes were prepared as previously described (Castel et al., 2006). Briefly, cerebral hemispheres from newborn Wistar rats were collected in DMEM/F12 (2:1; v/v) culture medium supplemented with 2 mM glutamine, 1% insulin, 5 mM HEPES, 0.4% glucose, and 1% of the antibiotic-antimycotic solution. Dissociated cells were resuspended in culture medium supplemented with 10% FBS, plated in 175-cm$^2$ flasks (Greiner Bio-one GmbH, Frickenhausen, Germany), and incubated at 37°C in a 5% $CO_2$/95% $O_2$ atmosphere. When cultures were confluent, astrocytes were isolated by shaking overnight the flasks with an orbital agitator and plated on 35-mm Petri dishes at a density of $0.3 \times 10^6$ cells/ml. All experiments were performed on 5- to 7-day-old secondary cultures.

### QUANTITATIVE RT-PCR ANALYSIS

Cultured cells were incubated at 37°C with fresh serum-free medium. At the end of the incubation, the culture medium was removed and the cells were washed twice with phosphate buffered saline (PBS; 0.1 M, pH 7.4). Total RNA was extracted by using Tri reagent (Sigma, St Quentin Fallavier, France) and purified using the NucleoSpin kit (Macherey-Nagel, Hoerd, France). cDNA was synthetized from 3–4 μg of total RNA with ImProm II Promega kit (Promega). Quantitative RT-PCR was performed on cDNA in the presence of a 1× Fast SYBR Green universal PCR Master mix (Applied Biosystems, Courtaboeuf, France) containing concentrations of dNTPs, $MgCl_2$, SYBR green reporter dye, AmpliTaq Gold DNA polymerase, and forward (5′-CCTTCTTGTTCTGCAACC-TGCTA-3′) and reverse (5′-CCGGACTCTCCGGTATCTGA-3′) SOD (GenBank accession no. NM_012880) primers, or forward (5′-CCACAGTCGCTGGAGAGTCA-3′) and reverse (5′-GTTTC-CCACAAGGTCCCAGTT-3′) catalase (GenBank accession no. NM_012520) primers, or forward (5′-CAGCCTCGTCTCATAGA-CAAGATG-3′) and reverse (5′- CAATGTCCACTTTGTCACAAG-AGAA-3′) glyceraldehyde-3-phosphate dehydrogenase (GADPH, GenBank accession no. NM_017008) primers (300 nM, each; Proligo, Paris, France), using the ABI Prism 7000 sequence detection system (Applied Biosystems). The amount of SOD and catalase cDNA in each sample was calculated by the comparative threshold cycle (Ct) method and expressed as $2^{-\Delta\Delta Ct}$ using GADPH as an internal control.

### MEASUREMENT OF ANTIOXIDANT ENZYME ACTIVITIES

Cultured cells were incubated at 37°C with fresh serum-free medium. At the end of the incubation, cells were washed twice with PBS and total cellular proteins were extracted by using the lysis buffer containing 50 mM Tris–HCl (pH 8.0), 10 mM EDTA, 100 μM phenylmethylsulfonyl fluoride, and 1% Triton X-100. The homogenate was centrifuged (16,000 *g*, 4°C, 20 min) and the cellular extract contained in the supernatant was stored at −20°C until enzyme activity determinations.

The activity of SOD was measured using a spectrophotometric assay, which consists in measuring epinephrine autoxidation induced by superoxide anion. Samples, prepared as described above, were incubated for 3 min with a mixture containing bovine catalase (0.4 U/μl), DL-epinephrine (5 mg/ml), and $Na_2CO_3/NaHCO_3$ buffer (62.5 mM, pH 10.2). The oxidation of epinephrine was measured at 480 nm with a Bio-Rad spectrophotometer (Bio-Rad Laboratories, Philadelphia, PA, USA).

The activity of catalase was determined on the basis of the decrease of $H_2O_2$. Samples, prepared as described above, were mixed with 30 mM $H_2O_2$ in PBS. The disappearance of $H_2O_2$ was measured at 240 nm for 180 s at 30 s intervals. Catalase activity was calculated using the extinction coefficient of 40/mM/cm for $H_2O_2$.

### STATISTICAL ANALYSIS

Data are presented as the mean ± SEM from three independent experiments performed in quadruplicate. Statistical analysis of the data was performed by using Student's *t*-test, ANOVA, followed by Bonferroni's test, and two-way ANOVA test. A *p*-value of 0.05 or less was considered as statistically significant.

## RESULTS

### ODN INCREASES SOD AND CATALASE mRNA LEVELS IN CULTURED ASTROCYTES

We have previously shown that picomolar concentrations of ODN suppress the inhibitory effects of 300 μM $H_2O_2$ on SOD and catalase activities in cultured rat astrocytes (Hamdi et al., 2011). To explore the mechanism involved in the effect of ODN on antioxidant enzyme systems we monitored SOD and catalase gene expression by quantitative PCR. Time-course experiments revealed that ODN (0.1 nM) significantly enhanced SOD and catalase mRNA levels within 2 min with a maximum effect after 10 min and 5 min of incubation, respectively (**Figure 1A**). Thereafter, the stimulatory effect of ODN on SOD and catalase expression gradually declined and vanished 60 and 30 min after the onset of ODN administration, respectively. Exposure of astrocytes to increasing concentrations of ODN (0.01 pM to 0.1 nM) induced a concentration-dependent increase of SOD and catalase mRNA levels (**Figure 1A**, inset). In contrast, incubation of astrocytes with graded concentrations of $H_2O_2$ (100–500 μM) dose-dependently decreased both SOD and catalase mRNA levels (**Figure 1B**). We next examined the effects of ODN/$H_2O_2$ co-incubation on enzyme expression. For moderate concentrations of $H_2O_2$ (100–300 μM), ODN (0.1 nM) restored SOD and catalase mRNA levels above control, whereas for higher concentrations of $H_2O_2$ (400 and 500 μM), ODN only partially prevented the decrease of SOD and catalase gene expression (**Figure 1B**).

### ODN BLOCKS $H_2O_2$-EVOKED INHIBITION OF SOD AND CATALASE mRNA LEVELS AND ACTIVITIES THROUGH ACTIVATION OF A METABOTROPIC RECEPTOR COUPLED TO THE PKA PATHWAY

We next examined the type of receptor of ODN involved in the stimulatory effects of ODN on endogenous antioxidant systems. Administration of the selective metabotropic receptor antagonist cyclo$_{1-8}$[DLeu$^5$]OP (1 μM) to cultured astrocytes did not induce any modification of SOD and catalase mRNA levels and activities, but totally abolished the effects of 0.1 nM ODN on $H_2O_2$-evoked inhibition of antioxidant enzyme gene transcription and activities. In contrast, the CBR antagonist flumazenil (1 μM) did not affect the protective action of ODN against the deleterious effect of $H_2O_2$ on endogenous antioxidant systems (**Figures 2A,B**).

Incubation of astrocytes with the selective protein kinase A (PKA) inhibitor H89 (20 μM) abrogated the effect of ODN on the inhibitory action of $H_2O_2$ on SOD and catalase mRNA levels and activities. In contrast, administration of the protein kinase C (PKC) inhibitor chelerythrine (0.1 μM) did not modify the effects of ODN (**Figures 3A,B**), indicating that only the PKA pathway is involved in the protective activity of ODN.

## DISCUSSION

Alteration of endogenous antioxidant systems, especially decrease of SOD and catalase activities, causes exacerbation of oxidative damages leading to apoptosis in various cell types, including astroglial cells (Giffard and Swanson, 2005; Lopez et al., 2007; Bi et al., 2008). Here, we demonstrate that ODN prevents the decrease of SOD and catalase mRNA levels and activities induced by $H_2O_2$ in cultured astrocytes, through activation of a metabotropic receptor positively coupled to the AC/PKA signaling pathway.

We have previously reported that, in cultured astrocytes, ODN at very low concentrations (in the picomolar range) stimulates SOD and catalase activities (Hamdi et al., 2011). The present study shows that, in the same range of concentrations, ODN induces a dose-dependent increase of SOD and catalase mRNA levels in cultured astroglial cells, indicating that ODN regulates not only enzyme activity but also gene transcription. Although SOD and catalase genes exhibit hallmarks of typical housekeeping genes, it has been shown that their promoters encompass consensus sequences for regulatory elements such as metal-responsive element, antioxidant responsive element, glucocorticoid-response element, and nuclear factor-κB (Nenoi et al., 2001; Zhu et al., 2001; Zelko et al., 2002), suggesting that these genes are actually regulated in the CNS. As a matter of fact, SOD and catalase gene expression is selectively increased by inflammatory mediators such as interleukin-1β, interferon (IFN)-γ, IFN-β, or lipopolysaccharides in astrocytes (Mokuno et al., 1994; Kifle et al., 1996; Vergara et al., 2010). Previous data have shown that ODN is specifically produced by astroglial cells (Tonon et al., 1990; Malagon et al., 1993; Compère et al., 2010) and that its release is regulated by various factors including agonists of formyl peptide receptors (Tokay et al., 2008) which are involved in inflammation. These observations suggest that ODN may act as an autocrine factor to finely regulate SOD and catalase gene expression in the brain.

Kinetic experiments indicate that the action of ODN on antioxidant enzyme gene transcription is very rapid but transient. Nevertheless, ODN exerts a protective effect against $H_2O_2$-reduced SOD and catalase mRNA levels. Similar time-response curves have already been observed on SOD and catalase activities, in cultured astrocytes (Hamdi et al., 2011). These data suggest that

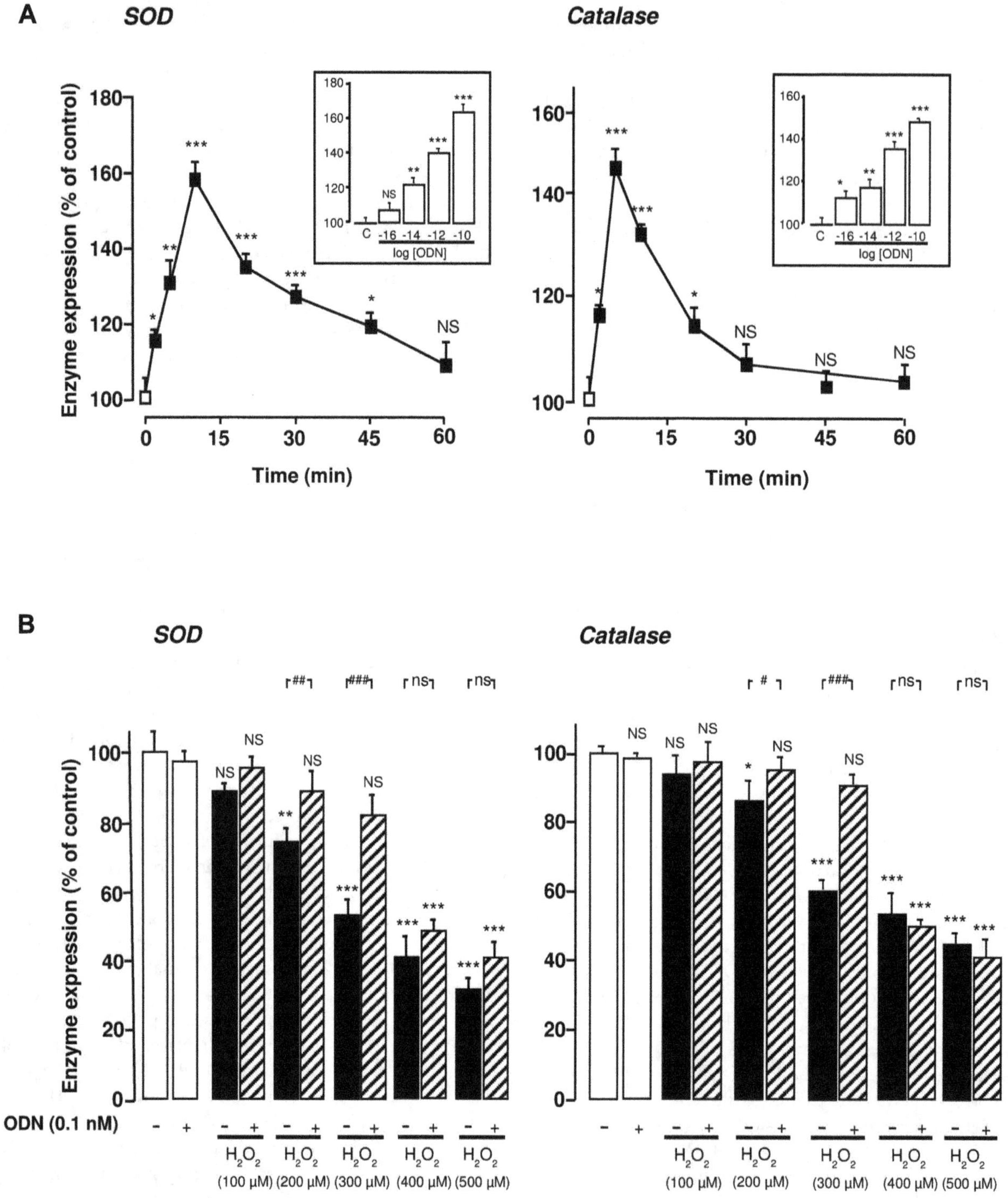


**FIGURE 1 | Protective effects of ODN against $H_2O_2$-evoked inhibition of SOD and catalase mRNA levels in cultured rat astrocytes. (A)** Effects of ODN on SOD and catalase mRNA levels. Astrocytes were incubated in the absence or presence of ODN (0.1 nM) for the times indicated. Inset, cells were treated for 10 min with increasing concentrations of ODN (0.01 pM to 0.1 nM). SOD and catalase mRNA levels were measured by quantitative RT-PCR. Data were corrected using the GAPDH signal as an internal control and the results are expressed as a percentage of controls. Each value is the mean (±SEM) of at least four different wells from three independent experiments. ANOVA followed by the Bonferroni's test. $^{*}p < 0.05$; $^{**}p < 0.01$; $^{***}p < 0.001$; NS, not statistically different vs. control. **(B)** Effects of ODN on $H_2O_2$-evoked inhibition of SOD and catalase mRNA levels. Cells were pre-incubated for 10 min in the absence or presence of 0.1 nM ODN, and then incubated for 1 h with medium alone or with graded concentrations of $H_2O_2$ (100–500 μM) in the absence or presence of ODN. The results are expressed as a percentage of control. Each value is the mean (±SEM) of at least four different wells from three independent experiments. Analyses similar to those in **(A)** were performed and symbols show the significance vs. $H_2O_2$-treated cells: $^{\#}p < 0.05$; $^{\#\#}p < 0.01$; $^{\#\#\#}p < 0.001$; ns, not statistically different.

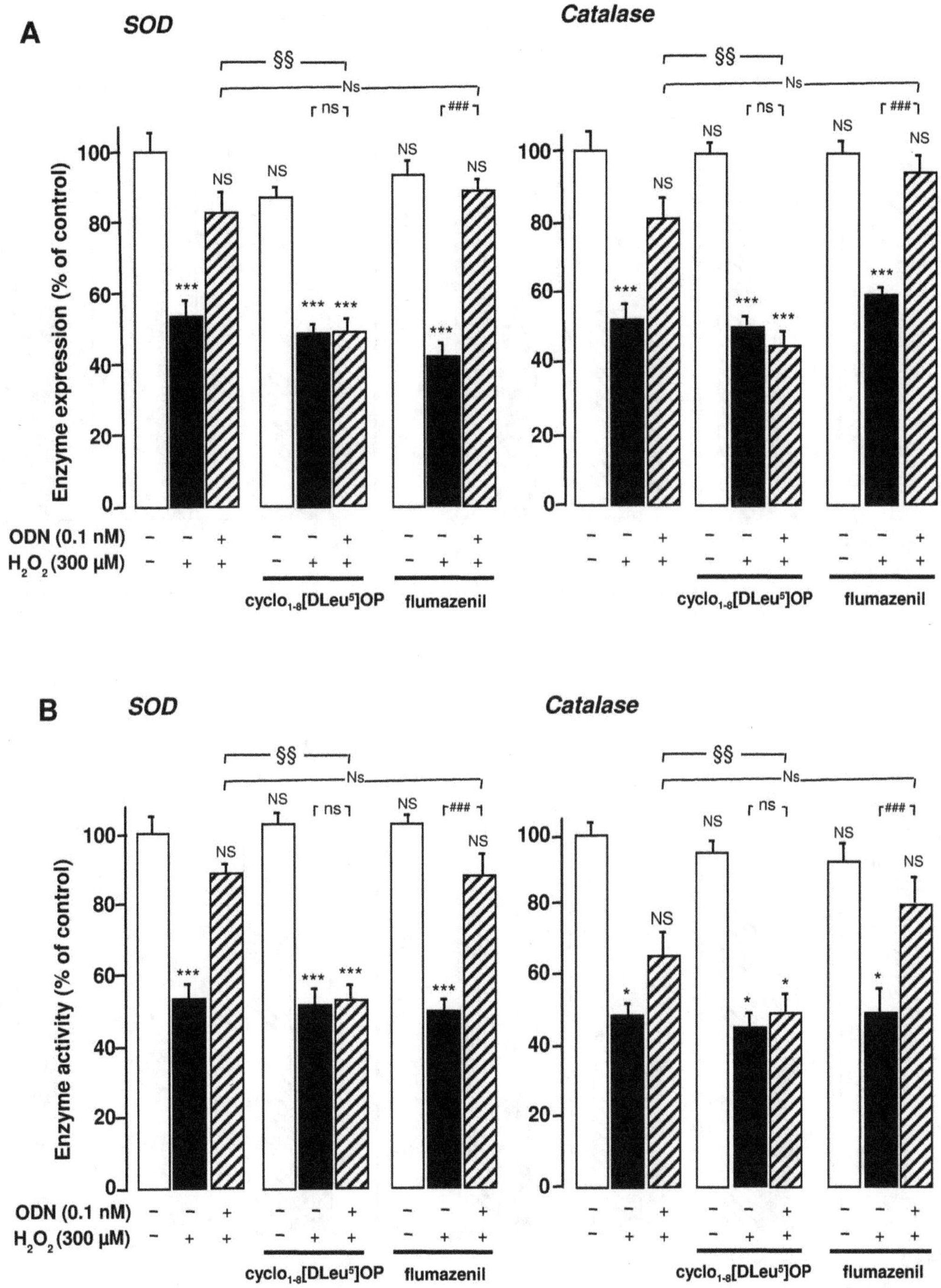


**FIGURE 2 | Involvement of the G protein-coupled receptor of ODN in its protective effects against the deleterious action of $H_2O_2$ on SOD and catalase in cultured rat astrocytes.** Astrocytes were pre-incubated for 30 min in the absence or presence of the metabotropic receptor antagonist cyclo$_{1-8}$ [Dleu$^5$] OP (1 μM) or the CBR antagonist flumazenil (1 μM) and then incubated for 1 h with medium alone or with 300 μM $H_2O_2$ without or with ODN (0.1 nM). **(A)** SOD and catalase mRNA levels were quantified as described in Figure 1. The results are expressed as a percentage of control. Each value is the mean (±SEM) of at least three different wells from three independent experiments. **(B)** The activity of SOD was measured using a spectrophotometric assay which consists in measuring epinephrine autoxidation induced by superoxide anion, and catalase activity was determined on the basis of the decomposition of $H_2O_2$. The results are expressed as a percentage of SOD or catalase activity with respect to control. Each value is the mean (±SEM) of at least four different dishes from three independent experiments. ANOVA followed by the Bonferroni's test: [(**A**, SOD) $F = 7.69$, $df = 40$; (**A**, catalase) $F = 8.58$, $df = 39$; (**B**, SOD) $F = 13.41$, $df = 44$; (**B**, catalase) $F = 7.58$, $df = 44$]; $^{*}p < 0.05$; $^{***}p < 0.001$; NS, not statistically different vs. control. $^{###}p < 0.001$; ns, not statistically different vs. $H_2O_2$-treated cells. Two-way ANOVA test: [(**A**, SOD) $F = 5$, $df = 17$; (**A**, catalase) $F = 8.13$, $df = 17$; (**B**, SOD) $F = 5.87$, $df = 20$; (**B**, catalase) $F = 2.79$, $df = 19$]; $^{§}p < 0.05$; $^{§§}p < 0.01$; Ns, not statistically different vs. ODN + $H_2O_2$-cotreated cells.

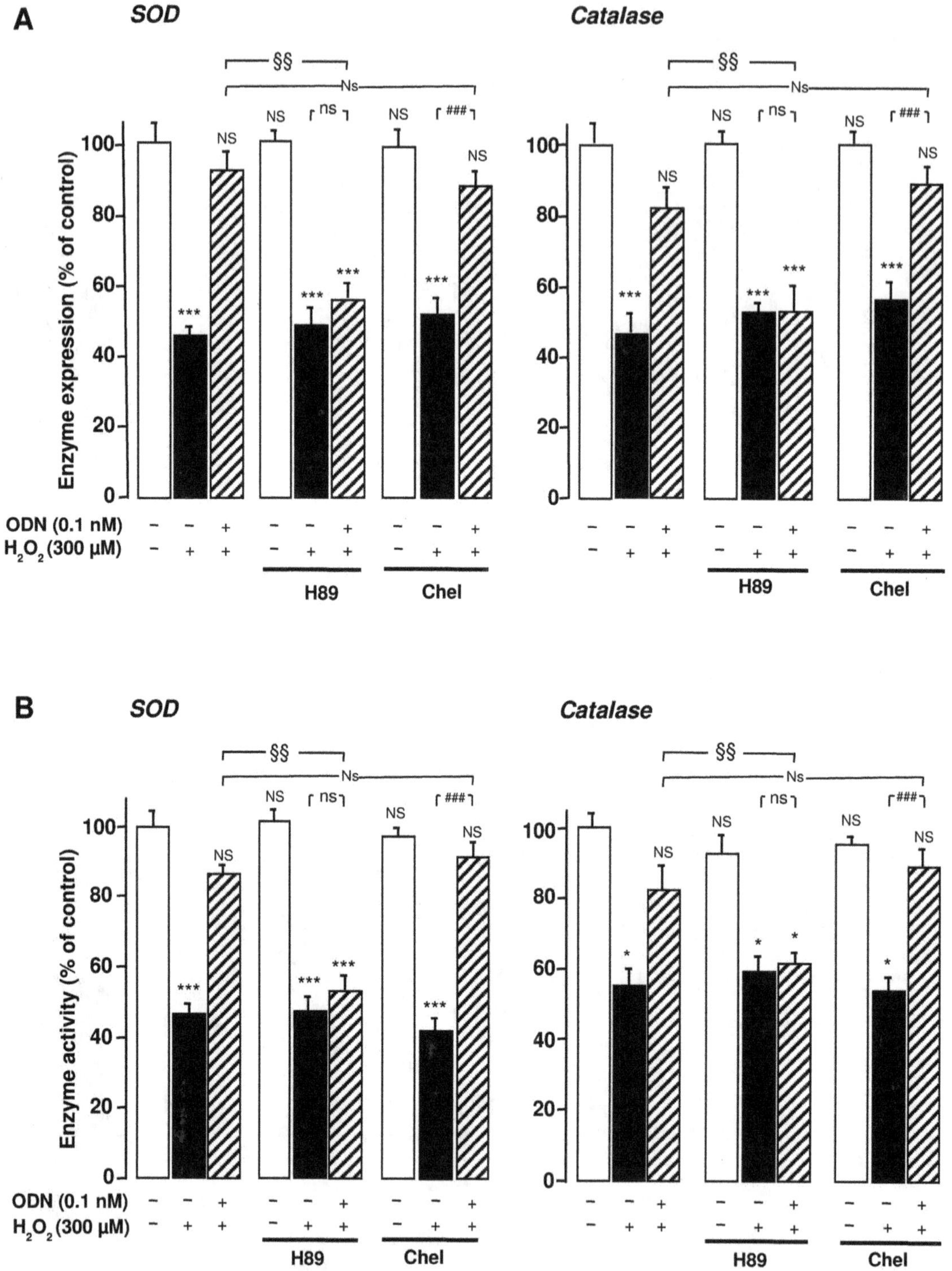


**FIGURE 3 | Protein kinase A-dependence of the protective effects of ODN on the expression and activities of SOD and catalase in cultured rat astrocytes.** Astrocytes were pre-treated for 30 min in the absence or presence of the PKA inhibitor H89 (20 μM) or the PKC inhibitor chelerythrine (Chel; 0.1 μM) and then incubated for 1 h with medium alone or with 300 μM $H_2O_2$ without or with ODN (0.1 nM). **(A)** SOD and catalase mRNA levels were quantified as described in Figure 1. The results are expressed as a percentage of controls. Each value is the mean (±SEM) of at least three different wells from three independent experiments. **(B)** The activity of SOD and catalase were quantified as described in Figure 2. The results are expressed as a percentage of SOD or catalase activity with respect to control. Each value is the mean (±SEM) of at least four different dishes from three independent experiments. ANOVA followed by the Bonferroni's test: [(**A**, SOD) $F = 7.49$, $df = 65$; (**A**, catalase) $F = 5.08$, $df = 53$; (**B**, SOD) $F = 12.37$, $df = 55$; (**B**, catalase) $F = 9.06$, $df = 60$]; $^{*}p < 0.05$; $^{***}p < 0.001$; NS, not statistically different vs. control. $^{###}p < 0.001$; ns, not statistically different vs. $H_2O_2$-treated cells. Two-way ANOVA test: [(**A**, SOD) $F = 2.40$, $df = 20$; (**A**, catalase) $F = 2.63$, $df = 17$; (**B**, SOD) $F = 6.97$, $df = 18$; (**B**, catalase) $F = 4.68$, $df = 24$]; $^{§}p < 0.05$; $^{§§}p < 0.01$; Ns, not statistically different vs. ODN + $H_2O_2$-cotreated cells.

ODN-induced rapid activation of antioxidant systems is required for the long-lasting inhibition of the deleterious effect of $H_2O_2$. That ODN-induced increase of transcription and activity of antioxidant enzymes is responsible, at least in part, for inhibition of cell death is consistent with previous data showing that SOD and catalase blockers suppress the protective effect of ODN against $H_2O_2$-induced astrocyte apoptosis (Hamdi et al., 2011). Furthermore, it has been reported that, in cultured astrocytes, overexpression of SOD is able to prevent ROS-induced alteration of mitochondrial integrity, caspase-3 activation and thus cells apoptosis (Yang et al., 2008).

Previous studies have shown that, in cultured astrocytes, ODN can interact with either CBR associated with the $GABA_A$ receptor (Gandolfo et al., 1999) or with a G protein-coupled receptor positively coupled to PLC (Patte et al., 1995; Leprince et al., 2001). Here, we found that the inhibitory effects of ODN on $H_2O_2$-evoked reduction of SOD and catalase mRNA levels and activities were suppressed by the ODN analog cyclo$_{1-8}$[DLeu$^5$]OP but were not affected by the specific CBR antagonist flumazenil. It has been reported that the cyclic analog of ODN exerts potent antagonistic activities on ODN-induced polyphosphoinositide turnover increase and intracellular calcium mobilization in rat astrocytes (Leprince et al., 2001). Thus, these data indicate that the antioxidant action of ODN is mediated through the activation of the G protein-coupled receptor.

We next investigated the signaling cascade involved in the effect of ODN on endogenous antioxidant systems. ODN blockage of $H_2O_2$-evoked inhibition of SOD and catalase gene transcription and enzyme activities was totally abrogated by the PKA inhibitor H89, while the PKC inhibitor chelerythrine had no effect. That, the ODN G protein-coupled receptor could stimulate the AC/PKA transduction cascade is in agreement with recent data indicating that ODN increases the production of cAMP in astrocytes (Hamdi et al., 2012). Altogether, these observations indicate that the antioxidant action of ODN against $H_2O_2$-induced oxidative stress can be specifically ascribed to the activation of the AC/PKA signaling pathway. Consistent with this notion, it has been shown that the SOD and catalase promoters contain a cAMP-responsive element-like sequence (Das et al., 1995; Zelko et al., 2002; Colombo and Moncada, 2009) and that siRNA knockdown of cAMP-responsive element-binding protein (CREB) or inhibition of CREB phosphorylation blocks the expression of SOD in the rat hypothalamus (Hsieh et al., 2008) and the expression of catalase in human vascular endothelial cells (Colombo and Moncada, 2009), respectively. The fact that ODN provokes ERK phosphorylation via a cAMP-dependent pathway in astrocytes (Hamdi et al., 2012), strongly suggests that the stimulatory effect of ODN on SOD and catalase expression can also be ascribed to activation of the ERK-type MAP kinase transduction pathway.

The protective effect of ODN against $H_2O_2$-reduced antioxidant enzyme expression and activities might have a physiopathological significance in neurodegenerative diseases and stroke. CNS is sensitive to oxidative stress due to its high metabolic rate and high levels of unsaturated lipids so that up-regulation of antioxidant enzyme systems in astroglial cells could be beneficial against cell death observed during and after ischemia and neurodegenerative diseases. In agreement with this hypothesis, we have recently shown that the endozepine ODN exerts a potent protective action against apoptosis induced by oxidative stress in astrocytes (Hamdi et al., 2011, 2012) and that the anti-apoptotic effect of ODN is attributable to activation of the antioxidant enzymes that act as scavengers of $H_2O_2$ and ROS (Hamdi et al., 2011). The fact that the glioprotective action of ODN is likely mediated through the metabotropic receptor is of particular interest. Previous data indicate that ODN induces a wide range of activities through activation of CBR (Tonon et al., 2006). In particular, ODN has been initially described as an anxiogenic peptide (De Mateos-Verchere et al., 1998). Since cyclic analog of ODN do not recognize CBR (Leprince et al., 2001), the development of specific cyclic agonists that would selectively mimic the glioprotective effect of ODN might prove useful for the treatment of ischemia and neurodegenerative diseases.

In conclusion, the present study has demonstrated that the endozepine ODN, acting through a metabotropic receptor sensitive to the cyclo$_{1-8}$[DLeu$^5$]OP antagonist, exerts a potent antioxidant action against $H_2O_2$-induced oxidative stress in astrocytes. This antioxidant effect of ODN is attributable to activation of both gene expression and activities of enzymatic antioxidant systems and can be ascribed to the stimulation of the AC/PKA transduction pathway.

## ACKNOWLEDGMENTS

Yosra Hamdi and Hadhemi Kaddour were recipients of fellowships from the University of Tunis El Manar and a France-Tunisia exchange program CMCU-Utique. Seyma Bahdoudi and Salma Douiri were recipients of fellowships from the University of Tunis El Manar and a France-Tunisia exchange program Inserm-DGRS. This study was supported by the Research Unit UR/11ES09, a CMCU-Utique program (to Mohamed Amri and Marie-Christine Tonon; grant number 07G0822), an Inserm-DGRS program (to Mohamed Amri and Marie-Christine Tonon; grant number M 10/M), Inserm (U982), the Institute for Medical Research and Innovation (IRIB) and the Région Haute-Normandie.

## REFERENCES

Alfonso, J., Le Magueresse, C., Zuccotti, A., Khodosevich, K., and Monyer, H. (2012). Diazepam binding inhibitor promotes progenitor proliferation in the postnatal SVZ by reducing GABA signaling. *Cell Stem Cell* 10, 76–87.

Bi, J., Jiang, B., Liu, J. H., Lei, C., Zhang, X. L., and An, L. J. (2008). Protective effects of catalpol against $H_2O_2$-induced oxidative stress in astrocytes primary cultures. *Neurosci. Lett.* 442, 224–227.

Burgi, B., Lichtensteiger, W., Lauber, M. E., and Schlumpf, M. (1999). Ontogeny of diazepam binding inhibitor/-acyl-CoA binding protein mRNA and peripheral benzodiazepine receptor mRNA expression in the rat. *J. Neuroendocrinol.* 11, 85–100.

Castel, H., Diallo, M., Chatenet, D., Leprince, J., Desrues, L., Schouft, M. T., et al. (2006). Biochemical and functional characterization of high-affinity urotensin II receptors in rat cortical astrocytes. *J. Neurochem.* 99, 582–595.

Chen, Y., Chan, P. H., and Swanson, R. A. (2001). Astrocytes overexpressing Cu,Zn superoxide dismutase have increased resistance to oxidative injury. *Glia* 33, 343–347.

Colombo, S. L., and Moncada, S. (2009). AMPKα1 regulates the antioxidant status of vascular endothelial cells. *Biochem. J.* 421, 163–169.

Compère, V., Lanfray, D., Castel, H., Morin, F., Leprince, J., Dureuil, B., et al. (2010). Acute food deprivation reduces expression of diazepam-binding inhibitor, the precursor of the anorexigenic octadecaneuropeptide ODN, in mouse glial cells. *J. Mol. Endocrinol.* 44, 295–299.

Compère, V., Li, S., Leprince, J., Tonon, M. C., Vaudry, H., and Pelletier, G. (2003). Effect of intracerebroventricular administration of the octadecaneuropeptide on the expression of pro-opiomelanocortin, neuropeptide Y and corticotropin-releasing hormone mRNAs in rat hypothalamus. *J. Neuroendocrinol.* 15, 197–203.

Compère, V., Li, S., Leprince, J., Tonon, M. C., Vaudry, H., and Pelletier, G. (2004). *In vivo* action of a new octadecaneuropeptide (ODN) antagonist on gonadotropin-releasing hormone gene expression in the male rat brain. *Neuroscience* 125, 411–415.

Das, K. C., Lewis-Molock, Y., and White, C. W. (1995). Activation of NF-κB and elevation of MnSOD gene expression by thiol reducing agents in lung adenocarcinoma (A549) cells. *Am. J. Physiol.* 269, L588–L602.

De Mateos-Verchere, J. G., Leprince, J., Tonon, M. C., Vaudry, H., and Costentin, J. (1998). The octadecaneuropeptide ODN induces anxiety in rodents: possible involvement of a shorter biologically active fragment. *Peptides* 19, 841–848.

Desagher, S., Glowinski, J., and Premont, J. (1996). Astrocytes protect neurons from hydrogen peroxide toxicity. *J. Neurosci.* 16, 2553–2562.

Do Rego, J. L., Mensah-Nyagan, A. G., Beaujean, D., Leprince, J., Tonon, M. C., Luu-The, V., et al. (2001). The octadecaneuropeptide ODN stimulates neurosteroid biosynthesis through activation of central-type benzodiazepine receptors. *J. Neurochem.* 76, 128–138.

Do Rego, J. C., Orta, M. H., Leprince, J., Tonon, M. C., Vaudry, H., and Costentin, J. (2007). Pharmacological characterization of the receptor mediating the anorexigenic action of the octadecaneuropeptide: evidence for an endozepinergic tone regulating food intake. *Neuropsychopharmacology* 32, 1641–1648.

Dong, E., Matsumoto, K., Tohda, M., and Watanabe, H. (1999). Involvement of diazepam binding inhibitor and its fragment octadecaneuropeptide in social isolation stress-induced decrease in pentobarbital sleep in mice. *Life Sci.* 64, 1779–1784.

Dringen, R., Kussmaul, L., Gutterer, J. M., Hirrlinger, J., and Hamprecht, B. (1999). The glutathione system of peroxide detoxification is less efficient in neurons than in astroglial cells. *J. Neurochem.* 72, 2523–2530.

Emerit, J., Edeas, M., and Bricaire, F. (2004). Neurodegenerative diseases and oxidative stress. *Biomed. Pharmacother.* 58, 39–46.

Ferrero-Gutierrez, A., Perez-Gomez, A., Novelli, A., and Fernandez-Sanchez, M. T. (2008). Inhibition of protein phosphatases impairs the ability of astrocytes to detoxify hydrogen peroxide. *Free Radic. Biol. Med.* 44, 1806–1816.

Ferrero, P., Santi, M. R., Conti-Tronconi, B., Costa, E., and Guidotti, A. (1986). Study of an octadecaneuropeptide derived from diazepam binding inhibitor (DBI): biological activity and presence in rat brain. *Proc. Natl. Acad. Sci. U.S.A.* 83, 827–831.

Gandolfo, P., Patte, C., Thoumas, J. L., Leprince, J., Vaudry, H., and Tonon, M. C. (1999). The endozepine ODN stimulates [3H]thymidine incorporation in cultured rat astrocytes. *Neuropharmacology* 38, 725–732.

Garcia, A. G., Rodriguez-Rocha, H., Madayiputhiya, N., Pappa, A., Panayiotidis, M. I., and Franco, R. (2012). Biomarkers of protein oxidation in human disease. *Curr. Mol. Med.* 12, 681–697

Giffard, R. G., and Swanson, R. A. (2005). Ischemia-induced programmed cell death in astrocytes. *Glia* 50, 299–306.

Guidotti, A., Forchetti, C. M., Corda, M. G., Konkel, D., Bennett, C. D., and Costa, E. (1983). Isolation, characterization, and purification to homogeneity of an endogenous polypeptide with agonistic action on benzodiazepine receptors. *Proc. Natl. Acad. Sci. U.S.A.* 80, 3531–3535.

Hamdi, Y., Kaddour, H., Vaudry, D., Bahdoudi, S., Douiri, S., Leprince, J., et al. (2012). The octadecaneuropeptide ODN protects astrocytes against hydrogen peroxide-induced apoptosis via a PKA/MAPK-dependent mechanism. *PLoS ONE* 7: e42498. doi: 10.1371/journal.pone.0042498.

Hamdi, Y., Masmoudi-Kouki, O., Kaddour, H., Belhadj, F., Gandolfo, P., Vaudry, D., et al. (2011). Protective effect of the octadecaneuropeptide on hydrogen peroxide-induced oxidative stress and cell death in cultured rat astrocytes. *J. Neurochem.* 118, 416–428.

Hayashi, M., Miyata, R., and Tanuma, N. (2012). Oxidative stress in developmental brain disorders. *Adv. Exp. Med. Biol.* 724, 278–290.

Hsieh, Y. S., Yang, S. F., Chu, S. C., Ho, Y. J., Kuo, C. S., and Kuo, D. Y. (2008). Transcriptional interruption of cAMP response element binding protein modulates superoxide dismutase and neuropeptide Y-mediated feeding behavior in freely moving rats. *J. Neurochem.* 105, 1438–1449.

Kavaliers, M., and Hirst, M. (1986). An octadecaneuropeptide (ODN) derived from diazepam binding inhibitor increases aggressive interactions in mice. *Brain Res.* 383, 343–349.

Kifle, Y., Monnier, J., Chesrown, S. E., Raizada, M. K., and Nick, H. S. (1996). Regulation of the manganese superoxide dismutase and inducible nitric oxide synthase gene in rat neuronal and glial cells. *J. Neurochem.* 66, 2128–2135.

Leprince, J., Oulyadi, H., Vaudry, D., Masmoudi, O., Gandolfo, P., Patte, C., et al. (2001). Synthesis, conformational analysis and biological activity of cyclic analogs of the octadecaneuropeptide ODN. Design of a potent endozepine antagonist. *Eur. J. Biochem.* 268, 6045–6057.

Li, Y., Bao, Y., Jiang, B., Wang, Z., Liu, Y., Zhang, C., et al. (2008). Catalpol protects primary cultured astrocytes from in vitro ischemia-induced damage. *Int. J. Dev. Neurosci.* 26, 309–317.

Lindenau, J., Noack, H., Possel, H., Asayama, K., and Wolf, G. (2000). Cellular distribution of superoxide dismutases in the rat CNS. *Glia* 29, 25–34.

Lopez, M. V., Cuadrado, M. P., Ruiz-Poveda, O. M., Del Fresno, A. M., and Accame, M. E. (2007). Neuroprotective effect of individual ginsenosides on astrocytes primary culture. *Biochim. Biophys. Acta* 1770, 1308–1316.

Malagon, M., Vaudry, H., Van Strien, F., Pelletier, G., Gracia-Navarro, F., and Tonon, M. C. (1993). Ontogeny of diazepam-binding inhibitor-related peptides (endozepines) in the rat brain. *Neuroscience* 57, 777–786.

Manabe, Y., Toyoda, T., Kuroda, K., Imaizum, M., Yamamoto, T., and Fushiki, T. (2001). Effect of diazepam binding inhibitor (DBI) on the fluid intake, preference and the taste reactivity in mice. *Behav. Brain Res.* 126, 197–204.

Mokuno, K., Ohtani, K., Suzumura, A., Kiyosawa, K., Hirose, Y., Kawai, K., et al. (1994). Induction of manganese superoxide dismutase by cytokines and lipopolysaccharide in cultured mouse astrocytes. *J. Neurochem.* 63, 612–616.

Nenoi, M., Ichimura, S., Mita, K., Yukawa, O., and Cartwright, I. L. (2001). Regulation of the catalase gene promoter by Sp1, CCAAT-recognizing factors, and a WT1/Egr-related factor in hydrogen peroxide-resistant HP100 cells. *Cancer Res.* 61, 5885–5894.

Park, S. J., Kim, H. Y., Kim, H., Park, S. M., Joe, E. H., Jou, I., et al. (2009). Oxidative stress induces lipid-raft-mediated activation of Src homology 2 domain-containing protein-tyrosine phosphatase 2 in astrocytes. *Free Radic. Biol. Med.* 46, 1694–1702.

Patte, C., Vaudry, H., Desrues, L., Gandolfo, P., Strijdveen, I., Lamacz, M., et al. (1995). The endozepine ODN stimulates polyphosphoinositide metabolism in rat astrocytes. *FEBS Lett.* 362, 106–110.

Saha, R. N., and Pahan, K. (2007). Differential regulation of Mn-superoxide dismutase in neurons and astroglia by HIV-1 gp120: implications for HIV-associated dementia. *Free Radic. Biol. Med.* 42, 1866–1878.

Shibata, N., and Kobayashi, M. (2008). The role for oxidative stress in neurodegenerative diseases. *Brain Nerve* 60, 157–170.

Sokolova, T., Gutterer, J. M., Hirrlinger, J., Hamprecht, B., and Dringen, R. (2001). Catalase in astroglia-rich primary cultures from rat brain: immunocytochemical localization and inactivation during the disposal of hydrogen peroxide. *Neurosci. Lett.* 297, 129–132.

Tokay, T., Hachem, R., Masmoudi-Kouki, O., Gandolfo, P., Desrues, L., Leprince, J., et al.(2008). Beta-amyloid peptide stimulates endozepine release in cultured rat astrocytes through activation of *N*-formyl peptide receptors. *Glia* 56, 1380–1389.

Tonon, M. C., Desy, L., Nicolas, P., Vaudry, H., and Pelletier, G. (1990). Immunocytochemical localization of the endogenous benzodiazepine ligand octadecaneuropeptide (ODN) in the rat brain. *Neuropeptides* 15, 17–24.

Tonon, M. C., Leprince, J., Gandolfo, P., Compère, V., Pelletier, G., Malagon, M. M., et al. (2006). "Endozepines" in *Handbook of Biologically Active Peptides*, ed. A. J. Kastin (New York: Elsevier), 813–819.

Vergara, D., Martignago, R., Bonsegna, S., De Nuccio, F., Santino, A., Nicolardi, G., et al. (2010). IFN-beta reverses the lipopolysaccharide-induced proteome modifications in treated astrocytes. *J. Neuroimmunol.* 221, 115–120.

Wang, J., Ma, J. H., and Giffard, R. G. (2005). Overexpression of copper/zinc superoxide dismutase decreases ischemia-like astrocyte injury. *Free Radic. Biol. Med.* 38, 1112–1118.

Yang, C. S., Tzou, B. C., Liu, Y. P., Tsai, M. J., Shyue, S. K., and Tzeng, S. F. (2008). Inhibition of cadmium-induced oxidative injury in rat primary astrocytes by the addition of antioxidants and the reduction of intracellular calcium. *J. Cell. Biochem.* 103, 825–834.

Zelko, I. N., Mariani, T. J., and Folz, R. J. (2002). Superoxide dismutase multigene family: a comparison of the CuZn-SOD (SOD1), Mn-SOD (SOD2), and EC-SOD (SOD3) gene structures, evolution, and expression. *Free Radic. Biol. Med.* 33, 337–349.

Zhu, C. H., Huang, Y., Oberley, L. W., and Domann, F. E. (2001). A family of AP-2 proteins down-regulate manganese superoxide dismutase expression. *J. Biol. Chem.* 276, 14407–14413.

# 8

# Activation of PAC1 receptors in rat cerebellar granule cells stimulates both calcium mobilization from intracellular stores and calcium influx through N-type calcium channels

**Magali Basille-Dugay[1,2,3,4], Hubert Vaudry[1,2,3,4], Alain Fournier[4,5], Bruno Gonzalez[2,6] and David Vaudry[1,2,3,4]***

[1] INSERM U982, Laboratory of Neuronal and Neuroendocrine Differentiation and Communication, University of Rouen, Mont-Saint-Aignan, France
[2] Institute for Research and Innovation in Biomedicine, University of Rouen, Mont-Saint-Aignan, France
[3] PRIMACEN, University of Rouen, Mont-Saint-Aignan, France
[4] International Associated Laboratory Samuel de Champlain, University of Rouen, Mont-Saint-Aignan, France
[5] Institut National de la Recherche Scientifique-Institut Armand Frappier, University of Québec, Laval, QC, Canada
[6] Région INSERM ERI28, Laboratory of Microvascular Endothelium and Neonate Lesions, University of Rouen, Rouen, France

**Edited by:**
*Jae Young Seong, Korea University, South Korea*

**Reviewed by:**
*Hitoshi Hashimoto, Osaka University, Japan*
*Dora Reglodi, University of Pecs, Hungary*

***Correspondence:**
*David Vaudry, INSERM U982, Laboratory of Neuronal and Neuroendocrine Differentiation and Communication, International Associated Laboratory Samuel de Champlain, University of Rouen, 76821 Mont-Saint-Aignan, Rouen, France.*
*e-mail: david.vaudry@univ-rouen.fr*

High concentrations of pituitary adenylate cyclase-activating polypeptide (PACAP) and a high density of PACAP binding sites have been detected in the developing rat cerebellum. In particular, PACAP receptors are actively expressed in immature granule cells, where they activate both adenylyl cyclase and phospholipase C. The aim of the present study was to investigate the ability of PACAP to induce calcium mobilization in cerebellar granule neurons. Administration of PACAP-induced a transient, rapid, and monophasic rise of the cytosolic calcium concentration ($[Ca^{2+}]_i$), while vasoactive intestinal peptide was devoid of effect, indicating the involvement of the PAC1 receptor in the $Ca^{2+}$ response. Preincubation of granule cells with the $Ca^{2+}$ ATPase inhibitor, thapsigargin, or the D-myo-inositol 1,4,5-trisphosphate ($IP_3$) receptor antagonist, 2-aminoethoxydiphenyl borate, markedly reduced the stimulatory effect of PACAP on $[Ca^{2+}]_i$. Furthermore, addition of the calcium chelator, EGTA, or exposure of cells to the non-selective $Ca^{2+}$ channel blocker, $NiCl_2$, significantly attenuated the PACAP-evoked $[Ca^{2+}]_i$ increase. Preincubation of granule neurons with the N-type $Ca^{2+}$ channel blocker, ω-conotoxin GVIA, decreased the PACAP-induced $[Ca^{2+}]_i$ response, whereas the L-type $Ca^{2+}$ channel blocker, nifedipine, and the P- and Q-type $Ca^{2+}$ channel blocker, ω-conotoxin MVIIC, had no effect. Altogether, these findings indicate that PACAP, acting through PAC1 receptors, provokes an increase in $[Ca^{2+}]_i$ in granule neurons, which is mediated by both mobilization of calcium from $IP_3$-sensitive intracellular stores and activation of N-type $Ca^{2+}$ channel. Some of the activities of PACAP on proliferation, survival, migration, and differentiation of cerebellar granule cells could thus be mediated, at least in part, through these intracellular and/or extracellular calcium fluxes.

**Keywords: pituitary adenylate cyclase-activating polypeptide, cerebellum, granule cells, calcium, cytoplasmic calcium stores, calcium channels, autoradiography**

## INTRODUCTION

Pituitary adenylate cyclase-activating polypeptide (PACAP) is a 38- or 27-amino acid peptide that was isolated from hypothalamic extracts for its ability to stimulate cAMP formation in anterior pituitary cells (Miyata et al., 1989). PACAP belongs to a superfamily of peptides that originate from a common ancestral sequence and have evolved through exon and gene duplications. In particular, PACAP27 exhibits 68% identity with vasoactive intestinal peptide (VIP). The sequence of PACAP has been very well conserved during evolution, suggesting that it may exert vital physiological activities (Vaudry et al., 2009). Indeed, numerous studies have shown that PACAP is widely expressed throughout the body and regulates a large array of biological functions, both in the central nervous system and in peripheral organs (Reglodi et al., 2012).

Three PACAP/VIP receptors, which belong to the class B family of seven-transmembrane G protein-coupled receptors, have been cloned and termed respectively PAC1, VPAC1, and VPAC2, according to their relative affinity for PACAP and VIP (Harmar et al., 2012). PAC1 recognizes PACAP27 and PACAP38 with 1000-fold higher affinity than VIP while, VPAC1 and VPAC2 exhibit similar affinity for both PACAP and VIP (Cauvin et al., 1990). All three receptors can activate a variety of second messengers including cAMP, cGMP, $IP_3$, or calcium, depending on the receptor types, splice variants, G proteins, and other intracellular components expressed by each cell type (Vaudry et al., 2009). This cellular context plays a crucial role in determining the effects of PACAP, as differential expression of PAC1 splice variants is sufficient to

**Abbreviations:** 2APB, 2-aminoethoxydiphenyl borate; $Ca^{2+}$, calcium; $[Ca^{2+}]_i$, intracellular calcium concentration; EGTA, ethylene glycol-bis(β-aminoethylether)-N,N,N′,N′-tetraacetic acid; P, postnatal day; PACAP, pituitary adenylate cyclase-activating polypeptide; PACAP27, 27-amino acid form of PACAP; PACAP38, 38-amino acid form of PACAP; VIP, vasoactive intestinal peptide.

trigger opposite activities on neuronal precursor proliferation (Nicot and DiCicco-Bloom, 2001).

It was initially shown that PACAP can increase calcium ion concentration in pituitary gonadotrope, somatotrope, and somatolactotrope cells (Canny et al., 1992; Gracia-Navarro et al., 1992; Matsuda et al., 2008). PACAP also induces calcium mobilization in chromaffin cells (Watanabe et al., 1992), hippocampal neurons (Tatsuno et al., 1992), folliculo-stellate cells (Yada et al., 1993), and type-2 astrocytes (Tatsuno and Arimura, 1994). Several transduction pathways are clearly involved in the effect of PACAP on calcium fluxes. For instance, in somatotrope cells, PACAP activates calcium mobilization in a cAMP- and protein kinase-A-dependent manner (Rawlings et al., 1993) while in gonadotrope cells, PACAP increases calcium through an inositol trisphosphate-dependent mechanism (Rawlings et al., 1994). Calcium mobilization induced by PACAP is essential for stimulation of acetylcholine (Masuo et al., 1993), catecholamine (Isobe et al., 1993), and insulin (Yada et al., 1994) release. Besides triggering neurosecretion, calcium influx also activates a variety of transcription factors that control gene expression involved in long-lasting changes of neuronal function. For instance, cAMP-dependent calcium mobilization is required for the ability of PACAP to regulate astrocyte differentiation (Cebolla et al., 2008).

In suprachiasmatic neurons, PACAP activates L-type calcium channel conductance by activating the MAPK pathway (Dziema and Obrietan, 2002). In this model, PACAP can either induce transient calcium mobilization (Dziema and Obrietan, 2002) or increase the amplitude and/or frequency of spontaneous calcium spikes (Michel et al., 2006). In cultured granule cells, some studies report that PACAP fails to increase calcium levels (Aoyagi and Takahashi, 2001) while others indicate that PACAP induces calcium mobilization (Mei, 1999). In cerebellar tissue slices, PACAP has no effect on the frequency of calcium transients but decreases the amplitude of calcium oscillations in granule cells (Cameron et al., 2007). Since PACAP exerts important neurodevelopmental and neuroprotective activities in the cerebellum (Botia et al., 2007), and since calcium plays a pivotal role in the control of cell proliferation, migration, and differentiation of granule cells (Sato et al., 2005), the aim of the present study was to investigate the ability of PACAP to induce calcium mobilization in cerebellar granule neurons and to characterize the channels involved.

## MATERIALS AND METHODS

### ANIMALS

Wistar rats were obtained from a colony raised at the University of Rouen in an accredited animal facility (approval B.76-451-04), according to the French recommendations for the care and use of laboratory animals. All experiments were performed in accordance with the French Ministry of Agriculture and the European Communities Council Directive 2010/63/UE of September 22, 2010 (approval number N/01-12-11/24/12-14) under the supervision of authorized investigators (David Vaudry, Magali Basille-Dugay). Animals were housed in a temperature-controlled room (22 ± 1°C) under a 12-h light/dark cycle and with *ad libitum* access to food and water. Pups, of both sexes, were killed by decapitation at postnatal day 8 (P8) and the cerebella were quickly dissected out.

### REAGENTS

The 38-amino acid form of PACAP (PACAP38) was synthesized by solid phase methodology as previously described (Jolivel et al., 2009). PACAP27 and VIP were obtained from PolyPeptide Laboratories (Strasbourg, France). Fluo-3 acetoxymethylester (Fluo-3/AM) was from Molecular Probes (Invitrogen, Cergy Pontoise, France). Thapsigargin, ethylene glycol-bis(β-aminoethylether)-N,N,N′,N′-tetraacetic acid (EGTA), nifedipine, ω-conotoxin GVIA, and ω-conotoxin MVIIC were purchased from Sigma-Aldrich (Saint-Quentin Fallavier, France). 2-aminoethoxydiphenyl borate (2APB) was from Fisher Scientific (Illkirch, France).

### CELL CULTURE

Granule cell suspensions were prepared from cerebella of P8 rats, as previously described (Kaddour et al., 2013). For calcium experiments, dispersed cells were seeded on poly-L-lysine-coated glass coverslips in Falcon 3001 dishes at a density of $1 \times 10^6$ cells/mL in a cultured medium consisting of 75% DMEM and 25% Ham's F12 supplemented with 10% fetal bovine serum, 25 mM KCl, and 1% antibiotic antimycotic solution. Cells were grown at 37°C in a humidified incubator with an atmosphere of 5% $CO_2$/95% air. After 20 h, cytosine arabinoside, a mitotic inhibitor, was added at a final concentration of 5 μM to avoid replication of non-neuronal cells. In these conditions, the culture mainly contains cerebellar granule cells and contaminant cells are mostly astrocytes, which can be recognized based on their morphology (Levi et al., 1989).

### CALCIUM MEASUREMENT

Forty-eight hours after plating, granule cells were loaded at 37°C for 45 min with 5 μM fluo-3/AM diluted in culture medium. Then, the calcium-dye-probe was washed off and replaced with a Ringer's solution containing 10 mM Hepes, 120 mM NaCl, 2 mM KCl, 1.8 mM $CaCl_2$, 1 mM $MgCl_2$, and 6 mM glucose (pH 7.4). Under certain conditions, pharmacological agents were added in the Ringer's solution 30 min before mounting the glass coverslip on the stage of a Nikon inverted microscope (Eclipse TE200) equipped with a Nikon 60x, 1.4 NA, oil-immersion objective. Fluo-3/AM was excited with the 488-nm laser line, and the emitted fluorescence was recorded with a 500-nm long-pass filter on a Noran OZ confocal laser-scanning microscope (Noran Instruments, Middleton, WI, USA), equipped with a standard argon/kripton laser for illumination. Images were acquired as a time series of scan of the same focal plane (512 × 480 pixels at 7.5 images/s) and data processing was carried out using the Intervision software (Noran Instruments). The cells were continuously perifused with Ringer's solution at constant flow rate (2 mL/min) and temperature (37°C). The perifusion system was also used to deliver test substances at the vicinity of the cultured neuroblasts. Any modification of fluorescence directly reflects a change of intracellular calcium concentration ($[Ca^{2+}]_i$). To determine the increase of $[Ca^{2+}]_i$, the value of the peak amplitude as well as the area under the curve (AUC) of each response profile were calculated by using the PRISM Software (GraphPad Software, San Diego, CA, USA). Results are expressed as histograms showing (i) the distribution of cells according to the amplitude of their response to PACAP and (ii) the mean AUCs of their $[Ca^{2+}]_i$ increase.

## BINDING STUDIES

PACAP27 was radioiodinated by means of the lactoperoxidase technique as previously described (Basille et al., 1994). The radioligand was purified by reverse-phase HPLC on a Vydac $C_{18}$ column (25 × 0.46 cm; Sigma-Aldrich), using a gradient of acetonitrile/water containing 0.1% TFA. The specific radioactivity of the tracer was approximately 800 Ci/mmol.

Twenty-μm-thick sections or granule cells from P8 rat cerebella cultured for 1 day were preincubated at 20°C in 50 mM Tris buffer (pH 7.4) supplemented with 1% bovine serum albumin (BSA), 32 mM saccharose, 5 mM $MgCl_2$, and 0.5 μg/mL bacitracin, for 30 or 10 min, respectively. Sections or cells were incubated with [$^{125}$I]PACAP27 (40 or 400 pM, respectively) at 20°C for 1 h in the same buffer, supplemented with 2% BSA. To visualize non-specific

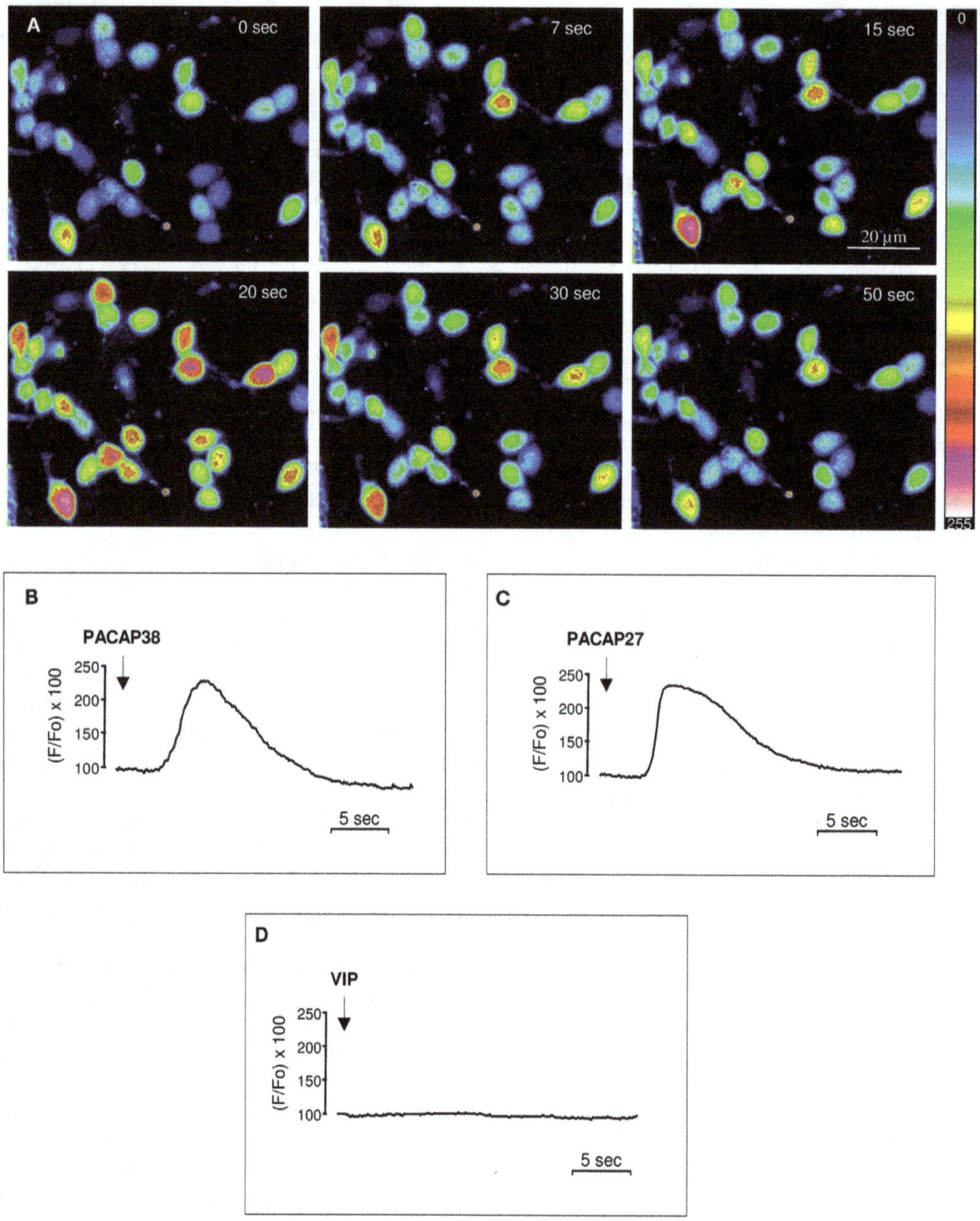


**FIGURE 1 | Effect of PACAP38, PACAP27, or VIP on [$Ca^{2+}$]$_i$ in cultured cerebellar granule cells.** **(A)** Time series of pseudocolor images illustrating the [$Ca^{2+}$]$_i$ changes in cultured granule cells loaded with the $Ca^{2+}$-sensitive dye fluo-3/AM after infusion of $10^{-6}$ M PACAP38 at the vicinity of the cells. The pseudocolor scale indicates the corresponding [$Ca^{2+}$]$_i$ changes expressed in arbitrary units. **(B–D)** Typical profiles illustrating the time-course of the variation of the fluorescence ratio evoked by a single application of $10^{-6}$ M PACAP38 **(B)**, PACAP27 **(C)**, or VIP **(D)** on [$Ca^{2+}$]$_i$ in cultured granule cells. The arrows indicate the onset of peptide application.

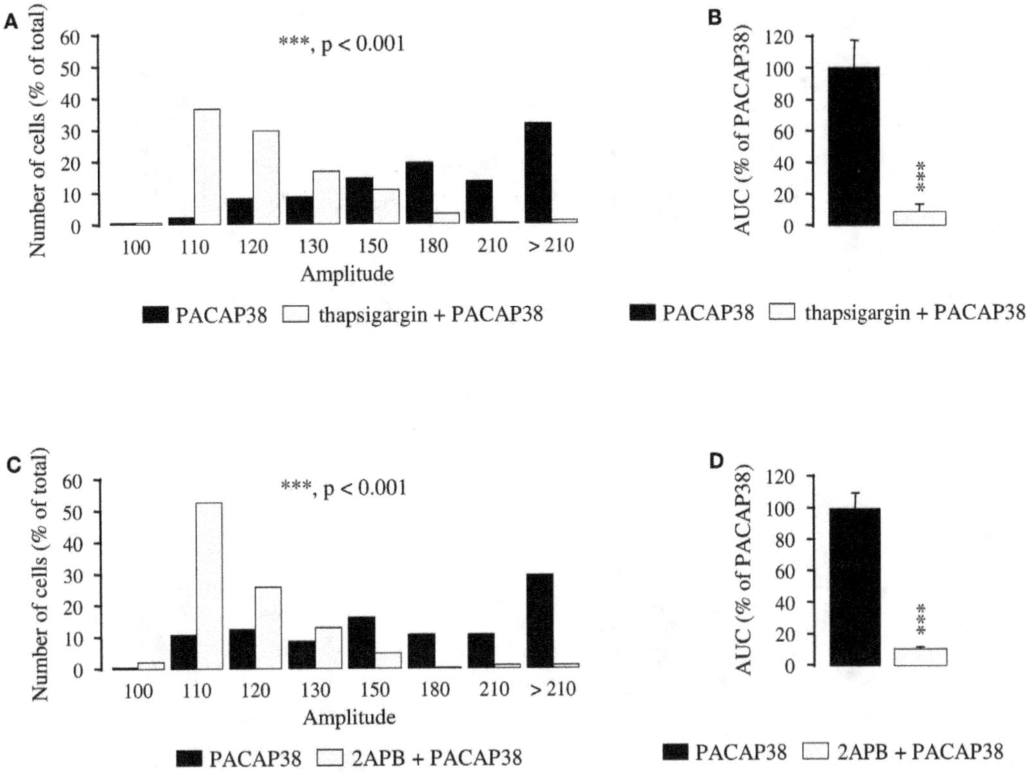


**FIGURE 2 | Involvement of intracellular calcium stores in the mechanism of action of PACAP38 in cerebellar granule cells. (A–D)** Effect of a single application of $10^{-6}$ M PACAP38 on the amplitude **(A,C)** and the area under the curve **(B,D)** of the $[Ca^{2+}]_i$ response in the absence (black bars) or presence (white bars) of $10^{-6}$ M thapsigargin, a $Ca^{2+}$ ATPase inhibitor, or $10^{-5}$ M 2APB, a membrane permeable D-myo-inositol 1,4,5-trisphosphate receptor antagonist. Thapsigargin and 2APB were added 15 and 30 min before application of the pulse of PACAP, respectively. **(A,C)** Histograms showing the distribution of granule cells according to the amplitude of their response to PACAP. Each graph represents the analysis of a least 50 cells from 3 different cultures. 2APB, 2-aminoethoxydiphenyl borate; AUC, area under the curve. $***p < 0.001$.

binding, slices, or cells were incubated with the radioligand in the presence of $10^{-6}$ M PACAP38. At the end of the incubation, sections, or cells were washed with cold Tris buffer and dried under an air stream. Finally, slices were apposed onto Hyperfilm-3H (GE Healthcare, Les Ulis, France) for 6 days and the radioactivity associated with the cells was counted in a gamma-counter (LKB, Wallac, Rockville, MI, USA). Tissue slices were photographed by means of a computer-assisted image-analysis station (Samba, Grenoble, Lyon).

### STATISTICAL ANALYSIS

Data are expressed as mean ± SEM values from at least three independent experiments. Statistical analyses were conducted with the PRISM software.

## RESULTS

### EFFECT OF PACAP38, PACAP27, AND VIP ON $[Ca^{2+}]i$

Perifusion of cultured cerebellar granule cells with $10^{-6}$ M PACAP38 provoked a marked increase of $[Ca^{2+}]_i$ in more than 90% of the cells (**Figure 1A**). In all responding cells $[Ca^{2+}]_i$ increased rapidly, i.e., within less than 5 s following PACAP infusion, and reached a maximum after 15–20 s, but the amplitude of the response was variable depending on the cell (**Figure 1A**). The response profile determined as the ratio between the fluo-3 fluorescence intensity under resting conditions and after exposure to test substances, revealed that both PACAP38 and PACAP27 ($10^{-6}$ M) induced a transient, rapid, and monophasic increase in $[Ca^{2+}]_i$ followed by gradual return to baseline (**Figures 1B,C**) while application of vehicle had no effect. Conversely, administration of $10^{-6}$ M VIP did not induce any modification of the $[Ca^{2+}]_i$ level (**Figure 1D**). When the same cells were exposed to a second pulse of PACAP, the stimulatory effect of the peptide on $[Ca^{2+}]_i$ was totally abolished (data not shown).

### CONTRIBUTION OF INTRACELLULAR $Ca^{2+}$ POOLS IN THE PACAP38-EVOKED INCREASE OF $[Ca^{2+}]i$

Preincubation of granule cells with the $Ca^{2+}$ ATPase inhibitor thapsigargin ($10^{-6}$ M; 15 min) induced a substantial reduction of the amplitude of the $[Ca^{2+}]_i$ response to $10^{-6}$ M PACAP38 in most cells ($p < 0.001$; **Figure 2A**). Indeed, in the absence of thapsigargin, more than 80% of the responding cells exhibited at least a 50% increase of their fluorescence intensity whereas in the presence of the inhibitor, 80% of the cells exhibited an increase of their fluorescence intensity that was lower than 30% (**Figure 2A**). As shown in **Figure 2B**,

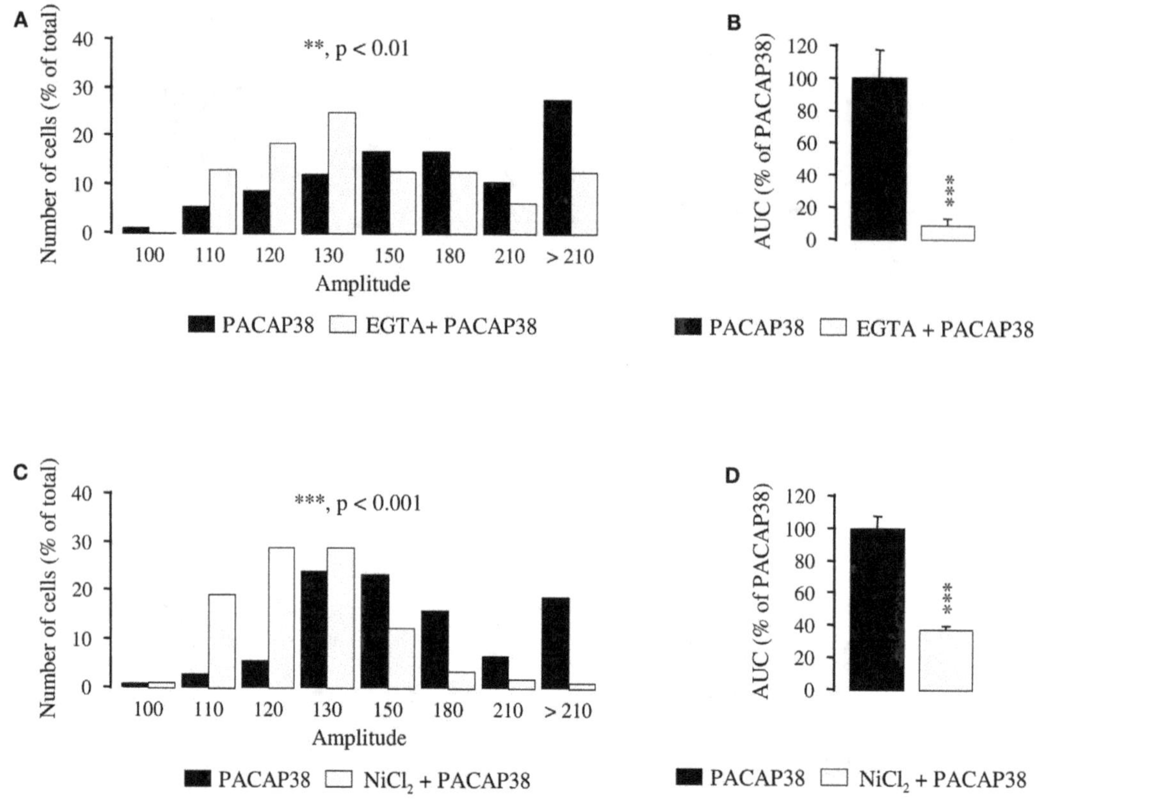


**FIGURE 3 | Involvement of calcium influx in the mechanism of action of PACAP38 in cerebellar granule cells. (A–D)** Effect of a single application of $10^{-6}$ M PACAP38 on the amplitude **(A,C)** and the area under the curve **(B,D)** of the $[Ca^{2+}]_i$ response in the absence (black bars) or presence (white bars) of 6 mM EGTA, a $Ca^{2+}$ chelator, or 3 mM $NiCl_2$, a blocker of voltage-operated calcium channels. EGTA and $NiCl_2$ were added to the incubation medium 10 min before application of the pulse of PACAP. **(A,C)** Histograms showing the distribution of granule cells according to the amplitude of their response to PACAP. Each graph represents the analysis of a least 50 cells from 3 different cultures. AUC, area under the curve; EGTA, ethylene glycol-bis(β-aminoethylether)-N,N,N′,N′-tetraacetic acid; $NiCl_2$, nickel chloride. $^{**}p < 0.01$, $^{***}p < 0.001$.

thapsigargin reduced by 86% the mean AUC of the PACAP38-evoked $[Ca^{2+}]_i$ response ($p < 0.001$). Preincubation of granule cells with the permeable D-myo-inositol 1,4,5-trisphosphate receptor antagonist 2APB ($10^{-5}$ M) markedly reduced the $[Ca^{2+}]_i$ response to $10^{-6}$ M PACAP38. In the presence of 2APB, more than 90% of responding cells exhibited an increase of their fluorescence intensity that was lower than 30% ($p < 0.001$; **Figure 2C**). As shown in **Figure 2D**, 2APB reduced by 89% the mean AUC of the PACAP38-evoked $[Ca^{2+}]_i$ response ($p < 0.001$).

### CONTRIBUTION OF EXTRACELLULAR $Ca^{2+}$ IN THE PACAP38-EVOKED STIMULATION OF $[Ca^{2+}]i$

Preincubation of granule cells with the calcium chelator EGTA (6 mM; 10 min), significantly attenuated the amplitude of the $[Ca^{2+}]_i$ response to $10^{-6}$ M PACAP38 ($p < 0.01$; **Figure 3A**) and diminished by 91% the AUC of the PACAP38-evoked $[Ca^{2+}]_i$ increase ($p < 0.001$; **Figure 3B**). Similarly, a 10-min preincubation with 3 mM $NiCl_2$, a blocker of voltage-operated calcium channels (VOCCs), significantly reduced the amplitude of the $[Ca^{2+}]_i$ peak in response to $10^{-6}$ M PACAP38 ($p < 0.001$; **Figure 3C**). Indeed, while 90% of the responding cells had a ratio of fluorescence intensity greater than 130 in the absence of $NiCl_2$, 79% of them had an amplitude lower than 130 in the presence of the VOCC blocker (**Figure 3C**). Furthermore, addition of $NiCl_2$ to the Ringer's solution reduced by 62% the AUC of the PACAP38-evoked $[Ca^{2+}]_i$ response ($p < 0.001$; **Figure 3D**).

### ABSENCE OF EFFECT OF EGTA ON [125I]PACAP27 BINDING

To verify that EGTA did not influence PACAP binding on its recognition sites, autoradiography experiments were carried out using $[^{125}I]$PACAP27 as a radioligand. As previously reported $[^{125}I]$PACAP27 binding was observed in the external granule cell layer of P8 rat cerebella (**Figure 4A**). Addition of $10^{-6}$ M PACAP38 to the incubation medium completely displaced $[^{125}I]$PACAP27 binding (**Figure 4B**). In the presence of 6 mM EGTA, specific binding of $[^{125}I]$PACAP27 on cerebellar tissue slices was not impaired (**Figure 4C**) and displacement of $[^{125}I]$PACAP27 binding by PACAP38 was not affected (**Figure 4D**). Binding experiments were also performed on 1-day-old cultured granule cells with $[^{125}I]$PACAP27 as a radioligand and it appeared that 6 mM EGTA did not modify the specific binding of $[^{125}I]$PACAP27 on cultured cells (**Figure 4E**).

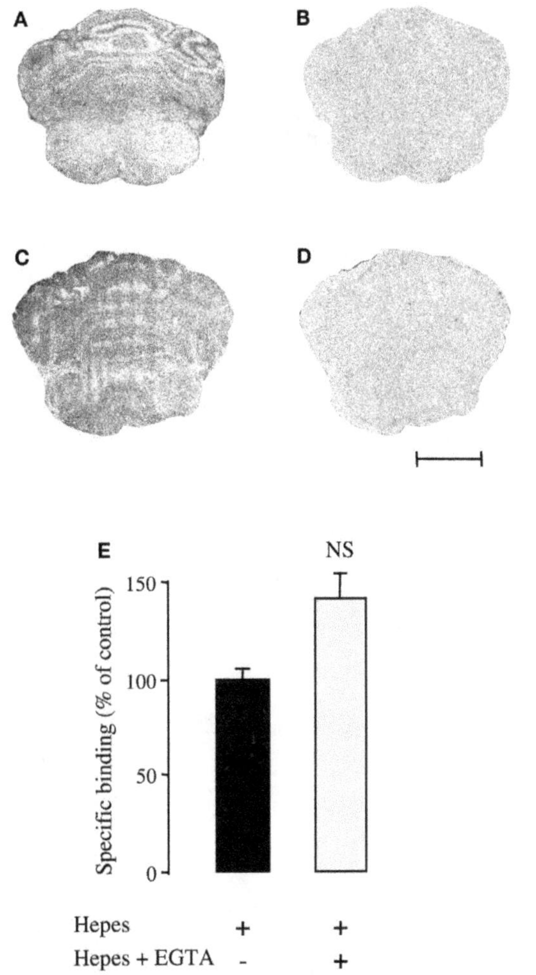


**FIGURE 4 | Effect of the $Ca^{2+}$ chelator EGTA (6 mM) on [$^{125}$I]PACAP27 binding to cerebellar tissue slices or cerebellar granule cells. (A–D)** Autoradiographic visualization of [$^{125}$I]PACAP27 binding sites in the absence **(A,C)** or presence of $10^{-6}$ M PACAP38 **(B,D)** in consecutive sections of P8 rat cerebellum. Scale bar = 1.7 mm. **(E)** Histograms showing specific binding of [$^{125}$I]PACAP27 in the absence (black bars) or presence (white bars) of 6 mM EGTA on cultured cerebellar granule cells. EGTA, ethylene glycol-bis(β-aminoethylether)-N,N,N′,N′-tetraacetic acid. NS, not significantly different from Hepes buffer.

## INVOLVEMENT OF N-TYPE CALCIUM CHANNELS IN THE PACAP38-EVOKED STIMULATION OF [$Ca^{2+}$]i

To determine which type of $Ca^{2+}$ channel is responsible for the stimulatory effect of PACAP38 on calcium influx, selective blockers of VOCCs were used. A 30-min incubation of cultured granule cells with the L-type $Ca^{2+}$ channel blocker nifedipine ($10^{-5}$ M; **Figures 5A,B**) or the P- and Q-type $Ca^{2+}$ channel blocker ω-conotoxin MVIIC ($10^{-6}$ M; **Figures 5C,D**) did not significantly modify the amplitude of the [$Ca^{2+}$]$_i$ response to $10^{-6}$ M PACAP38 ($p > 0.05$; **Figures 5A,C**). Consistent with these observations, nifedipine, and ω-conotoxin MVIIC did not impair the AUCs of the PACAP38-induced [$Ca^{2+}$]$_i$ rise ($p > 0.05$; **Figures 5B,D**). In contrast, preincubation of cells with the N-type $Ca^{2+}$ channel blocker ω-conotoxin GVIA ($10^{-6}$ M; 30 min; **Figures 5E,F**) provoked a significant decrease of the amplitude of the [$Ca^{2+}$]$_i$ increase induced by $10^{-6}$ M PACAP38, with 76 and 52% of responding cells exhibiting a ratio of fluorescence intensity greater than 130 in the absence or presence of ω-conotoxin GVIA, respectively ($p < 0.001$; **Figure 5E**). Furthermore, ω-conotoxin GVIA reduced by 46% the AUC of the PACAP38-evoked [$Ca^{2+}$]$_i$ response ($p < 0.001$; **Figure 5F**).

## DISCUSSION

The respective contribution of extracellular and intracellular $Ca^{2+}$ pools in PACAP-induced [$Ca^{2+}$]$_i$ increase in cerebellar neuroblasts has not been previously investigated. Because primary cultures of rat cerebellar granule cells are mainly composed of a single population of cells, the effect of PACAP on the [$Ca^{2+}$]$_i$ response could be monitored on a large number of neurons. Thus, we found that, in 90% of granule cells, infusion of $10^{-6}$ M PACAP38 or PACAP27 induced a transient, rapid, and monophasic [$Ca^{2+}$]$_i$ rise, similar to the PACAP-induced $Ca^{2+}$ response observed in neural NG108-15 cells (Holighaus et al., 2011) but different from that observed in rat pancreatic acinar AR42J cells (Barnhart et al., 1997) or human neuroblastoma NB-OK-1 cells (Delporte et al., 1993) in which the initial peak is followed by a plateau phase that lasts for approximately 2–3 min before the return of [$Ca^{2+}$]$_i$ to baseline level. These differences could be explained by the diversity of the PACAP receptor subtype repertoire expressed in each cell type and by the different intracellular signaling systems involved. For instance, in rat gonadotrophs, PACAP stimulates $Ca^{2+}$ oscillations through activation of VPAC1 coupled to a PTX-insensitive G protein and phospholipase C-β (Hezareh et al., 1996) whereas, in cerebellar neurons, in which VIP failed to affect [$Ca^{2+}$]$_i$, the ability of PACAP to induce [$Ca^{2+}$]$_i$ rise can be ascribed to activation of the PAC1 receptor, as previously reported in primary cultures of rat cortical neurons and astrocytes (Grimaldi and Cavallaro, 1999). In neural NG108-15 cells, the PACAP38-evoked [$Ca^{2+}$]$_i$ response is mainly mediated by the PAC1 hop1 splice variant (Mustafa et al., 2007; Holighaus et al., 2011), an isoform also expressed in granule neurons (Kienlen-Campard et al., 1997). Interestingly, this hop isoform has been reported to be mandatory for calcium influx in cortical precursors (Yan et al., 2013). In β-islet cells, the PAC1 TM4 splice variant increases [$Ca^{2+}$]$_i$ by stimulating $Ca^{2+}$ influx *via* a L-type $Ca^{2+}$ channel without activating adenylyl cyclase or phospholipase C in response to PACAP (Chatterjee et al., 1996). In cerebellar granule cells, the TM4 splice variant is expressed at a very low level (Chatterjee et al., 1996) and is thus probably not functionally relevant considering the strong activation of the cAMP pathway evoked by PACAP (Basille et al., 1993, 1995).

It has previously been demonstrated that, in cerebellar granule neurons, PACAP activates the phospholipase C pathway (Basille et al., 1995). We have thus explored the possible contribution of intracellular $Ca^{2+}$ stores in the stimulatory effect of PACAP on [$Ca^{2+}$]$_i$. The results showed that depletion of the endoplasmic reticulum $Ca^{2+}$ store with the $Ca^{2+}$ ATPase inhibitor thapsigargin reduced the amplitude and the AUC of the PACAP-evoked [$Ca^{2+}$]$_i$ response in cerebellar neurons. Consistent with the notion that intracellular $Ca^{2+}$ from $IP_3$-sensitive $Ca^{2+}$ pools could play an important role in the mechanism of action of PACAP, incubation of the cells with 2APB, a cell permeable D-myo-inositol

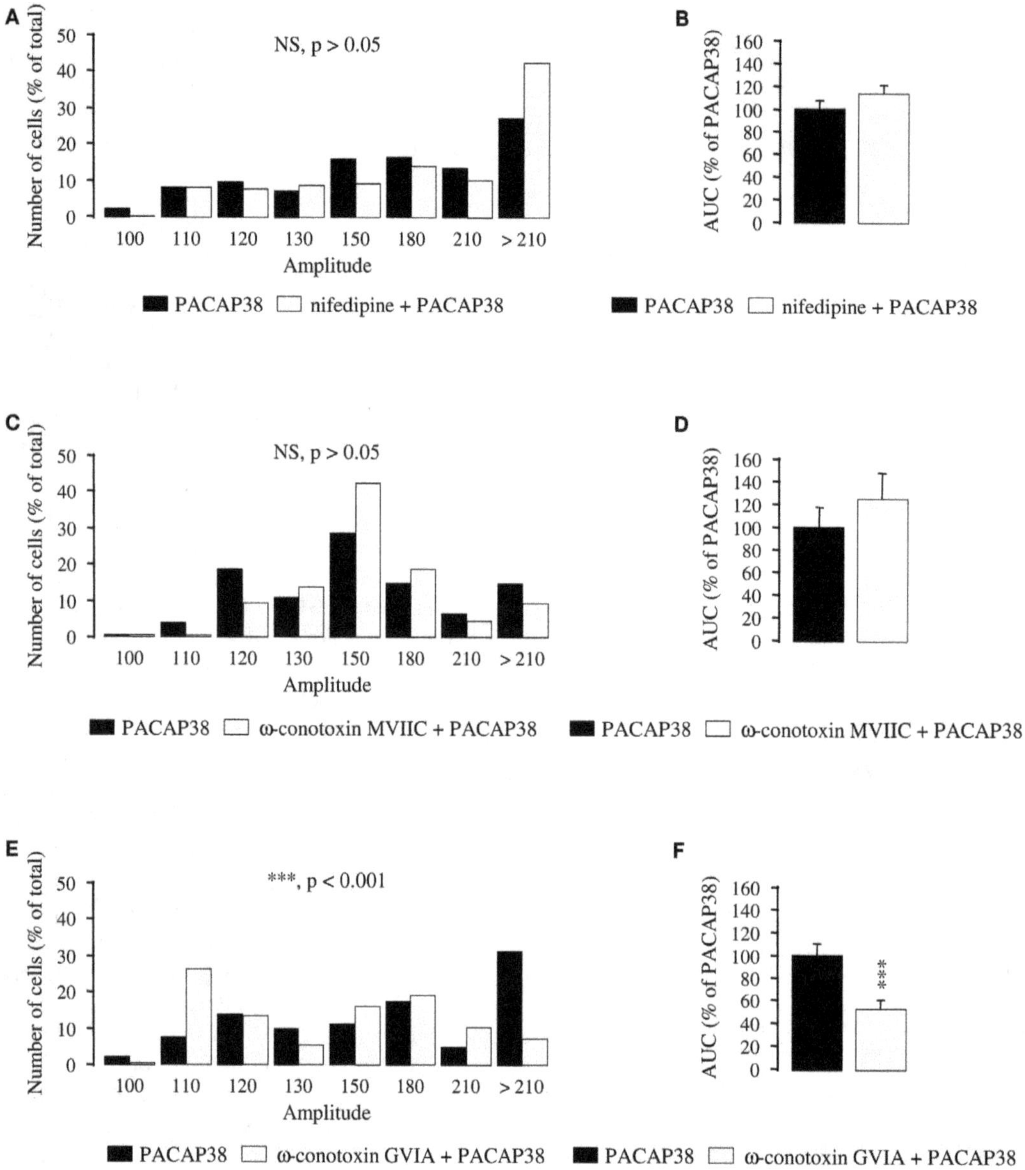


**FIGURE 5 | Effect of selective blockers of voltage-operated calcium channels on calcium influx induced by PACAP38 in cerebellar granule cells.** **(A–F)** Histograms showing the effect of a single application of $10^{-6}$ M PACAP38 on the amplitude **(A,C,E)** and the area under the curve **(B,D,F)** of the $[Ca^{2+}]_i$ response in the absence (black bars) or presence (white bars) of $10^{-5}$ M of the L-type $Ca^{2+}$ channel blocker nifedipine **(A,B)**, $10^{-6}$ M of the P- and Q-type $Ca^{2+}$ channel blocker ω-conotoxin MVIIC **(C,D)**, or $10^{-6}$ M of the N-type $Ca^{2+}$ channel blocker ω-conotoxin GVIA **(E,F)**. Nifedipine, ω-conotoxin MVIIC, and ω-conotoxin GVIA were added to the incubation medium 30 min before application of the pulse of PACAP38. **(A,C,E)** Histograms showing the distribution of granule cells according to the amplitude of their response to PACAP. Each graph represents the analysis of a least 50 cells from 3 different cultures. AUC, area under the curve; NS, not significantly different from the PACAP38; $***p < 0.001$.

1,4,5-trisphosphate receptor antagonist, decreased the $[Ca^{2+}]_i$ response to PACAP. Such a contribution of intracellular $Ca^{2+}$ stores to the PACAP-evoked $[Ca^{2+}]_i$ response has already been reported in rat gonadotrophs (Rawlings et al., 1994), in rat acinar AR42J cells (Barnhart et al., 1997), and in human neutrophils (Harfi and Sariban, 2006).

Alongside, suppression of extracellular $Ca^{2+}$ by EGTA or exposure of cells to the non-selective $Ca^{2+}$ channel blocker $NiCl_2$, also attenuated the stimulatory effect of PACAP38 on $[Ca^{2+}]_i$, indicating that $Ca^{2+}$ influx is also required for the transient phase of the $[Ca^{2+}]_i$ increase. Recruitment of both intracellular and extracellular sources of $Ca^{2+}$ after activation of PAC1 receptors has already been reported in several models including the rat acinar cell line AR42J (Barnhart et al., 1997), the human neuroblastoma cell line NB-OK-1 (Delporte et al., 1993), and primary cultures of rat cortical neurons (Grimaldi and Cavallaro, 1999). To determine which type of $Ca^{2+}$ channel was responsible for the stimulatory effect of PACAP on calcium influx, selective blockers of VOCCs were used. Preincubation of granule cells with the N-type $Ca^{2+}$ channel blocker ω-conotoxin GVIA decreased the PACAP-evoked $[Ca^{2+}]_i$ response, whereas the L-type $Ca^{2+}$ channel blocker nifedipine and the P- and Q-type $Ca^{2+}$ channel blocker ω-conotoxin MVIIC had no effect. These findings contrast with previous data showing the involvement of L-type $Ca^{2+}$ channels in the stimulatory effect of PACAP on human neutrophils (Harfi et al., 2005), on porcine somatotrope cells (Martinez-Fuentes et al., 1998) or on bovine adrenal chromaffin cells (Tanaka et al., 1996) and the implication of T-type $Ca^{2+}$ channels in mouse adrenal chromaffin cells (Hill et al., 2011). Nevertheless, other factors acting on cerebellar granule neurons, such as IGF-1, have already been shown to regulate N-type $Ca^{2+}$-channels (Blair and Marshall, 1997).

$Ca^{2+}$ is an essential intracellular messenger required for numerous cellular functions (Carafoli et al., 2001). For instance, during development, modifications of intracellular $Ca^{2+}$ concentrations have been shown to regulate proliferation (Owens et al., 2000), migration (Komuro and Rakic, 1992), differentiation (Benquet et al., 2002; Ronn et al., 2002), and apoptosis (Turner et al., 2002) of immature neurons. Various studies suggest that, depending on the pool involved, $Ca^{2+}$ can exert different effects on immature neurons. For instance, in rat cortical neurons, $Ca^{2+}$ release from intracellular stores is implicated in neurite elongation, while $Ca^{2+}$ influx regulates dendritic branching (Ramakers et al., 2000). In the immature cerebellum, a transient elevation of intracellular $Ca^{2+}$ levels increases the migration rate of granule neuroblasts (Komuro and Rakic, 1996) and the thapsigargin-sensitive $Ca^{2+}$ store plays an essential role in growth and maturation of cerebellar granule cells (Yao et al., 1999). Even though the implication of $Ca^{2+}$ on granule cell development is now well established, the neurotrophic factors able to control $Ca^{2+}$ levels in cerebellar neuroblasts are not yet clearly identified. Nevertheless, peptides acting on G protein-coupled receptors are thought to be important mediators to control neurite outgrowth and growth cone guidance in cerebellar granule cells through a $Ca^{2+}$-dependent pathway (Xiang et al., 2002).

Granule cells are, by far, the major population of interneurons in the cerebellum and they represent the main source of glutamate, the second most abundant population being GABA-ergic neurons (Voogd and Glickstein, 1998). Previous studies have demonstrated that plasticity of granule cells can be modulated by neuropeptides (Cote et al., 1999; Yacubova and Komuro, 2002). In particular, in cerebellar granule cells, PACAP has been shown to inhibit proliferation (Nicot et al., 2002), stop migration (Cameron et al., 2007), protect from apoptosis (Vaudry et al., 2000), and promote differentiation (Gonzalez et al., 1997). *In vivo*, PACAP receptors are expressed by precursors of cerebellar granule cells in the external granule cell layer (Basille et al., 1993) and PACAP administration increases the number of mature neurons in the post-migratory internal granule cell layer (Vaudry et al., 1999). The implication of adenylyl cyclase and MAP kinases in the effects of PACAP have been extensively investigated (Villalba et al., 1997; Vaudry et al., 1998; Nicot et al., 2002) but the contribution of PACAP-induced $Ca^{2+}$ increase in maturation of cerebellar neuroblasts is still poorly understood. So far, it has only been shown that calcium is involved in the inhibitory effect of PACAP on granule cell migration (Cameron et al., 2007). However, it is well established that potassium depolarization-induced $Ca^{2+}$ entry is essential for granule cell survival (Gallo et al., 1987), suggesting that the antiapoptotic effect of PACAP may involve calcium mobilization. As reported with cortical neurons, PACAP may induce BDNF expression in a $Ca^{2+}$-dependent manner to indirectly promote granule cell survival (Shintani et al., 2005; Kokubo et al., 2009). The stimulation of granule cell proliferation by calcium influx is suppressed by nifedipine but not by ω-conotoxin GVIA (Borodinsky and Fiszman, 1998), suggesting that the ability of PACAP to block granule cell division does not depend on calcium regulation. Consistent with this latter hypothesis, it has been shown that, in cortical neurons, PACAP inhibits cell proliferation through activation of the cAMP signaling pathway (Nicot and DiCicco-Bloom, 2001). Finally, potassium depolarization and NMDA treatment require calcium influx to induce neurofilament assembly in cerebellar granule cells (Bui et al., 2003), supporting the idea that PACAP-induced neurite outgrowth also requires calcium mobilization.

Altogether, these data indicate that some of the activities of PACAP on cerebellar granule cell proliferation, survival, migration, and differentiation involve, at least in part, intracellular and/or extracellular calcium mobilization, but further investigations are needed to decipher the precise role of calcium in each process.

## ACKNOWLEDGMENTS

The authors want to thank Dr. Arnaud Arabo, Mrs. Huguette Lemonnier, and Mr. Donovan Liot for skillful technical assistance. David Vaudry and Hubert Vaudry are Affiliated Professors at the Institut National de la Recherche Scientifique – Institut Armand Frappier. This study was supported by grants from INSERM (U982), the Interreg TC2N project, the LARC-Neuroscience network, and the Région Haute-Normandie.

## REFERENCES

Aoyagi, K., and Takahashi, M. (2001). Pituitary adenylate cyclase-activating polypeptide enhances Ca(2+)-dependent neurotransmitter release from PC12 cells and cultured cerebellar granule cells without affecting intracellular Ca(2+) mobilization. *Biochem. Biophys. Res. Commun.* 286, 646–651.

Barnhart, D. C., Sarosi, G. A. Jr., and Mulholland, M. W. (1997). PACAP-38 causes phospholipase C-dependent calcium signaling in rat acinar cell line. *Surgery* 122, 465–474.

Basille, M., Gonzalez, B. J., Desrues, L., Demas, M., Fournier, A., and Vaudry, H. (1995). Pituitary adenylate cyclase-activating polypeptide (PACAP) stimulates adenylyl cyclase and phospholipase C activity in rat cerebellar neuroblasts. *J. Neurochem.* 65, 1318–1324.

Basille, M., Gonzalez, B. J., Fournier, A., and Vaudry, H. (1994). Ontogeny of pituitary adenylate cyclase-activating polypeptide (PACAP) receptors in the rat cerebellum: a quantitative autoradiographic study. *Brain Res. Dev. Brain Res.* 82, 81–89.

Basille, M., Gonzalez, B. J., Leroux, P., Jeandel, L., Fournier, A., and Vaudry, H. (1993). Localization and characterization of PACAP receptors in the rat cerebellum during development: evidence for a stimulatory effect of PACAP on immature cerebellar granule cells. *Neuroscience* 57, 329–338.

Benquet, P., Le Guen, J., Pichon, Y., and Tiaho, F. (2002). Differential involvement of Ca(2+) channels in survival and neurite outgrowth of cultured embryonic cockroach brain neurons. *J. Neurophysiol.* 88, 1475–1490.

Blair, L. A., and Marshall, J. (1997). IGF-1 modulates N and L calcium channels in a PI 3-kinase-dependent manner. *Neuron* 19, 421–429.

Borodinsky, L. N., and Fiszman, M. L. (1998). Extracellular potassium concentration regulates proliferation of immature cerebellar granule cells. *Brain Res. Dev. Brain Res.* 107, 43–48.

Botia, B., Basille, M., Allais, A., Raoult, E., Falluel-Morel, A., Galas, L., et al. (2007). Neurotrophic effects of PACAP in the cerebellar cortex. *Peptides* 28, 1746–1752.

Bui, C. J., Beaman-Hall, C. M., and Vallano, M. L. (2003). Ca2+ and CaM kinase regulate neurofilament expression. *Neuroreport* 14, 2073–2077.

Cameron, D. B., Galas, L., Jiang, Y., Raoult, E., Vaudry, D., and Komuro, H. (2007). Cerebellar cortical-layer-specific control of neuronal migration by pituitary adenylate cyclase-activating polypeptide. *Neuroscience* 146, 697–712.

Canny, B. J., Rawlings, S. R., and Leong, D. A. (1992). Pituitary adenylate cyclase-activating polypeptide specifically increases cytosolic calcium ion concentration in rat gonadotropes and somatotropes. *Endocrinology* 130, 211–215.

Carafoli, E., Santella, L., Branca, D., and Brini, M. (2001). Generation, control, and processing of cellular calcium signals. *Crit. Rev. Biochem. Mol. Biol.* 36, 107–260.

Cauvin, A., Buscail, L., Gourlet, P., De Neef, P., Gossen, D., Arimura, A., et al. (1990). The novel VIP-like hypothalamic polypeptide PACAP interacts with high affinity receptors in the human neuroblastoma cell line NB-OK. *Peptides* 11, 773–777.

Cebolla, B., Fernandez-Perez, A., Perea, G., Araque, A., and Vallejo, M. (2008). DREAM mediates cAMP-dependent, Ca2+-induced stimulation of GFAP gene expression and regulates cortical astrogliogenesis. *J. Neurosci.* 28, 6703–6713.

Chatterjee, T. K., Sharma, R. V., and Fisher, R. A. (1996). Molecular cloning of a novel variant of the pituitary adenylate cyclase-activating polypeptide (PACAP) receptor that stimulates calcium influx by activation of L-type calcium channels. *J. Biol. Chem.* 271, 32226–32232.

Cote, F., Do, T. H., Laflamme, L., Gallo, J. M., and Gallo-Payet, N. (1999). Activation of the AT(2) receptor of angiotensin II induces neurite outgrowth and cell migration in microexplant cultures of the cerebellum. *J. Biol. Chem.* 274, 31686–31692.

Delporte, C., Van Praet, A., Herchuelz, A., Winand, J., and Christophe, J. (1993). Contrasting effects of PACAP and carbachol on [Ca2+]i and inositol phosphates in human neuroblastoma NB-OK-1 cells. *Peptides* 14, 1111–1118.

Dziema, H., and Obrietan, K. (2002). PACAP potentiates L-type calcium channel conductance in suprachiasmatic nucleus neurons by activating the MAPK pathway. *J. Neurophysiol.* 88, 1374–1386.

Gallo, V., Kingsbury, A., Balazs, R., and Jorgensen, O. S. (1987). The role of depolarization in the survival and differentiation of cerebellar granule cells in culture. *J. Neurosci.* 7, 2203–2213.

Gonzalez, B. J., Basille, M., Vaudry, D., Fournier, A., and Vaudry, H. (1997). Pituitary adenylate cyclase-activating polypeptide promotes cell survival and neurite outgrowth in rat cerebellar neuroblasts. *Neuroscience* 78, 419–430.

Gracia-Navarro, F., Lamacz, M., Tonon, M. C., and Vaudry, H. (1992). Pituitary adenylate cyclase-activating polypeptide stimulates calcium mobilization in amphibian pituitary cells. *Endocrinology* 131, 1069–1074.

Grimaldi, M., and Cavallaro, S. (1999). Functional and molecular diversity of PACAP/VIP receptors in cortical neurons and type I astrocytes. *Eur. J. Neurosci.* 11, 2767–2772.

Harfi, I., Corazza, F., D'Hondt, S., and Sariban, E. (2005). Differential calcium regulation of proinflammatory activities in human neutrophils exposed to the neuropeptide pituitary adenylate cyclase-activating protein. *J. Immunol.* 175, 4091–4102.

Harfi, I., and Sariban, E. (2006). Mechanisms and modulation of pituitary adenylate cyclase-activating protein-induced calcium mobilization in human neutrophils. *Ann. N. Y. Acad. Sci.* 1070, 322–329.

Harmar, A. J., Fahrenkrug, J., Gozes, I., Laburthe, M., May, V., Pisegna, J. R., et al. (2012). Pharmacology and functions of receptors for vasoactive intestinal peptide and pituitary adenylate cyclase-activating polypeptide. *Br. J. Pharmacol.* 166, 4–17.

Hezareh, M., Schlegel, W., and Rawlings, S. R. (1996). PACAP and VIP stimulate Ca2+ oscillations in rat gonadotrophs through the PACAP/VIP type 1 receptor (PVR1) linked to a pertussis toxin-insensitive G-protein and the activation of phospholipase C-beta. *J. Neuroendocrinol.* 8, 367–374.

Hill, J., Chan, S. A., Kuri, B., and Smith, C. (2011). Pituitary adenylate cyclase-activating peptide (PACAP) recruits low voltage-activated T-type calcium influx under acute sympathetic stimulation in mouse adrenal chromaffin cells. *J. Biol. Chem.* 286, 42459–42469.

Holighaus, Y., Mustafa, T., and Eiden, L. E. (2011). PAC1hop, null and hip receptors mediate differential signaling through cyclic AMP and calcium leading to splice variant-specific gene induction in neural cells. *Peptides* 32, 1647–1655.

Isobe, K., Nakai, T., and Takuwa, Y. (1993). Ca(2+)-dependent stimulatory effect of pituitary adenylate cyclase-activating polypeptide on catecholamine secretion from cultured porcine adrenal medullary chromaffin cells. *Endocrinology* 132, 1757–1765.

Jolivel, V., Basille, M., Aubert, N., de Jouffrey, S., Ancian, P., Le Bigot, J. F., et al. (2009). Distribution and functional characterization of pituitary adenylate cyclase-activating polypeptide receptors in the brain of non-human primates. *Neuroscience* 160, 434–451.

Kaddour, H., Hamdi, Y., Vaudry, D., Basille, M., Desrues, L., Leprince, J., et al. (2013). The octadecaneuropeptide ODN prevents 6-hydroxydopamine-induced apoptosis of cerebellar granule neurons through a PKC-MAPK-dependent pathway. *J. Neurochem.* 125, 620–633.

Kienlen-Campard, P., Crochemore, C., Rene, F., Monnier, D., Koch, B., and Loeffler, J. P. (1997). PACAP type I receptor activation promotes cerebellar neuron survival through the cAMP/PKA signaling pathway. *DNA Cell Biol.* 16, 323–333.

Kokubo, M., Nishio, M., Ribar, T. J., Anderson, K. A., West, A. E., and Means, A. R. (2009). BDNF-mediated cerebellar granule cell development is impaired in mice null for CaMKK2 or CaMKIV. *J. Neurosci.* 29, 8901–8913.

Komuro, H., and Rakic, P. (1992). Selective role of N-type calcium channels in neuronal migration. *Science* 257, 806–809.

Komuro, H., and Rakic, P. (1996). Intracellular Ca2+ fluctuations modulate the rate of neuronal migration. *Neuron* 17, 275–285.

Levi, A. C., DeMattei, M., Ravazzani, R., Corvetti, G., Golden, G. T., and Fariello, R. G. (1989). Effects of 1-methyl-4-phenyl-1,2,3,6-tetrahydropyridine (MPTP) on ultrastructure of nigral neuromelanin in *Macaca fascicularis*. *Neurosci. Lett.* 96, 271–276.

Martinez-Fuentes, A. J., Castano, J. P., Malagon, M. M., Vazquez-Martinez, R., and Gracia-Navarro, F. (1998). Pituitary adenylate cyclase-activating polypeptides 38 and 27 increase cytosolic free Ca2+ concentration in porcine somatotropes through common and distinct mechanisms. *Cell Calcium* 23, 369–378.

Masuo, Y., Matsumoto, Y., Tokito, F., Tsuda, M., and Fujino, M. (1993). Effects of vasoactive intestinal polypeptide (VIP) and pituitary adenylate cyclase activating polypeptide (PACAP) on the spontaneous release of acetylcholine from the rat hippocampus by brain microdialysis. *Brain Res.* 611, 207–215.

Matsuda, K., Nejigaki, Y., Satoh, M., Shimaura, C., Tanaka, M., Kawamoto, K., et al. (2008). Effect of pituitary adenylate cyclase-activating polypeptide (PACAP) on prolactin and somatolactin release from the goldfish pituitary in vitro. *Regul. Pept.* 145, 72–79.

Mei, Y. A. (1999). High-voltage-activated calcium current and its modulation by dopamine D4 and pituitary adenylate cyclase activating polypeptide receptors in cerebellar granule cells. *Zhongguo Yao Li Xue Bao* 20, 3–9.

Michel, S., Itri, J., Han, J. H., Gniotczynski, K., and Colwell, C. S. (2006). Regulation of glutamatergic signalling by PACAP in the mammalian suprachiasmatic nucleus. *BMC Neurosci.* 7:15. doi:10.1186/1471-2202-7-15

Miyata, A., Arimura, A., Dahl, R. R., Minamino, N., Uehara, A., Jiang, L., et al. (1989). Isolation of a novel 38 residue-hypothalamic polypeptide which stimulates adenylate cyclase in pituitary cells. *Biochem. Biophys. Res. Commun.* 164, 567–574.

Mustafa, T., Grimaldi, M., and Eiden, L. E. (2007). The hop cassette of the PAC1 receptor confers coupling to Ca2+ elevation required for pituitary adenylate cyclase-activating polypeptide-evoked neurosecretion. *J. Biol. Chem.* 282, 8079–8091.

Nicot, A., and DiCicco-Bloom, E. (2001). Regulation of neuroblast mitosis is determined by PACAP receptor isoform expression. *Proc. Natl. Acad. Sci. U.S.A.* 98, 4758–4763.

Nicot, A., Lelievre, V., Tam, J., Waschek, J. A., and DiCicco-Bloom, E. (2002). Pituitary adenylate cyclase-activating polypeptide and sonic hedgehog interact to control cerebellar granule precursor cell proliferation. *J. Neurosci.* 22, 9244–9254.

Owens, D. F., Flint, A. C., Dammerman, R. S., and Kriegstein, A. R. (2000). Calcium dynamics of neocortical ventricular zone cells. *Dev. Neurosci.* 22, 25–33.

Ramakers, G. M., Pasinelli, P., van Beest, M., van der Slot, A., Gispen, W. H., and De Graan, P. N. (2000). Activation of pre- and postsynaptic protein kinase C during tetraethylammonium-induced long-term potentiation in the CA1 field of the hippocampus. *Neurosci. Lett.* 286, 53–56.

Rawlings, S. R., Canny, B. J., and Leong, D. A. (1993). Pituitary adenylate cyclase-activating polypeptide regulates cytosolic Ca2+ in rat gonadotropes and somatotropes through different intracellular mechanisms. *Endocrinology* 132, 1447–1452.

Rawlings, S. R., Demaurex, N., and Schlegel, W. (1994). Pituitary adenylate cyclase-activating polypeptide increases [Ca2]i in rat gonadotrophs through an inositol trisphosphate-dependent mechanism. *J. Biol. Chem.* 269, 5680–5686.

Reglodi, D., Kiss, P., Szabadfi, K., Atlasz, T., Gabriel, R., Horvath, G., et al. (2012). PACAP is an endogenous protective factor-insights from PACAP-deficient mice. *J. Mol. Neurosci.* 48, 482–492.

Ronn, L. C., Dissing, S., Holm, A., Berezin, V., and Bock, E. (2002). Increased intracellular calcium is required for neurite outgrowth induced by a synthetic peptide ligand of NCAM. *FEBS Lett.* 518, 60–66.

Sato, M., Suzuki, K., Yamazaki, H., and Nakanishi, S. (2005). A pivotal role of calcineurin signaling in development and maturation of postnatal cerebellar granule cells. *Proc. Natl. Acad. Sci. U.S.A.* 102, 5874–5879.

Shintani, N., Suetake, S., Hashimoto, H., Koga, K., Kasai, A., Kawaguchi, C., et al. (2005). Neuroprotective action of endogenous PACAP in cultured rat cortical neurons. *Regul. Pept.* 126, 123–128.

Tanaka, K., Shibuya, I., Nagamoto, T., Yamashita, H., and Kanno, T. (1996). Pituitary adenylate cyclase-activating polypeptide causes rapid Ca2+ release from intracellular stores and long lasting Ca2+ influx mediated by Na( influx-dependent membrane depolarization in bovine adrenal chromaffin cells. *Endocrinology* 137, 956–966.

Tatsuno, I., and Arimura, A. (1994). Pituitary adenylate cyclase-activating polypeptide (PACAP) mobilizes intracellular free calcium in cultured rat type-2, but not type-1, astrocytes. *Brain Res.* 662, 1–10.

Tatsuno, I., Yada, T., Vigh, S., Hidaka, H., and Arimura, A. (1992). Pituitary adenylate cyclase activating polypeptide and vasoactive intestinal peptide increase cytosolic free calcium concentration in cultured rat hippocampal neurons. *Endocrinology* 131, 73–81.

Turner, C. P., Pulciani, D., and Rivkees, S. A. (2002). Reduction in intracellular calcium levels induces injury in developing neurons. *Exp. Neurol.* 178, 21–32.

Vaudry, D., Falluel-Morel, A., Bourgault, S., Basille, M., Burel, D., Wurtz, O., et al. (2009). Pituitary adenylate cyclase-activating polypeptide and its receptors: 20 years after the discovery. *Pharmacol. Rev.* 61, 283–357.

Vaudry, D., Gonzalez, B. J., Basille, M., Anouar, Y., Fournier, A., and Vaudry, H. (1998). Pituitary adenylate cyclase-activating polypeptide stimulates both c-fos gene expression and cell survival in rat cerebellar granule neurons through activation of the protein kinase A pathway. *Neuroscience* 84, 801–812.

Vaudry, D., Gonzalez, B. J., Basille, M., Fournier, A., and Vaudry, H. (1999). Neurotrophic activity of pituitary adenylate cyclase-activating polypeptide on rat cerebellar cortex during development. *Proc. Natl. Acad. Sci. U.S.A.* 96, 9415–9420.

Vaudry, D., Gonzalez, B. J., Basille, M., Pamantung, T. F., Fontaine, M., Fournier, A., et al. (2000). The neuroprotective effect of pituitary adenylate cyclase-activating polypeptide on cerebellar granule cells is mediated through inhibition of the CED3-related cysteine protease caspase-3/CPP32. *Proc. Natl. Acad. Sci. U.S.A.* 97, 13390–13395.

Villalba, M., Bockaert, J., and Journot, L. (1997). Pituitary adenylate cyclase-activating polypeptide (PACAP-38) protects cerebellar granule neurons from apoptosis by activating the mitogen-activated protein kinase (MAP kinase) pathway. *J. Neurosci.* 17, 83–90.

Voogd, J., and Glickstein, M. (1998). The anatomy of the cerebellum. *Trends Cogn. Sci. (Regul. Ed.)* 2, 307–313.

Watanabe, T., Masuo, Y., Matsumoto, H., Suzuki, N., Ohtaki, T., Masuda, Y., et al. (1992). Pituitary adenylate cyclase activating polypeptide provokes cultured rat chromaffin cells to secrete adrenaline. *Biochem. Biophys. Res. Commun.* 182, 403–411.

Xiang, Y., Li, Y., Zhang, Z., Cui, K., Wang, S., Yuan, X. B., et al. (2002). Nerve growth cone guidance mediated by G protein-coupled receptors. *Nat. Neurosci.* 5, 843–848.

Yacubova, E., and Komuro, H. (2002). Stage-specific control of neuronal migration by somatostatin. *Nature* 415, 77–81.

Yada, T., Sakurada, M., Ihida, K., Nakata, M., Murata, F., Arimura, A., et al. (1994). Pituitary adenylate cyclase activating polypeptide is an extraordinarily potent intra-pancreatic regulator of insulin secretion from islet beta-cells. *J. Biol. Chem.* 269, 1290–1293.

Yada, T., Vigh, S., and Arimura, A. (1993). Pituitary adenylate cyclase activating polypeptide (PACAP) increases cytosolic-free calcium concentration in folliculo-stellate cells and somatotropes of rat pituitary. *Peptides* 14, 235–239.

Yan, Y., Zhou, X., Pan, Z., Ma, J., Waschek, J. A., and Dicicco-Bloom, E. (2013). Pro- and anti-mitogenic actions of pituitary adenylate cyclase-activating polypeptide in developing cerebral cortex: potential mediation by developmental switch of PAC1 receptor mRNA isoforms. *J. Neurosci.* 33, 3865–3878.

Yao, C. J., Lin, C. W., and Lin-Shiau, S. Y. (1999). Roles of thapsigargin-sensitive Ca2+ stores in the survival of developing cultured neurons. *J. Neurochem.* 73, 457–465.

# 9

# Role of calcitonin gene-related peptide in cerebral vasospasm, and as a therapeutic approach to subarachnoid hemorrhage

**_Stelios Kokkoris[1], Peter Andrews[2]* and David J. Webb[3]_**

[1] *Intensive Care Unit, Western General Hospital, Edinburgh, UK*
[2] *Centre for Clinical Brain Sciences, University of Edinburgh, Edinburgh, UK*
[3] *Clinical Pharmacology Unit, British Heart Foundation Centre for Cardiovascular Science, Queen's Medical Research Institute, University of Edinburgh, Edinburgh, UK*

***Edited by:***
*Hubert Vaudry, University of Rouen, France*

***Reviewed by:***
*Akiyoshi Takahashi, Kitasato University, Japan*
*Jo G. De Mey, Maastricht University, Netherlands*

****Correspondence:***
*Peter Andrews, Centre for Clinical Brain Sciences, University of Edinburgh, Edinburgh, UK.*
*e-mail: p.andrews@ed.ac.uk*

Calcitonin gene-related peptide (CGRP) is one of the most potent microvascular vasodilators identified to date. Vascular relaxation and vasodilation is mediated via activation of the CGRP receptor. This atypical receptor is made up of a G protein-coupled receptor called calcitonin receptor-like receptor (CLR), a single transmembrane protein called receptor activity-modifying protein (RAMP), and an additional protein that is required for $G\alpha_S$ coupling, known as receptor component protein (RCP). Several mechanisms involved in CGRP-mediated relaxation have been identified. These include nitric oxide (NO)-dependent endothelium-dependent mechanisms or cAMP-mediated endothelium-independent pathways; the latter being more common. Subarachnoid hemorrhage (SAH) is associated with cerebral vasoconstriction that occurs several days after the hemorrhage and is often fatal. The vasospasm occurs in 30–40% of patients and is the major cause of death from this condition. The vasoconstriction is associated with a decrease in CGRP levels in nerves and an increase in CGRP levels in draining blood, suggesting that CGRP is released from nerves to oppose the vasoconstriction. This evidence has led to the concept that exogenous CGRP may be beneficial in a condition that has proven hard to treat. The present article reviews: (a) the pathophysiology of delayed ischemic neurologic deficit after SAH (b) the basics of the CGRP receptor structure, signal transduction, and vasodilatation mechanisms and (c) the studies that have been conducted so far using CGRP in both animals and humans with SAH.

**Keywords: GPCR, CGRP, subarachnoid hemorrhage, cerebral vasospasm, G proteins**

## INTRODUCTION

In the US, over 30,000 persons each year experience a subarachnoid hemorrhage (SAH). Whereas intracranial aneurysms are found in 2–5% of all autopsies, the incidence of rupture is only 2–20/100,000 individuals/year (Ingall et al., 2000). SAH is more frequent in women than men (3:2 ratio) over the age of 40, but the reverse is the case in those younger than 40 (The ACROSS Group, 2000; Ohkuma et al., 2002). Peak rupture rates occur between the ages of 50 and 60 years (The ACROSS Group, 2000; Ohkuma et al., 2002). Intracranial aneurysms account for approximately 85% of cases of non-traumatic SAH, whereas 10% have the pattern of non-aneurysmal perimesencephalic hemorrhage, a relatively harmless condition (van Gijn et al., 2007). The other causes include bleeding from other vascular malformations, moyamoya syndrome, coagulopathy, and, rarely, extension of an intracerebral hematoma (van Gijn et al., 2007). In up to 15%, no source of bleeding is identified (Kim et al., 2012). Approximately 10–15% of patients die before receiving medical treatment from the initial bleed or its immediate complications (Huang and van Gelder, 2002) and over 40% of hospitalized patients die within 1 month of the event (Ingall et al., 2000). Those that survive the initial bleed are at risk for a number of secondary insults including rebleeding (Winn et al., 1977; Ohkuma et al., 2001), hydrocephalus, and cerebral vasospasm (van Gijn et al., 2007).

Calcitonin gene-related peptide (CGRP) is one of the most potent microvascular vasodilator peptides identified to date. In the cerebral circulation, CGRP is released from sensory fibers originating in the trigeminal ganglia and acts to dilate cerebral vessels (McCulloch et al., 1986). CGRP has been found to be at least 1,000 times more potent than acetylcholine, substance P, ATP, adenosine, and 5-hydroxytriptamine, and 10–100 times more potent than the β-adrenergic agonist isoprenaline. Consequently, a dose of 15 pmol injected into human skin produces an erythema that lasts for 5–6 h (Brain et al., 1985). As we discuss later, CGRP has a particularly potent vasodilator activity in the cerebral circulation, rendering it a promising agent for the treatment of SAH-triggered cerebral vasospasm.

In the present review, we summarize the etiology and therapy of cerebral vasospasm, the biology of CGRP and its receptors, and review the role of CGRP as a treatment in SAH-associated vasospasm in both animals and humans.

## CEREBRAL VASOSPASM AFTER SAH

### DEFINITIONS

Throughout the literature, authors have used various means of defining vasospasm including terms like angiographic vasospasm, symptomatic vasospasm, and delayed cerebral ischemia (DCI). Angiographic vasospasm is a narrowing of the lumen of the major cerebral arteries, which is usually focal but may be diffuse. Vasospasm has its onset usually on day 3 after SAH, is maximal at days 6–8, and usually lasts for 2–3 weeks (Wilkins, 1990). Symptomatic vasospasm is characterized by the insidious onset of confusion and decreased level of consciousness, followed by focal motor and/or speech impairments. It is mainly a diagnosis of exclusion, when clinical deterioration occurs and hydrocephalus, rebleeding, hypoxia, and metabolic abnormalities have been ruled out. DCI is defined as symptomatic vasospasm, infarction attributable to vasospasm, or both (Frontera et al., 2009). Although about 70% of patients may develop arterial narrowing, only 30% will manifest neurological deficits. The outcome of DCI itself is death in about one-third and permanent deficit in another third (Dorsch, 1995). In the present review the term vasospasm is defined as arterial vessel narrowing.

### VASOSPASM PATHOPHYSIOLOGY

#### *Nitric oxide*

Loss of the biological effect of nitric oxide (NO) is considered to play a pivotal permissive role in the development of cerebral vasospasm. The principal effect of NO on cerebral vessels is the relaxation of vascular smooth muscle cells, with decreased bioavailability of NO being implicated in the formation of SAH-induced vasospasm. The depletion of NO has been assumed to occur via several mechanisms in the setting of SAH. First, due to its high affinity for hemoglobin (Hb), NO is scavenged by Hb released during the breakdown of subarachnoid blood (Goretski and Hollocher, 1988; Ignarro, 1990). Second, it is possible that the production of NO is decreased in SAH, as a result of the down-regulation of endothelial NO synthase (eNOS) and neuronal NOS (nNOS; Pluta, 2005). This is supported by studies that revealed the down-regulation/dysfunction of eNOS, and loss of nNOS in spastic arteries after SAH (Hino et al., 1996; Pluta et al., 1996), as well as the finding that levels of asymmetric dimethylarginine (ADMA), an endogenous inhibitor of eNOS, are elevated in the setting of cerebral vasospasm (Jung et al., 2004). Third, NO may reverse the effects of the potent vasoconstrictor endothelin-1 (ET-1; Thomas et al., 1997). Therefore, in the setting of decreased NO levels, the balance of vasodilator and vasoconstrictor influences is altered, and the relatively increased actions of ET-1 can potentiate cerebral vasospasm.

#### *Endothelin-1*

ET-1 is an extremely potent vasoconstrictor. In the brain, it is primarily produced by endothelial cells in response to ischemia, though it can also be produced by neurons, astrocytes, and activated leukocytes (Fassbender et al., 2000; Chow et al., 2002; Dumont et al., 2003). Levels of ET-1 are high in the plasma and cerebrospinal fluid (CSF) of SAH patients, correlate with the persistence of cerebral vasospasm (Seifert et al., 1995; Juvela, 2000), and decline in the absence of vasospasm (Seifert et al., 1995). Conversely, the administration of ET-1 antagonists or endothelin converting enzyme inhibitors prevents vasospasm (Kwan et al., 2002; Macdonald et al., 2008). Lastly, ET-1 induces NADPH oxidase expression and oxidative stress in human endothelial cells (Duerrschmidt et al., 2000).

#### *Inflammation*

Expression of adhesion molecules facilitates leukocyte adherence to the endothelium. Adhesion molecules, such as ICAM-1, VCAM-1, and E-selectin, have been found to be elevated in the CSF of patients with SAH and in blood vessel walls exposed to clot (Polin et al., 1998; Dumont et al., 2003). Leukocytes can contribute to vasospasm by promoting free radical formation that may evoke endothelial dysfunction (Grisham et al., 1998; Sullivan et al., 2000), and by producing a variety of vasoactive substances, including ET-1 and cytokines (Fassbender et al., 2000). Several cytokines have been found to be up-regulated in cerebral vasospasm, including TNF-alpha, IL-1, IL-6, and IL-8 (Hirashima et al., 1997; Fassbender et al., 2001; Takizawa et al., 2001).

#### *Oxidative stress*

Oxyhemoglobin (OxyHb) may catalyze generation of reactive oxygen species (ROS). Free radicals are considered to play a pivotal role in cerebral vasospasm through various mechanisms. First, they can initiate lipid peroxidation, whose products, lipid peroxides, are capable of producing vasospasm and damaging the structure of arteries (Lin et al., 2006). Second, it has been hypothesized that ROS can activate the protein kinase C (PKC) pathway directly and indirectly, through enhancement of the metabolism of membrane phospholipids resulting from peroxidative damage. This, in turn, can lead to vasospasm (Asano and Matsui, 1999). Other possible vasoactive compounds are bilirubin oxidation products (BOXes). Once bilirubin is formed, it is subsequently oxidized into BOXes, reaching maximum concentrations during the peak vasospasm period of 4–11 days. They are thought to be potentiators of cerebral vasospasm once it has been initiated, rather than primary initiators (Clark and Sharp, 2006).

#### *Hemoglobin*

A large body of evidence suggests that OxyHb, the ferrous form of hemoglobin, released from lysed erythrocytes, is a mediator of vasospasm. More specifically, OxyHb causes prolonged contraction of isolated cerebral arteries (Toda et al., 1991), and intracisternal injections of this agent result in cerebral vasospasm (Macdonald et al., 1991). Indeed, the presence of OxyHb in the CSF of patients after SAH and the extent of hemorrhage are correlated with the distribution, severity, and time course of vasospasm (Mayberg et al., 1990). Ferrous hemoglobin released from subarachnoid clot could lead to delayed arterial narrowing by a number of mechanisms, such as scavenging or decreased production of NO (Pluta, 2005), free radical production, modification of $K^+$ and $Ca^{2+}$ channels (Ishiguro et al., 2008), differential up-regulation of genes (Vikman et al., 2006), and activation of the Rho/Rho kinase and PKC pathways (Wickman et al., 2003).

#### *Intracellular $Ca^{2+}$*

Vasospasm can be regarded as an abnormal and prolonged contraction of vascular smooth muscle. The intracellular free $Ca^{2+}$

level plays a pivotal role in the regulation of smooth muscle contractility (Horowitz et al., 1996). Following SAH, changes have been reported in the electrical properties of smooth muscle cells of small diameter cerebral arteries leading to enhanced $Ca^{2+}$ influx, vasoconstriction, and decreased cerebral blood flow (Koide et al., 2011). Cerebral arteries from healthy animals express only L-type voltage-dependent $Ca^{2+}$ channels. Expression of an additional type of voltage-dependent $Ca^{2+}$ channels (R-type) occurs after SAH, leading to increased $Ca^{2+}$ channel density, increased $Ca^{2+}$ influx, and vasoconstriction (Ishiguro et al., 2005).

#### *Cortical spreading depolarization*

This is a pathogenetic process that has attracted much attention lately. The term "cortical spreading depolarization" describes the wave of near-complete neuronal depolarization and neuronal swelling in the brain that is ignited when passive cation influx across the cellular membranes exceeds ATP-dependent $Na^+$ and $Ca^{2+}$ pump activity. The cation influx is followed by water influx and shrinkage of the extracellular space by ~70% (Dreier et al., 2009). Although the ignition of cortical spreading depolarization occurs passively, driven by electrical and diffusion forces, energy consumption paradoxically increases since $Na^+$ and $Ca^{2+}$ pumps are immediately activated to correct the intracellular $Na^+$ and $Ca^{2+}$ surge. As a consequence, regional cerebral blood flow increases during the neuronal depolarization phase. The opposite of this physiological hemodynamic response to cortical spreading depolarization is termed "the inverse hemodynamic response," and occurs when there is local dysfunction of the microvasculature. With the inverse response, severe microvascular spasm instead of vasodilatation is coupled to the neuronal depolarization phase, and the term "cortical spreading ischemia" describes the cortical spreading depolarization-induced perfusion deficit (Dreier et al., 2009).

#### *Neurogenic factors*

The cerebral arteries have sympathetic, parasympathetic, and sensory innervation. It has been postulated that SAH causes a derangement of neuronal regulatory mechanisms, which in turn leads to vascular smooth muscle contraction. The vasoconstriction is associated with a decrease in CGRP levels in cerebral perivascular nerves (Edvinsson et al., 1991) and an increase in CGRP levels in blood draining from the external jugular vein (Juul et al., 1990), suggesting that CGRP is released antidromically from trigeminal sensory perivascular nerves to oppose the vasoconstriction. This evidence has led to the concept that administration of CGRP may be beneficial in SAH-associated vasospasm. The molecular characteristics of CGRP and its use as a treatment option in SAH are reviewed in Sections "Calcitonin Gene-related Peptide Biology" and "Calcitonin Gene-related Peptide and SAH," respectively, of the present article.

### TREATMENT OF VASOSPASM

The management of vasospasm involves routine "prophylactic" measures as well as more aggressive interventions, reserved for situations where there are signs or symptoms of DCI.

#### *Hemodynamic therapy*

The use of triple-H therapy (hypervolemia, hypertension, and hemodilution) stems from numerous clinical observations noting improvement in patients' clinical symptoms following induced hypertension and volume expansion (Kosnik and Hunt, 1976; Kassell et al., 1982). The relative contribution of each component is debated. However, there are many uncertainties for the use of prophylactic hemodynamic therapy following SAH. Two studies randomly assigned normovolemic or hypervolemic therapy to patients and reported no difference in the incidence of DCI between groups (Lennihan et al., 2000; Egge et al., 2001).

#### *Nimodipine*

Nimodipine is safe, cost-effective, and reduces the risk of poor outcome and secondary ischemia (Neil-Dwyer et al., 1987; Welty, 1987; Kostron et al., 1988; Mee et al., 1988), but has very modest effects. It is used prophylactically in all patients with SAH. Its precise mechanism of action remains unclear. Despite being shown to reduce the incidence of DCI and cerebral infarction in clinical trials, it has negligible effects on angiographic vasospasm; nimodipine may be neuroprotective by blocking $Ca^{2+}$ influx at a neuronal level (Al-Tamimi et al., 2010).

#### *Intracisternal thrombolysis*

A meta-analysis looking at a total of 652 patients who were treated with intracisternal thrombolytics concluded that thrombolytic therapy had a statistically significant beneficial effect. However, the authors acknowledged the lack of large, randomized prospective trials (Amin-Hanjani et al., 2004).

#### *Endovascular techniques*

Endovascular techniques frequently play a role in the aggressive treatment of vasospasm. They include transluminal angioplasty and intra-arterial infusion of vasodilators (papaverin, nicardipine, verapamil, etc.; Brisman et al., 2006). Transluminal balloon angioplasty is very effective at reversing angiographic spasm of large proximal vessels and produces a sustained reversal of arterial narrowing (Brisman et al., 2006; Jestaedt et al., 2008). The optimal timing of angioplasty in relation to medical therapy is uncertain. Major complications occur in ~5% of procedures and include vessel rupture, occlusion, dissection, hemorrhagic infarction, and hemorrhage from unsecured aneurysms (Zwienenberg-Lee et al., 2006).

#### *Statins*

Statins have been shown to possess cholesterol-lowering-independent pleiotropic effects in different clinical settings, including a decrease in the incidence and duration of severe vasospasm as well as a reduction in the mortality rate after SAH (Lynch et al., 2005; Tseng et al., 2005, 2007). Statins are thought to be beneficial in the prevention of cerebral vasospasm by down-regulating inflammation and up-regulating the expression of eNOS and therefore NO (Sugawara et al., 2011).

#### *Other treatments*

Clazosentan, an endothelin receptor A ($ET_A$) antagonist decreased the incidence of severe vasospasm, DCI and new infarcts seen on CT scans in a dose-dependent fashion. However, CONSCIOUS 1 study (a phase 2 trial) did not show a reduction in patient mortality, though the study was underpowered for this endpoint (the primary end point of this study was moderate or severe vasospasm within 14 days; Macdonald et al., 2008). CONSCIOUS 2 study (a phase 3 trial) included 1157 patients and its primary composite end point comprised all-cause mortality and vasospasm related morbidity. This study showed that clazosentan at 5 mg/h had no significant effect on mortality and vasospasm-related morbidity or functional outcome (Macdonald et al., 2011).

Erythropoietin (EPO) has also been examined in the setting of cerebral vasospasm. Apart from being potentially neuroprotective, EPO may play a role in preventing vasospasm by increasing the phosphorylation of eNOS (Santhanam et al., 2005), a potentially important mechanism for increasing NO production.

A recent randomized controlled trial (MASH 2) including 1204 patients did not show any benefit from intravenous (i.v.) magnesium sulfate administration in clinical outcome after aneurysmal SAH (Dorhout Mees et al., 2012).

Other drugs under investigation are tirilazad, a free radical scavenger (Haley et al., 1997), fasudil, a Rho-kinase inhibitor that inhibits vascular smooth muscle contraction (Shibuya et al., 1992), sodium nitrite, an NO donor (Pluta et al., 2005) and cisternal placement of prolonged-release nicardipine-loaded polymers (Kasuya et al., 2005).

## CALCITONIN GENE-RELATED PEPTIDE BIOLOGY

### CALCITONIN GENE-RELATED PEPTIDE

Calcitonin gene-related peptide is expressed in a subgroup of small neurons in the dorsal root, trigeminal, and vagal ganglia, which respond to noxious, thermal, or visceral input. These peptidergic neurons use L-glutamate as their primary neurotransmitter and project to the dorsal horn, trigeminal nucleus caudalis, or nucleus of the solitary tract. CGRP increases neurotransmitter release and neuronal responsiveness to noxious stimulation at all these levels, which leads to central sensitization underlying chronic pain states (Benarroch, 2011). CGRP can also be released antidromically in the periphery, eliciting vasodilatation as a component of neurogenic inflammation. CGRP may be involved in the pathophysiology of inflammatory and neuropathic pain. Involvement of CGRP in migraine headache has led to the development of CGRP antagonists for treatment of this disorder (Benarroch, 2011).

Calcitonin gene-related peptide is a 37-amino acid neuropeptide that was identified in 1982 by molecular biological techniques in the thyroid of aging rats and medullary thyroid carcinomas in humans, which were found to contain an alternative peptide product from the calcitonin gene (Amara et al., 1982). CGRP, in common with other members of this peptide family, is derived from the calcitonin gene. Other members of this family include adrenomedulin (AM), which is a potent vasodilator, amylin (AMY), which is important for maintaining glycemic control, and calcitonin, which contributes to calcium metabolism (Hay, 2007). CGRP exists in two forms, named αCGRP and βCGRP. While these two isoforms share the same biological activities, and differ by only three amino acids in the human (Steenbergh et al., 1985, 1986), they are formed from two distinct genes, which share >90% homology, at different sites on chromosome 11. CALC I gene forms calcitonin and αCGRP, whereas CALC II forms βCGRP (Alevizaki et al., 1986). αCGRP synthesis is caused by alternative splicing of the calcitonin gene (Amara et al., 1982; **Figure 1**). βCGRP is known to be transcribed from its own distinct gene (Steenbergh et al., 1985, 1986). The majority of CGRP within the body is αCGRP and primarily expressed in the peripheral and central nervous system. βCGRP is mainly expressed in the gut (Mulderry et al., 1988). However, it has also been identified in the central nervous system, pituitary, thyroid, and in medullary thyroid carcinoma as a major CGRP form together with αCGRP (Petermann et al., 1987).

Data from NMR studies suggest that CGRP consists of a characteristic N-terminal disulfide bridge-linked loop between cysteines $Cys_2$ and $Cys_7$, followed by an alpha-helix in amino acids $Val_8$-$Arg_{18}$ (Breeze et al., 1991). The next domain at residues 19–27 forms a hinge region (Conner et al., 2002). The C-terminus lies at residues 28–37, and contains two turn regions which form a putative binding epitope (Carpenter et al., 2001). It appears that the N-terminal cyclic portion of the CGRP molecule, containing a ring structure with a disulfide bond, is essential for agonistic activity (Maggi et al., 1990). It is interesting to note that the C-terminal fragment, $CGRP_{8-37}$, is devoid of any agonist activity at CGRP receptors, although it behaves as a competitive antagonist against the intact peptide (Chiba et al., 1989).

Calcitonin gene-related peptide is widely distributed in the central and peripheral nervous systems, primarily in sensory fibers that are closely associated with blood vessels (Uddman et al., 1986). CGRP is often co-localized with other peptides in these fibers, especially the tachykinin substance P (Uddman et al., 1986). In the cerebral circulation, CGRP is released from sensory fibers originating in the trigeminal ganglia and acts to dilate cerebral vessels (McCulloch et al., 1986). In the gut, CGRP is also released from spinal afferents, where it dilates mucosal blood vessels and may protect against the acidic environment (Holzer, 2000). CGRP-containing fibers also innervate coronary arteries of the heart (Gulbenkian et al., 1993).

The regulation of CGRP production is poorly understood. At a cellular level, nerve growth factor (NGF) up-regulates CGRP via the Ras/Raf/mitogen-activated protein kinase kinase-1 (MEK-1)/p42/p44 pathway (Freeland et al., 2000).

In the human circulation, CGRP has a half-life of approximately 7–10 min (Kraenzlin et al., 1985; Struthers et al., 1986). Regarding its metabolism, it seems that there is not an obvious mechanism, and it is probably broken down via a number of routes. First, mast cell tryptase has a potent effect in cleaving CGRP into inactive fragments, both *in vivo* and *in vitro.* More specifically, if both CGRP and substance P are released simultaneously, then CGRP could be inactivated by enzymes (tryptases), released by mast cells in response to substance P. This mechanism has been demonstrated in skin (Brain and Williams, 1988, 1989). Second, a matrix metalloproteinase II has the ability to metabolize CGRP and remove its vasodilator activity (Fernandez-Patron et al., 2000). Third, Sams-Nielsen et al. (2001) have provided evidence that CGRP is taken back up into sensory nerve terminals after repolarization *in vitro.* Finally, in the CSF, αCGRP is degraded by an endopeptidase that cleaves the peptide at the $Leu_{16}$-$Ser_{17}$ bond (Le Greves et al., 1989).

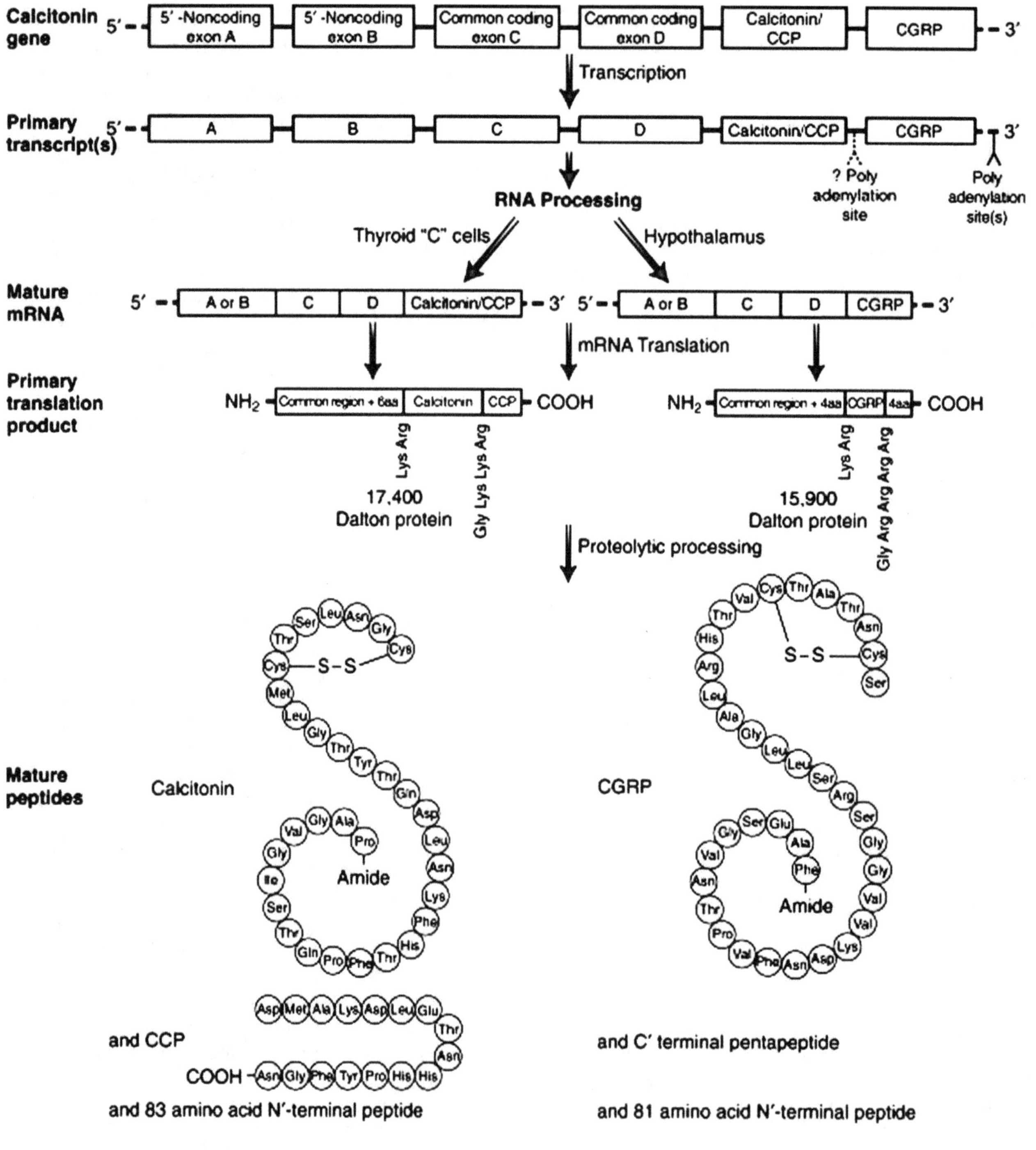


**FIGURE 1 | Tissue-specific expression of the calcitonin gene by alternative splicing.** Splicing of alternative exons leads to two different mRNAs. The mRNA encoding calcitonin is found predominantly in the thyroid C cell; the mRNA encoding a CGRP is found predominantly in the hypothalamus and other nervous tissue. CGRP, calcitonin gene related peptide; mRNA, messenger RNA; CCP, calcitonin carboxyl-terminal peptide. From Amara et al. (1982), with permission.

## STRUCTURE OF CGRP RECEPTORS

Many peptides, including the CGRP family, mediate their actions via G protein-coupled receptors (GPCR). The GPCRs form the largest family of cell-surface proteins that are capable of interacting with an extracellular stimulus and transducing that stimulus to produce a reaction inside a cell (Pierce et al., 2002). All GPCRs have seven transmembrane spanning domains, an extracellular N-terminus and an intracellular C-terminus and can be divided into three families based on signature amino acid sequences. Family A is the largest and generally binds small molecules and short peptides. Receptors in this class have been studied extensively, including photoreceptor rhodopsin, as well as adrenergic and olfactory receptors. Family B receptors bind larger peptides in the range of 27 to approximately 50 amino acids (secretin, glucagons, VIP, etc.). These receptors mediate the actions of CGRP and related peptides (Poyner et al., 2002; Hoare, 2005). Family C receptors include glutamate and $GABA_B$ receptors (Pierce et al., 2002).

Calcitonin receptor-like receptor (CLR), which belongs to family B of the GPCRs, comprises the main functional unit of the CGRP receptor (**Figure 2**). It was not until McLatchie's work (McLatchie et al., 1998) was published that it was recognized that a novel family of single transmembrane domain proteins, called receptor activity-membrane proteins (RAMP), were required to allow CLR to bind peptide and transduce signal. Three RAMPs have been identified so far ($RAMP_1$, $RAMP_2$, and $RAMP_3$). Each RAMP has a single transmembrane-spanning domain, a short intracellular C-terminal tail (~9 amino acids) and a long extracellular-terminus (~100 amino acids; McLatchie et al., 1998). As a result of CLR and calcitonin receptor (CTR) interactions with RAMP, the International Union of Pharmacology (IUPHAR) nomenclature recognizes that CGRP interacts with $CLR/RAMP_1$ ($CGRP_1$) receptors, whereas AM interacts with $CLR/RAMP_2$ ($AM_1$) or $CLR/RAMP_3$ ($AM_2$) receptors. The CTR without RAMP is sufficient for calcitonin binding, but CTR with RAMP 1, 2, or 3 are $AMY_1$, $AMY_2$, and $AMY_3$ receptors, respectively (Poyner et al., 2002). The discovery of RAMPs has led to evolution of our understanding of how receptor diversity is implemented, providing a novel mechanism for generating receptor subtypes within a subset of family B GPCRs (Sexton et al., 2006).

The primary function of CLR is thought to be related to ligand binding, whereas the RAMP molecule plays a crucial role in receptor trafficking to the membrane and determination of receptor pharmacology. The RAMP family regulate the glycosylation and transport of the CLR. However, they are not CGRP receptors by themselves (McLatchie et al., 1998; Sexton et al., 2009). Terminal glycosylation of the receptor and transit from the endoplasmic reticulum/Golgi apparatus to the cell surface require interaction of CLR with RAMP (Sexton et al., 2009).

Calcitonin gene-related peptide receptor activation is known to involve several crucial elements, in common with other GPCRs, such as the presence of a proline "kink" in transmembrane helix (TM)6 (Conner et al., 2005), and a putative 'DRY' motif equivalent (Conner et al., 2007), similar to family A GPCRs. There is also evidence suggesting stabilization of the CLR interaction with G "alpha" s ($G\alpha_s$) by another 17kDa intracellular membrane protein, called RCP (Evans et al., 2000).

The existence of two receptors, $CGRP_1$ and $CGRP_2$, was originally proposed in the late 1980s, with the $CGRP_1$ receptor being the predominant mediator of cardiovascular effects. This receptor classification was developed as a consequence of pharmacological studies carried out with different agonists and antagonists in a range of tissue preparations, especially the positive inotropic effect in the guinea pig or rat atrium for determination of $CGRP_1$ receptor activity, and the inhibition of electrically evoked twitch responses in the rat vas deferens for determination of $CGRP_2$ receptor activity (Dennis et al., 1989, 1990; Dumont et al., 1997). In general, receptors that can be antagonized by the 30-amino acid fragment of CGRP, $CGRP_{8-37}$, with an approximate $pA_2$ value of 7.0 are designated as $CGRP_1$ receptors, while those that $CGRP_{8-37}$ block with a $pA_2$ of 6.0 or less are classified as $CGRP_2$ receptors (Quirion et al., 1992; Poyner, 1995). However, it is questionable whether the $CGRP_2$ receptor is a single receptor type or whether it is, in fact, explained by multiple molecular entities (Hay, 2007).

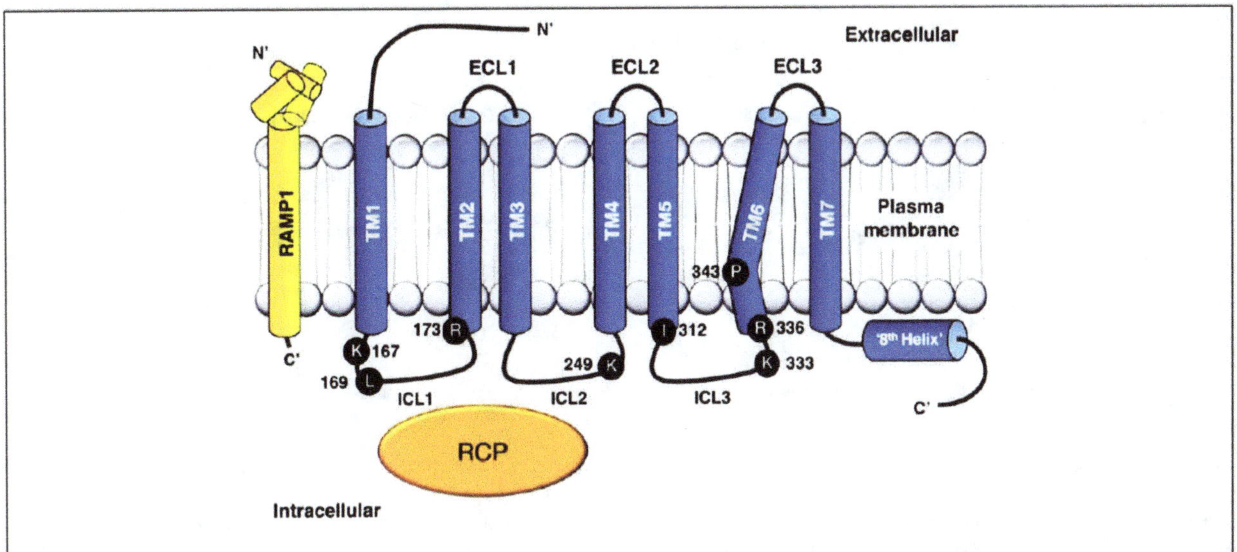


**FIGURE 2 | Structure of CGRP receptor.** CGRP receptor components and important residues for receptor signaling and internalization. The CGRP receptor is formed by CLR (blue), RAMP1 (yellow), and RCP (orange). Functionally important residues are shown as single letter abbreviations. CGRP, calcitonin gene-related peptide; CLR, calcitonin receptor-like receptor; RAMP, receptor activity-modifying protein; RCP, receptor component protein; C′, C-terminal; EC, extracellular loop; ICL, intracellular loop; N′, N-terminal; TM, transmembrane. From Walker et al. (2010), with permission.

In contrast, $CGRP_1$ is a well-defined receptor type consisting of CLR and $RAMP_1$.

### SIGNAL TRANSDUCTION OF CGRP RECEPTOR

Several mechanisms involved in CGRP-mediated vasorelaxation have been identified. These mechanisms include either NO-dependent endothelium-dependent mechanisms or cAMP-mediated endothelium-independent pathways. The most common pathway is NO- and endothelium-independent. Activation of the CGRP receptor is generally accepted to result in $G\alpha_s$-mediated activation of adenylate cyclase, with a subsequent increase in cAMP and activation of protein kinase A (PKA). In the absence of endothelium, CGRP is able to cause relaxation, suggesting it must directly act on the smooth muscle cells to stimulate adenylate cyclase (Edvinsson et al., 1985, 1998; Crossman et al., 1990). The resulting rise in cAMP then activates PKA, which phosphorylates and opens up ATP-sensitive $K^+$ channels, thus leading to relaxation (**Figure 3A**; Nelson et al., 1990).

Endothelium-independent relaxation to CGRP occurs in the majority of tissues examined to date. Exceptions include the rat aorta, where the relaxation to CGRP occurs only in the presence of an intact endothelium and is attenuated by inhibitors of NO synthase, implying an NO-dependent mechanism (Brain et al., 1985; Gray and Marshall, 1992a,b). A significant increase in both cAMP and cGMP occurs and is also dependent on the presence of endothelium (Gray and Marshall, 1992a). This implicates the release of NO from the endothelium, which then relaxes the smooth muscle cells through activation of guanylate cyclase and accumulation of cGMP. Moreover, it has been shown that cAMP is able to stimulate eNOS activity, leading to increased synthesis and release of NO (Ferro et al., 1999; Queen et al., 2000). The activation of eNOS via cAMP is probably mediated via PKA, as a study demonstrated that various protein kinases can phosphorylate and activate eNOS (Butt et al., 2000). It is a possibility that CGRP causes an increase in cAMP in endothelial cells, which leads to PKA activation. PKA, in turn, activates eNOS, which results in NO release, and thus relaxation of the smooth muscle (**Figure 3A**).

There is some evidence for $G\alpha_{i/o}$ signaling by the CGRP receptor, which is traditionally identified by sensitivity to pertussis toxin (PTX; **Figure 3B**). The CGRP-mediated stimulation of $Ca^{2+}$ transients in rat nodose neurons and the activation of c-Jun N-terminal kinase (JNK) in SK-N-MC cells (which express endogenous CGRP receptors) both displayed PTX sensitivity (Wiley et al., 1992; Disa et al., 2000).

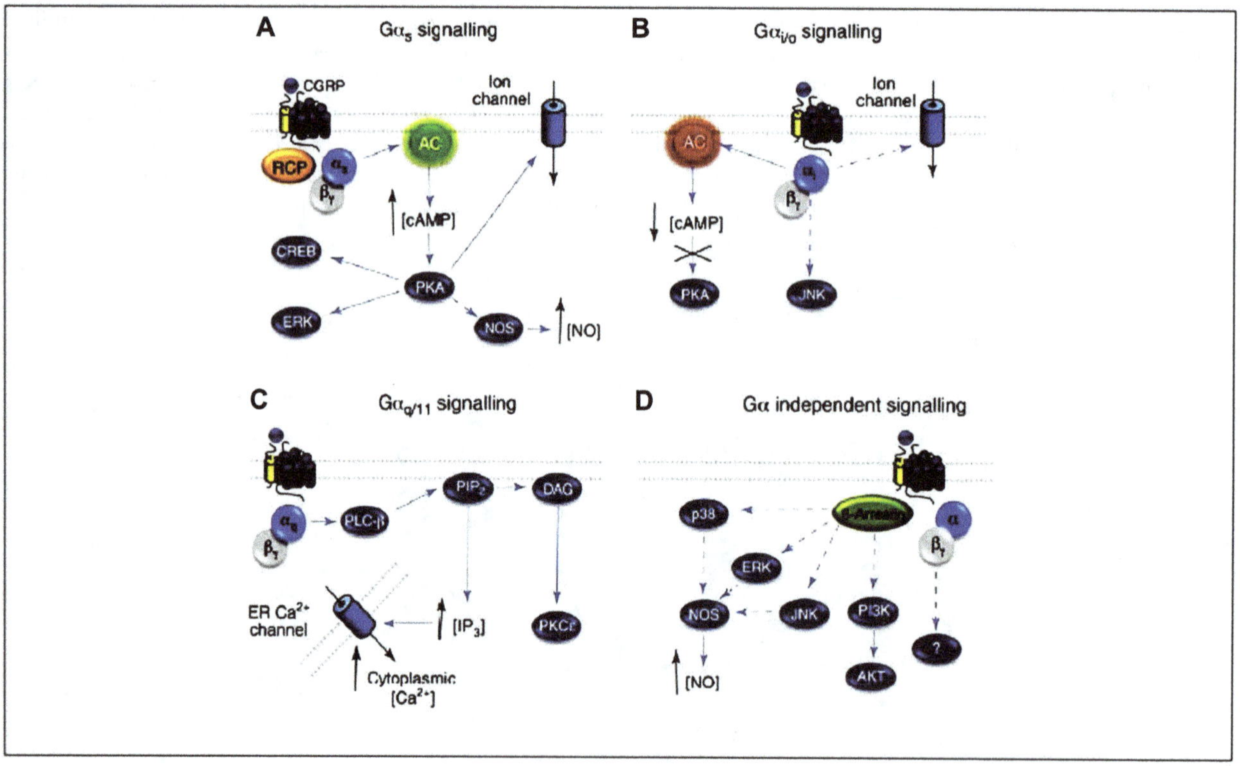


**FIGURE 3 | CGRP receptor-mediated intracellular signaling. (A)** $G\alpha_s$ signaling increases AC (green) activity, elevating intracellular cAMP, activating PKA and subsequently many potential downstream effectors. **(B)** The CGRP receptor might also couple to $G\alpha_{i/o}$, reducing AC (red) activity, decreasing intracellular cAMP and reducing PKA activity. **(C)** CGRP signaling via $G\alpha_q$ activates PLC-b, which cleaves $PIP_2$ into $IP_3$ and DAG, resulting in elevated intracellular $Ca^{2+}$ and PKC activation. **(D)** The CGRP receptor might also utilize Ga-independent signaling, and $G_{\beta\gamma}$- or b-arrestin-mediated signaling pathways. Arrows represent reported pathways; broken arrows represent potential or inferred pathways. CGRP, calcitonin gene-related peptide; CLR, calcitonin receptor-like receptor; Gα, α subunit of the G protein; NO, nitric oxide; NOS, nitric oxide synthase; AC, adenylyl cyclase; cAMP, cyclic adenosine monophosphate; PKA, protein kinase A; PKC, protein kinase C; RCP, receptor component protein; AC, adenylate cyclase; ER, endoplasmic reticulum; $PIP_2$, phosphatidylinositol 4,5-bisphosphate; DAG, diacylglycerol. From Walker et al. (2010), with permission.

The CGRP receptor may also be able to stimulate intracellular activity through a different G protein. Aiyar et al. (1999) reported that CGRP was able to activate phospholipase C (PLC) in HEK293 cells, leading to an increase in intracellular $Ca^{2+}$ via inositol trisphosphate (IP3) activity. This increase in $Ca^{2+}$ occurred concurrently with the stimulation of adenylyl cyclase and accumulation of cAMP. Activation of PLC is considered to occur through $G_{q/11\alpha}$, rather than through $G\alpha_s$, suggesting that the activated CGRP receptor is able to interact with both types of G protein. If this mechanism is present in endothelial cells, it provides an alternative explanation for CGRP activation of eNOS (which is traditionally considered to be dependent on $Ca^{2+}$/calmodulin for activation), independently of cAMP accumulation. The possibility that CGRP receptors may be coupled to phosphatidylinositol turnover is supported by another study that found this secondary messenger pathway in skeletal muscle (Laufer and Changeux, 1989; **Figure 3C**).

Recently, Meens et al. (2012) reported that activated CGRP receptors induce cyclic nucleotide-independent relaxation of vascular smooth muscle cells in mesenteric resistance arteries and terminate arterial effects of ET-1 via $G_{\beta\gamma}$. More specifically, CGRP receptor activation causes cAMP production but the relaxation of rat mesenteric resistance arteries induced by activation of this receptor involves $G_{\beta\gamma}$ and is not dependent on cAMP (**Figure 3D**).

Another study by Meens et al. (2010) discovered that CGRP released from peri-arterial sensory motor nerves terminates long-lasting vasoconstrictor effects of ET-1 by promoting dissociation of ET-1/$ET_A$-receptor complexes.

The CGRP receptor can also potentially activate other downstream signaling molecules, such as PKC and mitogen-activated protein kinase (MAPK) cascades, such as p38, JNK, and extracellular receptor activated kinase 1/2 (ERK ½; Walker et al., 2010). CGRP receptor signaling is regulated by desensitization, internalization, and trafficking, which, as with other GPCRs, involves GPCR kinases (GRK), β arrestin, and clathrin- and dynamin-dependent endocytosis (Walker et al., 2010). Padilla et al. (2007) proposed a mechanism by which endosomal endothelin converting enzyme-1 (ECE-1) degrades CGRP in endosomes to disrupt the peptide/receptor/β-arrestin complex, freeing internalized receptors from β-arrestins and promoting recycling and resensitization, resulting in long-lasting vascular relaxing response to CGRP.

## CALCITONIN GENE-RELATED PEPTIDE AND SAH

### PRELIMINARY OBSERVATIONAL STUDIES

An animal study of experimental SAH in rats revealed that the sensory innervation of the cerebral circulation by CGRP-containing fibers appeared to be reduced after SAH (estimated by the number of fibers present), and there was also a larger vasodilating response to CGRP in basilar arteries after SAH as compared to vessels from control animals. The reduction in CGRP could be due to release of the transmitter from the perivascular nerve terminals caused by blood in the subarachnoid space (Edvinsson et al., 1990).

In another study (Edvinsson et al., 1991), the proximal parts of the middle cerebral artery (MCA) were collected within 24 h after death from five humans suffering SAH (5–10 days beforehand) and from six subjects dying from myocardial infarction. In humans who had died from SAH the level of CGRP was nearly not detectable, being in contrast to that seen in age and sex matched subjects who had died of myocardial infarction. The trigemino-cerebrovascular system was suggested by the authors to act as an anti-vasoconstrictor system by releasing stored peptides, CGRP being the most likely candidate.

Juul et al. (1995) measured CGRP levels with specific radioimmunoassays (RIA) in patients with SAH, after operation with aneurysm clipping and nimodipine treatment. They used samples taken either from the external jugular vein ($n = 20$) or from the CSF ($n = 14$) during the postoperative course. They also used samples from healthy volunteers. The degree of vasoconstriction in the patients was monitored with Doppler ultrasound recordings. CGRP concentrations from the external jugular vein were significantly higher than from controls. Also, the CGRP level was measurable in SAH CSF but not in CSF of controls.

Others (Tran Dinh et al., 1994) showed that the basal level of endogenous CGRP in CSF was 0.77 nmol/L in rabbits. The CGRP concentration peaked at 14 nmol/L within 30 min, and at 8 nmol/L within 24 h, after SAH. They further showed that 3 days after SAH the CGRP concentration in CSF declined to 3.5 nmol/L.

Nozaki et al. (1989a) produced a model of SAH by a single injection of fresh autologous arterial blood into the cisterna magna of dogs. Then, they examined changes of CGRP immunoreactivity immunohistochemically in perivascular nerve fibers of the large pial arteries. CGRP in cerebrovascular nerve fibers was suppressed after SAH. The suppression was first detected on the third day after SAH, and was most marked during the 7th to 14th day. CGRP, however, recovered to a normal level by the 42nd day after SAH.

Arienta et al. (1991) isolated the basilar artery from five rabbits subjected to SAH and five control animals. A mild or severe vasospasm was observed in the basilar artery about 15 min after injection of blood in the cisterna magna, while fluorescence immunohistochemistry revealed a marked decrease of the perivascular nerves containing CGRP in the animals of the experimental group, as compared to the control group.

### EFFECTS OF CGRP ADMINISTRATION ON CEREBRAL VASOSPASM AFTER EXPERIMENTAL SAH IN ANIMALS (Table 1)

Nozaki et al. (1989b) produced experimental SAH in 30 dogs by injecting autologous arterial blood into the cisterna magna. They used two models of injection: in the first, single-injection model, 1 ml/kg of blood was injected on day 0, while 0.5 ml/kg of blood was injected successively 48 h apart in the second, double-injection model, on day 0 and day 2. The diameter of the basilar artery was measured by angiography. The most marked constriction of the basilar artery was seen on day 3 after SAH in the single-injection model and on day 7 in the double-injection model. When $10^{-10}$ mol/kg of CGRP was administered intracisternally (i.c.) on day 3 in the single-injection model, cerebral vasospasm reversed completely. The effect began to appear 5 min after CGRP administration, continued for 4 h, and disappeared by 24 h after the administration. When CGRP was administered at doses of $10^{-11}$ to $2 \times 10^{-10}$ mol/kg on day 7 after SAH in the double-injection model, the cerebral vasospasm was reversed in a dose-dependent manner: $2 \times 10^{-10}$ mol/kg of CGRP reversed the vasospasm completely. The effect began to appear 5 min after the CGRP

**Table 1 | Studies of CGRP administration after experimental SAH in animals.**

| Reference | Animal model | Total sample size (intervention/ control) | Way of CGRP administration | CGRP dose | Results | Adverse events |
|---|---|---|---|---|---|---|
| Nozaki et al. (1989b) | Dog | 30 (22/8) | i.c. | $2 \times 10^{-10}$ mol/kg | Vasospasm was reversed completely | AP and HR slightly increased |
| Imaizumi et al. (1996) | Rabbit | 16 (8/8) | i.c. | $10^{-10}$ mol/kg | Basilar artery dilated from 73 to 117%, significantly larger than 67% in control ($p < 0.01$) | None |
| Toshima et al. (1992) | Rabbit | 41 (17/24) | i.c./i.v. | 100 ng/kg/min i.c./ 100 ng/kg/min i.v. | Basilar artery diameter in either i.v. or i.c. CGRP groups was significantly greater than that of the respective control group | AP drop in i.v. CGRP administration |
| Ahmad et al. (1996) | Rabbit | 45 (22/23) | i.c. slow-release tablet | 24 or 153 μg | Vasospasm was completely reversed | None |
| Inoue et al. (1996) | Monkey | 10 (5/5) | i.c. slow-release tablet | 1,200 μg | Cerebral vasospasm was significantly ameliorated | None |
| Toyoda et al. (2000) | Rabbit | 16 (8/8) | i.c. adenovirus-mediated CGRP gene transfer | NA | Arterial diameter was similar before and after SAH in CGRP group | None |
| Satoh et al. (2002) | Dog | 20 (8/12) | i.c. adenovirus-mediated CGRP gene transfer | NA | Vasospasm was significantly reduced compared with the control group | None |

*i.c., intra-cisternal; i.v., intravenous; AP, arterial pressure; HR, heart rate; SAH, subarachnoid hemorrhage; NA, non-applicable.*

administration, continued for 4 h, and disappeared by 24 h. Of note, when the amounts of CGRP mentioned above were administered i.c., both mean arterial blood pressure and heart rate were only slightly increased and returned to the previous levels within several minutes.

In a similar study by Imaizumi et al. (1996), experimental SAH was produced by i.c. injection of arterial blood in rabbits. The animals were treated with intrathecal administration of CGRP 3 days after SAH. The degree of vasospasm and the effect of CGRP were evaluated angiographically by measuring the basilar artery diameter. The basilar artery constricted to 73% of the pre-SAH values 3 days after SAH. Fifteen minutes after $10^{-10}$ mol/kg CGRP injection, the basilar artery dilated from 73 to 117% ($n = 8$), which was significantly larger than 67.1% in the vehicle group ($n = 8$; $p < 0.01$). At 6 h after $10^{-10}$ mol/kg CGRP injection, the basilar artery was still dilated to 90% ($p < 0.05$). In the $10^{-11}$ mol/kg CGRP group, the basilar artery was dilated to 87% ($p < 0.05$) 15 min after the injection. The injection of $10^{-12}$ mol/kg CGRP had no significant effect. The dilatory effect in the $10^{-10}$ mol/kg CGRP group was demonstrated up to 6 h after injection. Arterial blood pressure was stable after injection of CGRP.

Toshima et al. (1992) produced SAH in 41 rabbits by injecting i.c. autologous blood. The animals were randomly assigned to five groups and were sacrificed on day 2 post-SAH. Group 1 was the control group. Immediately prior to sacrifice, group 2 and 3 animals received a 2-h i.c. injection of vehicle or CGRP (100 ng/kg/min), respectively. Group 4 and 5 animals received a 2-h i.v. injection of vehicle or CGRP (100 ng/kg/min), respectively. The diameter of basilar artery in group 3 (i.c. CGRP) was significantly larger than that in group 2 (i.c. vehicle, $p < 0.001$). Similarly, the diameter of basilar artery in group 5 (i.v. CGRP) was significantly greater than that in group 4 (i.v. vehicle, $p < 0.01$). Although no significant difference was observed in mean arterial blood pressure between groups 2 and 3 (i.c. groups), there was a significant difference between i.v. groups 4 and 5 (lower in group 5, $p < 0.01$).

Ahmad et al. (1996) implanted a CGRP slow-release tablet i.c., containing either 24 or 153 μg of human αCGRP, 24 h after experimental SAH was induced in rabbits. Following implantation, the CGRP level in the CSF remained elevated for 5 days. The implantation of the tablet almost completely ameliorated angiographic vasospasm. Moreover, no significant systemic hypotension or neurological adverse event was associated with the treatment.

In a similar approach, Inoue et al. (1996) investigated the efficacy of a CGRP slow-release tablet for the prevention of cerebral vasospasm after SAH in monkeys. Experimental SAH was produced by the method of Espinosa et al. (1984). The animal underwent a right frontotemporal craniectomy under sterile conditions. The dura mater was opened, and the arachnoid membrane was microsurgically incised until the ipsilateral internal carotid

**Table 2 | Studies of CGRP administration after aneurysmal SAH in humans.**

| Reference | Sample size/ patient type | Study design | Way of CGRP administration | Dose | Primary outcome | Results | Adverse events |
|---|---|---|---|---|---|---|---|
| Juul et al. (1994) | 5/ postoperative course after SAH | Not randomized, not controlled study | i.v. infusion | 0.6 μg/min | H.I. | Significant reduction in H.I. during CGRP infusion compared to that before infusion | HR increase during CGRP infusion |
| Johnston et al. (1990) | 15/ neurological deficit after surgical clipping of the aneurysm | Multicenter randomized placebo-controlled study | i.v. infusion | 0.035 μg/min, doubled every 10 min, max 1.15 μg/min | Modified GCS | Of the nine patients who showed a treatment preference, eight favored CGRP ($p < 0.05$) | None |
| European CGRP in SAH study (1992) | 117/ ischemic neurological deficit after operation for the aneurysm | Multicenter randomized placebo-controlled study | i.v. infusion | 0.6 μg/min | Glasgow outcome scale | Relative risk of a bad outcome in CGRP-treated compared with controls 0.88 (95% CI: 0.6–1.26) | 2/3 of the patients included in the CGRP group had reduced AP and did not complete treatment |

*i.v., intravenous; AP, arterial pressure; HR, heart rate; SAH, subarachnoid hemorrhage; H.I., hemodynamic index; GCS, Glasgow coma scale.*

artery (ICA) and proximal portions of the MCA and anterior cerebral artery (ACA) were exposed. An autologous blood clot (1 ml/kg) was then placed around the exposed arteries to produce experimental SAH. For animals in the CGRP ($n = 5$) and placebo ($n = 5$) groups, a total of three tablets (total drug 1200 μg) were ipsilaterally placed under the frontal and temporal lobes at the time of SAH production. In the control group, cerebral vasospasm developed on day 7 (56% as an average of the ICA, MCA, and ACA). In the CGRP group, vasospasm was significantly ameliorated on average (75%, $p < 0.02$). The CGRP concentration in CSF was measurable only on day 7 for the CGRP group (6.5 nmol/L). No significant untoward reactions were recorded.

Toyoda et al. (2000) sought to determine whether adenovirus-mediated gene transfer *in vivo* of CGRP, ameliorates cerebral vasoconstriction after experimental SAH. Arterial blood was injected into the cisterna magna of rabbits to mimic SAH 5 days after injection of adenovirus or vehicle. After injection of adenovirus ($n = 8$), there was a 400-fold increase in CGRP in CSF. In rabbits treated with vehicle (controls, $n = 8$), basilar artery diameter after SAH was 25% smaller than before SAH ($p < 0.0005$). In rabbits treated with adenovirus, arterial diameter was similar before and after SAH. Furthermore, treatment of rabbits with adenovirus after experimental SAH prevented spasm of the basilar artery 2 days after SAH.

Likewise, Satoh et al. (2002) investigated whether a delayed treatment with adenovirus encoding CGRP gene, 2 days after experimental SAH, reduces cerebral vasospasm in a double-hemorrhage model (on days 0 and 2) of severe vasospasm in dogs. Severe vasospasm was observed in control SAH dogs ($n = 12$) on day 7, and the mean basilar artery diameter was 53% of baseline. In the group treated with adenovirus ($n = 8$), vasospasm was significantly reduced (the basilar artery diameter was 78% of baseline, $p < 0.05$ compared with the control SAH group). High levels of CGRP were measured in CSF from dogs that received adenovirus (115-fold greater than baseline levels).

Intracisternal gene transfer of CGRP was initially thought to be more useful than i.v. infusion, because the local gene transfer might avoid systemic effects of CGRP and achieve its sustained release into the central nervous system. However, there are several concerns, such as the inflammatory process induced by adenovirus, the difficulty in approaching the target cells in the presence of a large subarachnoid blood clot, and its potential ability for cancerous transformation of the affected cells.

### EFFECTS OF CGRP ADMINISTRATION ON CEREBRAL VASOSPASM AFTER SAH IN HUMANS (Table 2)

Juul et al. (1994) investigated the effect of i.v. CGRP infusion at a rate of 0.6 μg/min in five patients with vasoconstriction in the postoperative course after SAH, where the hemodynamic index (ratio between middle cerebral and ICA mean velocities) was used as an indicator of vasoconstriction. A significant reduction was found in the hemodynamic index during the CGRP infusion as compared to that before infusion (4.3 vs. 6.2, $p < 0.05$). However, no significant change was observed in pulsatility index (another indicator of vasospasm, equal to the difference between the systolic and diastolic flow velocities divided by the mean flow velocity), blood pressure, or consciousness during CGRP infusion. A significant increase in heart rate was observed during the infusion, while blood pressure remained unaltered.

Johnston et al. (1990) undertook a multicenter, randomized, placebo-controlled trial to study the safety and efficacy of i.v. CGRP treatment to reverse neurological deficits after surgical clipping of a ruptured intracranial aneurysm. Patients were enrolled if they had postoperative neurological deficit. Patients received CGRP or placebo in random order, 24 h apart. Fifteen patients were eventually included in the study. Infusion started at a rate sufficient to deliver 0.035 μg/min CGRP, and was doubled every 10 min until either a clinical response was obtained or a maximum dose of 1.15 μg/min was reached at 1 h. If the neurological deficit had not deteriorated and the patient had no side-effects by that time, the maximum infusion rate was continued for another 20 min. Regarding neurological changes according to the modified Glasgow Coma Scale, five patients did not improve on either treatment, one improved on both, eight improved on CGRP but not on placebo, and one improved on placebo but not on CGRP. Of the nine patients who showed a treatment preference, eight (88.9%) favored CGRP ($p < 0.05$). The mean duration of neurological improvement was 25 min, after which patients returned to their previous neurological status. There was a significant decrease in both systolic and diastolic blood pressures during the infusion of CGRP.

A larger, multicenter, randomized controlled trial (European CGRP in SAH study, 1992) investigated the effect of a post-operative infusion of CGRP on outcome at 3 months. Patients with aneurysmal SAH who underwent surgery entered the trial if an ischemic neurological deficit developed after the operation. A total of 117 patients entered the study (62 patients received CGRP and 55 standard management). The CGRP-treated patients received the drug by i.v. infusion at a rate of 0.6 μg/min. If systemic hypotension developed, the infusion rate was reduced to 0.45 μg/min, then to 0.3 μg/min, if the hypotension was still apparent. CGRP treatment was given for at least 4 h; patients who showed a satisfactory neurological response continued to receive treatment for up to 10 days (minimum of 4 days). The percentage of patients with a good outcome was slightly but not significantly higher in the CGRP than in the control group. The relative risk of a bad outcome in CGRP-treated compared with control patients was 0.88 (95% CI: 0.60−1.28). Interestingly, only a third of patients randomized to receive CGRP completed treatment, so two-thirds included in the treatment group for the analyses had limited exposure to CGRP, mainly due to arterial hypotension.

## CONCLUSION

The pathogenesis of vasospasm after SAH is complex, multifactorial, and incompletely understood. CGRP has shown promising results both *in vitro* and *in vivo*, mainly in animal models of experimental SAH. However, there is a lack of studies in humans. Systemic hypotension induced by the i.v. administration of the drug seems to be a serious problem. The encouraging results from the i.c. application of CGRP in animals could warrant large studies in humans with CGRP instillation into the subarachnoid space, in order to avoid hypotension and achieve even more efficient dilatation of the cerebral arteries.

## REFERENCES


Ahmad, I., Imaizumi, S., Shimizu, H., Kaminuma, T., Ochiai, N., Tajima, M., et al. (1996). Development of calcitonin gene-related peptide slow-release tablet implanted in CSF space for prevention of cerebral vasospasm after experimental subarachnoid haemorrhage. *Acta Neurochir. (Wien)* 138, 1230–1240.

Aiyar, N., Disa, J., Stadel, J. M., and Lysko, P. G. (1999). Calcitonin gene-related peptide receptor independently stimulates 3′,5′-cyclic adenosine monophosphate and $Ca^{2+}$ signaling pathways. *Mol. Cell. Biochem.* 197, 179–185.

Al-Tamimi, Y. Z., Orsi, N. M., Quinn, A. C., Homer-Vanniasinkam, S., and Ross, S. A. (2010). A review of delayed ischemic neurologic deficit following aneurysmal subarachnoid hemorrhage: historical overview, current treatment, and pathophysiology. *World Neurosurg.* 73, 654–667.

Alevizaki, M., Shiraishi, A., Rassool, F. V., Ferrier, G. J., MacIntyre, I., and Legon, S. (1986). The calcitonin-like sequence of the beta CGRP gene. *FEBS Lett.* 206, 47–52.

Amara, S. G., Jonas, V., Rosenfeld, M. G., Ong, E. S., and Evans, R. M. (1982). Alternative RNA processing in calcitonin gene expression generates mRNAs encoding different polypeptide products. *Nature* 298, 240–244.

Amin-Hanjani, S., Ogilvy, C. S., and Barker, F. G. (2004). Does intracisternal thrombolysis prevent vasospasm after aneurysmal subarachnoid hemorrhage? A meta-analysis. *Neurosurgery* 54, 326–334.

Arienta, C., Balbi, S., Caroli, M., and Fumagalli, G. (1991). Depletion of calcitonin gene-related peptide in perivascular nerves during acute phase of posthemorrhagic vasospasm in the rabbit. *Brain Res. Bull.* 27, 605–609.

Asano, T., and Matsui, T. (1999). Antioxidant therapy against cerebral vasospasm following aneurysmal subarachnoid hemorrhage. *Cell Mol. Neurobiol.* 19, 31–44.

Benarroch, E. E. (2011). CGRP: sensory neuropeptide with multiple neurologic implications. *Neurology* 77, 281–287.

Brain, S. D., and Williams, T. J. (1988). Substance P regulates the vasodilator activity of calcitonin gene-related peptide. *Nature* 335, 73–75.

Brain, S. D., and Williams, T. J. (1989). Interactions between the tachykinins and calcitonin gene-related peptide lead to the modulation of oedema formation and blood flow in rat skin. *Br. J. Pharmacol.* 97, 77–82.

Brain, S. D., Williams, T. J., Tippins, J. R., Morris, H. R., and MacIntyre, I. (1985). Calcitonin gene-related peptide is a potent vasodilator. *Nature* 313, 54–56.

Breeze, A. L., Harvey, T. S., Bazzo, R., and Campbell, I. D. (1991). Solution structure of human calcitonin gene-related peptide by 1H NMR and distance geometry with restrained molecular dynamics. *Biochemistry* 30, 575–582.

Brisman, J. L., Eskridge, J. M., and Newell, D. W. (2006). Neurointerventional treatment of vasospasm. *Neurol. Res.* 28, 769–776.

Butt, E., Bernhardt, M., Smolenski, A., Kotsonis, P., Frohlich, L. G., Sickmann, A., et al. (2000). Endothelial nitric-oxide synthase (type III) is activated and becomes calcium independent upon phosphorylation by cyclic nucleotide-dependent protein kinases. *J. Biol. Chem.* 275, 5179–5187.

Carpenter, K. A., Schmidt, R., von Mentzer, B., Haglund, U., Roberts, E., and Walpole, C. (2001). Turn structures in CGRP C-terminal analogues promote stable arrangements of key residue side chains. *Biochemistry* 40, 8317–8325.

Chiba, T., Yamaguchi, A., Yamatani, T., Nakamura, A., Morishita, T., Inui, T., et al. (1989). Calcitonin gene-related peptide receptor antagonist human CGRP-(8−37). *Am. J. Physiol.* 256, E331–E335.

Chow, M., Dumont, A. S., and Kassell, N. F. (2002). Endothelin receptor antagonists and cerebral vasospasm: an update. *Neurosurgery* 51, 1333–1341.

Clark, J. F., and Sharp, F. R. (2006). Bilirubin oxidation products (BOXes) and their role in cerebral vasospasm after subarachnoid hemorrhage. *J. Cereb. Blood Flow Metab.* 26, 1223–1233.

Conner, A. C., Hay, D. L., Howitt, S. G., Kilk, K., Langel, U., Wheatley, M., et al. (2002). Interaction of calcitonin-gene-related peptide with its receptors. *Biochem. Soc. Trans.* 30, 451–455.

Conner, A. C., Hay, D. L., Simms, J., Howitt, S. G., Schindler, M., Smith, D. M., et al. (2005). A key role for transmembrane prolines in calcitonin receptor-like receptor agonist binding and signalling: implications for family B G-protein-coupled receptors. *Mol. Pharmacol.* 67, 20–31.

Conner, A. C., Simms, J., Barwell, J., Wheatley, M., and Poyner, D. R. (2007). Ligand binding and activation of the CGRP receptor. *Biochem. Soc. Trans.* 35, 729–732.

Crossman, D. C., Dashwood, M. R., Brain, S. D., McEwan, J., and Pearson, J. D. (1990). Action of calcitonin gene-related peptide upon bovine vascular endothelial and smooth muscle cells grown in isolation and co-culture. *Br. J. Pharmacol.* 99, 71–76.

Dennis, T., Fournier, A., Cadieux, A., Pomerleau, F., Jolicoeur, F. B., St Pierre, S., et al. (1990). hCGRP8-37, a calcitonin gene-related peptide antagonist revealing calcitonin gene-related peptide receptor heterogeneity in brain and periphery. *J. Pharmacol. Exp. Ther.* 254, 123–128.

Dennis, T., Fournier, A., St Pierre, S., and Quirion, R. (1989). Structure-activity profile of calcitonin gene-related peptide in peripheral and brain tissues. Evidence for receptor multiplicity. *J. Pharmacol. Exp. Ther.* 251, 718–725.

Disa, J., Parameswaran, N., Nambi, P., and Aiyar, N. (2000). Involvement of cAMP-dependent protein kinase and pertussis toxin-sensitive G-proteins in CGRP mediated JNK activation in human neuroblastoma cell line. *Neuropeptides* 34, 229–233.

Dorhout Mees, S. M., Algra, A., Vandertop, W. P., van Kooten, F., Kuijsten, H. A., Boiten, J., et al. (2012). Magnesium for aneurysmal subarachnoid haemorrhage (MASH-2): a randomised placebo-controlled trial. *Lancet* 380, 44–49.

Dorsch, N. W. (1995). Cerebral arterial spasm – a clinical review. *Br. J. Neurosurg.* 9, 403–412.

Dreier, J. P., Major, S., Manning, A., Woitzik, J., Drenckhahn, C., Steinbrink, J., et al. (2009). Cortical spreading ischaemia is a novel process involved in ischaemic damage in patients with aneurysmal subarachnoid haemorrhage. *Brain* 132, 1866–1881.

Duerrschmidt, N., Wippich, N., Goettsch, W., Broemme, H. J., and Morawietz, H. (2000). Endothelin-1 induces NAD(P)H oxidase in human endothelial cells. *Biochem. Biophys. Res. Commun.* 269, 713–717.

Dumont, A. S., Dumont, R. J., Chow, M. M., Lin, C. L., Calisaneller, T., Ley, K. F., et al. (2003). Cerebral vasospasm after subarachnoid hemorrhage: putative role of inflammation. *Neurosurgery* 53, 123–133.

Dumont, Y., Fournier, A., St-Pierre, S., and Quirion, R. (1997). A potent and selective CGRP2 agonist, [Cys(Et)2,7]hCGRP alpha: comparison in prototypical CGRP1 and CGRP2 in vitro bioassays. *Can. J. Physiol. Pharmacol.* 75, 671–676.

Edvinsson, L., Delgado-Zygmunt, T., Ekman, R., Jansen, I., Svendgaard, N. A., and Uddman, R. (1990). Involvement of perivascular sensory fibers in the pathophysiology of cerebral vasospasm following subarachnoid hemorrhage. *J. Cereb. Blood Flow Metab.* 10, 602–607.

Edvinsson, L., Ekman, R., Jansen, I., McCulloch, J., Mortensen, A., and Uddman, R. (1991). Reduced levels of calcitonin gene-related peptide-like immunoreactivity in human brain vessels after subarachnoid haemorrhage. *Neurosci. Lett.* 121, 151–154.

Edvinsson, L., Fredholm, B. B., Hamel, E., Jansen, I., and Verrecchia, C. (1985). Perivascular peptides relax cerebral arteries concomitant with stimulation of cyclic adenosine monophosphate accumulation or release of an endothelium-derived relaxing factor in the cat. *Neurosci. Lett.* 58, 213–217.

Edvinsson, L., Gulbenkian, S., Barroso, C. P., Cunha e Sa, M., Polak, J. M., Mortensen, A., et al. (1998). Innervation of the human middle meningeal artery: immunohistochemistry, ultrastructure, and role of endothelium for vasomotility. *Peptides* 19, 1213–1225.

Egge, A., Waterloo, K., Sjoholm, H., Solberg, T., Ingebrigtsen, T., and Romner, B. (2001). Prophylactic hyperdynamic postoperative fluid therapy after aneurysmal subarachnoid hemorrhage: a clinical, prospective, randomized, controlled study. *Neurosurgery* 49, 593–605.

Espinosa, F., Weir, B., Overton, T., Castor, W., Grace, M., and Boisvert, D. (1984). A randomized placebo-controlled double-blind trial of nimodipine after SAH in monkeys. Part 1: clinical and radiological findings. *J. Neurosurg.* 60, 1167–1175.

European CGRP in Subarachnoid Haemorrhage Study Group. (1992). Effect of calcitonin-gene-related peptide in patients with delayed postoperative cerebral ischaemia after aneurysmal subarachnoid haemorrhage. European CGRP in Subarachnoid Haemorrhage Study Group. *Lancet* 339, 831–834.

Evans, B. N., Rosenblatt, M. I., Mnayer, L. O., Oliver, K. R., and Dickerson, I. M. (2000). CGRP-RCP, a novel protein required for signal transduction at calcitonin gene-related peptide and adrenomedullin receptors. *J. Biol. Chem.* 275, 31438–31443.

Fassbender, K., Hodapp, B., Rossol, S., Bertsch, T., Schmeck, J., Schutt, S., et al. (2001). Inflammatory cytokines in subarachnoid haemorrhage: association with abnormal blood flow velocities in basal cerebral arteries. *J. Neurol. Neurosurg. Psychiatry* 70, 534–537.

Fassbender, K., Hodapp, B., Rossol, S., Bertsch, T., Schmeck, J., Schutt, S., et al. (2000). Endothelin-1 in subarachnoid hemorrhage: an acute-phase reactant produced by cerebrospinal fluid leukocytes. *Stroke* 31, 2971–2975.

Fernandez-Patron, C., Stewart, K. G., Zhang, Y., Koivunen, E., Radomski, M. W., and Davidge, S. T. (2000). Vascular matrix metalloproteinase-2-dependent cleavage of calcitonin gene-related peptide promotes vasoconstriction. *Circ. Res.* 87, 670–676.

Ferro, A., Queen, L. R., Priest, R. M., Xu, B., Ritter, J. M., Poston, L., et al. (1999). Activation of nitric oxide synthase by beta 2-adrenoceptors in human umbilical vein endothelium *in vitro*. *Br. J. Pharmacol.* 126, 1872–1880.

Freeland, K., Liu, Y. Z., and Latchman, D. S. (2000). Distinct signalling pathways mediate the cAMP response element (CRE)-dependent activation of the calcitonin gene-related peptide gene promoter by cAMP and nerve growth factor. *Biochem. J.* 345(Pt 2), 233–238.

Frontera, J. A., Fernandez, A., Schmidt, J. M., Claassen, J., Wartenberg, K. E., Badjatia, N., et al. (2009). Defining vasospasm after subarachnoid hemorrhage: what is the most clinically relevant definition? *Stroke* 40, 1963–1968.

Goretski, J., and Hollocher, T. C. (1988). Trapping of nitric oxide produced during denitrification by extracellular hemoglobin. *J. Biol. Chem.* 263, 2316–2323.

Gray, D. W., and Marshall, I. (1992a). Human alpha-calcitonin gene-related peptide stimulates adenylate cyclase and guanylate cyclase and relaxes rat thoracic aorta by releasing nitric oxide. *Br. J. Pharmacol.* 107, 691–696.

Gray, D. W., and Marshall, I. (1992b). Nitric oxide synthesis inhibitors attenuate calcitonin gene-related peptide endothelium-dependent vasorelaxation in rat aorta. *Eur. J. Pharmacol.* 212, 37–42.

Grisham, M. B., Granger, D. N., and Lefer, D. J. (1998). Modulation of leukocyte-endothelial interactions by reactive metabolites of oxygen and nitrogen: relevance to ischemic heart disease. *Free Radic. Biol. Med.* 25, 404–433.

Gulbenkian, S., Saetrum, O. O., Ekman, R., Costa, A. N., Wharton, J., Polak, J. M., et al. (1993). Peptidergic innervation of human epicardial coronary arteries. *Circ. Res.* 73, 579–588.

Haley, E. C. Jr., Kassell, N. F., Apperson-Hansen, C., Maile, M. H., and Alves, W. M. (1997). A randomized, double-blind, vehicle-controlled trial of tirilazad mesylate in patients with aneurysmal subarachnoid hemorrhage: a cooperative study in North America. *J. Neurosurg.* 86, 467–474.

Hay, D. L. (2007). What makes a CGRP2 receptor? *Clin. Exp. Pharmacol. Physiol.* 34, 963–971.

Hino, A., Tokuyama, Y., Weir, B., Takeda, J., Yano, H., Bell, G. I., et al. (1996). Changes in endothelial nitric oxide synthase mRNA during vasospasm after subarachnoid hemorrhage in monkeys. *Neurosurgery* 39, 562–567.

Hirashima, Y., Nakamura, S., Endo, S., Kuwayama, N., Naruse, Y., and Takaku, A. (1997). Elevation of platelet activating factor, inflammatory cytokines, and coagulation factors in the internal jugular vein of patients with subarachnoid hemorrhage. *Neurochem. Res.* 22, 1249–1255.

Hoare, S. R. (2005). Mechanisms of peptide and nonpeptide ligand binding to Class B G-protein-coupled receptors. *Drug Discov. Today* 10, 417–427.

Holzer, P. (2000). Local microcirculatory reflexes and afferent signalling in response to gastric acid challenge. *Gut* 47(Suppl. 4), iv46–iv48.

Horowitz, A., Menice, C. B., Laporte, R., and Morgan, K. G. (1996). Mechanisms of smooth muscle contraction. *Physiol. Rev.* 76, 967–1003.

Huang, J., and van Gelder, J. M. (2002). The probability of sudden death from rupture of intracranial aneurysms: a meta-analysis. *Neurosurgery* 51, 1101–1105.

Ignarro, L. J. (1990). Biosynthesis and metabolism of endothelium-derived nitric oxide. *Annu. Rev. Pharmacol. Toxicol.* 30, 535–560.

Imaizumi, S., Shimizu, H., Ahmad, I., Kaminuma, T., Tajima, M., and Yoshimoto, T. (1996). Effect of calcitonin gene-related peptide on delayed cerebral vasospasm after experimental subarachnoid hemorrhage in rabbits. *Surg. Neurol.* 46, 263–270.

Ingall, T., Asplund, K., Mahonen, M., and Bonita, R. (2000). A multinational comparison of subarachnoid hemorrhage epidemiology in the WHO MONICA stroke study. *Stroke* 31, 1054–1061.

Inoue, T., Shimizu, H., Kaminuma, T., Tajima, M., Watabe, K., and Yoshimoto, T. (1996). Prevention of cerebral vasospasm by calcitonin gene-related peptide slow-release tablet after subarachnoid hemorrhage in monkeys. *Neurosurgery* 39, 984–990.

Ishiguro, M., Murakami, K., Link, T., Zvarova, K., Tranmer, B. I., Morielli, A. D., et al. (2008). Acute and chronic effects of oxyhemoglobin on voltage-dependent ion channels in cerebral arteries. *Acta Neurochir. Suppl.* 104, 99–102.

Ishiguro, M., Wellman, T. L., Honda, A., Russell, S. R., Tranmer, B. I., and Wellman, G. C. (2005). Emergence of a R-type $Ca^{2+}$ channel (CaV 2.3) contributes to cerebral artery constriction after subarachnoid hemorrhage. *Circ. Res.* 96, 419–426.

Jestaedt, L., Pham, M., Bartsch, A. J., Kunze, E., Roosen, K., Solymosi, L., et al. (2008). The impact of balloon angioplasty on the evolution of vasospasm-related infarction after aneurysmal subarachnoid hemorrhage. *Neurosurgery* 62, 610–617.

Johnston, F. G., Bell, B. A., Robertson, I. J., Miller, J. D., Haliburn, C., O'Shaughnessy, D., et al. (1990). Effect of calcitonin-gene-related peptide on postoperative neurological deficits after subarachnoid haemorrhage. *Lancet* 335, 869–872.

Jung, C. S., Iuliano, B. A., Harvey-White, J., Espey, M. G., Oldfield, E. H., and Pluta, R. M. (2004). Association between cerebrospinal fluid levels of asymmetric dimethyl-L-arginine, an endogenous inhibitor of endothelial nitric oxide synthase, and cerebral vasospasm in a primate model of subarachnoid hemorrhage. *J. Neurosurg.* 101, 836–842.

Juul, R., Aakhus, S., Bjornstad, K., Gisvold, S. E., Brubakk, A. O., and Edvinsson, L. (1994). Calcitonin gene-related peptide (human alpha-CGRP) counteracts vasoconstriction in human subarachnoid haemorrhage. *Neurosci. Lett.* 170, 67–70.

Juul, R., Edvinsson, L., Gisvold, S. E., Ekman, R., Brubakk, A. O., and Fredriksen, T. A. (1990). Calcitonin gene-related peptide-LI in subarachnoid haemorrhage in man. Signs of activation of the trigemino-cerebrovascular system? *Br. J. Neurosurg.* 4, 171–179.

Juul, R., Hara, H., Gisvold, S. E., Brubakk, A. O., Fredriksen, T. A., Waldemar, G., et al. (1995). Alterations in perivascular dilatory neuropeptides (CGRP, SP, VIP) in the external jugular vein and in the cerebrospinal fluid following subarachnoid haemorrhage in man. *Acta Neurochir. (Wien)* 132, 32–41.

Juvela, S. (2000). Plasma endothelin concentrations after aneurysmal subarachnoid hemorrhage. *J. Neurosurg.* 92, 390–400.

Kassell, N. F., Peerless, S. J., Durward, Q. J., Beck, D. W., Drake, C. G., and Adams, H. P. (1982). Treatment of ischemic deficits from vasospasm with intravascular volume expansion and induced arterial hypertension. *Neurosurgery* 11, 337–343.

Kasuya, H., Onda, H., Sasahara, A., Takeshita, M., and Hori, T. (2005). Application of nicardipine prolonged-release implants: analysis of 97 consecutive patients with acute subarachnoid hemorrhage. *Neurosurgery* 56, 895–902.

Kim, Y. W., Lawson, M. F., and Hoh, B. L. (2012). Nonaneurysmal subarachnoid hemorrhage: an update. *Curr. Atheroscler. Rep.* 14, 328–334.

Koide, M., Nystoriak, M. A., Brayden, J. E., and Wellman, G. C. (2011). Impact of subarachnoid hemorrhage on local and global calcium signaling in cerebral artery myocytes. *Acta Neurochir. Suppl.* 110(Pt 1), 145–150.

Kosnik, E. J., and Hunt, W. E. (1976). Postoperative hypertension in the management of patients with intracranial arterial aneurysms. *J. Neurosurg.* 45, 148–154.

Kostron, H., Twerdy, K., and Grunert, V. (1988). The calcium entry blocker nimodipine improves the quality of life of patients operated on for cerebral aneurysms. A 5-year follow-up analysis. *Neurochirurgia (Stuttg.)* 31, 150–153.

Kraenzlin, M. E., Ch'ng, J. L., Mulderry, P. K., Ghatei, M. A., and Bloom, S. R. (1985). Infusion of a novel peptide, calcitonin gene-related peptide (CGRP) in man. Pharmacokinetics and effects on gastric acid secretion and on gastrointestinal hormones. *Regul. Pept.* 10, 189–197.

Kwan, A. L., Lin, C. L., Chang, C. Z., Winardi, D., Yen, C. P., Wu, S. C., et al. (2002). Oral administration of an inhibitor of endothelin-converting enzyme attenuates cerebral vasospasm following experimental subarachnoid haemorrhage in rabbits. *Clin. Sci. (Lond.)* 103(Suppl. 48), 414S–417S.

Laufer, R., and Changeux, J. P. (1989). Calcitonin gene-related peptide and cyclic AMP stimulate phosphoinositide turnover in skeletal muscle cells. Interaction between two second messenger systems. *J. Biol. Chem.* 264, 2683–2689.

Le Greves, P., Nyberg, F., Hokfelt, T., and Terenius, L. (1989). Calcitonin gene-related peptide is metabolized by an endopeptidase hydrolyzing substance P. *Regul. Pept.* 25, 277–286.

Lennihan, L., Mayer, S. A., Fink, M. E., Beckford, A., Paik, M. C., Zhang, H., et al. (2000). Effect of hypervolemic therapy on cerebral blood flow after subarachnoid hemorrhage: a randomized controlled trial. *Stroke* 31, 383–391.

Lin, C. L., Hsu, Y. T., Lin, T. K., Morrow, J. D., Hsu, J. C., Hsu. Y. H., et al. (2006). Increased levels of F2-isoprostanes following aneurysmal subarachnoid hemorrhage in humans. *Free Radic. Biol. Med.* 40, 1466–1473.

Lynch, J. R., Wang, H., McGirt, M. J., Floyd, J., Friedman, A. H., Coon, A. L., et al. (2005). Simvastatin reduces vasospasm after aneurysmal subarachnoid hemorrhage: results of a pilot randomized clinical trial. *Stroke* 36, 2024–2026.

Macdonald, R. L., Higashida, R. T., Keller, E., Mayer, S. A., Molyneux, A., Raabe, A., et al. (2011). Clazosentan, an endothelin receptor antagonist, in patients with aneurysmal subarachnoid haemorrhage undergoing surgical clipping: a randomised, double-blind, placebo-controlled phase 3 trial (CONSCIOUS-2). *Lancet Neurol.* 10, 618–625.

Macdonald, R. L., Kassell, N. F., Mayer, S., Ruefenacht, D., Schmiedek, P., Weidauer, S., et al. (2008). Clazosentan to overcome neurological ischemia and infarction occurring after subarachnoid hemorrhage (CONSCIOUS-1): randomized, double-blind, placebo-controlled phase 2 dose-finding trial. *Stroke* 39, 3015–3021.

Macdonald, R. L., Weir, B. K., Runzer, T. D., Grace, M. G., Findlay, J. M., Saito, K., et al. (1991). Etiology of cerebral vasospasm in primates. *J. Neurosurg.* 75, 415–424.

Maggi, C. A., Rovero, P., Giuliani, S., Evangelista, S., Regoli, D., and Meli, A. (1990). Biological activity of N-terminal fragments of calcitonin gene-related peptide. *Eur. J. Pharmacol.* 179, 217–219.

Mayberg, M. R., Okada, T., and Bark, D. H. (1990). The role of hemoglobin in arterial narrowing after subarachnoid hemorrhage. *J. Neurosurg.* 72, 634–640.

McCulloch, J., Uddman, R., Kingman, T. A., and Edvinsson, L. (1986). Calcitonin gene-related peptide: functional role in cerebrovascular regulation. *Proc. Natl. Acad. Sci. U.S.A.* 83, 5731–5735.

McLatchie, L. M., Fraser, N. J., Main, M. J., Wise, A., Brown, J., Thompson, N., et al. (1998). RAMPs regulate the transport and ligand specificity of the calcitonin-receptor-like receptor. *Nature* 393, 333–339.

Mee, E., Dorrance, D., Lowe, D., and Neil-Dwyer, G. (1988). Controlled study of nimodipine in aneurysm patients treated early after subarachnoid hemorrhage. *Neurosurgery* 22, 484–491.

Meens, M. J., Compeer, M. G., Hackeng, T. M., van Zandvoort, M. A., Janssen, B. J., and De Mey, J. G. (2010). Stimuli of sensory-motor nerves terminate arterial contractile effects of endothelin-1 by CGRP and dissociation of ET-1/ET(A)-receptor complexes. *PLoS ONE* 5, e10917. doi: 10.1371/journal.pone.0010917

Meens, M. J., Mattheij, N. J., van Loenen, P. B., Spijkers, L. J., Lemkens, P., Nelissen. J, et al. (2012). G-protein betagamma subunits in vasorelaxing and anti-endothelinergic effects of calcitonin gene-related peptide. *Br. J. Pharmacol.* 166, 297–308.

Mulderry, P. K., Ghatei, M. A., Spokes, R. A., Jones, P. M., Pierson, A. M., Hamid, Q. A., et al. (1988). Differential expression of alpha-CGRP and beta-CGRP by primary sensory neurons and enteric autonomic neurons of the rat. *Neuroscience* 25, 195–205.

Neil-Dwyer, G., Mee, E., Dorrance, D., and Lowe, D. (1987). Early intervention with nimodipine in subarachnoid haemorrhage. *Eur. Heart J.* 8(Suppl. K), 41–47.

Nelson, M. T., Huang, Y., Brayden, J. E., Hescheler, J., and Standen, N. B. (1990). Arterial dilations in response to calcitonin gene-related peptide involve activation of $K^+$ channels. *Nature* 344, 770–773.

Nozaki, K., Kikuchi, H., and Mizuno, N. (1989a). Changes of calcitonin gene-related peptide-like immunoreactivity in cerebrovascular nerve fibers in the dog after experimentally produced subarachnoid hemorrhage. *Neurosci. Lett.* 102, 27–32.

Nozaki, K., Uemura, Y., Okamoto, S., Kikuchi, H., and Mizuno, N. (1989b). Relaxant effect of calcitonin gene-related peptide on cerebral arterial spasm induced by experimental subarachnoid hemorrhage in dogs. *J. Neurosurg.* 71, 558–564.

Ohkuma, H., Fujita, S., and Suzuki, S. (2002). Incidence of aneurysmal subarachnoid hemorrhage in Shimokita, Japan, from 1989 to 1998. *Stroke* 33, 195–199.

Ohkuma, H., Tsurutani, H., and Suzuki, S. (2001). Incidence and significance of early aneurysmal rebleeding before neurosurgical or neurological management. *Stroke* 32, 1176–1180.

Padilla, B. E., Cottrell, G. S., Roosterman, D., Pikios, S., Muller, L., Steinhoff, M., et al. (2007). Endothelin-converting enzyme-1 regulates endosomal sorting of calcitonin receptor-like receptor and beta-arrestins. *J. Cell Biol.* 179, 981–997.

Petermann, J. B., Born, W., Chang, J. Y., and Fischer, J. A. (1987). Identification in the human central nervous system, pituitary, and thyroid of a novel calcitonin gene-related peptide, and partial amino acid sequence in the spinal cord. *J. Biol. Chem.* 262, 542–545.

Pierce, K. L., Premont, R. T., and Lefkowitz, R. J. (2002). Seven-transmembrane receptors. *Nat. Rev. Mol. Cell Biol.* 3, 639–650.

Pluta, R. M. (2005). Delayed cerebral vasospasm and nitric oxide: review, new hypothesis, and proposed treatment. *Pharmacol. Ther.* 105, 23–56.

Pluta, R. M., Dejam, A., Grimes, G., Gladwin, M. T., and Oldfield, E. H. (2005). Nitrite infusions to prevent delayed cerebral vasospasm in a primate model of subarachnoid hemorrhage. *JAMA* 293, 1477–1484.

Pluta, R. M., Thompson, B. G., Dawson, T. M., Snyder, S. H., Boock, R. J., and Oldfield, E. H. (1996). Loss of nitric oxide synthase immunoreactivity in cerebral vasospasm. *J. Neurosurg.* 84, 648–654.

Polin, R. S., Bavbek, M., Shaffrey, M. E., Billups, K., Bogaev, C. A., Kassell, N. F., et al. (1998). Detection of soluble E-selectin, ICAM-1, VCAM-1, and L-selectin in the cerebrospinal fluid of patients after subarachnoid hemorrhage. *J. Neurosurg.* 89, 559–567.

Poyner, D. (1995). Pharmacology of receptors for calcitonin gene-related peptide and amylin. *Trends Pharmacol. Sci.* 16, 424–428.

Poyner, D. R., Sexton, P. M., Marshall, I., Smith, D. M., Quirion, R., Born, W., et al. (2002). International Union of Pharmacology. XXXII. The mammalian calcitonin gene-related peptides, adrenomedullin, amylin, and calcitonin receptors. *Pharmacol. Rev.* 54, 233–246.

Queen, L. R., Xu, B., Horinouchi, K., Fisher, I., and Ferro, A. (2000). beta(2)-adrenoceptors activate nitric oxide synthase in human platelets. *Circ. Res.* 87, 39–44.

Quirion, R., Van Rossum, D., Dumont, Y., St-Pierre, S., and Fournier, A. (1992). Characterization of CGRP1 and CGRP2 receptor subtypes. *Ann. N. Y. Acad. Sci.* 657, 88–105.

Sams-Nielsen, A., Orskov, C., and Jansen-Olesen, I. (2001). Pharmacological evidence for CGRP uptake into perivascular capsaicin sensitive nerve terminals. *Br. J. Pharmacol.* 132, 1145–1153.

Santhanam, A. V., Smith, L. A., Akiyama, M., Rosales, A. G., Bailey, K. R., and Katusic, Z. S. (2005). Role of endothelial NO synthase phosphorylation in cerebrovascular protective effect of recombinant erythropoietin during subarachnoid hemorrhage-induced cerebral vasospasm. *Stroke* 36, 2731–2737.

Satoh, M., Perkins, E., Kimura, H., Tang, J., Chun, Y., Heistad, D. D., et al. (2002). Posttreatment with adenovirus-mediated gene transfer of calcitonin gene-related peptide to reverse cerebral vasospasm in dogs. *J. Neurosurg.* 97, 136–142.

Seifert, V., Loffler, B. M., Zimmermann, M., Roux, S., and Stolke, D. (1995). Endothelin concentrations in patients with aneurysmal subarachnoid hemorrhage. Correlation with cerebral vasospasm, delayed ischemic neurological deficits, and volume of hematoma. *J. Neurosurg.* 82, 55–62.

Sexton, P. M., Morfis, M., Tilakaratne, N., Hay, D. L., Udawela, M., Christopoulos, G., et al. (2006). Complexing receptor pharmacology: modulation of family B G protein-coupled receptor function by RAMPs. *Ann. N. Y. Acad. Sci.* 1070, 90–104.

Sexton, P. M., Poyner, D. R., Simms, J., Christopoulos, A., and Hay, D. L. (2009). Modulating receptor function through RAMPs: can they represent drug targets in themselves? *Drug Discov. Today* 14, 413–419.

Shibuya, M., Suzuki, Y., Sugita, K., Saito, I., Sasaki, T., Takakura, K., et al. (1992). Effect of AT877 on cerebral vasospasm after aneurysmal subarachnoid hemorrhage. Results of a prospective placebo-controlled double-blind trial. *J. Neurosurg.* 76, 571–577.

Steenbergh, P. H., Hoppener, J. W., Zandberg, J., Lips, C. J., and Jansz, H. S. (1985). A second human calcitonin/CGRP gene. *FEBS Lett.* 183, 403–407.

Steenbergh, P. H., Hoppener, J. W., Zandberg, J., Visser, A., Lips, C. J., and Jansz, H. S. (1986). Structure and expression of the human calcitonin/CGRP genes. *FEBS Lett.* 209, 97–103.

Struthers, A. D., Brown, M. J., Macdonald, D. W., Beacham, J. L., Stevenson, J. C., Morris, H. R., et al. (1986).

Human calcitonin gene related peptide: a potent endogenous vasodilator in man. *Clin. Sci. (Lond.)* 70, 389–393.

Sugawara, T., Ayer, R., Jadhav, V., Chen, W., Tsubokawa, T., and Zhang, J. H. (2011). Mechanisms of statin treatment in cerebral vasospasm. *Acta Neurochir. Suppl.* 110, 9–11.

Sullivan, G. W., Sarembock, I. J., and Linden, J. (2000). The role of inflammation in vascular diseases. *J. Leukoc. Biol.* 67, 591–602.

Takizawa, T., Tada, T., Kitazawa, K., Tanaka, Y., Hongo, K., Kameko, M., et al. (2001). Inflammatory cytokine cascade released by leukocytes in cerebrospinal fluid after subarachnoid hemorrhage. *Neurol. Res.* 23, 724–730.

The ACROSS Group. (2000). Epidemiology of aneurysmal subarachnoid hemorrhage in Australia and New Zealand: incidence and case fatality from the Australasian Cooperative Research on Subarachnoid Hemorrhage Study (ACROSS). *Stroke* 31, 1843–1850.

Thomas, J. E., Nemirovsky, A., Zelman, V., and Giannotta, S. L. (1997). Rapid reversal of endothelin-1-induced cerebral vasoconstriction by intrathecal administration of nitric oxide donors. *Neurosurgery* 40, 1245–1249.

Toda, N., Kawakami, M., and Yoshida, K. (1991). Constrictor action of oxyhemoglobin in monkey and dog basilar arteries *in vivo* and *in vitro*. *Am. J. Physiol.* 260, H420–H425.

Toshima, M., Kassell, N. F., Tanaka, Y., and Dougherty, D. A. (1992). Effect of intracisternal and intravenous calcitonin gene-related peptide on experimental cerebral vasospasm in rabbits. *Acta Neurochir. (Wien)* 119, 134–138.

Toyoda, K., Faraci, F. M., Watanabe, Y., Ueda, T., Andresen, J. J., Chu, Y., et al. (2000). Gene transfer of calcitonin gene-related peptide prevents vasoconstriction after subarachnoid hemorrhage. *Circ. Res.* 87, 818–824.

Tran Dinh, Y. R., Debdi, M., Couraud, J. Y., Creminon, C., Seylaz, J., and Sercombe, R. (1994). Time course of variations in rabbit cerebrospinal fluid levels of calcitonin gene-related peptide- and substance P-like immunoreactivity in experimental subarachnoid hemorrhage. *Stroke* 25, 160–164.

Tseng, M. Y., Czosnyka, M., Richards, H., Pickard, J. D., and Kirkpatrick, P. J. (2005). Effects of acute treatment with pravastatin on cerebral vasospasm, autoregulation, and delayed ischemic deficits after aneurysmal subarachnoid hemorrhage: a phase II randomized placebo-controlled trial. *Stroke* 36, 1627–1632.

Tseng, M. Y., Hutchinson, P. J., Czosnyka, M., Richards, H., Pickard, J. D., and Kirkpatrick, P. J. (2007). Effects of acute pravastatin treatment on intensity of rescue therapy, length of inpatient stay, and 6-month outcome in patients after aneurysmal subarachnoid hemorrhage. *Stroke* 38, 1545–1550.

Uddman, R., Edvinsson, L., Ekblad, E., Hakanson, R., and Sundler, F. (1986). Calcitonin gene-related peptide (CGRP): perivascular distribution and vasodilatory effects. *Regul. Pept.* 15, 1–23.

van Gijn, J., Kerr, R. S., and Rinkel, G. J. (2007). Subarachnoid haemorrhage. *Lancet* 369, 306–318.

Vikman, P., Beg, S., Khurana, T. S., Hansen-Schwartz, J., and Edvinsson, L. (2006). Gene expression and molecular changes in cerebral arteries following subarachnoid hemorrhage in the rat. *J. Neurosurg.* 105, 438–444.

Walker, C. S., Conner, A. C., Poyner, D. R., and Hay, D. L. (2010). Regulation of signal transduction by calcitonin gene-related peptide receptors. *Trends Pharmacol. Sci.* 31, 476–483.

Welty, T. E. (1987). Use of nimodipine for prevention and treatment of cerebral arterial spasm in patients with subarachnoid hemorrhage. *Clin. Pharm.* 6, 940–946.

Wickman, G., Lan, C., and Vollrath, B. (2003). Functional roles of the Rho/Rho kinase pathway and protein kinase C in the regulation of cerebrovascular constriction mediated by hemoglobin: relevance to subarachnoid hemorrhage and vasospasm. *Circ. Res.* 92, 809–816.

Wiley, J. W., Gross, R. A., and Macdonald, R. L. (1992). The peptide CGRP increases a high-threshold $Ca^{2+}$ current in rat nodose neurones via a pertussis toxin-sensitive pathway. *J. Physiol.* 455, 367–381.

Wilkins, R. H. (1990). Cerebral vasospasm. *Crit. Rev. Neurobiol.* 6, 51–77.

Winn, H. R., Richardson, A. E., and Jane, J. A. (1977). The long-term prognosis in untreated cerebral aneurysms: I. The incidence of late hemorrhage in cerebral aneurysm: a 10-year evaluation of 364 patients. *Ann. Neurol.* 1, 358–370.

# 10

# Diverse roles of neurotensin agonists in the central nervous system

**Mona Boules*, Zhimin Li, Kristin Smith, Paul Fredrickson and Elliott Richelson**

*Neuropsychopharmacology Laboratory, Department of Neuroscience, Mayo Clinic Florida, Jacksonville, FL, USA*

**Edited by:**
*Hubert Vaudry, University of Rouen, France*

**Reviewed by:**
*Sarah J. Spencer, RMIT University, Australia*
*Jean H. Costentin, University of Rouen, France*

***Correspondence:**
*Mona Boules, Neuropsychopharmacology Laboratory, Department of Neuroscience, Mayo Clinic, 4500 San Pablo Road, Jacksonville, FL 32224, USA.*
*e-mail: boules.mona@mayo.edu*

Neurotensin (NT) is a tridecapeptide that is found in the central nervous system (CNS) and the gastrointestinal tract. NT behaves as a neurotransmitter in the brain and as a hormone in the gut. Additionally, NT acts as a neuromodulator to several neurotransmitter systems including dopaminergic, sertonergic, GABAergic, glutamatergic, and cholinergic systems. Due to its association with such a wide variety of neurotransmitters, NT has been implicated in the pathophysiology of several CNS disorders such as schizophrenia, drug abuse, Parkinson's disease (PD), pain, central control of blood pressure, eating disorders, as well as, cancer and inflammation. The present review will focus on the role that NT and its analogs play in schizophrenia, endocrine function, pain, psychostimulant abuse, and PD.

**Keywords: neurotensin, endocrinology, schizophrenia, pain, psychostimulant abuse, central nervous system**

## INTRODUCTION

Neurotensin (NT) is a 13 amino acid neuropeptide (*p*Glu-Leu-Tyr-Glu-Asn-Lys-Pro-Arg-Arg-Pro-Tyr-Ile-Leu) that was first isolated from bovine hypothalamus by Carraway and Leeman (1973). It is abundant in gastrointestinal tract where it plays a role in gut motility. NT has also been detected in peripheral organs including: heart, liver, lung, pancreas, spleen, and small intestine. It is a paracrine and endocrine modulator of the cardiovascular system and of the digestive tract and acts as a growth factor on a variety of normal and cancerous cells. In addition, NT is widely distributed in the central nervous system (CNS), with the highest concentration in the amygdala, lateral septum, ventral tegmental area (VTA), and substantia nigra (SN).

In brain, NT plays a role in naloxone-independent antinociception (Clineschmidt et al., 1979), hypothermia (Bissette et al., 1976), control of anterior pituitary hormone secretion, and muscle relaxation (Kitabgi et al., 1992). NT also controls central blood pressure, and inflammation (St-Gelais et al., 2006 for review). The physiological functions of NT have been recently reviewed (Mustain et al., 2011).

Many literature reviews have presented the basic role of brain NT through its relationship with dopaminergic mesotelencephalic projection system and its modulating glutamatergic transmission and other signals (Seutin, 2005; Boules et al., 2006; Antonelli et al., 2007; Ferraro et al., 2008). The current review discusses the potential clinical function of NT and the potential clinical use of its analogs as novel therapy for neuropsychiatric disorders such as schizophrenia, addiction, Parkinson's disease (PD), and pain.

## NEUROTENSIN RECEPTORS

Neurotensin mediates its effects through three NT receptors (NTRs), the high affinity NTS1, the low affinity NTS2, and NTS3. Both NTS1 and NTS2 are G-protein coupled receptors, with seven-transmembrane domain. NTS1, the most studied NTR, is expressed in both neurons and glial cells and is broadly distributed in the CNS including medial septal nucleus, nucleus basalis magnocellularis, suprachiasmatic nucleus, SN, and VTA (Elde et al., 1990) as well as small dorsal root ganglion neurons of the spinal cord (Zhang et al., 1995). Activation of NTS1 induces excitatory effect through G-proteins, resulting in intracellular calcium influx. In turn, there is increased intracellular levels of cAMP, cGMP, and IP3; and increased activities of PLC, PKC, and Na+/K+-ATPase (Gilbert and Richelson, 1984; Watson et al., 1992; Yamada and Richelson, 1993; Hermans et al., 1994; Slusher et al., 1994; Poinot-Chazel et al., 1996; Lopez Ordieres and Rodriguez de Lores Arnaiz, 2000; Trudeau, 2000). NTS1 has a close association with dopaminergic and glutamatergic systems.

A high density of NTS1 receptors is co-localized with dopamine (DA) neurons in the ventral mesencephalon (Brouard et al., 1992; Nicot et al., 1995; Boudin et al., 1998). NT antagonizes DA effects at D2 receptors via NTS1/D2 receptor–receptor interaction (Jiang et al., 1994; Farkas et al., 1996). Several studies suggested that NTS1 receptors on mesencephalic DA neurons play an important role in sensitization to psychostimulant drugs and drug addiction (Binder et al., 2001a; Berod and Rostene, 2002; Panayi et al., 2005). Our recent work shows that (1) NTS1 knockout mice ($NTS1^{-/-}$) mice are spontaneously hyperactive and more sensitive to D-amphetamine-induced hyperactivity (Liang et al., 2010); (2) $NTS1^{-/-}$ mice have higher basal levels of DA and higher levels of amphetamine-induced DA release in striatum as compared with results for WT mice (Liang et al., 2010); and (3) $NTS1^{-/-}$ have abnormal D2/D1 ratio in striatum (Liang et al., 2010), leading to a decrease of D-amphetamine-induced glutamate and GABA release in striatum (Li et al., 2010b). The results suggest that NTS1 through possible modulation of DA receptor plays an important role in the dysregulation of striatal DA function which is thought to be secondary to a glutamate deficiency in schizophrenia through possible modulation of DA receptor. Additionally, a possible interaction between NTS1 and D1 receptor in medial prefrontal cortex (mPFC) has been proposed in one of our recent studies (Li et al.,

2010c). The same work also shows that there are significantly lower basal glutamate levels and lower density of *N*-methyl-D-aspartate (NMDA) receptor 2A subunit in the mPFC of NTS1 null mice as compared with results for WT mice (Li et al., 2010c). These data are consistent with the hypothesis that NTS1 is involved with the pathophysiology of the hypofunction of the glutamatergic system in schizophrenia.

The relationship between NTS1 and glutamatergic system has been investigated by Antonelli's group for years. Activation of NTS1 promotes and reinforces endogenous glutamate signaling in discrete brain regions by increasing the activation of PKC and leading to phosphorylation of the NMDA receptor. NTS1 receptors are highly expressed in nigro-striatal dopaminergic neurons, which degenerate in PD. It has been hypothesized (Antonelli et al., 2007) that in Parkinson's patients, possible elevated NT levels in the basal ganglia cause the NTS1 enhancement of excitotoxic glutamate signaling contributing to the DA neuron neurodegeneration in SN. However, paradoxically, NT or an NTS1 agonist has antiparkinson-like effect (Jolicoeur et al., 1991; Boules et al., 2001b). The discrepancy is likely due to different routes and time course of administration: local infusion in the striatum or SN for 60 min versus acute systemic i.p. administration. We have discussed previously that the effects of a NTR agonist given outside the brain cannot be predicted from studies in which a NTR agonist is injected into discrete areas of the brain (Richelson et al., 2003). Both groups agree that there is a critical role for NTS1 in PD.

NTS2 is localized mainly in the olfactory system, the cerebral and cerebellar cortices, the hippocampal formation, and selective hypothalamic nuclei, VTA, and SN. Importantly, strong expression of NTS2 receptors is in the areas related to pain, namely, the periaqueductal gray (PAG) and the rostral ventrolateral medulla (RVLM). Local administration of NT into the PAG and RVLM induces opioid-independent analgesia (Behbehani, 1992) through non-NTS1 dependent mechanisms (Dubuc et al., 1994). Antisense oligonucleotide knockdown of NTS2 receptor significantly decreases NT-induced analgesia, while oligodeoxynucleotides against NTS1 had no effect in this regard. These results are also supported by recent data from NT (Remaury et al., 2002) and the NTS2 receptor-selective agonist NT79 (Boules et al., 2010). Taken together it suggests that NTS2 plays an important role in pain.

NTS3/sortilin is a single transmembrane amino acid receptor, structurally unrelated to either NTS1 or NTS2. Its mRNA is expressed throughout the brain with high levels of expression in the SN, hippocampal formation, supraoptic nucleus, piriform and cerebral cortices, and medial and lateral septal nuclei (Mazella, 2001; Sarret et al., 2003). NTS3/sortilin participates in the modulation of NT intracellular sorting (hence the name "sortilin") and signaling processes (Sarret et al., 2003) and has been associated with the phosphatidylinositol 3-kinase and mitogen-activated protein kinase pathways in glial cells (Martin et al., 2003). NTS3/sortilin has been implicated in cell death in responsive cells including neurons. This is thought to be due to the ability of NTS3/sortilin to bind the unprocessed form of nerve growth factor (proNGF) (Nykjaer et al., 2004). Additionally, SorLA/LR11, a mosaic protein of the vacuolar protein sorting 10 protein (Vps10p) domain receptor family and the low density lipoprotein receptor (LDLR) family, represents the fourth NTR (NTS4). It has a similar structure as NTS3/sortilin, with a wide distribution in the brain, especially in the hippocampus, cerebellum, cingulate gyrus, entorhinal cortex, red nucleus, and oculomotor nucleus (Motoi et al., 1999). NTS4 may be involved in the intracellular trafficking and in termination of NT signaling (Jacobsen et al., 2001).

## NT AND NEUROTRANSMITTER SYSTEMS

Neurotensin acts as a primary neurotransmitter as well as a modulator of other neurotransmitter systems such as the dopaminergic, glutamatergic, GABAergic, cholinergic, and serotonergic systems (Rakovska et al., 1998; Ferraro et al., 2008; Petkova-Kirova et al., 2008). The functional and anatomical NT/DA interactions have been the most extensively studied and reviewed (Binder et al., 2001a; Jomphe et al., 2006; Fawaz et al., 2009; Thibault et al., 2011; Tanganelli et al., 2012).

### NEUROTENSIN AND DOPAMINE

As mentioned in the previous section, NT and DA are co-localized in a subpopulation of mesencephalic neuron within the VTA (Hokfelt et al., 1984; Seroogy et al., 1988; Bean and Roth, 1992). Additionally, NT-like immunoreactivity is highly expressed in areas enriched with DA cell bodies and nerve terminals such as SN, VTA, neostriatum, and nucleus accumbens (NA) (Quirion et al., 1982). NT also forms synaptic contacts with a subpopulation of tyrosine hydroxylase (TH) immunoreactive neurons (Woulfe and Beaudet, 1989). These data strongly indicate a modulatory function of NT on DA neurotransmission.

Neurotensin directly or indirectly (e.g., through glutamate release) modulates DA neurotransmission. NT can modulate DA through: (1) up-regulating TH gene expression (Burgevin et al., 1992a,b) or (2) decreasing the DA binding affinity for the DA $D_2$ receptors (Fuxe et al., 1992a; Li et al., 1995). NT also opposes DA $D_2$ receptor agonist-induced auto-inhibition of DA cell firing (Shi and Bunney, 1992). Allosteric receptor–receptor interactions between NT and DA $D_2$ receptors, as well as second messenger-dependent receptor alterations, such as phosphorylation and dephosphorylation, have also been implicated (see Fuxe et al., 1992b for review). It is important to mention that within the terminal fields, NT opposes the effects of DA both pre- and post-synaptically, leading either to an increase or to a decrease in DA transmission, depending on the intrinsic anatomical location of NTRs (for a more comprehensive review of the modulatory effects of NT on DA neurotransmission, we refer the reader to Binder et al. (2001a) and Kinkead and Nemeroff (2004).

### NT AND SEROTONIN

Neurotensin receptors are present on serotonergic neurons in the nucleus raphe magnus and dorsal raphe, where NT causes an increase in their firing rates (Jolas and Aghajanian, 1996; Li et al., 2001). Therefore, NT has been proposed to play a role in functions known to be affected by the serotonergic system including antinociception (Buhler et al., 2005; Boules et al., 2010), sleep-wake cycle (Jolas and Aghajanian, 1997), and stress (Corley et al., 2002).

### NT AND GLUTAMATE

There has been controversy regarding the effect of NT on glutamate release and modification of the glutamatergic and NMDA receptors. NT increases glutamate release in the striatum, globus pallidus, frontal cortex, and SN (Ferraro et al., 2011, 2012) implicating NT in conditions such as stroke, Alzheimer's disease, and PD.

Others have reported that systemic administration of NT analogs blocks ethanol-induced increases in glutamate levels in the striatum (Li et al., 2011), and decreases phencyclidine (PCP)-induced increases in glutamate in the prefrontal cortex (Li et al., 2010a). These data support the idea that the antipsychotic-like effects of NT may be mediated in part by its modulatory effect on glutamate.

## NT AND HYPOTHALAMIC-PITUITARY AXIS

### EFFECT OF NT ON HORMONE RELEASE

The presence of NT in the anterior pituitary gland and hypothalamus and its storage and release at the median eminence implicate NT and its receptors in neuroendocrine regulation (Rostene and Alexander, 1997). NT is thought to possess a paracrine or an autocrine role within the hypothalamus and the anterior pituitary (Bachelet et al., 1997; Bello et al., 2004). NT stimulates both directly and indirectly, the synthesis of corticotrophin releasing hormone (CRH), gonadotropin-releasing hormone (GnRH) (Cooke et al., 2009), growth hormone-releasing hormone (GHRH) (Blackburn et al., 1980), and prolactin secretion at anterior pituitary and median eminence (Memo et al., 1986).

#### *CRH-ACTH*

Neurotensin stimulates the activity of the hypothalamic-pituitary CRH-adrenocorticotropin hormone (ACTH) system. Central administration of NT increases ACTH and corticosterone in the presence of CRH receptor activation in the paraventricular nucleus (PVN) (Nussdorfer et al., 1992; Rowe et al., 1995). The modulatory action of NT on the pituitary-adrenocortical function in rats has been reported to be biphasic. The lower dose of NT exerts a stimulatory effect while the higher dose appears to have an inhibitory effect on both the pituitary-ACTH release and adrenocortical secretion (Malendowicz and Nussdorfer, 1994). NT also enhances the release of both CRH-ir and ACTH-ir in rat adrenal medulla (Mazzocchi et al., 1997).

#### *Gonadotropic hormones*

Many neurons in the anteroventral periventricular (AVPV) and medial preoptic nuclei (MPN) express estrogen receptors and project to GnRH neurons (Smith and Wise, 2001). Surprisingly, GnRH neurons do not seem to possess intracellular estrogen receptors (Herbison and Theodosis, 1993) and evidence suggests that other neurons mediate the stimulatory effects of estrogen on GnRH secretion (Shivers et al., 1983). Interestingly, GnRH neurons were found to express NTS1 receptors (Herbison and Theodosis, 1992) and GABA receptors (Herbison et al., 1993). The number of GnRH neurons expressing NTS1-mRNA peaks during proestrus suggesting that NT directly stimulates GnRH neurons contributing to luteinizing hormone (LH) surge (Smith and Wise, 2001). There has been some controversy regarding the role of NT on LH surge. While some report that the administration of NT directly into the medial preoptic area (where GnRH cell bodies reside) evokes pre-ovulatory GnRH/LH surge (Alexander et al., 1989a), others indicate that NT has no effect on GnRH-stimulated LH release (Leiva and Croxatto, 1994). The former group showed that immunoneutralization of NT in the preoptic region attenuates the LH surge induced by estrogen and progesterone treatment in ovariectomized rats (Alexander et al., 1989b). The effect of NT on LH secretion requires intact dopaminergic and alpha adrenergic systems (Akema and Kimura, 1989).

#### *Growth hormone*

Neurotensin is co-expressed with growth hormone (GH) releasing factor in the arcuate nucleus (Niimi et al., 1991) and modulates GH release. NT regulates GH secretion, in prepubertal children and adults (Bozzola et al., 1998a), as well as in neonates (Bozzola et al., 1998b), through the modulation of somatostatin release from the median eminence. In rats, estrogen plays a facilitatory role on NT-induced GH release that is independent of hypothalamic GHRH or somatostatin release (Ibanez et al., 1993).

#### *Prolactin*

With respect to prolactin release, NT has opposite actions, an inhibitory effect at the hypothalamic site and an excitatory effect at the pituitary. NT elevates plasma prolactin and GH levels in both normal and estrogen-progesterone pretreated male rats (Rivier et al., 1977). The inhibitory action of NT on prolactin release is mediated by the release of DA into the hypophyseal portal vein, which delivers the neurotransmitter to the anterior pituitary gland causing inhibition of prolactin release (Vijayan et al., 1988; McCann and Vijayan, 1992; Pan et al., 1992).

#### *Thyroid hormones*

Neurotensin also participates in the neuroendocrine control of the thyroid hormones by regulating thyroid releasing hormone (TRH) function and thyroid stimulating hormone (TSH) secretion. These data indicate that NT is involved in the metabolic actions of these hormones. The role of NT in the hypothalamic-anterior pituitary-thyroid axis and the functional cooperation between NT and thyroid hormones are excellently reviewed by Stolakis et al. (2010).

#### *Effect of NT on feeding*

In addition to its presence in the CNS NT is also found in neuroendocrine cells of the small bowel. There, NT participates in enteric digestive processes, gut motility, and intestinal inflammatory mechanisms. It also plays an important role in intestinal lipid metabolism, thus controlling appetite, weight status, and food intake (Kalafatakis and Triantafyllou, 2011). Additionally, NT exerts central control on blood glucose, feeding patterns, and body weight.

Centrally administered NT reduces appetite (Luttinger et al., 1982; Hawkins, 1986; Cooke et al., 2009), an effect that is mainly mediated by NTS1 (Remaury et al., 2002; Kim et al., 2008; Kim and Mizuno, 2010).

The anorectic effect of centrally administered NT is potentiated by peripheral injection of DA agonists, L-DOPA and bromocriptine, results suggesting that the effect of NT may be mediated by its ability to increase the activity of dopaminergic neurotransmission in the CNS (Hawkins et al., 1986).

Similar effects were shown for the NT agonist, PD149163, in rats and ob/ob mice (Feifel et al., 2010a) as well as the non-selective

NT agonist NT69L in Sprague-Dawley and in obese Zucker rats (Boules et al., 2000). The later study also showed that the effect of NT69L on food intake and body weight is due to functional interactions of NT with brain amines, and metabolic and endocrinological systems. NT69L transiently increases blood glucose and corticosterone levels and decreases TSH and T4 in Sprague-Dawley and in Zucker rats. NT69L also decreases norepinephrine in both the hypothalamus and NA, and increases DA, its metabolite 3,4-dihydroxyphenylacetic acid (DOPAC), and serotonin. These results indicate that feeding and energy expenditures are modulated by the interplay of hormones and neurotransmitters in the CNS (Brunetti et al., 2005).

Additionally, the effect of NT on feeding and body weight is also mediated, in part, by its action on the anorexigenic hormone leptin, which is secreted by adipocytes and regulates food intake by acting on hypothalamic neurons including NT-producing neurons (Beck et al., 1998; Sahu et al., 2001). Leptin together with insulin and α-melanocyte-stimulating hormones increase NT expression in the hypothalamus (Sahu, 1998; Cui et al., 2005). Similarly, the anorectic effect of leptin is at least partly mediated through central NTS1 and the leptin-NTS1 signaling pathway is involved in the regulation of food intake and the in the control of energy balance (Leinninger et al., 2011) since the lack of NTS1 reduces sensitivity to the anorectic action of leptin, causing hyperphagia and abnormal weight gain (Kim et al., 2008).

#### EFFECT OF HORMONES ON NT SYNTHESIS AND RELEASE IN HYPOTHALAMIC-PITUITARY AXIS

As NT modulates hypothalamic-pituitary axis (HPA) hormones, circulating hormones influence NT synthesis in the hypothalamus and anterior pituitary, results that suggest that NT mediates feedback effects of the hormones on neuroendocrine cells (Rostene and Alexander, 1997). Estrogen and progesterone regulate the activity of NT-synthesizing neurosecretory cells located in the hypothalamic arcuate nucleus (Alexander, 1999). Estrogen increases the secretion of NT at the median eminence and alters NT binding and NTS1-mRNA expression in the rostral preoptic nucleus (Moyse et al., 1988; Alexander, 1993; Watanobe and Takebe, 1993; Alexander and Leeman, 1994). GHRH neurosecretory cells synthesize NT under basal conditions (Niimi et al., 1991) and GH injection increases NT plasma levels in human (Schimpff et al., 1994).

Neurotensin's endocrine activity, and its modulatory effects on several neurotransmitter systems, kindled many studies suggesting that NT plays a role in the pathophysiology of several CNS disorders including PD, schizophrenia, and psychostimulant and nicotine addiction as well as pain and eating disorders (Caceda et al., 2006).

## NT AND NEUROPSYCHIATRIC DISORDERS

#### SCHIZOPHRENIA

Schizophrenia is a devastating psychotic disorder that affects approximately 1% of the population worldwide. The onset of illness usually occurs relatively early in life with most patients experiencing long-lasting adverse effects accompanied by severe impairment (reviewed in Carpenter and Buchanan (1994). The disease is manifested by positive symptoms (delusions, hallucinations, and an altered perception of reality), and negative symptoms (apathy, cognitive blunting, and social withdrawal), as well as a disorganization of thought and behavior. Many schizophrenic patients have difficulty holding a job or caring for themselves, placing a significant burden on their families and society. Additionally, increased mortality is associated with schizophrenia as patients experience a 20% shorter lifespan than the general population and are at an increased risk for committing suicide (Newman and Bland, 1991; Goff et al., 2001).

The exact cause(s) for the pathophysiology and progression of schizophrenia are not known; however it is generally accepted that associated symptoms are syndromal in nature, rather than manifestations of a single disease (Carpenter et al., 1999). These symptoms are likely caused by several compounding biochemical abnormalities and influenced by both genetics and environment. Theories as to the origin of these abnormalities focus on the dopaminergic system, but have more recently been expanded to include the serotonergic, γ-aminobutyric acid-ergic, and glutamatergic systems, as well as the NT system.

One of the earliest and most studied theories is the DA hypothesis of schizophrenia (Carlsson, 1988; Toda and Abi-Dargham, 2007; Howes and Kapur, 2009). While this theory originally emphasized general hyperdopaminergia as a causative factor in schizophrenia (Snyder, 1976), more recent versions focus on the balance of DA within discreet regions of the brain. The current theory predicts that hyperactive subcortical mesolimbic DA projections (resulting in hyperstimulation of $D_2$ receptors) are the main cause for positive symptoms, while hypoactive mesocortical DA projections to the PFC (resulting in hypostimulation of $D_1$ receptors) are the main cause for negative symptoms and cognitive impairment (Weinberger, 1987; Toda and Abi-Dargham, 2007). There is strong evidence for a close relationship between the dopaminergic system and NT (Nemeroff, 1986; Kitabgi et al., 1989), suggesting a role for NT in the pathophysiology of schizophrenia.

##### *Neurotensin and schizophrenia*

A role for NT in schizophrenia has been hypothesized for over three decades (Nemeroff, 1980). Specifically, the NT system is closely associated with the dopaminergic system, and deficits in NT neurotransmission have been implicated in the pathophysiology of schizophrenia. Schizophrenics have a 40% decrease in NTRs in the entorhinal cortex (Wolf et al., 1995), and schizophrenics with decreased NT concentrations in their cerebral spinal fluid have significantly higher levels of pretreatment psychopathology (Sharma et al., 1997).

NT receptors have been detected on DA cell bodies in the SN and VTA (Palacios and Kuhar, 1981; Szigethy and Beaudet, 1989) and NTR activation has an excitatory effect on midbrain DA neurons (Pinnock, 1985; Seutin et al., 1989; Mercuri et al., 1993). NT can inhibit DA $D_2$ autoreceptor function, thus relieving auto-inhibition of DA transmission (Jomphe et al., 2006) thereby increasing DA release, firing rate, and the synthesis of the rate limiting enzyme for DA synthesis, TH (Binder et al., 2001b). Because of this close association of NT with dopaminergic neurons and its neuromodulatory effects on the dopaminergic system, NT is hypothesized to be therapeutic in the treatment of schizophrenia. Central administration of NT does in fact cause antipsychotic-like effects (Jolicoeur et al., 1993), and therefore a great interest exists for developing NT-mimetics for the treatment of neuropsychiatric diseases, such as schizophrenia.

### *The potential role of NT as an antipsychotic drug*

Several lines of evidence suggest that antipsychotics, the traditional treatment for schizophrenia, act through the induction of endogenous NT (Kinkead et al., 1999): (1) all clinically effective antipsychotic drugs affect in some way the NT system of rats. The therapeutic potency of typical APDs is derived mainly from their ability to antagonize DA $D_2$ receptors with high affinity (Creese et al., 1976). Typical antipsychotics are associated with extrapyramidal side effects (ESP) characterized by movement disorders including tardive dyskinesia, dystonic reactions, and Parkinsonism. Alternatively, it is suggested that atypical APDs have a higher affinity for 5-$HT_{2A}$ relative to DA $D_2$ receptors (Meltzer et al., 1989; Nordstrom et al., 1995; Kapur et al., 1998; Gefvert et al., 2001). They are characterized by enhanced antipsychotic efficacy and lower risk of EPS (Meltzer et al., 1989). Both typical and atypical antipsychotics, those associated with little or no EPS, increase NT mRNA in specific regions of the brain after both acute and chronic treatment (Govoni et al., 1980; Merchant et al., 1991, 1992; Merchant and Dorsa, 1993). (2) These effects are selective for drugs with antipsychotic efficacy, and are not seen with other classes of psychotropic drugs. (3) Typical and atypical antipsychotic drugs differentially affect the NT system. Typical antipsychotics act on both the mesolimbic and nigro-striatal NT systems. By contrast, the actions of atypical antipsychotics on NT are thought to be restricted to the mesolimbic system, the region thought to be the site of therapeutic effect in schizophrenia. (4) Centrally administered NT elicits similar behavioral effects as systemically administered atypical antipsychotic drugs. It is hypothesized that the increase in NT neurotransmission in the mesolimbic system mediates the therapeutic effects of APDs, while the increase in NT neurotransmission in the nigrostriatum underlies the propensity to cause ESP (Binder et al., 2001b; Caceda et al., 2006). Interestingly, the pattern of increase in NT mRNA expression, NT tissue content and release (Kinkead et al., 1999) is similar to that of the immediate early genes, c-fos, FosB, and ΔFos B, after acute and chronic administration of typical and atypical APDs (Binder et al., 2001b).

The ability of a compound to inhibit climbing induced by apomorphine (a DA agonist), hyperactivity induced by amphetamine (indirect DA agonist), and to prevent the disruption of prepulse inhibition (PPI) induced by amphetamine [1-(2,5-dimethoxy-4-iodophenyl)-2-aminopropane] (DOI) (5-$HT_{2A}$ agonist), and dizocilpine (non-competitive NMDA antagonist) are tests used to predict antipsychotic-like activity of a drug. These tests also distinguish between typical and atypical antipsychotic-like effects (Merchant and Dorsa, 1993; Arnt et al., 1995) (see review by Geyer and Ellenbroek, 2003). The ability of a compound to block apomorphine-induced climbing over oro-facial stereotypies (sniffing and licking) induced by high doses of apomorphine, suggests atypicality of that compound (Gerhardt et al., 1985).

Neurotensin has been shown to prevent the disruption of amphetamine- and apomorphine-induced PPI (Feifel et al., 1997), as well as attenuate apomorphine-induced climbing (Jolicoeur et al., 1993), and amphetamine- and apomorphine-induced hyperactivity without affecting stereotypy (Jolicoeur et al., 1983). For these reasons it is hypothesized that NT transmission is integral to the mechanism of action of antipsychotic drugs and that NT can serve as an endogenous antipsychotic-like compound (reviewed in Kinkead et al., 1999; Binder et al., 2001b; Kinkead and Nemeroff, 2002).

### *The behavioral effects of neurotensin analogs in animal models of schizophrenia*

As discussed above, there is strong evidence to support NT as an endogenous antipsychotic drug. However, NT is easily degraded by peptidases and cannot cross the blood-brain barrier. In an effort to study more easily the effects of NT, our group has developed an extensive series of NT(8–13) analogs that can be delivered peripherally, and that elicit effects similar to centrally administered NT. These NT analogs have demonstrated antipsychotic-like activity similar to endogenous NT as determined by behavioral tests in rats. Most of our work has been with NT69L and NT79. NT69L binds human NTS1 and human NTS2 with high affinity. By contrast, NT79 preferentially binds to NTS2, as its binding affinity for the human NTS2 is approximately 25-fold higher than that for human NTS1. NT69L (Cusack et al., 2000), NT79 (Boules et al., 2010), and another analog NT77L (Boules et al., 2001c) are each modified from NT at amino acid positions located in the C-terminal 8–13 sequence. Additionally, PD149163, which is a reduced amide bond NT(8–13) mimetic shows antipsychotic-like activity.

PD149163 has strong affinity for NTRs ($K_i = 31.2$ nM in newborn mouse brain membranes) and improved metabolic stability (Wustrow et al., 1995), a factor that promotes central activity after systemic administration (Banks et al., 1995).

**Table 1** shows the structures of some NT analogs.

NT69L elicits similar neurochemical and behavioral effects as endogenous NT (for review, see Boules et al., 2003a). Intraperitoneal delivery of NT69L selectively inhibits stereotyped apomorphine-induced climbing at an $ED_{50}$ of 16 μg/kg, without affecting licking or sniffing at any dose given (Cusack et al., 2000). Additionally, NT69L does not cause catalepsy (muscle rigidity) at any dose given, but reverses haloperidol-induced catalepsy with an $ED_{50}$ of 0.2 mg/kg (Cusack et al., 2000). Catalepsy in rats has been used as a predictor of EPS potential of APDs in humans.

NT69L significantly increases both amphetamine- and dizocilpine-induced decreases in PPI with acute administration with an $ED_{50}$ of 0.08 and 0.05 mg/kg respectively (Shilling et al., 2003; Boules et al., 2010), as well as with chronic administration (Briody et al., 2010). Additionally, NT69L blocks PCP-induced hyperactivity (Li et al., 2010a), a test that may reflect both positive and negative symptoms of schizophrenia (Snyder, 1980; Javitt and Zukin, 1991). These results demonstrate that NT69L has properties similar to those of atypical APDs.

NT77 is also thought to have antipsychotic-like properties, although less potently than NT69L, based on similar rat behavioral studies (Boules et al., 2001c). NT77L selectively blocks apomorphine-induced climbing with an $ED_{50}$ of 5.6 mg/kg without affecting sniffing or licking behavior at any dose. NT77L moderately prevents/reverses the cataleptic effect of haloperidol ($ED_{50}$ 5.6 mg/kg) while it does not cause catalepsy itself at any dose. The effects of NT77L on PPI have yet to be tested.

Like NT69L and NT77L, NT79 also selectively blocks apomorphine-induced climbing without affecting sniffing or licking behavior at any dose. Similarly, NT79 significantly blocks amphetamine-induced hyperactivity as well as prevents the disruption of PPI induced by both amphetamine and DOI (Boules et al., 2010). PD149163 antagonizes the reduction in PPI of the rat startle reflex produced by amphetamine and dizocilpine (Feifel et al., 1999), blocks the disruption in PPI induced by the 5-$HT_{2A}$ agonist DOI (Feifel et al., 2003), and inhibits conditioned avoidance responding, which is a highly validated test for screening APD in rats, without causing catalepsy (Holly et al., 2011). These analogs show promise for use in the treatment of schizophrenic symptoms with a lower potential for adverse side effects. The antipsychotic effects of NT analogs are summarized in **Table 2**.

Studies with the use of knockout mice lacking NT or NTR subtypes suggest a role for NTS1 in the antipsychotic-like effect of NT. NT knockout mice have reduced PPI and are not sensitive to the PPI-disrupting effects of amphetamine as compared to wild type mice. These data indicate the importance of endogenous NT in the effects of amphetamine on PPI (Mechanic et al., 2009). Additionally, the use of NTS1- and NTS2-knockout (NTS1$^{-/-}$ and NTS2$^{-/-}$) mice revealed hyper-dopaminergic state in the NTS1$^{-/-}$ mice similar to the excessive striatal DA activity reported in schizophrenia (Liang et al., 2010). Furthermore, the NTS1$^{-/-}$ show changes in behavior, prefrontal cortex neurotransmitters, and protein expression that are similar to wild type mice treated with the psychomimetic PCP, an animal model for schizophrenia (Li et al., 2010c). The involvement of NTS1 in the antipsychotic-like effect of NT has been further demonstrated by the use of NT agonists. Administration of the NT agonists, NT69L and NT-2, reversed apomorphine-induced climbing in wild type but not in NTS1$^{-/-}$ mice (Mechanic et al., 2009). Likewise, PD149163 significantly facilitates PPI and decreases the acoustic startle response in wild type but not in NTS1$^{-/-}$ mice (Feifel et al., 2010b).

## PAIN

### *NT and pain*

Neurotensin and NTRs modulate nociception at several different levels (Dobner, 2005). In fact, on a molar basis, NT is more potent than is morphine as an antinociceptive agent (Nemeroff et al., 1979; al-Rodhan et al., 1991). Central administration of NT induces an analgesic response in both the hot plate (HP) and acetic acid-induced writhing tests in rats (Clineschmidt and McGuffin, 1977; Clineschmidt et al., 1979, 1982). NT also produces a long-lasting antinociceptive effect in the tail-flick (TF) assay following intra rostroventral medulla (RVM) administration (Fang et al., 1987). These results indicate that NT can influence nociceptive transmission at several different points in the descending pain modulatory circuitry in the brain. There is also limited evidence that NT may affect nociception transmission directly in the spinal cord (Dobner, 2006). Intrathecal NT administration increased both HP and aversive (hypertonic saline) response latencies, but had no significant analgesic effect in the TF (Hylden and Wilcox, 1983). In addition, intrathecal injection of either NT or one of our novel NT(8–13) into the spinal cord of rats modifies pain perception in a rodent model of persistent (Roussy et al., 2006) and of neuropathic pain (Dansereau et al., 2006).

### *NT receptor subtypes and pain*

The effect of NT on pain modulation is dose-dependent and receptor-selective (Urban and Smith, 1993). NT not only inhibits but also facilitates pain transmission in a dose-dependent manner. High doses (nanomolar range) of the peptide injected into the

**Table 1 | Structures of NT analogs.**

| | 1 | 2 | 3 | 4 | 5 | 6 | 7 | 8 | 9 | 10 | 11 | 12 | 13 |
|---|---|---|---|---|---|---|---|---|---|---|---|---|---|
| NT | *p*-Glu | l-Leu | l-Tyr | l-Glu | l-Asn | l-Lys | l-Pro | l-Arg | l-Arg | l-Pro | l-Tyr | l-Ile | l-Leu |
| NT69L | – | – | – | – | – | – | – | *N*-methyl-Arg | l-Lys | l-Pro | l-neo-Trp | Tert-Leu- | l-Leu |
| NT72 | | | | | | | | | d-Lys | l-Pto | l-neo-trp | tert- | l-Leu |
| NT77L | – | – | – | – | – | – | – | l-Arg | d-Orn | l-Pro | l-neo-Trp | tert-Leu | l-Leu |
| NT79 | – | – | – | – | – | – | – | *N*-methyl-Arg | l-Arg | l-Pro | d-3,1-Nal | tert-Leu | l-Leu |
| PD149163 | | | | | | | | H-Lys-psi[CH2NH] | Lys | Pro | Trp | Tle | Leu-Oet |

**Table 2 | Antipsychotic effects of NT analogs.**

| Analog | Apomorphine-induced climbing | Reversal of Haloperidol-induced catalepsy | Amphetamine-induced decrease in PPI and hyperactivity | Dizocilpine/DOI-induced decrease in PPI | PCP-induced hyperactivity |
|---|---|---|---|---|---|
| NT69L | Y[1] | Y[2] | Y[3] | Y[4] | Y[5] |
| NT77L | Y[6] | Y[6] | | | |
| NT79 | Y[7] | Y[7] | Y[7] | Y[7] | |
| PD149163 | | | Y[8,9] | Y[10] | |

*Y = has an effect.*

*[1] Cusack et al. (2000), Mechanic et al. (2009); [2] Cusack et al. (2000); [3] Boules et al. (2001a), Shilling et al. (2003), Briody et al. (2010); [4] Shilling et al. (2003), Secchi et al. (2009); [5] Li et al. (2010a); [6] Boules et al. (2001c); [7] Boules et al. (2010); [8] Feifel et al. (2008); [9] Feifel et al. (1999), Shilling et al. (2004); [10] Feifel et al. (1999), Feifel et al. (2003), Shilling et al. (2004).*

RVM have an antinociceptive effect as measured by the TF latency (TFL) in response to heat stimulus. In contrast, lower doses (picomolar range) have been shown to reduce latencies in the HP and TF tests, facilitate spinal nociception response, and increase the visceromotor response to noxious heat and visceral stimulation respectively (Urban and Smith, 1993, 1994).

The basis of the opposing actions of NT and its dose-dependent modulation is most probably due to separate and distinct NTR subtype with varying affinity for the peptide (Smith et al., 1997), as well as the involvement of separate and distinct neuronal pathways that modulate pain at the spinal level (Smith et al., 1997). Evidence suggests that both NTS1 and NTS2 mediate the antinociceptive effects of NT, depending upon the antinociceptive test and possibly, the species of rodent used. NTS1 and NTS2 modulate pain-induced behavioral responses by acting on distinct spinal and/or supra-spinal neural circuits (Roussy et al., 2008). Contradictory results have been reported regarding the NTR subtype mediating the antinociceptive effects of NT.

***NTS1 and pain.*** Reports on mice lacking the NTS1 gene reveal that NT and NT analogs fail to induce antinociception in the HP test (Pettibone et al., 2002). Consistent with the knockout mice studies, our group showed that the inhibition of NTS1 synthesis with the use of antisense peptide nucleic acids (PNAs) targeting the NTS1 gene also results in loss of the analgesic properties of NT in the HP test (Tyler et al., 1998b), results that implicate NTS1 in thermal analgesia. Conversely, other evidence that argues against the involvement of NTS1 in the analgesic effect of NT has been reported and summarized by Dubuc et al. (1999a). Thus, as summarized by this group, the analgesic effects of NT are not antagonized by the NTS1-selective antagonist SR48692 (Dubuc et al., 1994), the binding affinity of NT analogs to NTS1 does not correlate with their analgesic effects (Labbe-Jullie et al., 1994), and the administration of antisense oligonucleotides targeted to NTS1 does not reduce NT-induced analgesia in the writhing test in mice (Dubuc et al., 1999b). With respect to formalin-induced pain, Roussy et al. (2010) concluded that NTS1 is important for modulation of persistent pain following systemic administration of morphine in NTS1$^{-/-}$ mice.

***NTS2 and pain.*** NTS2 has also been implicated in the analgesic effects of NT (Dubuc et al., 1999b; Remaury et al., 2002; Yamauchi et al., 2003; Maeno et al., 2004; Sarret et al., 2005; Bredeloux et al., 2006). Dubuc et al. showed, with the use of NTS2 oligonucleotides, that NTS2 plays an important role in the writhing test. These data were supported by a close correlation between NT analog binding affinity at NTS2 and potency of the analog-induced analgesia in mice (Dubuc et al., 1999b). Maeno et al. (2004) working with mice, suggested that NTS2 plays an important role in thermal nociception. The role of NTS2 in mediating NT-induced analgesia has been based on observations using NTS2 antisense oligodeoxynucleotides and the NTS2 ligand levocabastine (Bredeloux et al., 2006). NTS2 has also been implicated in mediating visceral antinociception (Dubuc et al., 1999a).

### NT analogs and pain

As mentioned, NT must be administered directly into the brain to exert its effect since it gets degraded by peptidases (Tyler-McMahon et al., 2000a; Boules et al., 2005). Our laboratory has been testing our brain-penetrating stable analogs of NT(8–13) in several animal models of pain.

Studies by our group and others show that NT analogs are effective in treating thermal, visceral (acetic acid-induced writhing), and persistent inflammatory (formalin-induced) pain (Tyler-McMahon et al., 2000b; Bredeloux et al., 2008; Boules et al., 2009, 2010; Mechanic et al., 2009). However, as previously stated, evidence suggests that the analgesic efficacy of NT analogs varies with their selectivity for NTS1 and NTS2, the pain model, and, probably, animal species.

Intrathecal injection of the NTS1-selective agonist, PD149163, and the non-selective NT agonist NT69L significantly reduced pain-evoked responses during the inflammatory phase of the formalin test (Roussy et al., 2008). The same analogs also produced potent antiallodynic and antihyperalgesic effects in nerve injured rats, a model of neuropathic pain (Guillemette et al., 2012). Systemic injection of NT analogs NT69L, NT72 (NTS1-selective), and NT77 causes analgesia in the HP test (Tyler et al., 1998a, 1999; Boules et al., 2001c; Smith et al., 2011) with synergy to morphine (Boules et al., 2009). Additionally, NT69L and NT72, significantly reduce acetic acid-induced writhing (Smith et al., 2012).

Supporting the role of NTS2 in antinociception, intrathecal injection of NTS2 agonists levocabastine and JMV431 significantly inhibit the aversive behavior induced by formalin (Roussy et al., 2009) and induced dose-dependent antinociceptive response in the TF test (Sarret et al., 2005).

Interestingly, the NTS2-selective analog, NT79, is ineffective in reducing thermal pain, but blocks acetic acid-induced writhing in rats (Boules et al., 2010), without causing tolerance to its analgesic effects (Smith et al., 2012). It is also interesting that NT79 does not cause hypothermia. Since the NTS1-selective (NT72), and non-selective (NT69L) NT agonists attenuate visceral nociception, it is suggested that both NTR subtypes are involved in mediating visceral analgesia and their roles appear to be NT analog dependent (Smith et al., 2012). Additionally, the NTS2-selective analog, NT79, reduces formalin-induced pain and does so in synergy with morphine (Boules et al., 2011a). Further evidence for the involvement of NTS2 in reducing persistent pain comes with the use of knockout mice. Lafrance et al. (2010) demonstrated that mice lacking NTS2 exhibit significantly lower stress-induced analgesia following cold-water swim stress as compared to their wild type littermates. **Table 3** summarizes the analgesic effects of NT analogs.

### Analgesic synergy between NT and morphine

Morphine is a $\mu$-opioid receptor agonist that is widely used for the treatment of many types of chronic pain. However, morphine and other opioids are usually associated with some serious side effects. Additionally, tolerance develops to their analgesic effects, but not to all the side effects, and this tolerance requires dosage increases over time, to attain a consistent level of analgesia. Increasing morphine dosage increases the potential for serious undesired side effects, such as respiratory depression.

Neurotensin exerts a potent $\mu$-opioid-independent, antinociceptive effects in a variety of analgesic screening tests, including tail-flick, HP, and writhing induced by acetic acid (Clineschmidt et al., 1979, 1982; al-Rodhan et al., 1991; Wustrow et al., 1995;

**Table 3 | Analgesic effects of NT analogs.**

| Analog | Hot plate | Writhing | Formalin | NP |
|---|---|---|---|---|
| NT69L | Y[1] | Y[2] | Y[3] | Y[4] |
| NT72 | Y[2] | Y[2] | | |
| NT77 | Y[5] | | | |
| NT79 | N[6] | Y[6] | Y[7] | Y[8] |
| PD149163 | | | Y[9] | Y[4] |

*Y = has an effect; N = has no effect.*

*[1]Tyler-McMahon et al. (2000b), Boules et al. (2009), Smith et al. (2011); [2]Smith et al. (2012); [3]Roussy et al. (2008), Roussy et al. (2009); [4]Guillemette et al. (2012); [5]Boules et al. (2001c); [6]Boules et al. (2010); [7]Boules et al. (2011a); [8]Boules et al. (2012); [9]Roussy et al. (2008), Roussy et al. (2009).*

Sarhan et al., 1997). Both NTS2 and μ-opioid receptors have been found in the same brain structures involved in pain perception (Basbaum and Fields, 1984; Asselin et al., 2001) and neurotensinergic system seems to play an important role in the non-opioid form of stress-induced analgesia (Seta et al., 2001; Gui et al., 2004; Lafrance et al., 2010).

The functional analgesic interaction between endogenous NT and the opioid system has been further illustrated by Tershner and Helmstetter. These authors show that the antinociception induced by the μ-opioid receptor activation in the amygdala is partly dependent on the recruitment of NTRs in the ventral PAG (Tershner and Helmstetter, 2000). Additionally, mice rendered tolerant to morphine showed a reduced analgesic effect to NT (Luttinger et al., 1983) and morphine analgesia was considerably reduced in NTS1-deficient mice. These data indicate that the NTS1 actively participates in μ-opioid analgesia (Roussy et al., 2010). Conversely, opioid receptor antagonists do not block NT-mediated antinociception (Clineschmidt et al., 1982; al-Rodhan et al., 1991), but the perfusion of morphine in the PAG increases the extracellular levels of NT-ir in a naloxone-dependent manner (Stiller et al., 1997).

The use of adjuncts such as the NMDA receptor antagonist ketamine in combination with opioids to enhance their efficacy at low doses, and attenuate the occurrence of tolerance has been reported (Lutfy et al., 1996; Nishiyama, 2000). However, serious motor impairment is observed at doses of ketamine that are antinociceptive in the rat and in human, and ketamine can be psychotomimetic. Additionally, long-term exposure of ketamine on spinal tissue leads to tissue necrosis (Vranken et al., 2005). Studies in our laboratory show analgesic synergism between NT analogs and morphine in the use of HP (Boules et al., 2009), in acetic acid-induced writhing, and in formalin-induced pain (Boules et al., 2011a). These studies provide novel potential use for NT analogs in combination with morphine (and perhaps other opioids) to improve the pharmacological treatment of pain while minimizing specific adverse effects of each of the drugs at a higher dose.

### NT AND PSYCHOSTIMULANT ABUSE

Psychostimulants, including nicotine, amphetamine, and cocaine, are drugs that may be employed to improve cognitive and motor function, but can be highly addictive. The mesocorticolimbic system, to which NT colocalizes with DA and other neurotransmitters, provides the anatomic substrate for psychostimulant dependence and craving (McBride et al., 1999; Di Chiara, 2000). NT acts as a neurotransmitter as well as a modulator of DA and other monoamine neurotransmitter systems and has been linked through several lines of evidence to psychostimulant effects (Richelson et al., 2003).

Behavioral sensitization to psychostimulants, an animal model of addiction, is a process by which repeated administration of the same dose of a drug produces increasing degrees of locomotor effects (Domino, 2001). This process is thought to be due to changes in the NA. Initiation of sensitization is associated with changes in the NA shell, and maintenance of sensitization with changes in the NA core (Iyaniwura et al., 2001; Balfour, 2004). Behavioral sensitization models human acquisition of psychostimulant addiction and risk of relapse (Miller et al., 2001; De Vries et al., 2002).

Locomotor sensitization depends on activation of the mesolimbic DA system with additional long-term influences on glutamate, GABA, κ-opioid, and other neurotransmitter systems (Pierce and Kalivas, 1997; Hahn et al., 2000). DA neurons originating in the VTA and projecting to the shell and core of the NA lead to the initiation and expression of sensitization, respectively (Pierce and Kalivas, 1997). NT colocalizes with DA neurons and acts as a modulator of DA effects (Binder et al., 2001a). When injected into the VTA, NT causes hyperactivity and DA release in the NA, similar to the effects of psychostimulants (Kalivas and Duffy, 1990; Kalivas, 1994). However, NT injected into the NA reduces the response to psychostimulants, an effect similar to that of brain-penetrating NT analogs given extracranially (Ervin et al., 1981; Robledo et al., 1993; Richelson et al., 2003).

The NT agonist NT69L, given intraperitoneally, blocks the acute locomotor effects of cocaine and D-amphetamine (Boules et al., 2001a), and blocks both the initiation and expression of sensitization to nicotine after subcutaneous administration (Fredrickson et al., 2003a,b). This is one line of evidence suggesting NT agonists may be effective for treatment of nicotine, amphetamine, and cocaine addiction. Curiously, the NT antagonist SR48692 when administered chronically decreased locomotor sensitization to cocaine (Felszeghy et al., 2007).

How then can a NTR agonist and a NTR antagonist have similar effects in this particular animal model of addiction? Although further research is needed, several lines of evidence bear on this question. Repeated doses of the NT antagonist were required to produce the intended effect on sensitization. Classically, chronic receptor blockade can lead to up-regulation of the receptor, thus making the agonist more effective. Chronic blockade of the receptors may also lead to increased NT synthesis and release. Another approach to this question is with animals lacking NTRs. Studies with SR48692 would predict that mice lacking NTS1 would not sensitize to psychostimulants. However, such null mice are more sensitive to an acute injection of D-amphetamine and had an enhanced response to the sensitizing effects of this psychostimulant as compared to wild type mice (Boules et al., 2006).

The NT agonist NT69L attenuates intravenous (IV) self-administration of nicotine in rats (Boules et al., 2011b). Once animals acquired stable responding to nicotine they were pretreated with either NT69L or saline. Pretreatment with NT69L attenuated nicotine self-infusion under FR1 (fixed ratio of 1) and FR5 schedules of reinforcement. Control rats that were response-independent "yoked" as well as rats that self-infused saline showed minimal responses, indicating that nicotine served as a reinforcer. The stimulant and reinforcing effects of nicotine are attributed to stimulation of the mesolimbic DA system (Stein et al., 1998; Di Chiara, 2000; George et al., 2000). In this study, nicotine self-infusion increased TH, DA $D_1$, and DA $D_2$ receptor mRNA in the VTA, consistent with increased burst firing. NT69L antagonized these effects. In the PFC, an area implicated with learning, NT69L increased TH and DA $D_1$ mRNA. TH and DA $D_1$ mRNA levels were also increased in the striatum in response to the NT agonist. Taken together these results show that the NT agonist NT69L attenuated nicotine self-administration and suggest the drug would reduce craving and withdrawal symptoms (for example, cognitive complaints that are common during nicotine withdrawal).

Is there abuse potential for NT agonists? Although NT mimics the effects of psychostimulants when injected directly into the VTA, it blocks certain stimulant effects when injected into the NA. NT analogs given extracranially (native NT is degraded by peptidases when given peripherally) also block locomotor effects of stimulants, and attenuate nicotine self-administration in rats. Rats do not self administer NT. Therefore, the preponderance of evidence argues against an abuse or addiction potential for NT analogs. This conclusion is supported by data in rhesus monkeys; the animals did not self-infuse NT69L (Fantegrossi et al., 2005).

Although questions remain, a growing body of data supports a key role for NT in regulation of responses to psychostimulants. To the extent animal models are predictive, and NT agonists show promise for the treatment of human addiction. The relative contributions of NTS1 and NTS2 receptors in these models have not been extensively explored, and further research may lead to development of agonists which retain efficacy with fewer side effects such as hypothermia and hypotension.

### NT AND PARKINSON'S DISEASE

Studies show that plasma NT concentrations are consistently higher in PD patients as compared to controls and untreated as compared to treated patients (Schimpff et al., 2001). PD patients also have a twofold increase in NT content in both zona compacta and zona reticulate of the SN compared to that for controls (Fernandez et al., 1995). Brains from PD patients have fewer dopaminergic neurons and very low expression of NTS1 (Yamada and Richelson, 1995). Similar results were reported in an animal model for PD, where MPTP treated mice had significantly lower [$^3$H] NT and [$^3$H] mazindol binding in the striatum and SN, results indicating severe reduction in NTRs and DA uptake sites respectively. These data suggest that the dysfunction in NTRs may be involved in the degradation processes causing PD. Caceda et al. (2006) suggested that the increase in striatal and nigral NT tissue concentrations, as well as in CSF and plasma levels may be due either to a compensatory mechanism for the loss of DA neurons to preserve motor function and/or to a dysregulation of NT neurotransmission on striatal output favoring the striatopallidal pathway (Caceda et al., 2006). Injection of NT resulted in a dose related attenuation of muscular rigidity and tremors caused by bilateral injection of the neurotoxin 6-hydroxydopamine in the medial forebrain bundle (Jolicoeur et al., 1991). In addition, we showed that injection of the NT agonist, NT69L, attenuated the amphetamine and apomorphine rotatory behavior caused by the unilateral injection of the same drug in the nigro-striatal pathway (Boules et al., 2001b).

## POTENTIAL SIDE EFFECTS OF NT AGONISTS

### HYPOTHERMIA

Neurotensin (Bissette et al., 1976) and NT agonists (Tyler-McMahon et al., 2000b; Boules et al., 2001c, 2003a; Feifel et al., 2010a) elicit hypothermia in rodents. Hypothermia is mediated by NTS1. This has been established with the use of NTS1$^{-/-}$ and NTS2$^{-/-}$ mice (Remaury et al., 2002; Mechanic et al., 2009). Additionally, NTS2-selective analogs do not induce hypothermia (Boules et al., 2010), results that provide further proof for the involvement of NTS1 receptor subtype in mediating hypothermia. Interestingly, studies show potential therapeutic use for the NT agonist-induced hypothermia. The administration of the NT agonist ABS-201 immediately or up to 60 min after stroke attack significantly reduced infarct formation and brain cell death in an animal model of focal ischemia (Choi et al., 2012). In addition, it was effective in promoting long-term functional recovery in post-stroke animals (Choi et al., 2012). Similar studies on regulated hypothermia induced by the NT agonists reduce oxidative stress in the brain during reperfusion from asphyxial cardiac arrest (Katz et al., 2004a). Also, lowering body temperature with a NT agonist provided a better neurologic outcome than brief external cooling in a rat model of near drowning (Katz et al., 2004b). Consistent with these results, hypothermia induced by the NT analog JMV-449 had a neuroprotective effect in a mouse model of permanent distal middle cerebral artery occlusion (Torup et al., 2003).

### HYPOTENSION

Intracerebroventricular (ICV) or IV injections of NT induces a dose-dependent drop in arterial blood pressure in anesthetized rats. The drop in blood pressure is of rapid onset (30–60 s) and of short duration (1–4 min) (Rioux et al., 1981). Interestingly, the hypotensive effect of NT is not accompanied by any alteration in cardiac actions (Rosell et al., 1976; Rioux et al., 1981).

### DEVELOPMENT OF TOLERANCE

Animal studies show that tolerance develops to some but not all the effects of NT analogs. Tolerance develops to the hypothermia, thermal analgesia, and anticataleptic effect of NTS1 agonists (Boules et al., 2003b). Conversely, tolerance does not occur to the NT agonist's effects on the reversal of amphetamine- and cocaine-induced locomotor activity (Boules et al., 2003b; Hadden et al., 2005; Feifel et al., 2008), the reversal of apomorphine-induced climbing (Boules et al., 2003b), and the reversal of amphetamine or DOI-induced disruption of PPI (Feifel et al., 2007; Briody et al., 2010).

Interestingly, NTS2 seem to play an important role in the development of tolerance of NT69L-mediated hypothermia and thermal analgesia (Smith et al., 2011), while tolerance to its analgesic and anticataleptic effects the NTS2 analog NT79 does not occur (Boules et al., 2010).

Thus, the development of tolerance depends on the NT analog, their selectivity to the NTR subtypes, the paradigm being tested and the dosing regimen (Wang et al., 2005; Feifel et al., 2008).

## CONCLUSION

The association of NT with several neurotransmitter and endocrine systems suggests its involvement in a wide range of physiologic processes throughout the body and implicates it in the pathology of many neuropsychiatric diseases. Furthermore, the development of NT analogs that can be administered systemically may provide therapy for the treatment of several disorders including schizophrenia, pain, and psychostimulant abuse. Additionally, the use of NT analogs and genetically modified animals will allow further understanding of the molecular role of NT in health and disease.

## ACKNOWLEDGMENTS

This work was supported by Mayo Foundation for Medical Education and Research, the Siragusa Foundation Career Development Award in Neuroscience Research, and grant number 2KF01 from the Florida Department of Health to Mona Boules.

## REFERENCES


Akema, T., and Kimura, F. (1989). Inhibition by catecholaminergic blockers of the neurotensin-induced enhancement of luteinizing hormone secretion in the ovariectomized estrogen-primed rat. *Neuroendocrinology* 50, 688–692.

Alexander, M. J. (1993). Estrogen-regulated synthesis of neurotensin in neurosecretory cells of the hypothalamic arcuate nucleus in the female rat. *Endocrinology* 133, 1809–1816.

Alexander, M. J. (1999). Colocalization of neurotensin messenger ribonucleic acid (mRNA) and progesterone receptor mRNA in rat arcuate neurons under estrogen-stimulated conditions. *Endocrinology* 140, 4995–5003.

Alexander, M. J., and Leeman, S. E. (1994). Estrogen-inducible neurotensin immunoreactivity in the preoptic area of the female rat. *J. Comp. Neurol.* 345, 496–509.

Alexander, M. J., Mahoney, P. D., Ferris, C. F., Carraway, R. E., and Leeman, S. E. (1989a). Evidence that neurotensin participates in the central regulation of the preovulatory surge of luteinizing hormone in the rat. *Endocrinology* 124, 783–788.

Alexander, M. J., Dobner, P. R., Miller, M. A., Bullock, B. P., Dorsa, D. M., and Leeman, S. E. (1989b). Estrogen induces neurotensin/neuromedin N messenger ribonucleic acid in a preoptic nucleus essential for the preovulatory surge of luteinizing hormone in the rat. *Endocrinology* 125, 2111–2117.

al-Rodhan, N. R., Richelson, E., Gilbert, J. A., McCormick, D. J., Kanba, K. S., Pfenning, M. A., et al. (1991). Structure-antinociceptive activity of neurotensin and some novel analogues in the periaqueductal gray region of the brainstem. *Brain Res.* 557, 227–235.

Antonelli, T., Fuxe, K., Tomasini, M. C., Mazzoni, E., Agnati, L. F., Tanganelli, S., et al. (2007). Neurotensin receptor mechanisms and its modulation of glutamate transmission in the brain: relevance for neurodegenerative diseases and their treatment. *Prog. Neurobiol.* 83, 92–109.

Arnt, J., Sanchez, C., Lenz, S. M., Madsen, U., and Krogsgaard-Larsen, P. (1995). Differentiation of in vivo effects of AMPA and NMDA receptor ligands using drug discrimination methods and convulsant/anticonvulsant activity. *Eur. J. Pharmacol.* 285, 289–297.

Asselin, M. L., Dubuc, I., Coquerel, A., and Costentin, J. (2001). Localization of neurotensin NTS2 receptors in rat brain, using. *Neuroreport* 12, 1087–1091.

Bachelet, C. M., Scarceriaux, V., Rostene, W., and Pelaprat, D. (1997). Evidence for neurotensin autoreceptors and relationship of neurotensin and its receptors with tyrosine hydroxylase-positive neurons in rat primary hypothalamic cultures. *Eur. J. Neurosci.* 9, 1483–1487.

Balfour, D. J. (2004). The neurobiology of tobacco dependence: a preclinical perspective on the role of the dopamine projections to the nucleus accumbens [corrected]. *Nicotine Tob. Res.* 6, 899–912.

Banks, W. A., Wustrow, D. J., Cody, W. L., Davis, M. D., and Kastin, A. J. (1995). Permeability of the blood-brain barrier to the neurotensin8-13 analog NT1. *Brain Res.* 695, 59–63.

Basbaum, A. I., and Fields, H. L. (1984). Endogenous pain control systems: brainstem spinal pathways and endorphin circuitry. *Annu. Rev. Neurosci.* 7, 309–338.

Bean, A. J., and Roth, R. H. (1992). Dopamine-neurotensin interactions in mesocortical neurons. Evidence from microdialysis studies. *Ann. N. Y. Acad. Sci.* 668, 43–53.

Beck, B., Stricker-Krongrad, A., Richy, S., and Burlet, C. (1998). Evidence that hypothalamic neurotensin signals leptin effects on feeding behavior in normal and fat-preferring rats. *Biochem. Biophys. Res. Commun.* 252, 634–638.

Behbehani, M. M. (1992). Physiological mechanisms of the analgesic effect of neurotensin. *Ann. N. Y. Acad. Sci.* 668, 253–265.

Bello, A. R., Reyes, R., Hernandez, G., Negrin, I., Gonzalez, M., Tramu, G., et al. (2004). Developmental expression of neurotensin in thyrotropes and gonadotropes of male and female rats. *Neuroendocrinology* 79, 90–99.

Berod, A., and Rostene, W. (2002). Neurotensin: an endogenous psychostimulant? *Curr. Opin. Pharmacol.* 2, 93–98.

Binder, E. B., Kinkead, B., Owens, M. J., and Nemeroff, C. B. (2001a). Neurotensin and dopamine interactions. *Pharmacol. Rev.* 53, 453–486.

Binder, E. B., Kinkead, B., Owens, M. J., and Nemeroff, C. B. (2001b). The role of neurotensin in the pathophysiology of schizophrenia and the mechanism of action of antipsychotic drugs. *Biol. Psychiatry* 50, 856–872.

Bissette, G., Nemeroff, C. B., Loosen, P. T., Prange, A. J., and Lipton, M. A. (1976). Hypothermia and intolerance to cold induced by intracisternal administration of the hypothalamic peptide neurotensin. *Nature* 262, 607–609.

Blackburn, A. M., Fletcher, D. R., Adrian, T. E., and Bloom, S. R. (1980). Neurotensin infusion in man: pharmacokinetics and effect on gastrointestinal and pituitary hormones. *J. Clin. Endocrinol. Metab.* 51, 1257–1261.

Boudin, H., Pelaprat, D., Rostene, W., Pickel, V. M., and Beaudet, A. (1998). Correlative ultrastructural distribution of neurotensin receptor proteins and binding sites in the rat substantia nigra. *J. Neurosci.* 18, 8473–8484.

Boules, M., Cusack, B., Zhao, L., Fauq, A., McCormick, D. J., and Richelson, E. (2000). A novel neurotensin peptide analog given extracranially decreases food intake and weight in rodents. *Brain Res.* 865, 35–44.

Boules, M., Fredrickson, P., and Richelson, E. (2003a). Current topics: brain penetrating neurotensin analog. *Life Sci.* 73, 2785–2792.

Boules, M., McMahon, B., Wang, R., Warrington, L., Stewart, J., Yerbury, S., et al. (2003b). Selective tolerance to the hypothermic and anticataleptic effects of a neurotensin analog that crosses the blood-brain barrier. *Brain Res.* 987, 39–48.

Boules, M., Fredrickson, P., and Richelson, E. (2005). Neurotensin agonists as an alternative to antipsychotics. *Expert Opin. Investig. Drugs* 14, 359–369.

Boules, M., Fredrickson, P., and Richelson, E. (2006). Bioactive analogs of neurotensin. *Peptides* 27, 2523–2533.

Boules, M., Johnston, H., Tozy, J., Smith, K., Li, Z., and Richelson, E. (2011a). Analgesic synergy of NTS2 receptor agonist (NT79) and morphine. *Behav. Pharmacol.* 22, 573–581.

Boules, M., Oliveros, A., Liang, Y., Williams, K., Shaw, A., Robinson, J., et al. (2011b). A neurotensin analog, NT69L, attenuates intravenous nicotine self-administration in rats. *Neuropeptides* 45, 9–16.

Boules, M., Liang, Y., Briody, S., Miura, T., Fauq, I., Oliveros, A., et al. (2010). NT79: a novel neurotensin analog with selective behavioral effects. *Brain Res.* 1308, 35–46.

Boules, M., Shaw, A., Liang, Y., Barbut, D., and Richelson, E. (2009). NT69L, a novel analgesic, shows synergy with morphine. *Brain Res.* 1294, 22–28.

Boules, M., Warrington, L., Fauq, A., McCormick, D., and Richelson, E. (2001a). A novel neurotensin analog blocks cocaine- and D-amphetamine-induced hyperactivity. *Eur. J. Pharmacol.* 426, 73–76.

Boules, M., Warrington, L., Fauq, A., McCormick, D., and Richelson, E. (2001b). Antiparkinson-like effects of a novel neurotensin analog in unilaterally 6-hydroxydopamine lesioned rats. *Eur. J. Pharmacol.* 428, 227–233.

Boules, M., McMahon, B., Warrington, L., Stewart, J., Jackson, J., Fauq, A., et al. (2001c). Neurotensin analog selective for hypothermia over antinociception and exhibiting atypical neuroleptic-like properties. *Brain Res.* 919, 1–11.

Boules, M., Cai, S., Li, Z., Shukoor, N., and Richelson, E. (2012). NTS2 receptors: novel targets for neuropathic pain management. *Biol. Psychiatry* 71, 302S.

Bozzola, M., Thome, A. N., Giraldi, E., Lhiaubet, A. M., and Schimpff, R. M. (1998a). Plasma neurotensin levels in prepubertal children and adults: possible involvement in the regulation of growth hormone secretion. *J. Pediatr. Endocrinol. Metab.* 11, 615–621.

Bozzola, M., Ntodou-Thome, A., Bona, G., Autelli, M., Magnani, M. L., Radetti, G., et al. (1998b). Possible role of plasma neurotensin on growth hormone regulation in neonates. *J. Pediatr. Endocrinol. Metab.* 11, 607–613.

Bredeloux, P., Cavelier, F., Dubuc, I., Vivet, B., Costentin, J., and Martinez, J. (2008). Synthesis and biological effects of c(Lys-Lys-Pro-Tyr-Ile-Leu-Lys-Lys-Pro-Tyr-Ile-Leu) (JMV2012), a new analogue of neurotensin that crosses the blood-brain barrier. *J. Med. Chem.* 51, 1610–1616.

Bredeloux, P., Costentin, J., and Dubuc, I. (2006). Interactions between NTS2 neurotensin and opioid receptors on two nociceptive responses assessed on the hot plate test in mice. *Behav. Brain Res.* 175, 399–407.

Briody, S., Boules, M., Oliveros, A., Fauq, I., and Richelson, E. (2010). Chronic NT69L potently prevents drug-induced disruption of prepulse inhibition without causing tolerance. *Behav. Brain Res.* 207, 118–124.

Brouard, A., Pelaprat, D., Dana, C., Vial, M., Lhiaubet, A. M., and Rostene, W. (1992). Mesencephalic dopaminergic neurons in primary cultures express functional neurotensin receptors. *J. Neurosci.* 12, 1409–1415.

Brunetti, L., Di Nisio, C., Orlando, G., Ferrante, C., and Vacca, M. (2005). The regulation of feeding: a cross talk between peripheral and central signalling. *Int. J. Immunopathol. Pharmacol.* 18, 201–212.

Buhler, A. V., Choi, J., Proudfit, H. K., and Gebhart, G. F. (2005). Neurotensin activation of the NTR1 on spinally-projecting serotonergic neurons in the rostral ventromedial medulla is antinociceptive. *Pain* 114, 285–294.

Burgevin, M. C., Castel, M. N., Quarteronet, D., Chevet, T., and Laduron, P. M. (1992a). Neurotensin increases tyrosine hydroxylase messenger RNA-positive neurons in substantia nigra after retrograde axonal transport. *Neuroscience* 49, 627–633.

Burgevin, M. C., Laduron, P. M., Quarteronnet, D., Chevet, T., and Castel, M. N. (1992b). Striatal injection of neurotensin increases tyrosine hydroxylase mRNA in substantia nigra. *Ann. N. Y. Acad. Sci.* 668, 311–313.

Caceda, R., Kinkead, B., and Nemeroff, C. B. (2006). Neurotensin: role in psychiatric and neurological diseases. *Peptides* 27, 2385–2404.

Carlsson, A. (1988). The current status of the dopamine hypothesis of schizophrenia. *Neuropsychopharmacology* 1, 179–186.

Carpenter, W. T. Jr., and Buchanan, R. W. (1994). Schizophrenia. *N. Engl. J. Med.* 330, 681–690.

Carpenter, W. T., Kirkpatrick, B., and Buchanan, R. W. (1999). Schizophrenia: syndromes and diseases. *J. Psychiatr. Res.* 33, 473–475.

Carraway, R., and Leeman, S. E. (1973). The isolation of a new hypotensive peptide, neurotensin, from bovine hypothalami. *J. Biol. Chem.* 248, 6854–6861.

Choi, K. E., Hall, C. L., Sun, J. M., Wei, L., Mohamad, O., Dix, T. A., et al. (2012). A novel stroke therapy of pharmacologically induced hypothermia after focal cerebral ischemia in mice. *FASEB J.* 26, 2799–2810.

Clineschmidt, B. V., Martin, G. E., and Veber, D. F. (1982). Antinocisponsive effects of neurotensin and neurotensin-related peptides. *Ann. N. Y. Acad. Sci.* 400, 283–306.

Clineschmidt, B. V., and McGuffin, J. C. (1977). Neurotensin administered intracisternally inhibits responsiveness of mice to noxious stimuli. *Eur. J. Pharmacol.* 46, 395–396.

Clineschmidt, B. V., McGuffin, J. C., and Bunting, P. B. (1979). Neurotensin: antinocisponsive action in rodents. *Eur. J. Pharmacol.* 54, 129–139.

Cooke, J. H., Patterson, M., Patel, S. R., Smith, K. L., Ghatei, M. A., Bloom, S. R., et al. (2009). Peripheral and central administration of xenin and neurotensin suppress food intake in rodents. *Obesity (Silver Spring)* 17, 1135–1143.

Corley, K. C., Phan, T. H., Daugherty, W. P., and Boadle-Biber, M. C. (2002). Stress-induced activation of median raphe serotonergic neurons in rats is potentiated by the neurotensin antagonist, SR 48692. *Neurosci. Lett.* 319, 1–4.

Creese, I., Burt, D. R., and Snyder, S. H. (1976). Dopamine receptor binding predicts clinical and pharmacological potencies of antischizophrenic drugs. *Science* 192, 481–483.

Cui, H., Cai, F., and Belsham, D. D. (2005). Anorexigenic hormones leptin, insulin, and alpha-melanocyte-stimulating hormone directly induce neurotensin (NT) gene expression in novel NT-expressing cell models. *J. Neurosci.* 25, 9497–9506.

Cusack, B., Boules, M., Tyler, B. M., Fauq, A., McCormick, D. J., and Richelson, E. (2000). Effects of a novel neurotensin peptide analog given extracranially on CNS behaviors mediated by apomorphine and haloperidol. *Brain Res.* 856, 48–54.

Dansereau, M. A., Roussy, G., Belleville, K., Beaudet, N., Richelson, E., et al. (2006). *Potent Antinociceptive Effects of NTS1 Agonists in a Model of Neuropathic Pain.* Neuroscience Meeting Planner. Society for Neuroscience, Atlanta, GA.

De Vries, T. J., Schoffelmeer, A. N., Binnekade, R., Raaso, H., and Vanderschuren, L. J. (2002). Relapse to cocaine- and heroin-seeking behavior mediated by dopamine D2 receptors is time-dependent and associated with behavioral sensitization. *Neuropsychopharmacology* 26, 18–26.

Di Chiara, G. (2000). Role of dopamine in the behavioural actions of nicotine related to addiction. *Eur. J. Pharmacol.* 393, 295–314.

Dobner, P. R. (2005). Multitasking with neurotensin in the central nervous system. *Cell. Mol. Life Sci.* 62, 1946–1963.

Dobner, P. R. (2006). Neurotensin and pain modulation. *Peptides* 27, 2405–2414.

Domino, E. F. (2001). Nicotine induced behavioral locomotor sensitization. *Prog. Neuropsychopharmacol. Biol. Psychiatry* 25, 59–71.

Dubuc, I., Costentin, J., Terranova, J. P., Barnouin, M. C., Soubrie, P., Le Fur, G., et al. (1994). The nonpeptide neurotensin antagonist, SR 48692, used as a tool to reveal putative neurotensin receptor subtypes. *Br. J. Pharmacol.* 112, 352–354.

Dubuc, I., Remande, S., and Costentin, J. (1999a). The partial agonist properties of levocabastine in neurotensin-induced analgesia. *Eur. J. Pharmacol.* 381, 9–12.

Dubuc, I., Sarret, P., Labbe-Jullie, C., Botto, J. M., Honore, E., Bourdel, E., et al. (1999b). Identification of the receptor subtype involved in the analgesic effect of neurotensin. *J. Neurosci.* 19, 503–510.

Feifel, D., Melendez, G., Murray, R. J., Tina Tran, D. N., Rullan, M. A., and Shilling, P. D. (2008). The reversal of amphetamine-induced locomotor activation by a selective neurotensin-1 receptor agonist does not exhibit tolerance. *Psychopharmacology (Berl.)* 200, 197–203.

Elde, R., Schalling, M., Ceccatelli, S., Nakanishi, S., and Hokfelt, T. (1990). Localization of neuropeptide receptor mRNA in rat brain: initial observations using probes for neurotensin and substance P receptors. *Neurosci. Lett.* 120, 134–138.

Ervin, G. N., Birkemo, L. S., Nemeroff, C. B., and Prange, A. J. (1981). Neurotensin blocks certain amphetamine-induced behaviours. *Nature* 291, 73–76.

Fang, F. G., Moreau, J. L., and Fields, H. L. (1987). Dose-dependent antinociceptive action of neurotensin microinjected into the rostroventromedial medulla of the rat. *Brain Res.* 420, 171–174.

Fantegrossi, W. E., Ko, M. C., Woods, J. H., and Richelson, E. (2005). Antinociceptive, hypothermic, hypotensive, and reinforcing effects of a novel neurotensin receptor agonist, NT69L, in rhesus monkeys. *Pharmacol. Biochem. Behav.* 80, 341–349.

Farkas, R. H., Chien, P. Y., Nakajima, S., and Nakajima, Y. (1996). Properties of a slow nonselective cation conductance modulated by neurotensin and other neurotransmitters in midbrain dopaminergic neurons. *J. Neurophysiol.* 76, 1968–1981.

Fawaz, C. S., Martel, P., Leo, D., and Trudeau, L. E. (2009). Presynaptic action of neurotensin on dopamine release through inhibition of D(2) receptor function. *BMC Neurosci.* 10:96. doi:10.1186/1471-2202-10-96

Feifel, D., Goldenberg, J., Melendez, G., and Shilling, P. D. (2010a). The acute and subchronic effects of a brain-penetrating, neurotensin-1 receptor agonist on feeding, body weight and temperature. *Neuropharmacology* 58, 195–198.

Feifel, D., Pang, Z., Shilling, P. D., Melendez, G., Schreiber, R., and Button, D. (2010b). Sensorimotor gating in neurotensin-1 receptor null mice. *Neuropharmacology* 58, 173–178.

Feifel, D., Melendez, G., Priebe, K., and Shilling, P. D. (2007). The effects of chronic administration of established and putative antipsychotics on natural prepulse inhibition deficits in Brattleboro rats. *Behav. Brain Res.* 181, 278–286.

Feifel, D., Melendez, G., and Shilling, P. D. (2003). A systemically administered neurotensin agonist blocks disruption of prepulse inhibition produced by a serotonin-2A agonist. *Neuropsychopharmacology* 28, 651–653.

Feifel, D., Reza, T. L., and Robeck, S. L. (1997). Pro-dopamine effects of neurotensin on sensorimotor gating deficits. *Peptides* 18, 1457–1460.

Feifel, D., Reza, T. L., Wustrow, D. J., and Davis, M. D. (1999). Novel antipsychotic-like effects on prepulse inhibition of startle produced by a neurotensin agonist. *J. Pharmacol. Exp. Ther.* 288, 710–713.

Felszeghy, K., Espinosa, J. M., Scarna, H., Berod, A., Rostene, W., and Pelaprat, D. (2007). Neurotensin receptor antagonist administered during cocaine withdrawal decreases locomotor sensitization and conditioned place preference. *Neuropsychopharmacology* 32, 2601–2610.

Fernandez, A., Jenner, P., Marsden, C. D., and De Ceballos, M. L. (1995). Characterization of neurotensin-like immunoreactivity in human basal ganglia: increased neurotensin levels in substantia nigra in Parkinson's disease. *Peptides* 16, 339–346.

Ferraro, L., Beggiato, S., Tomasini, M. C., Fuxe, K., Tanganelli, S., and Antonelli, T. (2011). Neurotensin regulates cortical glutamate transmission by modulating N-methyl-D-aspartate receptor functional activity: an in vivo microdialysis study. *J. Neurosci. Res.* 89, 1618–1626.

Ferraro, L., O'Connor, W. T., Beggiato, S., Tomasini, M. C., Fuxe, K., Tanganelli, S., et al. (2012). Striatal NTS1, dopamine D2 and NMDA receptor regulation of pallidal GABA and glutamate release – a dual-probe microdialysis study in the intranigral 6-hydroxydopamine unilaterally lesioned rat. *Eur. J. Neurosci.* 35, 207–220.

Ferraro, L., Tomasini, M. C., Mazza, R., Fuxe, K., Fournier, J., Tanganelli, S., et al. (2008). Neurotensin receptors as modulators of glutamatergic transmission. *Brain Res. Rev.* 58, 365–373.

Fredrickson, P., Boules, M., Yerbury, S., and Richelson, E. (2003a). Blockade of nicotine-induced locomotor sensitization by a novel neurotensin analog in rats. *Eur. J. Pharmacol.* 458, 111–118.

Fredrickson, P., Boules, M., Yerbury, S., and Richelson, E. (2003b). Novel neurotensin analog blocks the initiation and expression of nicotine-induced locomotor sensitization. *Brain Res.* 979, 245–248.

Fuxe, K., Agnati, L. F., von Euler, G., Tanganelli, S., O'Connor, W. T., Ferre, S., et al. (1992a). Neuropeptides, excitatory amino acid and adenosine A2 receptors regulate D2 receptors via intramembrane receptor–receptor interactions. Relevance for Parkinson's disease and schizophrenia. *Neurochem. Int.* 20(Suppl.), 215S–224S.

Fuxe, K., Von Euler, G., Agnati, L. F., Merlo Pich, E., O'Connor, W. T., Tanganelli, S., et al. (1992b). Intramembrane interactions between neurotensin receptors and dopamine D2 receptors as a major mechanism for the neuroleptic-like action of neurotensin. *Ann. N. Y. Acad. Sci.* 668, 186–204.

Gefvert, O., Lundberg, T., Wieselgren, I. M., Bergstrom, M., Langstrom, B., Wiesel, F., et al. (2001). D(2) and 5HT(2A) receptor occupancy of different doses of quetiapine in schizophrenia: a PET study. *Eur. Neuropsychopharmacol.* 11, 105–110.

George, T. P., Verrico, C. D., Picciotto, M. R., and Roth, R. H. (2000). Nicotinic modulation of mesoprefrontal dopamine neurons: pharmacologic and neuroanatomic characterization. *J. Pharmacol. Exp. Ther.* 295, 58–66.

Gerhardt, S., Gerber, R., and Liebman, J. M. (1985). SCH 23390 dissociated from conventional neuroleptics in apomorphine climbing and primate acute dyskinesia models. *Life Sci.* 37, 2355–2363.

Geyer, M. A., and Ellenbroek, B. (2003). Animal behavior models of the mechanisms underlying antipsychotic atypicality. *Prog. Neuropsychopharmacol. Biol. Psychiatry* 27, 1071–1079.

Gilbert, J. A., and Richelson, E. (1984). Neurotensin stimulates formation of cyclic GMP in murine neuroblastoma clone N1E-115. *Eur. J. Pharmacol.* 99, 245–246.

Goff, D. C., Heckers, S., and Freudenreich, O. (2001). Schizophrenia. *Med. Clin. North Am.* 85, 663–689.

Govoni, S., Hong, J. S., Yang, H. Y., and Costa, E. (1980). Increase of neurotensin content elicited by neuroleptics in nucleus accumbens. *J. Pharmacol. Exp. Ther.* 215, 413–417.

Gui, X., Carraway, R. E., and Dobner, P. R. (2004). Endogenous neurotensin facilitates visceral nociception and is required for stress-induced antinociception in mice and rats. *Neuroscience* 126, 1023–1032.

Guillemette, A., Dansereau, M. A., Beaudet, N., Richelson, E., and Sarret, P. (2012). Intrathecal administration of NTS1 agonists reverses nociceptive behaviors in a rat model of neuropathic pain. *Eur. J. Pain.* 16, 473–484.

Hadden, M. K., Orwig, K. S., Kokko, K. P., Mazella, J., and Dix, T. A. (2005). Design, synthesis, and evaluation of the antipsychotic potential of orally bioavailable neurotensin (8-13) analogues containing non-natural arginine and lysine residues. *Neuropharmacology* 49, 1149–1159.

Hahn, B., Stolerman, I. P., and Shoaib, M. (2000). Kappa-opioid receptor modulation of nicotine-induced behaviour. *Neuropharmacology* 39, 2848–2855.

Hawkins, M. F. (1986). Central nervous system neurotensin and feeding. *Physiol. Behav.* 36, 1–8.

Hawkins, M. F., Barkemeyer, C. A., and Tulley, R. T. (1986). Synergistic effects of dopamine agonists and centrally administered neurotensin on feeding. *Pharmacol. Biochem. Behav.* 24, 1195–1201.

Herbison, A. E., Robinson, J. E., and Skinner, D. C. (1993). Distribution of estrogen receptor-immunoreactive cells in the preoptic area of the ewe: co-localization with glutamic acid decarboxylase but not luteinizing hormone-releasing hormone. *Neuroendocrinology* 57, 751–759.

Herbison, A. E., and Theodosis, D. T. (1992). Localization of oestrogen receptors in preoptic neurons containing neurotensin but not tyrosine hydroxylase, cholecystokinin or luteinizing hormone-releasing hormone in the male and female rat. *Neuroscience* 50, 283–298.

Herbison, A. E., and Theodosis, D. T. (1993). Absence of estrogen receptor immunoreactivity in somatostatin (SRIF) neurons of the periventricular nucleus but sexually dimorphic colocalization of estrogen receptor and SRIF immunoreactivities in neurons of the bed nucleus of the stria terminalis. *Endocrinology* 132, 1707–1714.

Hermans, E., Gailly, P., Octave, J. N., and Maloteaux, J. M. (1994). Rapid desensitization of agonist-induced calcium mobilization in transfected PC12 cells expressing the rat neurotensin receptor. *Biochem. Biophys. Res. Commun.* 198, 400–407.

Hokfelt, T., Everitt, B. J., Fuxe, K., Kalia, M., Agnati, L., Johansson, O., et al. (1984). Transmitter and peptide systems in areas involved in the control of blood pressure. *Clin. Exp. Hypertens. A* 6, 23–41.

Holly, E. N., Ebrecht, B., and Prus, A. J. (2011). The neurotensin-1 receptor agonist PD149163 inhibits conditioned avoidance responding without producing catalepsy in rats. *Eur. Neuropsychopharmacol.* 21, 526–531.

Howes, O. D., and Kapur, S. (2009). The dopamine hypothesis of schizophrenia: version III – the final common pathway. *Schizophr. Bull.* 35, 549–562.

Hylden, J. L., and Wilcox, G. L. (1983). Antinociceptive action of intrathecal neurotensin in mice. *Peptides* 4, 517–520.

Ibanez, R., Mallo, F., Benitez, L., Alvarez, C. V., Sanchez-Franco, F., and Dieguez, C. (1993). Effect of neurotensin on growth hormone release in vivo. *Life Sci.* 53, 227–232.

Iyaniwura, T. T., Wright, A. E., and Balfour, D. J. (2001). Evidence that mesoaccumbens dopamine and locomotor responses to nicotine in the rat are influenced by pretreatment dose and strain. *Psychopharmacology (Berl.)* 158, 73–79.

Jacobsen, L., Madsen, P., Jacobsen, C., Nielsen, M. S., Gliemann, J., and Petersen, C. M. (2001). Activation and functional characterization of the mosaic receptor SorLA/LR11. *J. Biol. Chem.* 276, 22788–22796.

Javitt, D. C., and Zukin, S. R. (1991). Recent advances in the phencyclidine model of schizophrenia. *Am. J. Psychiatry* 148, 1301–1308.

Jiang, Z. G., Pessia, M., and North, R. A. (1994). Neurotensin excitation of rat ventral tegmental neurones. *J. Physiol. (Lond.)* 474, 119–129.

Jolas, T., and Aghajanian, G. K. (1996). Neurotensin excitation of serotonergic neurons in the dorsal raphe nucleus of the rat in vitro. *Eur. J. Neurosci.* 8, 153–161.

Jolas, T., and Aghajanian, G. K. (1997). Neurotensin and the serotonergic system. *Prog. Neurobiol.* 52, 455–468.

Jolicoeur, F. B., De Michele, G., Barbeau, A., and St-Pierre, S. (1983). Neurotensin affects hyperactivity but not stereotypy induced by pre and post synaptic dopaminergic stimulation. *Neurosci. Biobehav. Rev.* 7, 385–390.

Jolicoeur, F. B., Gagne, M. A., Rivest, R., Drumheller, A., and St-Pierre, S. (1993). Atypical neuroleptic-like behavioral effects of neurotensin. *Brain Res. Bull.* 32, 487–491.

Jolicoeur, F. B., Rivest, R., St-Pierre, S., and Drumheller, A. (1991). Antiparkinson-like effects of neurotensin in 6-hydroxydopamine lesioned rats. *Brain Res.* 538, 187–192.

Jomphe, C., Lemelin, P. L., Okano, H., Kobayashi, K., and Trudeau, L. E. (2006). Bidirectional regulation of dopamine D2 and neurotensin NTS1 receptors in dopamine neurons. *Eur. J. Neurosci.* 24, 2789–2800.

Kalafatakis, K., and Triantafyllou, K. (2011). Contribution of neurotensin in the immune and neuroendocrine modulation of normal and abnormal enteric function. *Regul. Pept.* 170, 7–17.

Kalivas, P. W. (1994). Blockade of neurotensin-induced motor activity by inhibition of protein kinase. *Psychopharmacology (Berl.)* 114, 175–180.

Kalivas, P. W., and Duffy, P. (1990). Effect of acute and daily neurotensin and enkephalin treatments on extracellular dopamine in the nucleus accumbens. *J. Neurosci.* 10, 2940–2949.

Kapur, S., Zipursky, R. B., Remington, G., Jones, C., DaSilva, J., Wilson, A. A., et al. (1998). 5-HT2 and D2 receptor occupancy of olanzapine in schizophrenia: a PET investigation. *Am. J. Psychiatry* 155, 921–928.

Katz, L. M., Young, A. S., Frank, J. E., Wang, Y., and Park, K. (2004a). Regulated hypothermia reduces brain oxidative stress after hypoxic-ischemia. *Brain Res.* 1017, 85–91.

Katz, L. M., Young, A., Frank, J. E., Wang, Y., and Park, K. (2004b). Neurotensin-induced hypothermia improves neurologic outcome after hypoxic-ischemia. *Crit. Care Med.* 32, 806–810.

Kim, E. R., Leckstrom, A., and Mizuno, T. M. (2008). Impaired anorectic effect of leptin in neurotensin receptor 1-deficient mice. *Behav. Brain Res.* 194, 66–71.

Kim, E. R., and Mizuno, T. M. (2010). Role of neurotensin receptor 1 in the regulation of food intake by neuromedins and neuromedin-related peptides. *Neurosci. Lett.* 468, 64–67.

Kinkead, B., Binder, E. B., and Nemeroff, C. B. (1999). Does neurotensin mediate the effects of antipsychotic drugs? *Biol. Psychiatry* 46, 340–351.

Kinkead, B., and Nemeroff, C. B. (2002). Neurotensin: an endogenous antipsychotic? *Curr. Opin. Pharmacol.* 2, 99–103.

Kinkead, B., and Nemeroff, C. B. (2004). Neurotensin, schizophrenia, and antipsychotic drug action. *Int. Rev. Neurobiol.* 59, 327–349.

Kitabgi, P., De Nadai, F., Labbe-Jullie, C., Dubuc, I., Nouel, D., Costentin, J., et al. (1992). Functional and pharmacological aspects of central neuropeptidergic transmission mediated by neurotensin and neuromedin n. *Clin. Neuropharmacol.* 15(Suppl. 1) (Pt A), 313A–314A.

Kitabgi, P., Herve, D., Studler, J. M., Tramu, G., Rostene, W., and Tassin, J. P. (1989). Neurotensin/dopamine interactions. *Encephale* 15, 91–94.

Labbe-Jullie, C., Deschaintres, S., Gully, D., Le Fur, G., and Kitabgi, P. (1994). Effect of the nonpeptide neurotensin antagonist, SR 48692, and two enantiomeric analogs, SR 48527 and SR 49711, on neurotensin binding and contractile responses in guinea pig ileum and colon. *J. Pharmacol. Exp. Ther.* 271, 267–276.

Lafrance, M., Roussy, G., Belleville, K., Maeno, H., Beaudet, N., Wada, K., et al. (2010). Involvement of NTS2 receptors in stress-induced analgesia. *Neuroscience* 166, 639–652.

Leinninger, G. M., Opland, D. M., Jo, Y. H., Faouzi, M., Christensen, L., Cappellucci, L. A., et al. (2011). Leptin action via neurotensin neurons controls orexin, the mesolimbic dopamine system and energy balance. *Cell Metab.* 14, 313–323.

Leiva, L. A., and Croxatto, H. B. (1994). Comparison of the effect of hypothalamic neuropeptides upon luteinizing hormone secretion by cultured rat anterior pituitary cells. *Biol. Res.* 27, 113–121.

Li, A. H., Yeh, T. H., Tan, P. P., Hwang, H. M., and Wang, H. L. (2001). Neurotensin excitation of serotonergic neurons in the rat nucleus raphe magnus: ionic and molecular mechanisms. *Neuropharmacology* 40, 1073–1083.

Li, X. M., Ferraro, L., Tanganelli, S., O'Connor, W. T., Hasselrot, U., Ungerstedt, U., et al. (1995). Neurotensin peptides antagonistically regulate postsynaptic dopamine D2 receptors in rat nucleus accumbens: a receptor binding and microdialysis study. *J. Neural Transm. Gen. Sect.* 102, 125–137.

Li, Z., Boules, M., and Richelson, E. (2011). NT69L blocks ethanol-induced increase of dopamine and glutamate levels in striatum of mouse. *Neurosci. Lett.* 487, 322–324.

Li, Z., Boules, M., Williams, K., Peris, J., and Richelson, E. (2010a). The novel neurotensin analog NT69L blocks phencyclidine (PCP)-induced increases in locomotor activity and PCP-induced increases in monoamine and amino acids levels in the medial prefrontal cortex. *Brain Res.* 1311, 28–36.

Li, Z., Liang, Y., Boules, M., Gordillo, A., and Richelson, E. (2010b). Effect of amphetamine on extracellular concentrations of amino acids in striatum in neurotensin subtype 1 and 2 receptor null mice: a possible interaction between neurotensin receptors and amino acid systems for study of schizophrenia. *Neuropharmacology* 58, 1174–1178.

Li, Z., Boules, M., Williams, K., Gordillo, A., Li, S., and Richelson, E. (2010c). Similarities in the behavior and molecular deficits in the frontal cortex between the neurotensin receptor subtype 1 knockout mice and chronic phencyclidine-treated mice: relevance to schizophrenia. *Neurobiol. Dis.* 40, 467–477.

Liang, Y., Boules, M., Li, Z., Williams, K., Miura, T., Oliveros, A., et al. (2010). Hyperactivity of the dopaminergic system in NTS1 and NTS2 null mice. *Neuropharmacology* 58, 1199–1205.

Lopez Ordieres, M. G., and Rodriguez de Lores Arnaiz, G. (2000). Neurotensin inhibits neuronal Na+, K+-ATPase activity through high affinity peptide receptor. *Peptides* 21, 571–576.

Lutfy, K., Shen, K. Z., Woodward, R. M., and Weber, E. (1996). Inhibition of morphine tolerance by NMDA receptor antagonists in the formalin test. *Brain Res.* 731, 171–181.

Luttinger, D., Burgess, S. K., Nemeroff, C. B., and Prange, A. J. (1983). The effects of chronic morphine treatment on neurotensin-induced antinociception. *Psychopharmacology (Berl.)* 81, 10–13.

Luttinger, D., King, R. A., Sheppard, D., Strupp, J., Nemeroff, C. B., and Prange, A. J. (1982). The effect of neurotensin on food consumption in the rat. *Eur. J. Pharmacol.* 81, 499–503.

Maeno, H., Yamada, K., Santo-Yamada, Y., Aoki, K., Sun, Y. J., Sato, E., et al. (2004). Comparison of mice deficient in the high- or low-affinity neurotensin receptors, Ntsr1 or Ntsr2, reveals a novel function for Ntsr2 in thermal nociception. *Brain Res.* 998, 122–129.

Malendowicz, L. K., and Nussdorfer, G. G. (1994). Modulatory action of neurotensin on the pituitary-adrenocortical function in rats: evidence for an acute dose-dependent biphasic effect. *Life Sci.* 55, 201–205.

Martin, S., Vincent, J. P., and Mazella, J. (2003). Involvement of the neurotensin receptor-3 in the neurotensin-induced migration of human microglia. *J. Neurosci.* 23, 1198–1205.

Mazella, J. (2001). Sortilin/neurotensin receptor-3: a new tool to investigate neurotensin signaling and cellular trafficking? *Cell. Signal.* 13, 1–6.

Mazzocchi, G., Malendowicz, L. K., Rebuffat, P., Gottardo, G., and Nussdorfer, G. G. (1997). Neurotensin stimulates CRH and ACTH release by rat adrenal medulla in vitro. *Neuropeptides* 31, 8–11.

McBride, W. J., Murphy, J. M., and Ikemoto, S. (1999). Localization of brain reinforcement mechanisms: intracranial self-administration and intracranial place-conditioning studies. *Behav. Brain Res.* 101, 129–152.

McCann, S. M., and Vijayan, E. (1992). Control of anterior pituitary hormone secretion by neurotensin. *Ann. N. Y. Acad. Sci.* 668, 287–297.

Mechanic, J. A., Sutton, J. E., Berson, A. E., Wu, X., Kwan, J., Schreiber, R., et al. (2009). Involvement of the neurotensin receptor 1 in the behavioral effects of two neurotensin agonists, NT-2 and NT69L: lack of hypothermic, antinociceptive and antipsychotic actions in receptor knockout mice. *Eur. Neuropsychopharmacol.* 19, 466–475.

Meltzer, H. Y., Matsubara, S., and Lee, J. C. (1989). Classification of typical and atypical antipsychotic drugs on the basis of dopamine D-1, D-2 and serotonin2 pKi values. *J. Pharmacol. Exp. Ther.* 251, 238–246.

Memo, M., Castelletti, L., Valerio, A., Missale, C., and Spano, P. F. (1986). Identification of neurotensin receptors associated with calcium channels and prolactin release in rat pituitary. *J. Neurochem.* 47, 1682–1688.

Merchant, K. M., Dobner, P. R., and Dorsa, D. M. (1992). Differential effects of haloperidol and clozapine on neurotensin gene transcription in rat neostriatum. *J. Neurosci.* 12, 652–663.

Merchant, K. M., and Dorsa, D. M. (1993). Differential induction of neurotensin and c-fos gene expression by typical versus atypical antipsychotics. *Proc. Natl. Acad. Sci. U.S.A.* 90, 3447–3451.

Merchant, K. M., Miller, M. A., Ashleigh, E. A., and Dorsa, D. M. (1991). Haloperidol rapidly increases the number of neurotensin mRNA-expressing neurons in neostriatum of the rat brain. *Brain Res.* 540, 311–314.

Mercuri, N. B., Stratta, F., Calabresi, P., and Bernardi, G. (1993). Neurotensin induces an inward current in rat mesencephalic dopaminergic neurons. *Neurosci. Lett.* 153, 192–196.

Miller, D. K., Wilkins, L. H., Bardo, M. T., Crooks, P. A., and Dwoskin, L. P. (2001). Once weekly administration of nicotine produces long-lasting locomotor sensitization in rats via a nicotinic receptor-mediated mechanism. *Psychopharmacology (Berl.)* 156, 469–476.

Motoi, Y., Aizawa, T., Haga, S., Nakamura, S., Namba, Y., and Ikeda,

K. (1999). Neuronal localization of a novel mosaic apolipoprotein E receptor, LR11, in rat and human brain. *Brain Res.* 833, 209–215.

Moyse, E., Miller, M. M., Rostene, W., and Beaudet, A. (1988). Effects of ovariectomy and estradiol replacement on the binding of 125I-neurotensin in rat suprachiasmatic nucleus. *Neuroendocrinology* 48, 53–60.

Mustain, W. C., Rychahou, P. G., and Evers, B. M. (2011). The role of neurotensin in physiologic and pathologic processes. *Curr. Opin. Endocrinol. Diabetes Obes.* 18, 75–82.

Nemeroff, C. B. (1980). Neurotensin: perchance an endogenous neuroleptic? *Biol. Psychiatry* 15, 283–302.

Nemeroff, C. B. (1986). The interaction of neurotensin with dopaminergic pathways in the central nervous system: basic neurobiology and implications for the pathogenesis and treatment of schizophrenia. *Psychoneuroendocrinology* 11, 15–37.

Nemeroff, C. B., Osbahr, A. J., Manberg, P. J., Ervin, G. N., and Prange, A. J. (1979). Alterations in nociception and body temperature after intracisternal administration of neurotensin, beta-endorphin, other endogenous peptides, and morphine. *Proc. Natl. Acad. Sci. U.S.A.* 76, 5368–5371.

Newman, S. C., and Bland, R. C. (1991). Mortality in a cohort of patients with schizophrenia: a record linkage study. *Can. J. Psychiatry* 36, 239–245.

Nicot, A., Rostene, W., and Berod, A. (1995). Differential expression of neurotensin receptor mRNA in the dopaminergic cell groups of the rat diencephalon and mesencephalon. *J. Neurosci. Res.* 40, 667–674.

Niimi, M., Takahara, J., Sato, M., and Kawanishi, K. (1991). Neurotensin and growth hormone-releasing factor-containing neurons projecting to the median eminence of the rat: a combined retrograde tracing and immunohistochemical study. *Neurosci. Lett.* 133, 183–186.

Nishiyama, T. (2000). Interaction between intrathecal morphine and glutamate receptor antagonists in formalin test. *Eur. J. Pharmacol.* 395, 203–210.

Nordstrom, A. L., Farde, L., Nyberg, S., Karlsson, P., Halldin, C., and Sedvall, G. (1995). D1, D2, and 5-HT2 receptor occupancy in relation to clozapine serum concentration: a PET study of schizophrenic patients. *Am. J. Psychiatry* 152, 1444–1449.

Nussdorfer, G. G., Malendowicz, L. K., Meneghelli, V., and Mazzocchi, G. (1992). Neurotensin enhances plasma adrenocorticotropin concentration by stimulating corticotropin-releasing hormone secretion. *Life Sci.* 50, 639–643.

Nykjaer, A., Lee, R., Teng, K. K., Jansen, P., Madsen, P., Nielsen, M. S., et al. (2004). Sortilin is essential for proNGF-induced neuronal cell death. *Nature* 427, 843–848.

Palacios, J. M., and Kuhar, M. J. (1981). Neurotensin receptors are located on dopamine-containing neurones in rat midbrain. *Nature* 294, 587–589.

Pan, J. T., Tian, Y., Lookingland, K. J., and Moore, K. E. (1992). Neurotensin-induced activation of hypothalamic dopaminergic neurons is accompanied by a decrease in pituitary secretion of prolactin and alpha-melanocyte-stimulating hormone. *Life Sci.* 50, 2011–2017.

Panayi, F., Colussi-Mas, J., Lambas-Senas, L., Renaud, B., Scarna, H., and Berod, A. (2005). Endogenous neurotensin in the ventral tegmental area contributes to amphetamine behavioral sensitization. *Neuropsychopharmacology* 30, 871–879.

Petkova-Kirova, P., Rakovska, A., Della Corte, L., Zaekova, G., Radomirov, R., and Mayer, A. (2008). Neurotensin modulation of acetylcholine, GABA, and aspartate release from rat prefrontal cortex studied in vivo with microdialysis. *Brain Res. Bull.* 77, 129–135.

Pettibone, D. J., Hess, J. F., Hey, P. J., Jacobson, M. A., Leviten, M., Lis, E. V., et al. (2002). The effects of deleting the mouse neurotensin receptor NTR1 on central and peripheral responses to neurotensin. *J. Pharmacol. Exp. Ther.* 300, 305–313.

Pierce, R. C., and Kalivas, P. W. (1997). A circuitry model of the expression of behavioral sensitization to amphetamine-like psychostimulants. *Brain Res. Brain Res. Rev.* 25, 192–216.

Pinnock, R. D. (1985). Neurotensin depolarizes substantia nigra dopamine neurones. *Brain Res.* 338, 151–154.

Poinot-Chazel, C., Portier, M., Bouaboula, M., Vita, N., Pecceu, F., Gully, D., et al. (1996). Activation of mitogen-activated protein kinase couples neurotensin receptor stimulation to induction of the primary response gene Krox-24. *Biochem. J.* 320, 145–151.

Quirion, R., Gaudreau, P., St-Pierre, S., and Rioux, F. (1982). Localization of neurotensin binding sites in rat kidney. *Peptides* 3, 765–769.

Rakovska, A., Giovannini, M. G., Della Corte, L., Kalfin, R., Bianchi, L., and Pepeu, G. (1998). Neurotensin modulation of acetylcholine and GABA release from the rat hippocampus: an in vivo microdialysis study. *Neurochem. Int.* 33, 335–340.

Remaury, A., Vita, N., Gendreau, S., Jung, M., Arnone, M., Poncelet, M., et al. (2002). Targeted inactivation of the neurotensin type 1 receptor reveals its role in body temperature control and feeding behavior but not in analgesia. *Brain Res.* 953, 63–72.

Richelson, E., Boules, M., and Fredrickson, P. (2003). Neurotensin agonists: possible drugs for treatment of psychostimulant abuse. *Life Sci.* 73, 679–690.

Rioux, F., Quirion, R., St-Pierre, S., Regoli, D., Jolicoeur, F. B., Belanger, F., et al. (1981). The hypotensive effect of centrally administered neurotensin in rats. *Eur. J. Pharmacol.* 69, 241–247.

Rivier, C., Brown, M., and Vale, W. (1977). Effect of neurotensin, substance P and morphine sulfate on the secretion of prolactin and growth hormone in the rat. *Endocrinology* 100, 751–754.

Robledo, P., Maldonado, R., and Koob, G. F. (1993). Neurotensin injected into the nucleus accumbens blocks the psychostimulant effects of cocaine but does not attenuate cocaine self-administration in the rat. *Brain Res.* 622, 105–112.

Rosell, S., Burcher, E., Chang, D., and Folkers, K. (1976). Cardiovascular and metabolic actions of neurotensin and (Gln4)-Neurotensin. *Acta Physiol. Scand.* 98, 484–491.

Rostene, W. H., and Alexander, M. J. (1997). Neurotensin and neuroendocrine regulation. *Front. Neuroendocrinol.* 18, 115–173.

Roussy, G., Beaudry, H., Lafrance, M., Belleville, K., Beaudet, N., Wada, K., et al. (2010). Altered morphine-induced analgesia in neurotensin type 1 receptor null mice. *Neuroscience.* 170, 1286–1294.

Roussy, G., Dansereau, M. A., Baudisson, S., Ezzoubaa, F., Belleville, K., Beaudet, N., et al. (2009). Evidence for a role of NTS2 receptors in the modulation of tonic pain sensitivity. *Mol. Pain* 5, 38–52.

Roussy, G., Dansereau, M. A., Belleville, K., Beaudet, N., Richelson, E., and Sarret, P. (2006). *NTS1-Preferring Agonists Produce Spinal Antinociception in a Formalin Tonic Pain Model.* Neuroscience Meeting Planner. Society for Neuroscience, Atlanta, GA.

Roussy, G., Dansereau, M. A., Dore-Savard, L., Belleville, K., Beaudet, N., Richelson, E., et al. (2008). Spinal NTS1 receptors regulate nociceptive signaling in a rat formalin tonic pain model. *J. Neurochem.* 105, 1100–1114.

Rowe, W., Viau, V., Meaney, M. J., and Quirion, R. (1995). Stimulation of CRH-mediated ACTH secretion by central administration of neurotensin: evidence for the participation of the paraventricular nucleus. *J. Neuroendocrinol.* 7, 109–117.

Sahu, A. (1998). Evidence suggesting that galanin (GAL), melanin-concentrating hormone (MCH), neurotensin (NT), proopiomelanocortin (POMC), and neuropeptide Y (NPY) are targets of leptin signaling in the hypothalamus. *Endocrinology* 139, 795–798.

Sahu, A., Carraway, R. E., and Wang, Y. (2001). Evidence that neurotensin mediates the central effect of leptin on food intake in rat. *Brain Res.* 888, 343–347.

Sarhan, S., Hitchcock, J. M., Grauffel, C. A., and Wettstein, J. G. (1997). Comparative antipsychotic profiles of neurotensin and a related systemically active peptide agonist. *Peptides* 18, 1223–1227.

Sarret, P., Esdaile, M. J., Perron, A., Martinez, J., Stroh, T., and Beaudet, A. (2005). Potent spinal analgesia elicited through stimulation of NTS2 neurotensin receptors. *J. Neurosci.* 25, 8188–8196.

Sarret, P., Krzywkowski, P., Segal, L., Nielsen, M. S., Petersen, C. M., Mazella, J., et al. (2003). Distribution of NTS3 receptor/sortilin mRNA and protein in the rat central nervous system. *J. Comp. Neurol.* 461, 483–505.

Schimpff, R. M., Avard, C., Fenelon, G., Lhiaubet, A. M., Tenneze, L., Vidailhet, M., et al. (2001). Increased plasma neurotensin concentrations in patients with Parkinson's disease. *J. Neurol. Neurosurg. Psychiatr.* 70, 784–786.

Schimpff, R. M., Bozzola, M., Lhiaubet, A. M., Spadaro, B., Tettoni, K., and Rostene, W. (1994). Effects of growth hormone administration on neurotensin release in children with growth delay. *Horm. Res.* 42, 95–99.

Secchi, R. L., Sung, E., Hedley, L. R., Button, D., and Schreiber, R. (2009). The neurotensin agonist NT69L improves sensorimotor gating deficits in rats induced by a glutamatergic antagonist but not by dopaminergic agonists. *Behav. Brain Res.* 202, 192–197.

Seroogy, K., Ceccatelli, S., Schalling, M., Hokfelt, T., Frey, P., Walsh, J., et al. (1988). A subpopulation of dopaminergic neurons in rat ventral mesencephalon contains both neurotensin and cholecystokinin. *Brain Res.* 455, 88–98.

Seta, K. A., Jansen, H. T., Kreitel, K. D., Lehman, M., and Behbehani, M. M. (2001). Cold water swim stress increases the expression of neurotensin mRNA in the lateral hypothalamus and medial preoptic regions of the rat brain. *Brain Res. Mol. Brain Res.* 86, 145–152.

Seutin, V. (2005). Dopaminergic neurones: much more than dopamine? *Br. J. Pharmacol.* 146, 167–169.

Seutin, V., Massotte, L., and Dresse, A. (1989). Electrophysiological effects of neurotensin on dopaminergic neurones of the ventral tegmental area of the rat in vitro. *Neuropharmacology* 28, 949–954.

Sharma, R. P., Janicak, P. G., Bissette, G., and Nemeroff, C. B. (1997). CSF neurotensin concentrations and antipsychotic treatment in schizophrenia and schizoaffective disorder. *Am. J. Psychiatry* 154, 1019–1021.

Shi, W. X., and Bunney, B. S. (1992). Roles of intracellular cAMP and protein kinase A in the actions of dopamine and neurotensin on midbrain dopamine neurons. *J. Neurosci.* 12, 2433–2438.

Shilling, P. D., Melendez, G., Priebe, K., Richelson, E., and Feifel, D. (2004). Neurotensin agonists block the prepulse inhibition deficits produced by a 5-HT(2A) and an alpha(1) agonist. *Psychopharmacology (Berl.)* 175, 353–359.

Shilling, P. D., Richelson, E., and Feifel, D. (2003). The effects of systemic NT69L, a neurotensin agonist, on baseline and drug-disrupted prepulse inhibition. *Behav. Brain Res.* 143, 7–14.

Shivers, B. D., Harlan, R. E., Morrell, J. I., and Pfaff, D. W. (1983). Absence of oestradiol concentration in cell nuclei of LHRH-immunoreactive neurones. *Nature* 304, 345–347.

Slusher, B. S., Zacco, A. E., Maslanski, J. A., Norris, T. E., McLane, M. W., Moore, W. C., et al. (1994). The cloned neurotensin receptor mediates cyclic GMP formation when coexpressed with nitric oxide synthase cDNA. *Mol. Pharmacol.* 46, 115–121.

Smith, D. J., Hawranko, A. A., Monroe, P. J., Gully, D., Urban, M. O., Craig, C. R., et al. (1997). Dose-dependent pain-facilitatory and -inhibitory actions of neurotensin are revealed by SR 48692, a nonpeptide neurotensin antagonist: influence on the antinociceptive effect of morphine. *J. Pharmacol. Exp. Ther.* 282, 899–908.

Smith, E., Boules, M., Williams, K., Fauq, A., and Richelson, E. (2011). The role of NTS2 in the development of tolerance to NT69L in mouse models for hypothermia and thermal analgesia. *Behav. Brain Res.* 224, 344–349.

Smith, K. E., Boules, M., Williams, K., and Richelson, E. (2012). NTS1 and NTS2 mediate analgesia following neurotensin analog treatment in a mouse model for visceral pain. *Behav. Brain Res.* 232, 93–97.

Smith, M. J., and Wise, P. M. (2001). Neurotensin gene expression increases during proestrus in the rostral medial preoptic nucleus: potential for direct communication with gonadotropin-releasing hormone neurons. *Endocrinology* 142, 3006–3013.

Snyder, S. H. (1976). The dopamine hypothesis of schizophrenia: focus on the dopamine receptor. *Am. J. Psychiatry* 133, 197–202.

Snyder, S. H. (1980). Phencyclidine. *Nature* 285, 355–356.

Stein, E. A., Pankiewicz, J., Harsch, H. H., Cho, J. K., Fuller, S. A., Hoffmann, R. G., et al. (1998). Nicotine-induced limbic cortical activation in the human brain: a functional MRI study. *Am. J. Psychiatry* 155, 1009–1015.

St-Gelais, F., Jomphe, C., and Trudeau, L. E. (2006). The role of neurotensin in central nervous system pathophysiology: what is the evidence? *J Psychiatry Neurosci* 31, 229–245.

Stiller, C. O., Gustafsson, H., Fried, K., and Brodin, E. (1997). Opioid-induced release of neurotensin in the periaqueductal gray matter of freely moving rats. *Brain Res.* 774, 149–158.

Stolakis, V., Kalafatakis, K., Botis, J., Zarros, A., and Liapi, C. (2010). The regulatory role of neurotensin on the hypothalamic-anterior pituitary axons: emphasis on the control of thyroid-related functions. *Neuropeptides* 44, 1–7.

Szigethy, E., and Beaudet, A. (1989). Correspondence between high affinity 125I-neurotensin binding sites and dopaminergic neurons in the rat substantia nigra and ventral tegmental area: a combined radioautographic and immunohistochemical light microscopic study. *J. Comp. Neurol.* 279, 128–137.

Tanganelli, S., Antonelli, T., Tomasini, M. C., Beggiato, S., Fuxe, K., and Ferraro, L. (2012). Relevance of dopamine D(2)/neurotensin NTS1 and NMDA/neurotensin NTS1 receptor interaction in psychiatric and neurodegenerative disorders. *Curr. Med. Chem.* 19, 304–316.

Tershner, S. A., and Helmstetter, F. J. (2000). Antinociception produced by mu opioid receptor activation in the amygdala is partly dependent on activation of mu opioid and neurotensin receptors in the ventral periaqueductal gray. *Brain Res.* 865, 17–26.

Thibault, D., Albert, P. R., Pineyro, G., and Trudeau, L. E. (2011). Neurotensin triggers dopamine D2 receptor desensitization through a protein kinase C and beta-arrestin1-dependent mechanism. *J. Biol. Chem.* 286, 9174–9184.

Toda, M., and Abi-Dargham, A. (2007). Dopamine hypothesis of schizophrenia: making sense of it all. *Curr Psychiatry Rep* 9, 329–336.

Torup, L., Borsdal, J., and Sager, T. (2003). Neuroprotective effect of the neurotensin analogue JMV-449 in a mouse model of permanent middle cerebral ischaemia. *Neurosci. Lett.* 351, 173–176.

Trudeau, L. E. (2000). Neurotensin regulates intracellular calcium in ventral tegmental area astrocytes: evidence for the involvement of multiple receptors. *Neuroscience* 97, 293–302.

Tyler, B. M., Douglas, C. L., Fauq, A., Pang, Y. P., Stewart, J. A., Cusack, B., et al. (1999). In vitro binding and CNS effects of novel neurotensin agonists that cross the blood-brain barrier. *Neuropharmacology* 38, 1027–1034.

Tyler, B. M., Groshan, K., Cusack, B., and Richelson, E. (1998a). In vivo studies with low doses of levocabastine and diphenhydramine, but not pyrilamine, antagonize neurotensin-mediated antinociception. *Brain Res.* 787, 78–84.

Tyler, B. M., McCormick, D. J., Hoshall, C. V., Douglas, C. L., Jansen, K., Lacy, B. W., et al. (1998b). Specific gene blockade shows that peptide nucleic acids readily enter neuronal cells in vivo. *FEBS Lett.* 421, 280–284.

Tyler-McMahon, B. M., Boules, M., and Richelson, E. (2000a). Neurotensin: peptide for the next millennium. *Regul. Pept.* 93, 125–136.

Tyler-McMahon, B. M., Stewart, J. A., Farinas, F., McCormick, D. J., and Richelson, E. (2000b). Highly potent neurotensin analog that causes hypothermia and antinociception. *Eur. J. Pharmacol.* 390, 107–111.

Urban, M. O., and Smith, D. J. (1993). Role of neurotensin in the nucleus raphe magnus in opioid-induced antinociception from the periaqueductal gray. *J. Pharmacol. Exp. Ther.* 265, 580–586.

Urban, M. O., and Smith, D. J. (1994). Localization of the antinociceptive and antianalgesic effects of neurotensin within the rostral ventromedial medulla. *Neurosci. Lett.* 174, 21–25.

Vijayan, E., Carraway, R., Leeman, S. E., and McCann, S. M. (1988). Use of antiserum to neurotensin reveals a physiological role for the peptide in rat prolactin release. *Proc. Natl. Acad. Sci. U.S.A.* 85, 9866–9869.

Vranken, J. H., Troost, D., Wegener, J. T., Kruis, M. R., and van der Vegt, M. H. (2005). Neuropathological findings after continuous intrathecal administration of S(+)-ketamine for the management of neuropathic cancer pain. *Pain* 117, 231–235.

Wang, R., Boules, M., Gollatz, E., Williams, K., Tiner, W., and Richelson, E. (2005). Effects of 5 daily injections of the neurotensin-mimetic NT69L on the expression of neurotensin receptors in rat brain. *Brain Res. Mol. Brain Res.* 138, 24–34.

Watanobe, H., and Takebe, K. (1993). In vivo release of neurotensin from the median eminence of ovariectomized estrogen-primed rats as estimated by push-pull perfusion: correlation with luteinizing hormone and prolactin surges. *Neuroendocrinology* 57, 760–764.

Watson, M. A., Yamada, M., Cusack, B., Veverka, K., Bolden-Watson, C., and Richelson, E. (1992). The rat neurotensin receptor expressed in Chinese hamster ovary cells mediates the release of inositol phosphates. *J. Neurochem.* 59, 1967–1970.

Weinberger, D. R. (1987). Implications of normal brain development for the pathogenesis of schizophrenia. *Arch. Gen. Psychiatry* 44, 660–669.

Wolf, S. S., Hyde, T. M., Saunders, R. C., Herman, M. M., Weinberger, D. R., and Kleinman, J. E. (1995). Autoradiographic characterization of neurotensin receptors in the entorhinal cortex of schizophrenic patients and control subjects. *J. Neural Transm. Gen. Sect.* 102, 55–65.

Woulfe, J., and Beaudet, A. (1989). Immunocytochemical evidence for direct connections between neurotensin-containing axons and dopaminergic neurons in the rat ventral midbrain tegmentum. *Brain Res.* 479, 402–406.

Wustrow, D. J., Davis, M. D., Akunne, H. C., Corbin, A. E., Wiley, J. N., Wise, L. D., et al. (1995). Reduced amine bond neurotensin 8-13 mimetics with potent in vivo activity. *Bioorg. Med. Chem. Lett.* 5, 997–1002.

Yamada, M., and Richelson, E. (1993). Role of signal transduction systems in neurotensin receptor downregulation induced by agonist in murine neuroblastoma clone N1E-115 cells. *J. Pharmacol. Exp. Ther.* 267, 128–133.

Yamada, M., and Richelson, E. (1995). Heterogeneity of melanized neurons expressing neurotensin receptor messenger RNA in the substantia nigra and the nucleus paranigralis of control and Parkinson's disease brain. *Neuroscience* 64, 405–417.

Yamauchi, R., Sonoda, S., Jinsmaa, Y., and Yoshikawa, M. (2003). Antinociception induced by beta-lactotensin, a neurotensin agonist peptide derived from beta-lactoglobulin, is mediated by NT2 and D1 receptors. *Life Sci.* 73, 1917–1923.

Zhang, X., Nicholas, A. P., and Hokfelt, T. (1995). Ultrastructural studies on peptides in the dorsal horn of the rat spinal cord – II. Co-existence of galanin with other peptides in local neurons. *Neuroscience* 64, 875–891.

# 11

# Gastrin-releasing peptide receptors in the central nervous system: role in brain function and as a drug target

**Rafael Roesler[1,2,3]* and Gilberto Schwartsmann[2,3,4]**

[1] Laboratory of Neuropharmacology and Neural Tumor Biology, Department of Pharmacology, Institute for Basic Health Sciences, Federal University of Rio Grande do Sul, Porto Alegre, Brazil
[2] Cancer Research Laboratory, University Hospital Research Center (CPE-HCPA), Federal University of Rio Grande do Sul, Porto Alegre, Brazil
[3] National Institute for Translational Medicine, Porto Alegre, Brazil
[4] Department of Internal Medicine, School of Medicine, Federal University of Rio Grande do Sul, Porto Alegre, Brazil

**Edited by:**
*Hubert Vaudry, University of Rouen, France*

**Reviewed by:**
*Hélène Volkoff, Memorial University of Newfoundland, Canada*
*Mitsuhiro Kawata, Kyoto Prefectural University of Medicine, Japan*

***Correspondence:**
*Rafael Roesler, Laboratory of Neuropharmacology and Neural Tumor Biology, Department of Pharmacology, Institute for Basic Health Sciences, Federal University of Rio Grande do Sul, 90050-170 Porto Alegre, Rio Grande do Sul, Brazil.*
*e-mail: rafael.roesler@pq.cnpq.br*

Neuropeptides acting on specific cell membrane receptors of the G protein-coupled receptor (GPCR) superfamily regulate a range of important aspects of nervous and neuroendocrine function. Gastrin-releasing peptide (GRP) is a mammalian neuropeptide that binds to the GRP receptor (GRPR, BB2). Increasing evidence indicates that GRPR-mediated signaling in the central nervous system (CNS) plays an important role in regulating brain function, including aspects related to emotional responses, social interaction, memory, and feeding behavior. In addition, some alterations in GRP or GRPR expression or function have been described in patients with neurodegenerative, neurodevelopmental, and psychiatric disorders, as well as in brain tumors. Findings from preclinical models are consistent with the view that the GRPR might play a role in brain disorders, and raise the possibility that GRPR agonists might ameliorate cognitive and social deficits associated with neurological diseases, while antagonists may reduce anxiety and inhibit the growth of some types of brain cancer. Further preclinical and translational studies evaluating the potential therapeutic effects of GRPR ligands are warranted.

**Keywords: gastrin-releasing peptide, gastrin-releasing peptide receptor, bombesin receptors, neuropeptide signaling, brain disorders**

## INTRODUCTION

Neuropeptide signaling regulates a variety of aspects of nervous and neuroendocrine function (Hökfelt et al., 2003; Salio et al., 2006). Neuropeptides act by activating specific cell membrane receptors that are members of the G protein-coupled receptor (GPCR) superfamily, leading to stimulation of downstream protein kinase signaling pathways and ultimately altering gene expression (Oh et al., 2006).

Gastrin-releasing peptide (GRP), a neuropeptide originally isolated from the porcine stomach, is a 27-amino acid peptide synthesized as a 148-amino acid precursor (PreproGRP) and subsequently metabolized posttranslationally (Spindel et al., 1984, 1990; Lebacq-Verheyden et al., 1988). GRP is the mammalian homolog of the amphibian 14-amino acid peptide bombesin, isolated from the skin of the European frog *Bombina bombina* in 1970 (Erspamer et al., 1970). GRP and bombesin display similar biological activities and share the same seven C-terminal amino acid sequence. Early experiments examining the effects of bombesin when administered in the brain showed that intracerebroventricular (i.c.v.) infusions of bombesin induced hypothermia and hyperglycemia in rats (Brown et al., 1977a,b). In peripheral tissues, the physiological functions of GRP include regulating gastrin and somatostatin release, gastric acid secretion, pancreatic secretion, gastrointestinal motility, lung development, and chemoattraction in immune system cells (Ruff et al., 1985; Schubert et al., 1991; Del Rio and De la Fuente, 1994; Niebergall-Roth and Singer, 2001; Ohki-Hamazaki et al., 2005; Gonzalez et al., 2008; Jensen et al., 2008b; Czepielewski et al., 2012). Another member of the bombesin-like peptide (BLP) family found in mammals is neuromedin B (NMB), the mammalian equivalent of ranatensin, which acts on the NMB receptor (NMBR; Minamino et al., 1983). An additional peptide originally named neuromedin C (NMC) is in fact a decapeptide of GRP (GRP-10, $GRP_{18-27}$; Minamino et al., 1984). Thus, BLPs in mammalian tissues have been increasingly shown to constitute a class of signaling peptides regulating a large range of physiological functions.

Gastrin-releasing peptide acts by binding to the GRP receptor (GRPR, also called BB2), a GPCR that binds preferentially to GRP and bombesin, with much lower affinity for NMB (Jensen and Gardner, 1981; Moody et al., 1988, 1992; von Schrenck et al., 1989, 1990; Ladenheim et al., 1990, 1992; Wang et al., 1992). Increasing evidence indicates that GRPR-mediated signal transduction in the central nervous system (CNS) plays an important role in regulating behavior, especially aspects related to emotional responses, social interaction, memory, and feeding. In addition, we have proposed that dysfunctions in GRPR expression and signaling might play a role in CNS disorders including anxiety, autism, memory dysfunction associated with neurodegenerative disorders, and brain tumors. Here we review the role of GRPRs in regulating brain function, and its potential as a drug target for CNS disorders.

## MOLECULAR ORGANIZATION OF THE GRPR

All mammalian bombesin receptors (GRPR, NMBR, and the orphan receptor BRS-3 or BB3) exhibit the characteristic seven transmembrane domain structure of GPCRs. This review will focus solely on the GRPR. For a comprehensive review of the classification, nomenclature, structure, expression, signaling, and functions of the different types of bombesin receptors, see Jensen et al. (2008b).

The GRPR, cloned from murine Swiss 3T3 cells in 1990 (Spindel et al., 1990; Battey et al., 1991), is a 384-amino acid protein in humans, mice, and rats. The chromosomal location for the GRPR gene (named *GRPR* in humans and *Grpr* in mice and rats) is at chromosome Xp22.2-p22.13 (human), X F4 (mouse), and Xq21 (rat; Jensen et al., 2008a; **Table 1**).

## GRPR SIGNALING

Experiments using different types of normal and tumor cells from humans and rodents have provided consistent evidence that the GRPR is directly coupled to the $G_q$ type of G protein, and GRPR activation leads to an increase in cellular $[Ca^{2+}]$ and stimulation of the phospholipase C (PLC)/protein kinase C (PKC) and extracellular signal-regulated protein kinase (ERK)/mitogen-activated protein kinase (MAPK) pathways (Hellmich et al., 1999; Chen and Kroog, 2004; Stangelberger et al., 2005). GRPR signaling also interacts with a range of other enzymes (e.g., phospholipases $A_2$ and D, tyrosine kinases, phosphatidylinositol 3-kinase – PI3K, and ciclooxigenase-2), growth factor receptor systems (including epidermal growth factor receptor, EGFR, and TrkB), and immediate-early genes (c-fos and c-jun; Szepeshazi et al., 1997; Chatzistamou et al., 2000; Thomas et al., 2005; Hohla et al., 2007; Ishola et al., 2007; Liu et al., 2007; Flores et al., 2008; de Farias et al., 2010; Czepielewski et al., 2012; Petronilho et al., 2012). Data on signaling mechanisms mediating GRPR actions specifically in the CNS will be discussed below.

**Table 1 | Molecular structure of the gastrin-releasing peptide receptor (GRPR).**

| GRPR (BB2) | | | | |
|---|---|---|---|---|
| Species | TM | AA | Chromosomal location | Gene name |
| Human | 7 | 384 | Xp22.2-p22.13 | *GRPR* |
| Rat | 7 | 384 | Xq21 | *Grpr* |
| Mouse | 7 | 384 | X F4 | *Grpr* |

Aminoacid sequence (*Homo sapiens*)

| | | | | |
|---|---|---|---|---|
| (1–60) | MALNDCFLLN | LEVDHFMHCN | ISSHSADLPV | NDDWSHPGIL |
| | YVIPAVYGVI | ILIGLIGNIT | | |
| (61–120) | LIKIFCTVKS | MRNVPNLFIS | SLALGDLLLL | ITCAPVDASR |
| | YLADRWLFGR | IGCKLIPFIQ | | |
| (121–180) | LTSVGVSVFT | LTALSADRYK | AIVRPMDIQA | SHALMKICLK |
| | AAFIWIISML | LAIPEAVFSD | | |
| (181–240) | LHPFHEESTN | QTFISCAPYP | HSNELHPKIH | SMASFLVFYV |
| | IPLSIISVYY | YFIAKNLIQS | | |
| (241–300) | AYNLPVEGNI | HVKKQIESRK | RLAKTVLVFV | GLFAFCWLPN |
| | HVIYLYRSYH | YSEVDTSMLH | | |
| (301–360) | FVTSICARLL | AFTNSCVNPF | ALYLLSKSFR | KQFNTQLLCC |
| | QPGLIIRSHS | TGRSTTCMTS | | |
| (361–384) | LKSTNPSVAT | FSLINGNICH | ERYV | |

*Structural data are from Spindel et al. (1990), Battey et al. (1991), Wada et al. (1991), and Jensen et al. (2008a). Modified from Roesler et al. (2012), with permission).*

## GRPR EXPRESSION IN THE CNS

Early studies investigating the presence of bombesin receptors binding sites in the mammalian CNS showed that bombesin could bind with high affinity to rat brain membranes (Moody et al., 1978). Subsequently, autoradiographic studies indicated that areas containing high densities of GRPRs include the olfactory bulb, nucleus accumbens, caudate putamen, central amygdala, dorsal hippocampus, as well as the paraventricular, central medial, and paracentral thalamic nuclei (Wolf et al., 1983; Wolf and Moody, 1985; Zarbin et al., 1985). A detailed immunohistochemical characterization of GRPR expression in the mouse brain showed high GRPR immunoreactivity in the basolateral and central nuclei of the amygdala (BLA and CeA, respectively), hippocampus, hypothalamus, brain stem, nucleus tractus solitarius (NTS), and several cortical areas. Importantly, GRPR expression was restricted to neuronal cell bodies and dendrites, and was not present in axons or glial cells (Kamichi et al., 2005). Thus, the pattern of GRPR location in the brain suggests that it is specifically involved in regulating synaptic transmission. In some rat brain areas, GRPR expression shows marked changes during development – specifically between postnatal (PN) days 1 and 16 – with its expression increasing in the dentate gyrus and decreasing in the caudate putamen and lateral cerebellar nucleus (Wada et al., 1992).

Regarding receptor ligands, the use of radioimmunoassay techniques allowed demonstrating the presence of endogenous BLPs in the rat brain, with high concentrations in brain areas including the NTS, amygdala, and hypothalamus (Moody and Pert, 1979; Moody et al., 1981). GRP mRNA has the highest density in forebrain areas and hypothalamus (Wada et al., 1990; Battey and Wada, 1991; for reviews, see Moody and Merali, 2004; Roesler et al., 2006a; Jensen et al., 2008b).

In the rodent spinal cord, GRPR expression is restricted to lamina I of the dorsal spinal cord, and GRP is expressed in a subset of dorsal root ganglion neurons including lumbar spinothalamic neurons (Sun and Chen, 2007; Fleming et al., 2012; Kozyrev et al., 2012). Importantly, the GRP system in the spinal cord is sexually dimorphic. In male rats, neurons in the L3 and L4 levels of the lumbar spinal cord project to the lower lumbar spinal cord (L5–L6 level) and release GRP onto somatic and autonomic centers containing GRPRs, whereas this system is vestigial in females (Sakamoto et al., 2008; Sakamoto, 2011). This has important implications for the control of male sexual reflexes by GRPR signaling (see below).

## GRPR REGULATION OF CNS FUNCTION

Evidence that GRPRs in the brain and spinal cord regulate several physiological functions has come mostly from *in vivo* studies using pharmacological or genetic manipulation of the GRPR in rats or mice. Below, we summarize relevant findings of selected studies focusing on GRPR regulation of memory, stress and anxiety responses, feeding, itching, and sexual behavior.

## SYNAPTIC PLASTICITY AND MEMORY

In the late 1980s, Flood and Morley (1988) demonstrated that systemic or i.c.v. injections of GRP or bombesin after learning modulated memory retention for a T-maze footshock avoidance task in mice. When i.c.v. infusions were used, both peptides facilitated memory consolidation, whereas systemic injections produced memory enhancement or impairment depending on the drug dose and training conditions. Consistently with these findings, bombesin given after training through systemic injections (Rashidy-Pour and Razvani, 1998) or infusions directly into the NTS (Williams and McGaugh, 1994) enhanced memory retention in rats.

Memory modulation by GRPRs seems to be particularly important for memories involving emotional arousal and fear. Thus, pretraining injections of the GRPR antagonist [Leu13-(psi-CH(2)NH)-Leu14]BN impaired memory for inhibitory avoidance conditioning in mice (Santo-Yamada et al., 2003), and injection of another selective GRPR antagonist, RC-3095, in rats impaired memory for inhibitory avoidance but not for a task with less emotional content, novel object recognition (Roesler et al., 2004b). Similar impairing effects of RC-3095 on inhibitory avoidance memory were obtained with systemic posttraining injections (Roesler et al., 2004c), pre- or posttraining intrahippocampal microinfusions (Roesler et al., 2003; Venturella et al., 2005; Dantas et al., 2006; Preissler et al., 2007), or posttraining infusions into the BLA (Roesler et al., 2004c). The effects of the GRPR antagonist followed a typical inverted U-shaped dose–response pattern, in which intermediate doses resulted in memory impairment, whereas higher doses had no effect or produced memory enhancement (Roesler et al., 2003, 2004b; Dantas et al., 2006). Conversely, intrahippocampal infusion of bombesin resulted in enhancement of inhibitory avoidance memory at intermediate doses and impairment at higher doses (Roesler et al., 2006b). In addition to influencing memory formation, pharmacological manipulation GRPRs in specific brain areas has been shown to regulate fear memory expression, extinction, and reconsolidation-like processes (Luft et al., 2006, 2008; Mountney et al., 2006, 2008; Merali et al., 2011). For example, infusion of the GRPR antagonist RC-3095 into the rat dorsal hippocampus after memory reactivation blocks the extinction and reconsolidation of fear memory (Luft et al., 2006, 2008; for a review, see Roesler et al., 2012).

The role of GRPRs in regulating fear memory and synaptic plasticity has also been revealed by genetic studies using GRPR knockout mice. Contextual and cued fear conditioning were enhanced by the genetic deletion of GRPR, whereas spatial in the Morris water maze was unaffected. The enhancement of fear memory in GRPR knockout mice was accompanied by enhanced synaptic plasticity measured by long-term potentiation (LTP) in the amygdala. In wild-type mice, GRPR was preferentially expressed in amygdalar inhibitory interneurons releasing gamma-aminobutyric acid (GABA), and GRP might be released as a co-transmitter from glutamatergic neurons to activate preferentially GRPRs located on GABAergic interneurons to stimulate inhibitory transmission within the amygdala and function as an inhibitory constraint for the formation of fear-motivated memories (Shumyatsky et al., 2002).

Additional studies recently found enhanced retention and impaired extinction of cued fear conditioning, associated with an increase in c-fos activity in the BLA and reduced c-fos in the prefrontal cortex, in GRPR knockout mice. However, these mice showed unaltered contextual fear conditioning, multiple-trial cued fear conditioning, and conditioned taste aversion (Chaperon et al., 2012; Martel et al., 2012). Together, these findings indicate that the GRPR acts as a negative regulator of synaptic plasticity in the BLA and specific types of fear conditioning. However, the use of first generation knockout mouse models might confound the interpretation of the results, given that they do not allow the investigation of separate phases of memory (encoding, consolidation, and expression), and knockout mice might have up-regulation of compensatory pathways and non-specific alterations in CNS development in response to gene ablation (reviewed in Roesler et al., 2012).

We have shown that a number of signal transduction mechanisms downstream of receptor activation are involved in mediating memory regulation by the GRPR. In the CA1 area of the dorsal hippocampus, memory enhancement induced by bombesin was prevented by inhibitors of PKC, MAPK, PKA, and PI3K (Roesler et al., 2006b, 2009, 2012), and potentiated by coinfusion of stimulators of the dopamine D1/D5 receptor (D1R)/cAMP/PKA pathway, namely the D1R agonist SKF 38393, the adenylyl cyclase activator forskolin, and the cAMP analog 8-Br-cAMP (Roesler et al., 2006b). These findings indicate that the PKC, MAPK, PI3K, and PKA pathways are critical in mediating memory modulation by hippocampal GRPRs, and that GRPR activation can interact with cAMP/PKA signaling in enhancing hippocampal memory formation (**Figure 1**). GRPRs in the rat brain also show functional interactions with other growth factor systems including basic fibroblast growth factor (bFGF/FGF-2), nerve growth factor (NGF), and brain-derived neurotrophic factor (BDNF; Kauer-Sant'Anna et al., 2007; Preissler et al., 2007).

## EMOTIONAL BEHAVIOR

Gastrin-releasing peptide and GRPR are highly expressed in brain regions, such as the amygdala, activated by stressful stimuli, and, as discussed above, GRPR signaling is likely to be a major regulator of memory associated with fear and emotional arousal. Merali and colleagues have shown that chronic stressor exposure leads to an elevation of GRP levels in the anterior pituitary in rats, and GRP release in the rat amygdala is increased in response to exposure to a shock. GRP may stimulate the release of adrenocorticotropic hormone (ACTH), playing a role in mediating the corticotropin-releasing hormone (CRH) stress response, and increasing the activity of the hypothalamic–pituitary–adrenal (HPA) axis. In addition, bombesin administration induces endocrine, autonomic, and behavioral effects associated with stress, and bombesin receptor antagonists attenuate the behavioral and neurochemical effects of stressors (Merali et al., 2002, 2009; Moody and Merali, 2004; Mountney et al., 2011). Moreover, we have shown that systemic administration of a GRPR antagonist can induce an anxiogenic-like effect in the elevated plus maze test in rats

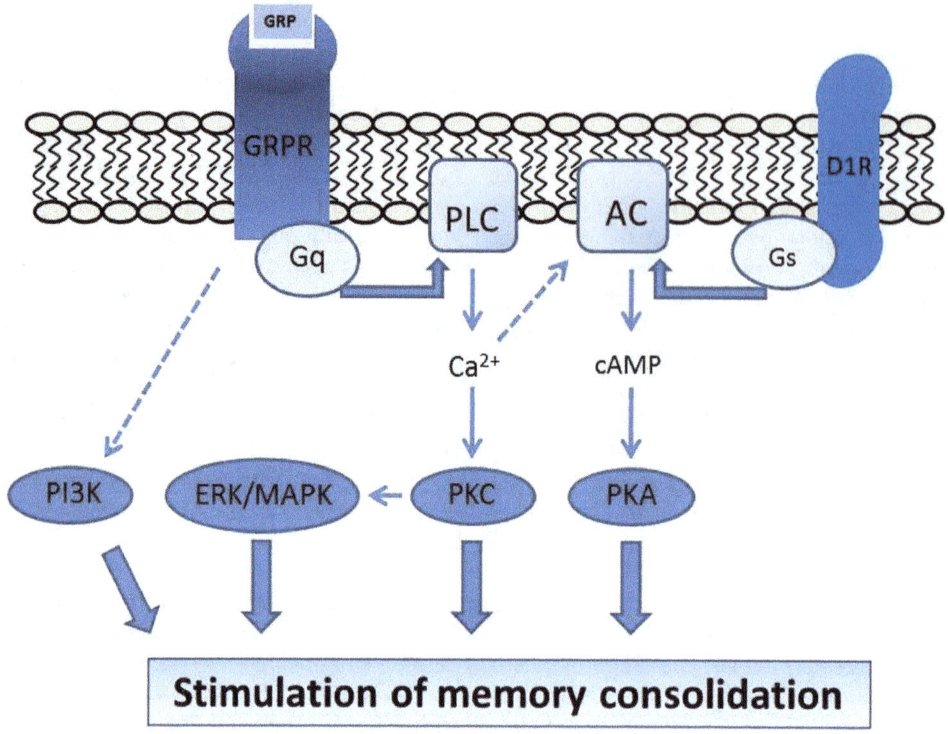


**FIGURE 1 | Proposed molecular mechanisms mediating GRPR regulation of brain function.** The stimulation of hippocampal memory consolidation by GRPR activation depends on PKC, MAPK, PKA, and PI3K, and is potentiated by activation of the D1R/cAMP/PKA pathway (Roesler et al., 2006a, 2009, 2012). GRPR activation at the postsynaptic membrane is coupled to $G_q$ protein activity and increases in $[Ca^{2+}]$, leading to stimulation of the PLC/PKC and ERK/MAPK pathways. D1R is coupled to the $G_S$ protein and adenylyl cyclase (AC) activation. The D1R-induced cAMP signal might be potentiated by $[Ca^{2+}]$-induced stimulation of $[Ca^{2+}]$-responsive types of AC (Wong et al., 1999; Chan and Wong, 2005; Roesler et al., 2006b, 2012), providing a possible mechanism for the requirement of cAMP/PKA signaling for GRPR influences on memory. Modified from Roesler et al. (2006b, 2012), with permission.

(Martins et al., 2005). Together, these data suggest that brain GRPRs might regulate emotional behavioral and responses to stress.

### FEEDING BEHAVIOR

It has been known for over 30 years that systemic or i.c.v. administration of bombesin or GRP in rats reduces the intake of liquid and solid food in rats (Gibbs et al., 1981). Similar effects on meal size are observed after systemic bombesin injections in mice and intravenous (i.v.) injections in baboons and humans (Gibbs, 1985). In addition, brief vena caval infusions of GRP and NMB in rats, given alone or together at the onset of the first nocturnal meal, significantly reduced meal size and duration (Rushing et al., 1996), and bombesin or GRP given systemically extended the duration of the intermeal interval (Thaw et al., 1998). The suppression of glucose intake induced by systemic administration of GRP or bombesin was blocked by infusion of a GRPR antagonist into the fourth ventricle in rats (Ladenheim et al., 1996), and was absent in GRPR knockout mice (Hampton et al., 1998; Ladenheim et al., 2002), indicating that central GRPRs are critical in mediating the effects of peripheral bombesin and GRP on feeding. In addition, GRPR knockout mice ate significantly more at each meal than wild-type controls (although total 24 h food consumption was equivalent), and showed elevated body weight compared with wild-type littermates beginning at 45 weeks of age (Ladenheim et al., 2002). The finding that systemic GRP potently reduced independent intake of both sucrose and milk from a bottle but did not affect intraoral intake of either solution indicated that the GRPR regulates the appetitive-related aspects of the feeding process (Rushing and Houpt, 1999). The amygdala is likely a key brain area involved in mediating the regulatory action of GRPRs on feeding: bilateral infusion of GRP into the central amygdala produced a transient inhibition of food intake, an effect that was prevented by the GRPR antagonist [Leu(13)-psi(CH(2)NH)-Leu(14)]BN (Fekete et al., 2002).

These findings provide strong support for a role of GRP/GRPR signaling in regulating feeding. It has been proposed that BLPs may also be released from the gastrointestinal tract in response to food ingestion, acting to bridge the gut and brain to inhibit further food intake. Conversely, the suppression of release of BLPs in the brain may trigger the initiation of a feeding episode (reviewed in Merali et al., 1999).

### SEXUAL BEHAVIOR

One of the most exciting recent developments in GRPR research was the identification by Sakamoto et al. (2008) of a sexually dimorphic GRPR system in the spinal cord that is crucial in regulating male sexual function. In male rats, but not in females or males with a dysfunctional androgen receptor gene, GRP-containing neurons in the upper lumbar spinal cord innervate lower lumbar regions controlling erection and ejaculation. Pharmacological stimulation of spinal GRP receptors restores penile reflexes and ejaculation after castration, whereas intrathecal administration of the GRPR antagonist RC-3095 inhibits penile reflexes and ejaculations. The inhibitory effect of castration on GRP expression in this spinal center suggests that androgen signaling plays a major role in regulating GRP expression in the male spinal cord (Sakamoto et al., 2009b). Moreover, exposure to traumatic stress decreases the local GRP content and reduces penile reflexes in male rats (Sakamoto et al., 2009a; Sakamoto, 2010). Thus, GRP/GRPR signaling has emerged as a new target for the understanding of psychogenic erectile dysfunction and the development of potential therapeutic approaches to masculine reproductive dysfunction (Sakamoto et al., 2008, 2009a,b; Sakamoto and Kawata, 2009; Sakamoto, 2010, 2011).

### ITCHING

Another function in which GRPRs in the spinal cord have been shown to play a major role is itching. GRPR knockout mice show normal thermal, mechanical, inflammatory, and pain responses, but reduced responses to pruritogenic stimuli, and GRP-induced pruritus in wild-type mice is blocked by intrathecal administration of a GRPR antagonist (Sun and Chen, 2007). The selective ablation of GRPR-expressing lamina I neurons in the mouse spinal cord of mice results in scratching deficits in response to itching stimuli, but does not affect pain behaviors (Sun et al., 2009). These findings allowed the identification of GRPR as a central molecular mediator of the itch sensation in the spinal cord (Sun and Chen, 2007; Sun et al., 2009).

A recent seminal study showed that the μ-opioid receptor (MOR) isoform MOR1D heterodimerizes with GRPR in the spinal cord to relay itch information. Blocking the association between MOR1D and GRPR attenuates morphine-induced scratching. Morphine triggers internalization of both GRPR and MOR1D, whereas GRP specifically triggers both GRPR internalization and morphine-independent scratching. These data suggest that opioid-induced itch is independent of opioid analgesia and occurs via cross-activation of GRPR signaling by MOR1D heterodimerization (Liu et al., 2011).

## POSSIBLE ROLE OF ALTERATIONS IN GRPR EXPRESSION AND SIGNALING IN THE PATHOGENESIS OF BRAIN DISORDERS

Since GRPRs are highly expressed in neurons in brain areas including the hippocampus and BLA, and regulate crucial aspects of behavior that can be altered in patients with CNS disorders, it is possible that deregulated GRPR signaling contribute to the pathogenesis of neurological and psychiatric diseases. Although a causative role of GRPR dysfunction in CNS disorders has not been directly established, some alterations in the levels of BLPs peptides or GRPR density or function have been observed in patients with psychiatric, neurodegenerative, and neurodevelopmental disorders. In addition, the use of preclinical models has provided further evidence indicating a role for the GRPR in some CNS pathologies. Based on these findings, we have put forward that the GRPR may be a novel molecular target for the development of therapeutic strategies for patients with neurological and psychiatric disorders (Roesler et al., 2004a, 2006a). **Table 2** summarizes the findings from studies examining possible alterations in GRP and GRPR content or signaling found in patients with brain disorders.

### NEURODEGENERATIVE DISORDERS

The concentration of BLPs was found to be significantly reduced in the caudate nucleus and globus pallidus of patients with Parkinson's disease (PD; Bissette et al., 1985). However, Stoddard et al. (1991) found no alterations in bombesin-like immunoreactivity in the adrenal medullary tissue of patients with PD, although the concentration of several other neuropeptides was reduced. A reduction in bombesin receptor density and altered bombesin-induced calcium signaling have been reported in fibroblasts from patients with Alzheimer's disease (AD; Ito et al., 1994; Gibson et al., 1997).

**Table 2 | Findings from selected studies examining possible alterations in the GRPR system in patients with CNS disorders. Modified from Roesler et al. (2006a), with permission.**

| CNS disorder | Main findings | Reference |
|---|---|---|
| Parkinson's disease | Reduced levels of BLPs peptides in caudate nucleus and globus pallidus | Bissette et al. (1985) |
| Parkinson's disease | Normal bombesin-like immunoreactivity in adrenal medullary tissue | Stoddard et al. (1991) |
| Alzheimer's disease | Reduced bombesin receptor density and enhanced bombesin-induced calcium release in fibroblasts | Ito et al. (1994) |
| Alzheimer's disease | Reduced bombesin-induced calcium mobilization in fibrobasts | Gibson et al. (1997) |
| Autism | X;8 translocation in the GRPR gene | Ishikawa-Brush et al. (1997) |
| Autism | No association with two polymorphic sites in the second exon of the GRPR gene | Marui et al. (2004) |
| Autism | C6S and L181F mutations in the GRPR gene | Seidita et al. (2008) |
| Schizophrenia | Reduced radioimmunoassay-detectable bombesin in the CSF | Gerner et al. (1985) |
| Schizophrenia | Reduced urinary levels of BLPs | Olincy et al. (1999) |
| Anxiety disorders | No association between GRP and GRPR genes and panic disorders | Hodges et al. (2009) |
| Eating disorders | Reduced GRP levels in the CSF of women who were recovered from bulimia nervosa | Frank et al. (2001) |
| Brain tumors | GRPR overexpression in glioma | Flores et al. (2010) |

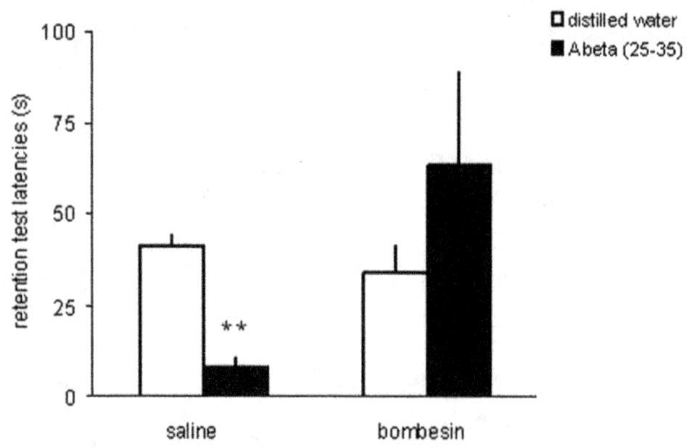


**FIGURE 2 | The GRPR agonist bombesin prevents memory impairment induced by beta-amyloid peptide in the rat hippocampus.** Data are mean ± SEM retention test step-down latencies (s), in an inhibitory avoidance conditioning, of rats given a bilateral infusion of the GRPR agonist bombesin (BB; 0.002 μg) or saline (SAL; control group) 10 min before being trained in IA, and beta-amyloid peptide (Abeta; 25–35) or distilled water (DW; controls) immediately after IA training. The number of animals was 8–14 per group. $^{**}P < 0.01$ compared to the control group treated with SAL and DW. Reproduced from Roesler et al. (2006b), with permission.

For example, in fibroblasts from patients with familial AD presenting the Swedish APP670/671 mutation, elevations in calcium induced by bombesin were reduced by 40% (Gibson et al., 1997).

Using the memory impairment produced by a microinfusion of a low dose of beta-amyloid peptide (25–35; Abeta) into the rat CA1 area of the dorsal hippocampus as a model of memory dysfunction associated with AD, we showed that an intrahippocampal infusion of bombesin completely prevented the Abeta-induced impairment in inhibitory avoidance memory (Roesler et al., 2006b; **Figure 2**). This finding provided preliminary preclinical evidence suggesting that pharmacological stimulation of the GRPR might rescue memory deficits associated with AD.

## NEURODEVELOPMENTAL DISORDERS

The first evidence suggesting that the GRPR might be a candidate gene in autism spectrum disorders (ASD) was the finding of a translocation breakpoint on the X chromosome in the first intron of the *GRPR* gene in a patient with autism accompanied by mental retardation and epilepsy (Ishikawa-Brush et al., 1997). Although a subsequent study investigating two polymorphic sites in the second exon of the *GRPR* gene in patients did not support the *GRPR* as a candidate locus for autism (Marui et al., 2004), more recently a possible role of C6S and L181F mutations of the *GRPR* gene in GRPR function and ASD was found in two patients (Seidita et al., 2008).

In order to examine the role of GRPR in CNS development and its possible involvement in ASD, we submitted rat pups to pharmacological GRPR blockade by systemic administration of RC-3095 from PN days 1–10, and examined long-lasting behavioral and molecular alterations produced by this treatment. Rats given neonatal RC-3095 showed pronounced deficits in social interaction (a hallmark of rodent models of ASD) when tested at PN days 30–35 (Presti-Torres et al., 2007; **Figure 3**) or PN day 60 (Presti-Torres et al., 2012). In addition, RC-3095-treated rats showed impaired 24-h retention of memory for inhibitory avoidance and novel object recognition, whereas body weight during development, open field behavior, and short-term memory were not affected (Presti-Torres et al., 2007, 2012). Neonatal GRPR blockade also reduced maternal odor preference, a behavioral measure of attachment behavior (Garcia et al., 2010). The impairment in social behavior induced by GRPR blockade was rescued by treatment with the atypical antipsychotic clozapine (Presti-Torres et al., 2012). Together, these findings suggest that GRPR blockade during CNS development can lead to specific behavioral alterations that are consistent with ASD, and support the possibility that abnormal GRPR expression or function during development might play a role in disease pathogenesis. Also, we have proposed that neonatal GRPR blockade in rats may serve as a novel animal model of ASD (Presti-Torres et al., 2007, 2012).

## OTHER NEUROPSYCHIATRIC DISORDERS

The findings from rodent studies discussed above, indicating that normal GRPR function during development might be important for behaviors related to social interaction, attachment, and cognition, and that clozapine rescues social behavior deficits produced by GRPR blockade, are also consistent with the possibility that GRPR signaling is altered in schizophrenia. In addition, we found that GRPR blockade by systemic injections of RC-3095 prevent apomorphine-induced stereotypy in mice and amphetamine-induced hyperlocomotion in rats, which are models of schizophrenic psychosis and mania (Meller et al., 2004; Kauer-Sant'Anna et al., 2007). In patients with schizophrenia, a reduction in the levels of radioimmunoassay-detectable bombesin in the cerebrospinal fluid (CSF; Gerner et al., 1985), and reduced urinary levels of BLPs (Olincy et al., 1999) have been found. Further studies using samples from patients and animal models are required to examine whether GRPR signaling is involved in schizophrenia.

As reviewed above, data from animal studies also consistently show that GRPRs in brain areas including the amygdala regulate memory related to fear and anxiety responses, raising the possibility that GRPR signaling plays a role in anxiety disorders (Moody and Merali, 2004; Roesler et al., 2012). For example, pharmacological manipulation of the GRPR in the hippocampus can affect extinction and reconsolidation of fear memory, which are preclinical models used in the investigation and screening of potential therapeutic strategies for post-traumatic stress disorder (PTSD) and other fear-related disorders (Luft et al., 2006, 2008). In postmortem analyses of brains from suicides compared to control subjects, Merali et al. (2006) reported discrete alterations in the levels of GRP and NMB. More recently, however, the possibility that GRP and GRPR are candidate genes in panic disorders was not confirmed in an association and linkage analysis (Hodges et al., 2009).

Anxiety disorders may show comorbidity with eating disorders, anorexia and bulimia nervosa. Given the important role of GRPR in regulating feeding behavior (see above), it is possible that it contributes to eating disorders. One study found significantly reduced GRP levels in the CSF of women who were recovered from bulimia nervosa, compared to women recovered from anorexia or healthy control women. The authors suggested that persistent alterations in GRP levels after recovery indicate that this alteration might be

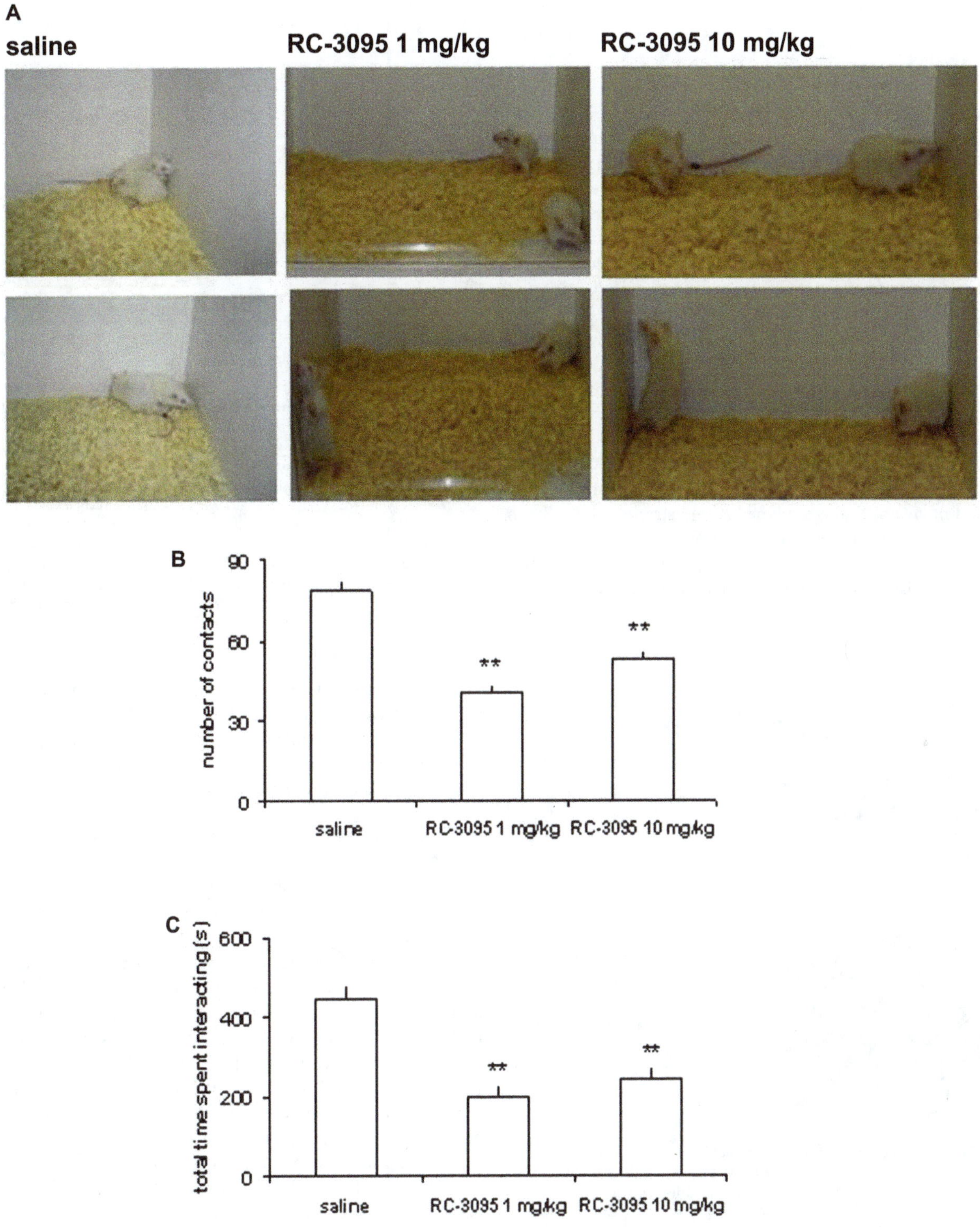


**FIGURE 3 | GRPR blockade during CNS development in rats results in long-lasting behavioral alterations associated with experimental models of autistic spectrum disorders (ASDs).** Rats were given intraperitoneal injections of saline (SAL; control group) or the GRPR antagonist RC-3095 (1 or 10 mg/kg) twice daily from postnatal days (PN) 1 to 10. A social behavior test was carried out at PN 30. **(A)** Representative photographs of rats given SAL or RC-3095 (1 or 10 mg/kg) during the social interaction test. **(B)** Mean ± SEM number of social contacts. **(C)** Mean ± SEM time spent engaged in social interaction (in seconds). The number of animals was 6–7 per group; $^{**}P < 0.01$ compared to the control group. Reproduced from Presti-Torres et al. (2007), with permission.

trait-related and contribute to episodic hyperphagia in patients with bulimia nervosa (Frank et al., 2001).

### BRAIN TUMORS

Gastrin-releasing peptide receptor overexpression has been demonstrated in many types of cancer (Cornelio et al., 2007), and we have recently shown widespread expression and a high content of GRPR in human glioma, the most common and lethal type of neurological cancer (Flores et al., 2010; **Figure 4**). GRPR activation by GRP or bombesin stimulates the growth of glioma cell lines (Moody et al., 1989; Pinski et al., 1994; Sharif et al., 1997; de Farias et al., 2008; Flores et al., 2008). We have recently shown that the stimulatory effect of GRPR activation on proliferation of glioma cells depends on PI3K signaling (Flores et al., 2008) and is potentiated by co-activation of the cAMP/PKA pathway (de Farias et al., 2008; reviewed in Roesler et al., 2010).

Gastrin-releasing peptide receptor antagonists inhibit the growth of human U-87MG and U-373MG gliomas xenografted into nude mice (Pinski et al., 1994; Kiaris et al., 1999). In addition, GRPR antagonism by RC-3095, alone or combined with temozolomide, significantly reduced the growth of C6 gliomas both *in vitro* and *in vivo*, with the combined administration of TMZ and RC-3095 being the most effective treatment (**Figure 5**; de Oliveira et al., 2009). These findings strongly suggest that targeting GRPR may be a promising strategy for the development of novel therapies against glioma. The GRPR might also regulate the growth of neuroblastoma (Kim et al., 2002; Qiao et al., 2008; Abujamra et al., 2009), although, in contrast, we could not find a role for GRPR in regulating the *in vitro* growth of medulloblastoma, the most common brain cancer of childhood (Schmidt et al., 2009).

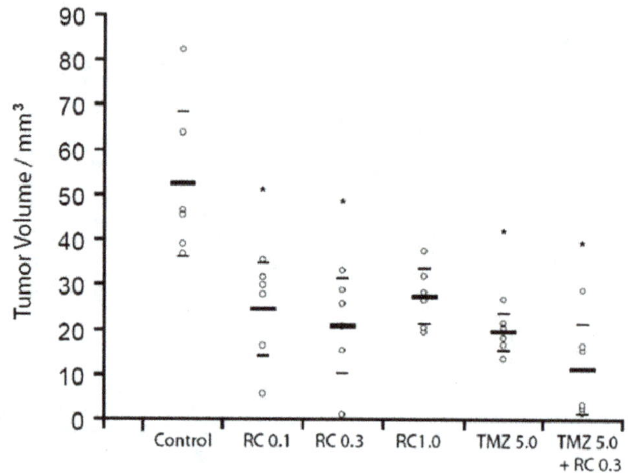


**FIGURE 5 | A GRPR antagonist inhibits the growth of experimental brain tumors.** Rats implanted with C6 experimental gliomas in the striatum were treated for seven consecutive days with intraperitoneal injections of the GRPR antagonist RC-3095 alone (0.1, 0.3, and 1.0 mg/kg twice a day), temozolomide (TMZ) alone (5 mg/kg once a day), or RC-3095 combined with TMZ. Control animals were injected with vehicle. Pharmacological treatments were initiated 10 days after tumor implantation. The number of animals was 6 rats per group. Tumor size was measured 20 days after tumor implantation. Data are shown as median (interquartile ranges) tumor volume ($mm^3$). Values for individual animals are shown by dots; $*P < 0.002$ compared to control animals. Reproduced from de Oliveira et al. (2009), with permission.

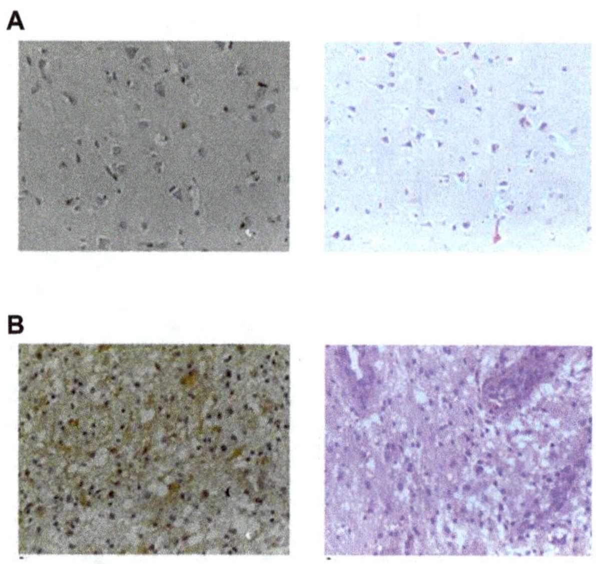


**FIGURE 4 | GRPR content in human normal brain tissue and brain tumors.** Representative sections of **(A)** normal brain and **(B)** astrocytoma grade IV from an immunohistochemical study of GRPR content from samples of patients with gliomas and normal brain samples. GRPR staining is shown in the right column (brown, ×400) and hematoxylin–eosin (HE) in the left column (×400). GRPR staining in the normal brain tissue is restricted to neuronal bodies and dendrites, whereas its presence in astrocytoma samples is widespread. Sections were incubated with anti-GRPR antibody, sequentially treated with biotinylated anti-rabbit IgG and streptavidin-biotin peroxidase solution, and then developed with diaminobenzidine as chromogen. Modified from Flores et al. (2010), with permission.

## GRPR LIGANDS AS CANDIDATE THERAPEUTIC DRUGS IN BRAIN DISORDERS

The evidence reviewed above indicates that the GRPR might be considered a novel molecular target in different types of CNS disorders, and raise the possibility that GRPR agonists might ameliorate cognitive and social deficits associated with neurological diseases, while antagonists may, for example, reduce anxiety and inhibit the growth of some types of brain cancer. Studies examining the effects of GRP administration on satiety and eating behavior in humans (Gutzwiller et al., 1994), as well as a phase I trial of the GRPR antagonist RC-3095 in patients with solid tumors (Schwartsmann et al., 2006) have suggested that GRP and peptidergic GRPR antagonists can be safely administered intravenously in human subjects. Thus, the potential therapeutic effect of GRPR ligands in preclinical models as well as in patients with CNS disorders warrants further investigation.

## ACKNOWLEDGMENTS

This work was supported by the National Council for Scientific and Technological Development (CNPq; grant number 303703/2009-1 to Rafael Roesler); the National Institute for Translational Medicine (INCT-TM); and the South American Office for Anticancer Drug Development.

## REFERENCES


Abujamra, A. L., Almeida, V. R., Brunetto, A. L., Schwartsmann, G., and Roesler, R. (2009). A gastrin-releasing peptide receptor antagonist stimulates Neuro2a neuroblastoma cell growth: prevention by a histone deacetylase inhibitor. *Cell Biol. Int.* 33, 899–903.

Battey, J., and Wada, E. (1991). Two distinct receptor subtypes for mammalian bombesin-like peptides. *Trends Neurosci.* 14, 524–528.

Battey, J. F., Way, J. M., Corjay, M. H., Shapira, H., Kusano, K., Harkins, R., et al. (1991). Molecular cloning of the bombesin/gastrin-releasing peptide receptor from Swiss 3T3 cells. *Proc. Natl. Acad. Sci. U.S.A.* 88, 395–399.

Bissette, G., Nemeroff, C. B., Decker, M. W., Kizer, J. S., Agid, Y., and Javoy-Agid, F. (1985). Alterations in regional brain concentrations of neurotensin and bombesin in Parkinson's disease. *Ann. Neurol.* 17, 324–328.

Brown, M., Rivier, J., and Vale, W. (1977a). Bombesin: potent effects on thermoregulation in the rat. *Science* 196, 998–1000.

Brown, M. R., Rivier, J., and Vale, W. W. (1977b). Bombesin affects the central nervous system to produce hyperglycemia in rats. *Life Sci.* 21, 1729–1734.

Chaperon, F., Fendt, M., Kelly, P. H., Lingenhoehl, K., Mosbacher, J., Olpe, H. R., et al. (2012). Gastrin-releasing peptide signaling plays a limited and subtle role in amygdala physiology and aversive memory. *PLoS ONE* 7:e34963. doi: 10.1371/journal.pone.0034963

Chan, A. S., and Wong, Y. H. (2005). Gq-mediated activation of c-Jun N-terminal kinase by the gastrin-releasing peptide-preferring bombesin receptor is inhibited upon costimulation of the Gs-coupled dopamine D1 receptor in COS-7 cells. *Mol. Pharmacol.* 68, 1354–1364.

Chatzistamou, I., Schally, A. V., Sun, B., Armatis, P., and Szepeshazi, K. (2000). Inhibition of growth of OV-1063 human epithelial ovarian cancers and c- jun and c- fos oncogene expression by bombesin antagonists. *Br. J. Cancer* 83, 906–913.

Chen, P. W., and Kroog, G. S. (2004). Alterations in receptor expression or agonist concentration change the pathways gastrin-releasing peptide receptor uses to regulate extracellular signal-regulated kinase. *Mol. Pharmacol.* 66, 1625–1634.

Cornelio, D., Roesler, R., and Schwartsmann, G. (2007). Gastrin-releasing peptide receptor as a molecular target in experimental anticancer therapy. *Ann. Oncol.* 18, 1457–1466.

Czepielewski, R. S., Porto, B. N., Rizzo, L. B., Roesler, R., Abujamra, A. L., Pinto, L. G., et al. (2012). Gastrin-releasing peptide receptor (GRPR) mediates chemotaxis in neutrophils. *Proc. Natl. Acad. Sci. U.S.A.* 109, 547–552.

Dantas, A. S., Luft, T., Henriques, J. A., Schwartsmann, G., and Roesler, R. (2006). Opposite effects of low and high doses of the gastrin-releasing peptide receptor antagonist RC-3095 on memory consolidation in the hippocampus: possible involvement of the GABAergic system. *Peptides* 27, 2307–2312.

de Farias, C. B., Lima, R. C., Lima, L. O., Flores, D. G., Meurer, L., Brunetto, A. L., et al. (2008). Stimulation of proliferation of U138-MG glioblastoma cells by gastrin-releasing peptide in combination with agents that enhance cAMP signaling. *Oncology* 75, 27–31.

de Farias, C. B., Rosemberg, D. B., Heinen, T. E., Koehler-Santos, P., Abujamra, A. L., Kapczinski, F., et al. (2010). BDNF/TrkB content and interaction with gastrin-releasing peptide receptor blockade in colorectal cancer. *Oncology* 79, 430–439.

de Oliveira, M. S., Cechim, G., Braganhol, E., Santos, D. G., Meurer, L., de Castro, C.G. Jr., et al. (2009). Anti-proliferative effect of the gastrin-release peptide receptor antagonist RC-3095 plus temozolomide in experimental glioblastoma models. *J. Neurooncol.* 93, 191–201.

Del Rio, M., and De la Fuente, M. (1994). Chemoattractant capacity of bombesin, gastrin-releasing peptide and neuromedin C is mediated through PKC activation in murine peritoneal leukocytes. *Regul. Pept.* 49, 185–193.

Erspamer, V., Erpamer, G. F., and Inselvini, M. (1970). Some pharmacological actions of alytesin and bombesin. *J. Pharm. Pharmacol.* 22, 875–876.

Fekete, E., Vígh, J., Bagi, E. E., and Lénárd, L. (2002). Gastrin-releasing peptide microinjected into the amygdala inhibits feeding. *Brain Res.* 955, 55–63.

Fleming, M. S., Ramos, D., Han, S. B., Zhao, J., Son, Y. J., and Luo, W. (2012). The majority of dorsal spinal cord gastrin releasing peptide is synthesized locally whereas neuromedin B is highly expressed in pain- and itch-sensing somatosensory neurons. *Mol. Pain* 8, 52.

Flood, J. F., and Morley, J. E. (1988). Effects of bombesin and gastrin-releasing peptide on memory processing. *Brain Res.* 460, 314–322.

Flores, D. G., de Farias, C. B., Leites, J., de Oliveira, M. S., Lima, R. C., Tamajusuku, A. S., et al. (2008). Gastrin-releasing peptide receptors regulate proliferation of C6 Glioma cells through a phosphatidylinositol 3-kinase-dependent mechanism. *Curr. Neurovasc. Res.* 5, 99–105.

Flores, D. G., Meurer, L., Uberti, A. F., Macedo, B. R., Lenz, G., Brunetto, A. L., et al. (2010). Gastrin-releasing peptide receptor content in human glioma and normal brain. *Brain Res. Bull.* 82, 95–98.

Frank, G. K., Kaye, W. H., Ladenheim, E. E., and McConaha, C. (2001). Reduced gastrin releasing peptide in cerebrospinal fluid after recovery from bulimia nervosa. *Appetite* 37, 9–14.

Garcia, V. A., Dornelles, A. S., Presti-Torres, J., Alcalde, L. A., Halmenschlager, L. H., Schwartsmann, G., et al. (2010). Neonatal gastrin-releasing peptide receptor blockade reduces maternal odor preference in rats. *Behav. Brain Res.* 214, 456–459.

Gerner, R. H., van Kammen, D. P., and Ninan, P. T. (1985). Cerebrospinal fluid cholecystokinin, bombesin and somatostatin in schizophrenia and normals. *Prog. Neuropsychopharmacol. Biol. Psychiatry* 9, 73–82.

Gibbs, J. (1985). Effect of bombesin on feeding behavior. *Life Sci.* 37, 147–153.

Gibbs, J., Kulkosky, P. J., and Smith, G. P. (1981). Effects of peripheral and central bombesin on feeding behavior of rats. *Peptides* 2(Suppl. 2), 179–183.

Gibson, G. E., Vestling, M., Zhang, H., Szolosi, S., Alkon, D., Lannfelt, L., et al. (1997). Abnormalities in Alzheimer's disease fibroblasts bearing the APP670/671 mutation. *Neurobiol. Aging* 18, 573–580.

Gonzalez, N., Moody, T. W., Igarashi, H., Ito, T., and Jensen, R. T. (2008). Bombesin-related peptides and their receptors: recent advances in their role in physiology and disease states. *Curr. Opin. Endocrinol. Diabetes Obes.* 15, 58–64.

Gutzwiller, J. P., Drewe, J., Hildebrand, P., Rossi, L., Lauper, J. Z., and Beglinger, C. (1994). Effect of intravenous human gastrin-releasing peptide on food intake in humans. *Gastroenterology* 106, 1168–1173.

Hampton, L. L., Ladenheim, E. E., Akeson, M., Way, J. M., Weber, H. C., Sutliff, V. E., et al. (1998). Loss of bombesin-induced feeding suppression in gastrin-releasing peptide receptor-deficient mice. *Proc. Natl. Acad. Sci. U.S.A.* 95, 3188–3192.

Hellmich, M. R., Ives, K. L., Udupi, V., Soloff, M. S., Greeley, G.H. Jr., Christensen, B. N., et al. (1999). Multiple protein kinase pathways are involved in gastrin-releasing peptide receptor-regulated secretion. *J. Biol. Chem.* 274, 23901–23909.

Hodges, L. M., Weissman, M. M., Haghighi, F., Costa, R., Bravo, O., Evgrafov, O., et al. (2009). Association and linkage analysis of candidate genes GRP, GRPR, CRHR1, and TACR1 in panic disorder. *Am. J. Med. Genet. B Neuropsychiatr. Genet.* 150B, 65–73.

Hökfelt, T., Bartfai, T., and Bloom, F. (2003). Neuropeptides: opportunities for drug discovery. *Lancet Neurol.* 2, 463–472.

Hohla, F., Schally, A. V., Kanashiro, C. A., Buchholz, S., Baker, B., Kannadka, C., et al. (2007). Growth inhibition of non-small-cell lung carcinoma by BN/GRP antagonist is linked with suppression of K-Ras, COX-2, and pAkt. *Proc. Natl. Acad. Sci. U.S.A.* 104, 18671–18676.

Ishikawa-Brush, Y., Powell. J. F., Bolton. P., Miller. A. P., Francis, F., Willard, H. F., et al. (1997). Autism and multiple exostoses associated with an X;8 translocation occurring within the GRPR gene and 3′ to the SDC2 gene. *Hum. Mol. Genet.* 6, 1241–1250.

Ishola, T. A., Kang, J., Qiao, J., Evers, B. M., and Chung, D. H. (2007). Phosphatidylinositol 3-kinase regulation of gastrin-releasing peptide-induced cell cycle progression in neuroblastoma cells. *Biochim. Biophys. Acta* 1770, 927–932.

Ito, E., Oka, K., Etcheberrigaray, R., Nelson, T. J., McPhie, D. L., Tofel-Grehl, B., et al. (1994). Internal $Ca^{2+}$ mobilization is altered in fibroblasts from patients with Alzheimer disease. *Proc. Natl. Acad. Sci. U.S.A.* 91, 534–538.

Jensen, R. T., Battey, J. F., Benya, R. V., and Spindel, E. R. (2008a). *Bombesin Receptors. IUPHAR Database (IUPHAR-DB).* Available at: http://www.iuphar-db.org/DATABASE/FamilyMenuForward?familyId=9 [accessed on October 1, 2012].

Jensen, R. T., Battey, J. F., Spindel, E. R., and Benya, R. V. (2008b). International Union of Pharmacology. LXVIII. Mammalian bombesin receptors: nomenclature, distribution, pharmacology, signaling, and functions in normal and disease states. *Pharmacol. Rev.* 60, 1–42.

Jensen, R. T., and Gardner, J. D. (1981). Identification and characterization of receptors for secretagogues on pancreatic acinar cells. *Fed. Proc.* 40, 2486–2496.

Kamichi, S., Wada, E., Aoki, S., Sekiguchi, M., Kimura, I., and Wada, K. (2005). Immunohistochemical localization of gastrin-releasing peptide receptor in the mouse brain. *Brain Res.* 1032, 162–170.

Kauer-Sant'Anna, M., Andreazza, A. C., Valvassori, S. S., Martins, M. R., Barbosa, L. M., Schwartsmann, G., et al. (2007). A gastrin-releasing peptide receptor antagonist blocks D-amphetamine-induced hyperlocomotion and increases hippocampal NGF and BDNF levels in rats. *Peptides* 28, 1447–1452.

Kiaris, H., Schally, A. V., Sun, B., Armatis, P., and Groot, K. (1999). Inhibition of growth of human malignant glioblastoma in nude mice by antagonists of bombesin/gastrin-releasing peptide. *Oncogene* 18, 7168–7173.

Kim, S., Hu, W., Kelly, D. R., Hellmich, M. R., Evers, B. M., and Chung, D. H. (2002). Gastrin-releasing peptide is a growth factor for human neuroblastomas. *Ann. Surg.* 235, 621–629.

Kozyrev, N., Lehman, M. N., and Coolen, L. M. (2012). Activation of gastrin-releasing peptide receptors in the lumbosacral spinal cord is required for ejaculation in male rats. *J. Sex. Med.* 9, 1303–1318.

Ladenheim, E. E., Hampton, L. L., Whitney, A. C., White, W. O., Battey, J. F., and Moran, T. H. (2002). Disruptions in feeding and body weight control in gastrin-releasing peptide receptor deficient mice. *J. Endocrinol.* 174, 273–281.

Ladenheim, E. E., Jensen, R. T., Mantey, S. A., McHugh, P. R., and Moran, T. H. (1990). Receptor heterogeneity for bombesin-like peptides in the rat central nervous system. *Brain Res.* 537, 233–240.

Ladenheim, E. E., Jensen, R. T., Mantey, S. A., McHugh, P. R., and Moran, T. H. (1992). Distinct distributions of bombesin receptor subtypes in the rat central nervous system. *Brain Res.* 593, 168–178.

Ladenheim, E. E., Taylor, J. E., Coy, D. H., Moore, K. A., and Moran, T. H. (1996). Hindbrain GRP receptor blockade antagonizes feeding suppression by peripherally administered GRP. *Am. J. Physiol.* 271(Pt 2), R180–R184.

Lebacq-Verheyden, A. M., Krystal, G., Sartor, O., Way, J., and Battey, J. F. (1988). The rat prepro gastrin releasing peptide gene is transcribed from two initiation sites in the brain. *Mol. Endocrinol.* 2, 556–563.

Liu, X., Carlisle, D. L., Swick, M. C., Gaither-Davis, A., Grandis, J. R., and Siegfried, J. M. (2007). Gastrin-releasing peptide activates Akt through the epidermal growth factor receptor pathway and abrogates the effect of gefitinib. *Exp. Cell Res.* 313, 1361–1372.

Liu, X. Y., Liu, Z. C., Sun, Y. G., Ross, M., Kim, S., Tsai, F. F., et al. (2011). Unidirectional cross-activation of GRPR by MOR1D uncouples itch and analgesia induced by opioids. *Cell* 147, 447–458.

Luft, T., Amaral, O. B., Schwartsmann, G., and Roesler, R. (2008). Transient disruption of fear-related memory by post-retrieval inactivation of gastrin-releasing peptide or *N*-methyl-D-aspartate receptors in the hippocampus. *Curr. Neurovasc. Res.* 5, 21–27.

Luft, T., Flores, D. G., Vianna, M. R., Schwartsmann, G., Roesler, R., and Izquierdo, I. (2006). A role for hippocampal gastrin-releasing peptide receptors in extinction of aversive memory. *Neuroreport* 17, 935–939.

Martel, G., Hevi, C., Wong, A., Zushida, K., Uchida, S., and Shumyatsky, G. P. (2012). Murine GRPR and stathmin control in opposite directions both cued fear extinction and neural activities of the amygdala and prefrontal cortex. *PLoS ONE* 7:e30942. doi: 10.1371/journal.pone.0030942

Martins, M. R., Reinke, A., Valvassori, S. S., Machado, R. A., Quevedo, J., Schwartsmann, G., et al. (2005). Non-associative learning and anxiety in rats treated with a single systemic administration of the gastrin-releasing peptide receptor antagonist RC-3095. *Peptides* 26, 2525–2529.

Marui, T., Hashimoto, O., Nanba, E., Kato, C., Tochigi, M., Umekage, T., et al. (2004). Gastrin-releasing peptide receptor (GRPR) locus in Japanese subjects with autism. *Brain Dev.* 26, 5–7.

Meller, C. A., Henriques, J. A., Schwartsmann, G., and Roesler, R. (2004). The bombesin/gastrin releasing peptide receptor antagonist RC-3095 blocks apomorphine but not MK-801-induced stereotypy in mice. *Peptides* 25, 585–588.

Merali, Z., Hayley, S., Kent, P., McIntosh, J., Bédard, T., and Anisman, H. (2009). Impact of repeated stressor exposure on the release of corticotropin-releasing hormone, arginine-vasopressin and bombesin-like peptides at the anterior pituitary. *Behav. Brain Res.* 198, 105–112.

Merali, Z., Kent, P., and Anisman, H. (2002). Role of bombesin-related peptides in the mediation or integration of the stress response. *Cell. Mol. Life Sci.* 59, 272–287.

Merali, Z., Kent, P., Du, L., Hrdina, P., Palkovits, M., Faludi, G., et al. (2006). Corticotropin-releasing hormone, arginine vasopressin, gastrin-releasing peptide, and neuromedin B alterations in stress-relevant brain regions of suicides and control subjects. *Biol. Psychiatry* 59, 594–602.

Merali, Z., McIntosh, J., and Anisman, H. (1999). Role of bombesin-related peptides in the control of food intake. *Neuropeptides* 33, 376–386.

Merali, Z., Mountney, C., Kent, P., and Anisman, H. (2011). Effects of intracerebral ventricular administration of gastrin-releasing peptide and its receptor antagonist RC-3095 on learned fear responses in the rat. *Behav. Brain Res.* 216, 519–524.

Minamino, N., Kangawa, K., and Matsuo, H. (1983). Neuromedin B: a novel bombesin-like peptide identified in porcine spinal cord. *Biochem. Biophys. Res. Commun.* 114, 541–548.

Minamino, N., Kangawa, K., and Matsuo, H. (1984). Neuromedin C: a bombesin-like peptide identified in porcine spinal cord. *Biochem. Biophys. Res. Commun.* 119, 14–20.

Moody, T. W., Getz, R., O'Donohue, T. L., and Rosenstein, J. M. (1988). Localization of receptors for bombesin-like peptides in the rat brain. *Ann. N. Y. Acad. Sci.* 547, 114–130.

Moody, T. W., and Merali, Z. (2004). Bombesin-like peptides and associated receptors within the brain: distribution and behavioral implications. *Peptides* 25, 511–520.

Moody, T. W., Mahmoud, S., Staley, J., Naldini, L., Cirillo, D., South, V., et al. (1989). Human glioblastoma cell lines have neuropeptide receptors for bombesin/gastrin-releasing peptide. *J. Mol. Neurosci.* 1, 235–242.

Moody, T. W., O'Donohue, T. L., and Jacobowitz, D. M. (1981). Biochemical localization and characterization of bombesin-like peptides in discrete regions of rat brain. *Peptides* 2, 75–79.

Moody, T. W., and Pert, C. B. (1979). Bombesin-like peptides in rat brain: quantitation and biochemical characterization. *Biochem. Biophys. Res. Commun.* 90, 7–14.

Moody, T. W., Pert, C. B., Rivier, J., and Brown, M. R. (1978). Bombesin: specific binding to rat brain membranes. *Proc. Natl. Acad. Sci. U.S.A.* 75, 5372–5376.

Moody, T. W., Staley, J., Zia, F., Coy, D. H., and Jensen, R. T. (1992). Neuromedin B binds with high affinity, elevates cytosolic calcium and stimulates the growth of small cell lung cancer cell lines. *J. Pharmacol. Exp. Ther.* 263, 311–317.

Mountney, C., Anisman, H., and Merali, Z. (2008). Effects of gastrin-releasing peptide agonist and antagonist administered to the basolateral nucleus of the amygdala on conditioned fear in the rat. *Psychopharmacology (Berl.)* 200, 51–58.

Mountney, C., Anisman, H., and Merali, Z. (2011). *In vivo* levels of corticotropin-releasing hormone and gastrin-releasing peptide at the basolateral amygdala and medial prefrontal cortex in response to conditioned fear in the rat. *Neuropharmacology* 60, 410–417.

Mountney, C., Sillberg, V., Kent, P., Anisman, H., and Merali, Z. (2006). The role of gastrin-releasing peptide on conditioned fear: differential cortical and amygdaloid responses in the rat. *Psychopharmacology (Berl.)* 189, 287–296.

Niebergall-Roth, E., and Singer, M. V. (2001). Central and peripheral neural control of pancreatic exocrine secretion. *J. Physiol. Pharmacol.* 52, 523–538.

Oh, D. Y., Kim, K., Kwon, H. B., and Seong, J. Y. (2006). Cellular and molecular biology of orphan G protein-coupled receptors. *Int. Rev. Cytol.* 252, 163–218.

Ohki-Hamazaki, H., Iwabuchi, M., and Maekawa, F. (2005). Development and function of bombesin-like peptides and their receptors. *Int. J. Dev. Biol.* 49, 293–300.

Olincy, A., Leonard, S., Young, D. A., Sullivan, B., and Freedman, R. (1999). Decreased bombesin peptide response to cigarette smoking in schizophrenia. *Neuropsychopharmacology* 20, 52–59.

Petronilho, F., Vuolo, F., Galant, L. S., Constantino, L., Tomasi, C. D., Giombelli, V. R., et al. (2012). Gastrin-releasing peptide receptor antagonism induces protection from lethal sepsis: involvement of toll-like receptor 4 signaling. *Mol. Med.* doi: 10.2119/molmed.2012.00083. [Epub ahead of print].

Pinski, J., Schally, A. V., Halmos, G., Szepeshazi, K., and Groot, K. (1994). Somatostatin analogues and bombesin/gastrin-releasing peptide antagonist RC-3095 inhibit the growth of human glioblastomas *in vitro* and *in vivo*. *Cancer Res.* 54, 5895–5901.

Preissler, T., Luft, T., Kapczinski, F., Quevedo, J., Schwartsmann, G., and Roesler, R. (2007). Basic fibroblast growth factor prevents the memory impairment induced by gastrin-releasing peptide receptor antagonism in area CA1 of the rat hippocampus. *Neurochem. Res.* 32, 1381–1386.

Presti-Torres, J., de Lima, M. N., Scalco, F. S., Caldana, F., Garcia, V. A., Guimarães, M. R., et al. (2007). Impairments of social behavior and memory after neonatal gastrin-releasing peptide receptor blockade in rats: implications for an animal model of neurodevelopmental disorders. *Neuropharmacology* 52, 724–732.

Presti-Torres, J., Garcia, V. A., Dornelles, A., Halmenschlager, L. H., Alcalde, L. A., Vedana, G., et al. (2012). Rescue of social behavior impairment by clozapine and alterations in the expression of neuronal receptors in a rat model of neurodevelopmental impairment induced by GRPR blockade. *J. Neural Transm.* 119, 319–327.

Qiao, J., Kang, J., Ishola, T. A., Rychahou, P. G., Evers, B. M., and Chung, D. H. (2008). Gastrin-releasing peptide receptor silencing suppresses the tumorigenesis and metastatic potential of neuroblastoma. *Proc. Natl. Acad. Sci. U.S.A.* 105, 12891–12896.

Rashidy-Pour, A., and Razvani, M. E. (1998). Unilateral reversible inactivations of the nucleus tractus solitarius and amygdala attenuate the effects of bombesin on memory storage. *Brain Res.* 814, 127–132.

Roesler, R., Brunetto, A. T., Abujamra, A. L., de Farias, C. B., Brunetto, A. L., and Schwartsmann, G. (2010). Current and emerging molecular targets in glioma. *Expert Rev. Anticancer Ther.* 10, 1735–1751.

Roesler, R., Henriques, J. A., and Schwartsmann, G. (2004a). Neuropeptides and anxiety disorders: bombesin receptors as novel therapeutic targets. *Trends Pharmacol. Sci.* 25, 241–242.

Roesler, R., Kopschina, M. I., Rosa, R. M., Henriques, J. A., Souza, D. O., and Schwartsmann, G. (2004b). RC-3095, a bombesin/gastrin-releasing peptide receptor antagonist, impairs aversive but not recognition memory in rats. *Eur. J. Pharmacol.* 486, 35–41.

Roesler, R., Lessa, D., Venturella, R., Vianna, M. R., Luft, T., Henriques, J. A., et al. (2004c). Bombesin/gastrin-releasing peptide receptors in the basolateral amygdala regulate memory consolidation. *Eur. J. Neurosci.* 19, 1041–1045.

Roesler, R., Henriques, J. A., and Schwartsmann, G. (2006a). Gastrin-releasing peptide receptor as a molecular target for psychiatric and neurological disorders. *CNS Neurol. Disord. Drug Targets* 5, 197–204.

Roesler, R., Luft, T., Oliveira, S. H., Farias, C. B., Almeida, V. R., Quevedo, J., et al. (2006b). Molecular mechanisms mediating gastrin-releasing peptide receptor modulation of memory consolidation in the hippocampus. *Neuropharmacology* 51, 350–357.

Roesler, R., Kent, P., Schröder, N., Schwartsmann, G., and Merali, Z. (2012). Bombesin receptor regulation of emotional memory. *Rev. Neurosci.* 23, 571–586.

Roesler, R., Meller, C. A., Kopschina, M. I., Souza, D. O., Henriques, J. A., and Schwartsmann, G. (2003). Intrahippocampal infusion of the bombesin/gastrin-releasing peptide antagonist RC-3095 impairs inhibitory avoidance retention. *Peptides* 24, 1069–1074.

Roesler, R., Valvassori, S. S., Castro, A. A., Luft, T., Schwartsmann, G., and Quevedo, J. (2009). Phosphoinositide 3-kinase is required for bombesin-induced enhancement of fear memory consolidation in the hippocampus. *Peptides* 30, 1192–1196.

Ruff, M., Schiffmann, E., Terranova, V., and Pert, C. B. (1985). Neuropeptides are chemoattractants for human tumor cells and monocytes: a possible mechanism for metastasis. *Clin. Immunol. Immunopathol.* 37, 387–396.

Rushing, P. A., Gibbs, J., and Geary, N. (1996). Brief, meal-contingent infusions of gastrin-releasing peptide1–27 and neuromedin B-10 inhibit spontaneous feeding in rats. *Physiol. Behav.* 60, 1501–1504.

Rushing, P. A., and Houpt, T. A. (1999). Gastrin-releasing peptide suppresses independent but not intraoral intake. *Peptides* 20, 737–741.

Sakamoto, H. (2010). The neurobiology of psychogenic erectile dysfunction in the spinal cord. *J. Androl.* 31, 519–526.

Sakamoto, H. (2011). Gastrin-releasing peptide system in the spinal cord mediates masculine sexual function. *Anat. Sci. Int.* 86, 19–29.

Sakamoto, H., and Kawata, M. (2009). Gastrin-releasing peptide system in the spinal cord controls male sexual behaviour. *J. Neuroendocrinol.* 21, 432–435.

Sakamoto, H., Matsuda, K., Zuloaga, D. G., Hongu, H., Wada, E., Wada, K., et al. (2008). Sexually dimorphic gastrin releasing peptide system in the spinal cord controls male reproductive functions. *Nat. Neurosci.* 11, 634–636.

Sakamoto, H., Matsuda, K., Zuloaga, D. G., Nishiura, N., Takanami, K., Jordan, C. L., et al. (2009a). Stress affects a gastrin-releasing peptide system in the spinal cord that mediates sexual function: implications for psychogenic erectile dysfunction. *PLoS ONE* 4:e4276. doi: 10.1371/journal.pone.0004276

Sakamoto, H., Takanami, K., Zuloaga, D. G., Matsuda, K., Jordan, C. L., Breedlove, S. M., et al. (2009b). Androgen regulates the sexually dimorphic gastrin-releasing peptide system in the lumbar spinal cord that mediates male sexual function. *Endocrinology* 150, 3672–3679.

Salio, C., Lossi, L., Ferrini, F., and Merighi, A. (2006). Neuropeptides as synaptic transmitters. *Cell Tissue Res.* 326, 583–598.

Santo-Yamada, Y., Yamada, K., Wada, E., Goto, Y., and Wada, K. (2003). Blockade of bombesin-like peptide receptors impairs inhibitory avoidance learning in mice. *Neurosci. Lett.* 340, 65–68.

Schmidt, A. L., de Farias, C. B., Abujamra, A. L., Kapczinski, F., Schwartsmann, G., Brunetto, A. L., et al. (2009). BDNF and PDE4, but not the GRPR, regulate viability of human medulloblastoma cells. *J. Mol. Neurosci.* 40, 303–310.

Schubert, M. L., Hightower, J., Coy, D. H., and Makhlouf, G. M. (1991). Regulation of acid secretion by bombesin/GRP neurons of the gastric fundus. *Am. J. Physiol.* 260, G156–G160.

Schwartsmann, G., DiLeone, L. P., Horowitz, M., Schunemann, D., Cancella, A., Pereira, A. S., et al. (2006). A phase I trial of the bombesin/gastrin-releasing peptide (BN/GRP) antagonist RC3095 in patients with advanced solid malignancies. *Invest. New Drugs* 24, 403–412.

Seidita, G., Mirisola, M., D'Anna, R. P., Gallo, A., Jensen, R. T., Mantey, S. A., et al. (2008). Analysis of the gastrin-releasing peptide receptor gene in Italian patients with autism spectrum disorders. *Am. J. Med. Genet. B Neuropsychiatr. Genet.* 147B, 807–813.

Sharif, T. R., Luo, W., and Sharif, M. (1997). Functional expression of bombesin receptor in most adult and pediatric human glioblastoma cell lines; role in mitogenesis and in stimulating the mitogen-activated protein kinase pathway. *Mol. Cell. Endocrinol.* 130, 119–130.

Shumyatsky, G. P., Tsvetkov, E., Malleret, G., Vronskaya, S., Hatton, M., Hampton, L., et al. (2002). Identification of a signaling network in lateral nucleus of amygdala important for inhibiting memory specifically related to learned fear. *Cell* 111, 905–918.

Spindel, E. R., Chin, W. W., Price, J., Rees, L. H., Besser, G. M., and Habener, J. F. (1984). Cloning and characterization of cDNAs encoding human gastrin-releasing peptide. *Proc. Natl. Acad. Sci. U.S.A.* 81, 5699–5703.

Spindel, E. R., Giladi, E., Brehm, P., Goodman, R. H., and Segerson, T. P. (1990). Cloning and functional characterization of a complementary DNA encoding the murine fibroblast bombesin/gastrin-releasing peptide receptor. *Mol. Endocrinol.* 4, 1956–1963.

Stangelberger, A., Schally, A. V., Varga, J. L., Zarandi, M., Cai, R. Z., Baker, B., et al. (2005). Inhibition of human androgen-independent PC-3 and DU-145 prostate cancers by antagonists of bombesin and growth hormone releasing hormone is linked to PKC, MAPK and c-jun intracellular signalling. *Eur. J. Cancer* 41, 2735–2344.

Stoddard, S. L., Tyce, G. M., Ahlskog, J. E., Zinsmeister, A. R., Nelson, D. K., and Carmichael, S. W. (1991). Decreased levels of [Met]enkephalin, neuropeptide Y, substance P, and vasoactive intestinal peptide in parkinsonian adrenal medulla. *Exp. Neurol.* 114, 23–27.

Sun, Y. G., and Chen, Z. F. (2007). A gastrin-releasing peptide receptor mediates the itch sensation in the spinal cord. *Nature* 448, 700–703.

Sun, Y. G., Zhao, Z. Q., Meng, X. L., Yin, J., Liu, X. Y., and Chen, Z. F. (2009). Cellular basis of itch sensation. *Science* 325, 1531–1534.

Szepeshazi, K., Schally, A. V., Halmos, G., Lamharzi, N., Groot, K., and Horvath, J. E.(1997). A single *in vivo* administration of bombesin antagonist RC-3095 reduces the levels and mRNA expression of epidermal growth factor receptors in MXT mouse mammary cancers. *Proc. Natl. Acad. Sci. U.S.A.* 94, 10913–10918.

Thaw, A. K., Smith, J. C., and Gibbs, J. (1998). Mammalian bombesin-like peptides extend the intermeal interval in freely feeding rats. *Physiol. Behav.* 64, 425–428.

Thomas, S. M., Grandis, J. R., Wentzel, A. L., Gooding, W. E., Lui, V. W., and Siegfried, J. M. (2005). Gastrin-releasing peptide receptor mediates activation of the epidermal growth factor receptor in lung cancer cells. *Neoplasia* 7, 426–431.

Venturella, R., Lessa, D., Luft, T., Roozendaal, B., Schwartsmann, G., and Roesler, R. (2005). Dexamethasone reverses the memory impairment induced by antagonism of hippocampal gastrin-releasing peptide receptors. *Peptides* 26, 821–825.

von Schrenck, T., Heinz-Erian, P., Moran, T., Mantey, S. A., Gardner, J. D., and Jensen, R. T. (1989). Neuromedin B receptor in esophagus: evidence for subtypes of bombesin receptors. *Am. J. Physiol.* 256, G747–G758.

von Schrenck, T., Wang, L. H., Coy, D. H., Villanueva, M. L., Mantey, S., and Jensen, R. T. (1990). Potent bombesin receptor antagonists distinguish receptor subtypes. *Am. J. Physiol.* 259, G468–G473.

Wada, E., Way, J., Lebacq-Verheyden, A. M., and Battey, J. F. (1990). Neuromedin B and gastrin-releasing peptide mRNAs are differentially distributed in the rat nervous system. *J. Neurosci.* 10, 2917–2930.

Wada, E., Way, J., Shapira, H., Kusano, K., Lebacq-Verheyden, A. M., Coy, D., et al. (1991). cDNA cloning, characterization, and brain region-specific expression of a neuromedin B-preferring bombesin receptor. *Neuron* 6, 421–430.

Wada, E., Wray, S., Key, S., and Battey, J. (1992). Comparison of gene expression for two distinct bombesin receptor subtypes in postnatal rat central nervous system. *Mol. Cell. Neurosci.* 3, 446–460.

Wang, L. H., Battey, J. F., Wada, E., Lin, J. T., Mantey, S., Coy, D. H., et al. (1992). Activation of neuromedin B-preferring bombesin receptors on rat glioblastoma c-6 cells increases cellular $Ca^{2+}$ and phosphoinositides. *Biochem. J.* 286, 641–648.

Williams, C. L., and McGaugh, J. L. (1994). Enhancement of memory processing in an inhibitory avoidance and radial maze task by post-training infusion of bombesin into the nucleus tractus solitarius. *Brain Res.* 654, 251–256.

Wolf, S. S., and Moody, T. W. (1985). Receptors for GRP/bombesin-like peptides in the rat forebrain. *Peptides* 6(Suppl. 1), 111–114.

Wolf, S. S., Moody, T. W., O'Donohue, T. L., Zarbin, M. A., and Kuhar, M. J. (1983). Autoradiographic visualization of rat brain binding sites for bombesin-like peptides. *Eur. J. Pharmacol.* 87, 163–164.

Wong, S. T., Athos, J., Figueroa, X. A., Pineda, V. V., Schaefer, M. L., Chavkin, C. C., et al. (1999). Calcium-stimulated adenylyl cyclase activity is critical for hippocampus-dependent long-term memory and late phase LTP. *Neuron* 23, 787–798.

Zarbin, M. A., Kuhar, M. J., O'Donohue, T. L., Wolf, S. S., and Moody, T. W. (1985). Autoradiographic localization of (125I-Tyr4)bombesin-binding sites in rat brain. *J. Neurosci.* 5, 429–437.

# 12

# Neuropeptide GPCRs in neuroendocrinology: the case of activity-dependent neuroprotective protein (ADNP)

***Illana Gozes****

*The Lily and Avraham Gildor Chair for the Investigation of Growth Factors, Department of Human Molecular Genetics and Biochemistry, Sagol School of Neuroscience, Adams Super Center for Brain Studies, Sackler Faculty of Medicine, Tel Aviv University, Tel Aviv, Israel*

**Correspondence: igozes@post.tau.ac.il*

***Edited by:***

*Hubert Vaudry, University of Rouen, France*

***Reviewed by:***

*Dora Reglodi, University of Pecs, Hungary*

*Terry Moody, National Cancer Institute, USA*

*Mario Delgado, Consejo Superior de Investigaciones Científicas, Spain*

## VASOACTIVE INTESTINAL PEPTIDE (VIP): NEUROPROTECTION AND SYNAPSE FORMATION

This review is a selected overview of the chosen subject. As, I have recently summarized my work on VIP (Gozes, 2008), I will describe here only selected topics focusing on the GPCR connection of the VIP-regulated protein, activity-dependent neuroprotective protein (ADNP) (Gozes, 2007).

In the mid 1980s we were the first to clone the gene encoding the 28 amino acid neuropeptide, vasoactive intestinal peptide (VIP) (Bodner et al., 1985). This allowed us to follow up VIP gene expression in the brain showing developmental increases at the time of postnatal synapse formation and glial expansion (Gozes et al., 1987). Given the increased expression of VIP at the time of synapse formation and glial expansion, we hypothesized a developmental role for the peptide—associated with synaptogenesis and neuroprotection. Follow-up studies by the laboratory of Douglas Brenneman indeed showed that VIP provided neuroprotection through glial cells (Brenneman et al., 1987). We teamed up to show together with the group of Ronald McKay that VIP enhances synapse formation through glial cell activation (Blondel et al., 2000).

Together with the late Frank Baldino, we showed extensive VIP mRNA expression in the brain, for example, in the suprachiasmatic nucleus (SCN) (Card et al., 1988), an area regulating diurnal rhythms. Our further studies utilizing our VIP hybrid antagonist showed that VIP function during development was required for maintenance of diurnal rhythmicity (Gozes et al., 1995). These findings were later confirmed by knocking out either VIP (Loh et al., 2011), or the VIP receptor VPAC2 (Harmar et al., 2002), which brings us to part of the subject of this review, GPCRs.

## VIP RECEPTORS

We have recently reviewed the current status of research on VIP receptors (Harmar et al., 2012). In short, VIP and pituitary adenylate cyclase-activating polypeptide (PACAP) are members of a superfamily of structurally related peptide hormones that includes glucagon, glucagon-like peptides, secretin, gastric inhibitory peptide (GIP) and growth hormone-releasing hormone (GHRH). VIP and PACAP exert their actions through three GPCRs—PAC1, VPAC1 and VPAC2—belonging to class B (also referred to as class II, or secretin receptor-like GPCRs). PAC1 receptors are selective for PACAP, whereas VPAC1 and VPAC2 respond to both VIP and PACAP with high affinity (Harmar et al., 2012). As indicated above, VPAC2 was associated with diurnal rhythmicity (Harmar et al., 2002) as well as astrogenesis (Zupan et al., 1998). Other functions, including association with cancer propagation and immunomodulation have been extensively reviewed (as cited above).

## VIP RECEPTORS AND NEUROPROTECTION, OUR POINT OF VIEW

Prior to the molecular cloning of VIP and PACAP receptors, binding and displacement assays coupled to functional assays suggested high affinity binding for VIP on glial cells (astrocytes)—associated with the release of neuroprotective proteins and low affinity binding to astrocytes, associated with cAMP formation (Gozes et al., 1991). With the available VPAC1, VPAC2, and PAC1 clones (including the alternatively spliced PAC1 receptors), we have used antisense oligodeoxynucleotides specific for each of the then known receptor subtypes to identify receptors involved in neuroprotection. Our data showed that one of the PAC1 splice variants, the hop2-like receptor is a receptor that mediates neuroprotection (Ashur-Fabian et al., 1997). The PAC1 cDNA was cloned from rat cerebral astrocytes. Using genetic manipulation we obtained the hop2 splice variant and expressed it in COS-7 cells. Results showed that VIP bound the cloned hop2 splice variant (Pilzer and Gozes, 2006). Stearyl-neurotensin (6–11) VIP (7–28) (SNH), an antagonist for VIP, was also found to bind hop2. Other studies have shown that this particular antagonist that we have developed (Gozes et al., 1995) binds to all know VIP receptors (Moody et al., 2002). In addition, VIP protected COS-7 cells expressing hop2 from oxidative stress. Parallel assays demonstrated that VIP increased cAMP accumulation in COS-7 cells expressing hop2. These results support the hypothesis that hop2 mediates some of the cytoprotective effects attributed to VIP (Pilzer and Gozes, 2006).

However, the study cited above did not address the requirement for astrocytes for VIP neuroprotection, suggesting additional players.

## VIP STIMULATE ASTROCYTE SECRETION OF GROWTH FACTORS

We teamed up together with Douglas Brenneman to isolate novel growth factors from VIP-stimulated astrocyte conditioned media. Our first attempt included sequential chromatography coupled to functional assays of neuroprotection, yielding activity-dependent neurotrophic factor (ADNF) (Brenneman and Gozes, 1996). This study took us to three directions: (1) identification of an active peptide site within ADNF—potential future therapeutic; (2) production of antibodies against ADNF as tools for functional studies and (3) use of the antibodies for expression cloning toward the identification of novel ADNF-like molecules, thus cloning ADNP (Bassan et al., 1999). We have further identified ADNP immunoreactivity in astrocyte conditioned medium, which was increased upon exposure to VIP (Furman et al., 2004).

## GPCR INVOLVEMENT IN ADNP EXPRESSION

Using VIP analogues specific for the VPAC1 and the VPAC2 receptors, we discovered that VIP-induced changes in ADNP expression in astrocytes via the VPAC2 receptor. The constitutive synthesis of ADNP and VPAC2 was shown to be age-dependent and increased as the astrocyte culture developed. The VIP-related peptide, PACAP also induced changes in ADNP expression. The apparent change-induced by VIP and PACAP on ADNP expression were developmentally dependent, and while stimulating expression in young astrocytes (Bassan et al., 1999), an inhibition was demonstrated in older cultures suggesting that VIP, PACAP, and the VPAC2 receptor may all contribute to the regulation of ADNP gene expression in the developing astrocyte (Zusev and Gozes, 2004).

Parallel studies by the discoverer of PACAP, the late Akira Arimura, showed that when PACAP38 was added to mouse neuroglial cultures, it induced ADNP mRNA expression in a bimodal fashion at subpico- and nanomolar concentrations with greater response at subpicomolar level. The response was attenuated by a PAC1 receptor antagonist at both concentrations and by a VPAC1 receptor antagonist at nanomolar concentration only. An IP3/PLC inhibitor attenuated the response at both concentrations of PACAP38, but a MAPK inhibitor had no effect. A PKA inhibitor suppressed the response at nanomolar concentration only. The findings suggest that ADNP expression is mediated through multiple receptors and signaling pathways that are regulated by different concentrations of PACAP (Nakamachi et al., 2006) as well as VIP. A further study showed that ADNP-immunoreactive cells in the cerebral cortex were multi-polar-shaped and co-immunostained with the astrocyte marker, glial fibrillary acidic protein (GFAP). ADNP-immunoreactive cells in the cerebellum were found to surround Purkinje cells and showed GFAP immunoreactivity. In contrast, ADNP-immunoreactive cells in the hippocampus and septum were round in shape and co-immunostained with neuron-specific enolase (NSE). Importantly, all of the ADNP-immunopositive cells co-localized with PAC1 immunoreactivity. The observations suggest that ADNP is expressed in both astrocytes and neurons, and that ADNP expression may be regulated in part by PACAP (Nakamachi et al., 2008).

Using bioinformatics analysis, we have identified an ADNP family member which we have named, ADNP2 (Zamostiano et al., 2001; Kushnir et al., 2008).

To evaluate the impact of VIP expression *in vivo* on ADNP and the related protein ADNP2, we examined gene expression in adult wild-type (VIP+/+) and VIP null (VIP−/−) offspring of VIP deficient mothers (VIP+/−) comparing them to wild-type offspring of wild-type mothers. Quantitative real time polymerase chain reaction (PCR) revealed regionally specific reductions of ADNP mRNA in the brains of VIP−/− mice compared with the brains of wild-type offspring of a wild-type mother. ADNP was significantly reduced in the cortex and hypothalamus of VIP−/− mice, but not in the hippocampus or thalamus. ADNP2 exhibited a similar pattern but reached a statistically significant reduction only in the hypothalamus. The RNA transcripts for ADNP and ADNP2 also tended to be reduced in the cortex and hippocampus of the wild-type littermates of the VIP−/− mice, indicating that the VIP genotype of the mother may have had an impact on the ADNP expression of her offspring, regardless of their own VIP genotype. Thus, VIP regulates brain ADNP expression in a regionally specific manner and both maternal and offspring VIP genotype may influence ADNP expression in the brain (Giladi et al., 2007).

## CLINICAL IMPLICATIONS

Recent genetic studies titled: duplications of the neuropeptide receptor gene VPAC2 confer significant risk for schizophrenia implicated the VPAC2 receptor in susceptibility to schizophrenia. Further studies implicated the PAC1 receptor and PACAP in post-traumatic stress disorder as recently reviewed (Harmar et al., 2012).

In this respect, we found deregulation of ADNP/ADNP2 in the postmortem hippocampus of schizophrenia patients (Dresner et al., 2011) and correlated with disease duration.

Other findings associated reduced ADNP expression to the progression of multiple sclerosis and increased pro-inflammatory markers (Braitch et al., 2009), and potential modulation by the ADNP derived drug candidate davunetide (NAP).

While VIP may present a dual function in the regulation of multiple sclerosis (Abad et al., 2010; Loh et al., 2011), it should be borne in mind that ADNP regulation, while in part associated with VIP and PACAP, is regulated by other control mechanisms. While VIP knockout exhibited a subtle phenotype (e.g., Abad et al., 2010; Loh et al., 2011) and VIP over expression, eventually led to down-regulation of activity with learning deficits (Gozes et al., 1993), ADNP knockout is lethal at embryonic time of brain formation, implicating ADNP as crucial for brain formation (Pinhasov et al., 2003; Mandel et al., 2007). Interestingly, VIP is suggested as a growth factor to the developing embryo (Gressens et al., 1993, 1994). Furthermore, partial ADNP deficiency leads to cognitive and social dysfunction (Vulih-Shultzman et al., 2007), similar to partial deficiency in VIP functions (Glowa et al., 1992; Gozes et al., 1993; Hill et al., 2007). This deficiency can be also associated with deficiency at the cellular level, with ADNP knockdown (or partial deficiency) associated with blocked neurite outgrowth (Mandel et al., 2008) and reduced glial neurotrophic milieu (Pascual and Guerri, 2007; Vulih-Shultzman et al., 2007) and with VIP blockade resulting in neuronal damage (Hill et al., 1994) and inhibition of synaptogenesis (Blondel et al., 2000).

In the case of ADNP, davunetide, an eight amino acid peptide snippet of ADNP is in phase 2/3 clinical trials in a severe neurodegeneration, progressive supranuclear palsy (PSP) (Gold et al., 2012).

## FUTURE PERSPECTIVE

While this review focused on VIP and ADNP, from my point of view, it should be taken into consideration that we have developed a family of peptide hybrids/fragments and lipophilic VIP analogs, agonists and antagonists (Gozes et al., 1995), with activities ranging from neurtrophism/neurodevelopment neuroprotection (Gozes et al., 1999) to stimulation of sexual/social function and cancer growth inhibition. The precise GPCR involvement in these analogues activities remains to be elucidated (Gourlet et al., 1998; Moody et al., 2002). Interestingly, ADNP expression was shown to be reduced as a consequence of ischemia in tissue culture, and this was inhibited by treatment with the neuroprotective lypophilic VIP analog Stearyl-Norleucine17 VIP(7–28) (SNV) (Sigalov et al., 2000), awaiting future development.

## ACKNOWLEDGMENTS

Current support is provided by AMN Foundation, Canadian Friends of Tel Aviv University—Montreal Circle of Friends, Joe and Grace Alter, Barbara and Don Seal, the Oberfeld family, the Adams family and Allon Therapeutics Inc. Illana Gozes is the incumbent of the Professorial Lily and Avraham Gildor Chair for the Investigation of Growth Factors, and the Director of the Adams Super Center for Brain Studies, and the Elton Laboratory at Tel Aviv University.

## REFERENCES

Abad, C., Tan, Y. V., Lopez, R., Nobuta, H., Dong, H., Phan, P., et al. (2010). Vasoactive intestinal peptide loss leads to impaired CNS parenchymal T-cell infiltration and resistance to experimental autoimmune encephalomyelitis. *Proc. Natl. Acad. Sci. U.S.A.* 107, 19555–19560.

Ashur-Fabian, O., Giladi, E., Brenneman, D. E., and Gozes, I. (1997). Identification of VIP/PACAP receptors on rat astrocytes using antisense oligodeoxynucleotides. *J. Mol. Neurosci.* 9, 211–222.

Bassan, M., Zamostiano, R., Davidson, A., Pinhasov, A., Giladi, E., Perl, O., et al. (1999). Complete sequence of a novel protein containing a femtomolar-activity-dependent neuroprotective peptide. *J. Neurochem.* 72, 1283–1293.

Blondel, O., Collin, C., McCarran, W. J., Zhu, S., Zamostiano, R., Gozes, I., et al. (2000). A glia-derived signal regulating neuronal differentiation. *J. Neurosci.* 20, 8012–8020.

Bodner, M., Fridkin, M., and Gozes, I. (1985). Coding sequences for vasoactive intestinal peptide and PHM-27 peptide are located on two adjacent exons in the human genome. *Proc. Natl. Acad. Sci. U.S.A.* 82, 3548–3551.

Braitch, M., Kawabe, K., Nyirenda, M., Gilles, L. J., Robins, R. A., Gran, B., et al. (2009). Expression of activity-dependent neuroprotective protein in the immune system: possible functions and relevance to multiple sclerosis. *Neuroimmunomodulation* 17, 120–125.

Brenneman, D. E., and Gozes, I. (1996). A femtomolar-acting neuroprotective peptide. *J. Clin. Invest.* 97, 2299–2307.

Brenneman, D. E., Neale, E. A., Foster, G. A., d'Autremont, S. W., and Westbrook, G. L. (1987). Nonneuronal cells mediate neurotrophic action of vasoactive intestinal peptide. *J. Cell Biol.* 104, 1603–1610.

Card, J. P., Fitzpatrick-McElligott, S., Gozes, I., and Baldino, F. Jr. (1988). Localization of vasopressin-, vasoactive intestinal polypeptide-, peptide histidine isoleucine- and somatostatin-mRNA in rat suprachiasmatic nucleus. *Cell Tissue Res.* 252, 307–315.

Dresner, E., Agam, G., and Gozes, I. (2011). Activity-dependent neuroprotective protein (ADNP) expression level is correlated with the expression of the sister protein ADNP2: deregulation in schizophrenia. *Eur. Neuropsychopharmacol.* 21, 355–361.

Furman, S., Steingart, R. A., Mandel, S., Hauser, J. M., Brenneman, D. E., and Gozes, I. (2004). Subcellular localization and secretion of activity-dependent neuroprotective protein in astrocytes. *Neuron Glia Biol.* 1, 193–199.

Giladi, E., Hill, J. M., Dresner, E., Stack, C. M., and Gozes, I. (2007). Vasoactive intestinal peptide (VIP) regulates activity-dependent neuroprotective protein (ADNP) expression *in vivo*. *J. Mol. Neurosci.* 33, 278–283.

Glowa, J. R., Panlilio, L. V., Brenneman, D. E., Gozes, I., Fridkin, M., and Hill, J. M. (1992). Learning impairment following intracerebral administration of the HIV envelope protein gp120 or a VIP antagonist. *Brain Res.* 570, 49–53.

Gold, M., Lorenzl, S., Stewart, A. J., Morimoto, B. H., Williams, D. R., and Gozes, I. (2012). Critical appraisal of the role of davunetide in the treatment of progressive supranuclear palsy. *Neuropsychiatr. Dis. Treat* 8, 85–93.

Gourlet, P., Rathe, J., De Neef, P., Cnudde, J., Vandermeers-Piret, M. C., Waelbroeck, M., et al. (1998). Interaction of lipophilic VIP derivatives with recombinant VIP1/PACAP and VIP2/PACAP receptors. *Eur. J. Pharmacol.* 354, 105–111.

Gozes, I. (2007). Activity-dependent neuroprotective protein: from gene to drug candidate. *Pharmacol. Ther.* 114, 146–154.

Gozes, I. (2008). VIP, from gene to behavior and back: summarizing my 25 years of research. *J. Mol. Neurosci.* 36, 115–124.

Gozes, I., Glowa, J., Brenneman, D. E., McCune, S. K., Lee, E., and Westphal, H. (1993). Learning and sexual deficiencies in transgenic mice carrying a chimeric vasoactive intestinal peptide gene. *J. Mol. Neurosci.* 4, 185–193.

Gozes, I., Lilling, G., Glazer, R., Ticher, A., Ashkenazi, I. E., Davidson, A., et al. (1995). Superactive lipophilic peptides discriminate multiple vasoactive intestinal peptide receptors. *J. Pharmacol. Exp. Ther.* 273, 161–167.

Gozes, I., McCune, S. K., Jacobson, L., Warren, D., Moody, T. W., Fridkin, M., et al. (1991). An antagonist to vasoactive intestinal peptide affects cellular functions in the central nervous system. *J. Pharmacol. Exp. Ther.* 257, 959–966.

Gozes, I., Perl, O., Giladi, E., Davidson, A., Ashur-Fabian, O., Rubinraut, S., et al. (1999). Mapping the active site in vasoactive intestinal peptide to a core of four amino acids: neuroprotective drug design. *Proc. Natl. Acad. Sci. U.S.A.* 96, 4143–4148.

Gozes, I., Shani, Y., and Rostene, W. H. (1987). Developmental expression of the VIP-gene in brain and intestine. *Brain Res.* 388, 137–148.

Gressens, P., Hill, J. M., Gozes, I., Fridkin, M., and Brenneman, D. E. (1993). Growth factor function of vasoactive intestinal peptide in whole cultured mouse embryos. *Nature* 362, 155–158.

Gressens, P., Hill, J. M., Paindaveine, B., Gozes, I., Fridkin, M., and Brenneman, D. E. (1994). Severe microcephaly induced by blockade of vasoactive intestinal peptide function in the primitive neuroepithelium of the mouse. *J. Clin. Invest.* 94, 2020–2027.

Harmar, A. J., Fahrenkrug, J., Gozes, I., Laburthe, M., May, V., Pisegna, J. R., et al. (2012). Pharmacology and functions of receptors for vasoactive intestinal peptide and pituitary adenylate cyclase-activating polypeptide: IUPHAR review 1. *Br. J. Pharmacol.* 166, 4–17.

Harmar, A. J., Marston, H. M., Shen, S., Spratt, C., West, K. M., Sheward, W. J., et al. (2002). The VPAC(2) receptor is essential for circadian function in the mouse suprachiasmatic nuclei. *Cell* 109, 497–508.

Hill, J. M., Hauser, J. M., Sheppard, L. M., Abebe, D., Spivak-Pohis, I., Kushnir, M., et al. (2007). Blockage of VIP during mouse embryogenesis modifies adult behavior and results in permanent changes in brain chemistry. *J. Mol. Neurosci.* 31, 183–200.

Hill, J. M., Mervis, R. F., Politi, J., McCune, S. K., Gozes, I., Fridkin, M., et al. (1994). Blockade of VIP during neonatal development induces neuronal damage and increases VIP and VIP receptors in brain. *Ann. N.Y. Acad. Sci.* 739, 211–225.

Kushnir, M., Dresner, E., Mandel, S., and Gozes, I. (2008). Silencing of the ADNP-family member, ADNP2, results in changes in cellular viability under oxidative stress. *J. Neurochem.* 105, 537–545.

Loh, D. H., Dragich, J. M., Kudo, T., Schroeder, A. M., Nakamura, T. J., Waschek, J. A., et al. (2011).

Effects of vasoactive intestinal peptide genotype on circadian gene expression in the suprachiasmatic nucleus and peripheral organs. *J. Biol. Rhythms* 26, 200–209.

Mandel, S., Rechavi, G., and Gozes, I. (2007). Activity-dependent neuroprotective protein (ADNP) differentially interacts with chromatin to regulate genes essential for embryogenesis. *Dev. Biol.* 303, 814–824.

Mandel, S., Spivak-Pohis, I., and Gozes, I. (2008). ADNP differential nucleus/cytoplasm localization in neurons suggests multiple roles in neuronal differentiation and maintenance. *J. Mol. Neurosci.* 35, 127–141.

Moody, T. W., Jensen, R. T., Fridkin, M., and Gozes, I. (2002). (N-stearyl, norleucine17) VIPhybrid is a broad spectrum vasoactive intestinal peptide receptor antagonist. *J. Mol. Neurosci.* 18, 29–35.

Nakamachi, T., Li, M., Shioda, S., and Arimura, A. (2006). Signaling involved in pituitary adenylate cyclase-activating polypeptide-stimulated ADNP expression. *Peptides* 27, 1859–1864.

Nakamachi, T., Ohtaki, H., Yofu, S., Dohi, K., Watanabe, J., Hayashi, D., et al. (2008). Pituitary adenylate cyclase-activating polypeptide (PACAP) type 1 receptor (PAC1R) co-localizes with activity-dependent neuroprotective protein (ADNP) in the mouse brains. *Regul. Pept.* 145, 88–95.

Pascual, M., and Guerri, C. (2007). The peptide NAP promotes neuronal growth and differentiation through extracellular signal-regulated protein kinase and Akt pathways, and protects neurons co-cultured with astrocytes damaged by ethanol. *J. Neurochem.* 103, 557–568.

Pilzer, I., and Gozes, I. (2006). VIP provides cellular protection through a specific splice variant of the PACAP receptor: a new neuroprotection target. *Peptides* 27, 2867–2876.

Pinhasov, A., Mandel, S., Torchinsky, A., Giladi, E., Pittel, Z., Goldsweig, A. M., et al. (2003). Activity-dependent neuroprotective protein: a novel gene essential for brain formation. *Brain Res. Dev. Brain Res.* 144, 83–90.

Sigalov, E., Fridkin, M., Brenneman, D. E., and Gozes, I. (2000). VIP-related protection against lodoacetate toxicity in pheochromocytoma (PC12) cells: a model for ischemic/hypoxic injury. *J. Mol. Neurosci.* 15, 147–154.

Vulih-Shultzman, I., Pinhasov, A., Mandel, S., Grigoriadis, N., Touloumi, O., Pittel, Z., et al. (2007). Activity-dependent neuroprotective protein snippet NAP reduces tau hyperphosphorylation and enhances learning in a novel transgenic mouse model. *J. Pharmacol. Exp. Ther.* 323, 438–449.

Zamostiano, R., Pinhasov, A., Gelber, E., Steingart, R. A., Seroussi, E., Giladi, E., et al. (2001). Cloning and characterization of the human activity-dependent neuroprotective protein. *J. Biol. Chem.* 276, 708–714.

Zupan, V., Hill, J. M., Brenneman, D. E., Gozes, I., Fridkin, M., Robberecht, P., et al. (1998). Involvement of pituitary adenylate cyclase-activating polypeptide II vasoactive intestinal peptide 2 receptor in mouse neocortical astrocytogenesis. *J. Neurochem.* 70, 2165–2173.

Zusev, M., and Gozes, I. (2004). Differential regulation of activity-dependent neuroprotective protein in rat astrocytes by VIP and PACAP. *Regul. Pept.* 123, 33–41.

# 13

# Somatostatinergic systems: an update on brain functions in normal and pathological aging

**_Guillaume Martel, Patrick Dutar, Jacques Epelbaum and Cécile Viollet*_**

*Inserm UMR894 - Center for Psychiatry and Neuroscience, Université Paris Descartes, Sorbonne Paris Cité, Paris, France*

**_Edited by:_**
*Hubert Vaudry, University of Rouen, France*

**_Reviewed by:_**
*Paola Bagnoli, University of Pisa, Italy*
*Kyriaki Thermos, University of Crete, Greece*

**_*Correspondence:_**
*Cécile Viollet, Inserm UMR894 - Center for Psychiatry and Neuroscience, Université Paris Descartes, Sorbonne Paris Cité, 2 ter rue d'Alésia, 75014 Paris, France.*
*e-mail: cecile.viollet@inserm.fr*

Somatostatin is highly expressed in mammalian brain and is involved in many brain functions such as motor activity, sleep, sensory, and cognitive processes. Five somatostatin receptors have been described: $sst_1$, $sst_2$ (A and B), $sst_3$, $sst_4$, and $sst_5$, all belonging to the G-protein-coupled receptor family. During the recent years, numerous studies contributed to clarify the role of somatostatin systems, especially long-range somatostatinergic interneurons, in several functions they have been previously involved in. New advances have also been made on the alterations of somatostatinergic systems in several brain diseases and on the potential therapeutic target they represent in these pathologies.

**Keywords: interneurons, SRIF, GPCR, sst, cortistatin, long-range, Alzheimer's disease**

## NEUROANATOMY OF SOMATOSTATINERGIC SYSTEM

### SOMATOSTATIN PEPTIDES IN THE BRAIN

Somatostatin$_{14}$ (SRIF, somatotropin release inhibiting factor) was serendipitously discovered in 1972 by Roger Guillemin and colleagues who were aiming to purify and characterize growth hormone (GH)-releasing hormone from sheep hypothalamus (Brazeau et al., 1973). Soon thereafter, an N-terminally extended peptide, SRIF$_{28}$, was purified from the gut. Both peptides, arising from a common propeptide encoded from a single gene, were found in the mammalian nervous system where SRIF$_{14}$ is the predominant form (for review, see Epelbaum, 1986).

Two brain SRIF-related bioactive peptides have been discovered later. Cortistatin (CST) has been cloned in 1996 (De Lecea et al., 1996) and shares 11 amino acids with SRIF (**Figure 1**). CST peptides are predicted to occur as 14-AA or 17-AA short forms in rodents and humans, respectively, and a 29-AA extended form in both species. CST is mainly restricted to the cerebral cortex and the hippocampus in the central nervous system (CNS). CST has been implicated in several brain functions such as learning and memory, regulation of sleep/wakefulness rhythms and it is suspected to have an anticonvulsant activity (for review, see de Lecea, 2008). Recently, bioinformatics analyses of evolutionary conserved sequences identified neuronostatin, a 13-AA amidated peptide also encoded by the somatostatin gene. Mostly found in pancreas, spleen, and brain, it is involved in metabolic, cardiovascular, and neuronal functions (Samson et al., 2008).

Somatostatin induces many transduction mechanisms in transfected systems (for review, see Lahlou et al., 2004; Olias et al., 2004), but deciphering the physiological actions of the native receptors *in situ* remains an intense field of study. The last decade showed increasing progress in understanding the role of SRIF in brain functions using molecular, pharmacological, and behavioral approaches. The development of innovative molecular, genetic, and imaging tools now allows to go a step further and to assess the cellular contribution of SRIF-expressing cells in neuronal networks *ex vivo* and soon *in vivo*. In this review we will give an overview of the latest findings concerning SRIF systems in brain, report some recent data concerning their synaptic actions and their physiological roles within the brain, in normal or pathological conditions.

### SOMATOSTATINERGIC NETWORKS IN THE BRAIN

Somatostatin is ubiquitously expressed in mammalian brain, including humans (**Figure 2A**). SRIF-immunoreactivity is found at high level in the mediobasal hypothalamus and median eminence, amygdala, preoptic area, hippocampus, striatum, cerebral cortex, sensory regions, and the brainstem (for review, see Epelbaum, 1986; Viollet et al., 2008).

Somatostatin peptide colocalizes with gamma-aminobutyric acid (GABA), a major inhibitory neurotransmitter and labels mostly non-glutamatergic cells in the brain. In order to target SRIF interneurons *in situ*, most recent studies took advantage of rodent models expressing the green fluorescent protein (GFP) under the control of the GAD67 promoter to visualize GABAergic populations more easily. In the GIN (GFP-expressing inhibitory neurons) strain (Oliva et al., 2000) nearly all GFP cells stained for SRIF while in the GAD67-GFP strain, SRIF immunohistochemistry labels 37% of total GFP cells (Ma et al., 2006). The recent development of specific Cre recombinase and knock-in inducible driver lines for SRIF (Taniguchi et al., 2011) opens promising avenues to study SRIF functions at the cellular level combined to optogenetic and imaging tools.

Previous immunohistochemical and tracing studies have identified two main categories of SRIF neurons: those acting locally in a given structure within microcircuits (interneurons) and those projecting to a distant structure (long-projecting neurons). Nevertheless, recent data using GFP transgenic mice revisit previous anatomical records by demonstrating that some formerly called interneurons also belonged to the projecting neurons category. The different kinds of GABAergic interneurons are classified

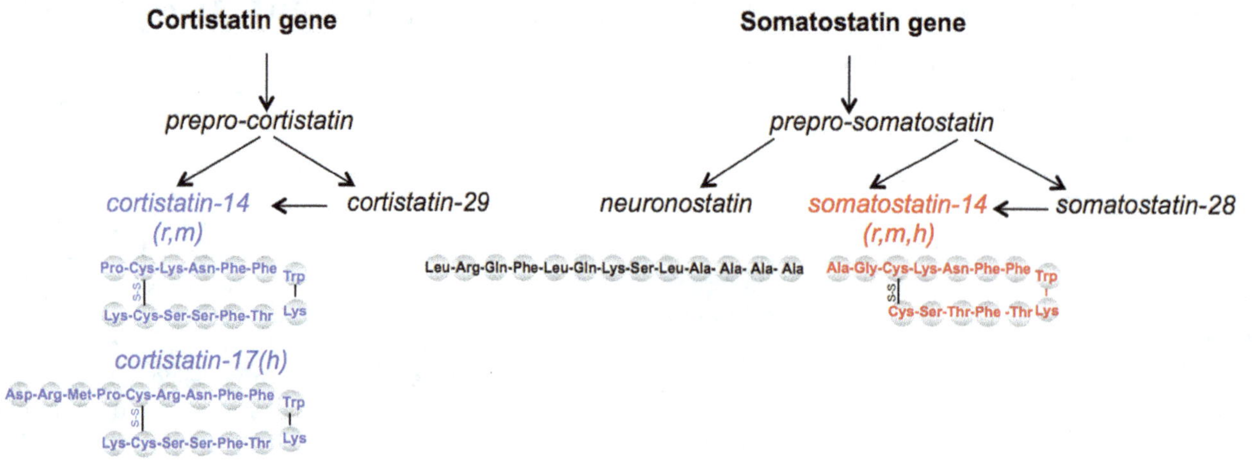


**FIGURE 1 | Schematic representation of somatostatin-related peptides.** $SRIF_{14}$ and $CST_{14}$ come from two distinct genes but bind the five mammalian sst receptors. Neuronostatin is encoded by the same gene as SRIF but does not bind SRIF receptors; its effects seem mediated through the melanocortin system. r, rat; m, mouse; h, human.

according to their molecular, physiological, and morphological properties. Immunohistochemical characterization of neuronal populations in rat cortex initially stated, based on calcium-binding proteins and peptides expressions that parvalbumin (PV), SRIF, calretinin, and cholecystokinin labeled four main non-overlapping chemical classes of interneurons (Xu et al., 2006). However, several studies later reported a significant colocalization of SRIF and calretinin in mouse brain (Xu et al., 2006; Kosaka and Kosaka, 2007; Lepousez et al., 2010a), pointing out species-dependent variations in the repertoire of calcium-binding proteins and neuropeptides. It seems that neuronal populations immunoreactive for calbindin or the neuropeptide Y strongly overlap with the somatostatinergic population in rats whereas calretinin is preferentially coexpressed with SRIF in the mouse.

Recent morphological and electrophysiological studies using GIN mice focused on SRIF-expressing populations in cortical circuits. In mouse cortex, parvalbumin- and SRIF-expressing neurons respectively constitute 40 and 30% of the total GABAergic neurons, calretinin being expressed in 50% of the somatostatinergic population (Rudy et al., 2011). The remaining cortical inhibitory interneurons, expressing ionotropic serotonergic receptor 5HT3a, include VIP- and NPY-positive subpopulations whose partial colocalization with SRIF has been reported (Gonchar et al., 2007; Xu et al., 2010; Rudy et al., 2011). SRIF-positive interneurons are homogeneously distributed in all cortical layers (2–6), as compared to PV-positive inhibitory interneurons that are concentrated in the upper part of the layer (Perrenoud et al., 2012).

The major class of SRIF interneurons, the Martinotti cells, have ascending axons that arborize and spread horizontally in layer 1, targeting the distal dendritic parts of excitatory pyramidal neurons (for review, see Viollet et al., 2008). Excitatory inputs onto Martinotti cells are generally strongly facilitating, allowing feedback inhibition of the excited pyramidal cell that increases as function of the rate and the duration of the presynaptic discharge (Kapfer et al., 2007; Silberberg and Markram, 2007). The relative distance between excitatory and interneurons inputs may also impact feedback selectivity and grade, inhibition being stronger for closer inputs. A recent study using a two-photon microscopy approach coupled to uncaged glutamate in cortical slices of GIN mouse mapped the inhibitory network between SRIF-positive interneurons and pyramidal cells at the single-cell resolution (Fino and Yuste, 2011). Whatever the pyramidal cell stimulated, it led to a dense innervation of the surrounding somatostatinergic interneurons, with activity related to the proximity of the cells. Notably, this inhibitory connectivity looked unspecific as all inhibitory interneurons were locally connected to every sampled pyramidal cells regardless whether these were connected among themselves or not. This dense circuit and the fact that somatostatinergic neurons electrically communicate via gap junctions (Ma et al., 2006; Hu et al., 2011) favors the hypothesis that the entire somatostatinergic population belongs to a same inhibitory cortical circuit, contradicting the hypothesis of specific inhibitory cortical subnetworks.

Additional classes of cortical SRIF inhibitory interneurons have been recently described according to their localization, intrinsic firing properties, expression of molecular markers, and connectivity (Gonchar et al., 2007; McGarry et al., 2010). On one hand, calretinin expression was proposed as a distinctive marker (Rudy et al., 2011), since its expression is associated to distinct neuronal morphology and connectivity in populations with distinct ontogenic origin (Sousa et al., 2009; Xu et al., 2010). On the other hand, two novel SRIF-positive subtypes were identified after cluster and principal component analysis of a whole range of morphological or electrophysiological parameters (McGarry et al., 2010). These cell types have some similarities to neurons labeled in a GABAergic-GFP strain distinct from GIN (X94 strain; Ma et al., 2006), such as the lack of expression in the layer 1, but they target different cortical layers. Future identification of their respective calcium-binding proteins and neuropeptides repertoire as well as their molecular phenotype will help to conciliate these independent classifications based on morphological and electrophysiological properties.

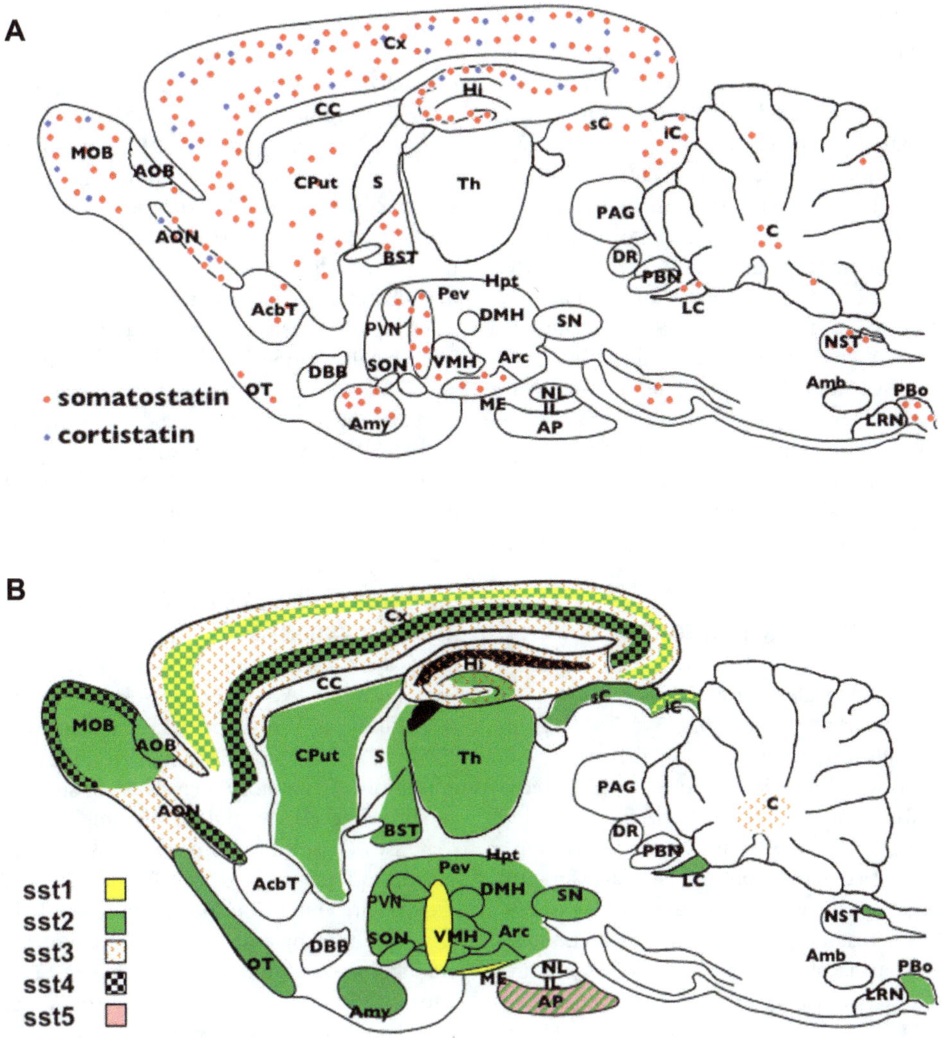


**FIGURE 2 | (A)** Schematic representation of somatostatin and cortistatin distribution in the mouse brain. **(B)** Schematic representation of somatostatin receptors distribution in the mouse brain. AcbT, nucleus accumbens; Amb, ambiguous nucleus; AP, anterior pituitary; AOB, accessory olfactory bulb; Amy, amygdala; Arc, arcuate nucleus; BNST, bed nucleus of the stria terminalis; CC, corpus callosum; CPut, caudate putamen; Cx, cortex; DBB, diagonal band of broca; DMH, dorsomedian hypothalamus; DR, dorsal raphe; iC, inferior colliculus; IL, intermediate lobe of the pituitary; Hi, hippocampus; Hpt, hypothalamus; LRN, lateral reticularis nucleus; ME, median eminence; MOB, main olfactory bulb; NL, neural lobe of the pituitary; NTS, nucleus of the solitary tract; OT, olfactory tubercle; PAG, periaqueductal gray; PBo, pre-Bötzinger nucleus; PeV, periventricular nucleus; PVN, paraventricular nucleus; sC, superior colliculus; S, septum; SON, supraoptic nucleus; SN, substantia nigra; Th, thalamus; VMH, ventromedian hypothalamus.

Somatostatin is found in most sensory systems, i.e., retina (Thermos, 2003; Cervia and Bagnoli, 2007). In the olfactory system, SRIF expression has also been described in sparse short-axon cells scattered in the deep part of the granule cell layer (the main site of intrinsic inhibitory neurons; Shipley and Ennis, 1996; Eyre et al., 2009) and in the peripheral glomerular layer (which receives sensory inputs) in some species (Hwang et al., 2004). Recently, a novel type of somatostatinergic interneurons has been described as predominant in the murine olfactory bulb and specific to this species (Lepousez et al., 2010a). SRIF-positive somata and dendritic fields are restricted to the layer of the olfactory bulb where intrinsic GABAergic interneurons and bulbar principal cells interact through dendrodendritic reciprocal synapses to initiate local gamma oscillations responsible for odor processing. Electron microscopy evidences suggest that SRIF-positive interneurons also establish reciprocal dendrodendritic synapses with the bulbar principal cells (mitral cells). SRIF-positive neurons have also been described downstream in the olfactory pathway; SRIF interneurons constitute a major GABAergic population in the pars principalis of the anterior olfactory nucleus and in the olfactory tubercle (Brunjes et al., 2011). In both piriform and entorhinal cortices, two cortical structures involved in the processing of odor coding, multipolar SRIF-positive interneurons displaying Martinotti-like morphological and electrical properties are found in the deep (Young and Sun, 2009; Saiz-Sanchez et al., 2010; Suzuki and Bekkers, 2010) and superficial (Saiz-Sanchez et al., 2010; Tahvildari et al., 2012) layers respectively.

As mentioned before, in addition to the somatostatinergic interneurons acting within microcircuits, long-projecting somatostatinergic cells have been described in several regions (Viollet et al., 2008). As glutamatergic pyramidal cells projections do, long-range inhibitory connections mediate communication between multiple brain areas. Long-range inhibitory terminals have a larger diameter and a thicker myelin layer than excitatory projection neurons, suggesting that inhibitory signal may precede the arrival of excitation in co-innervated cortical areas (Jinno et al., 2007). Long-range projecting SRIF-containing neurons are encountered in numerous brain areas (for review, see Viollet et al., 2008) such as the hippocampus (Jinno et al., 2007), the cerebral cortex (Tomioka et al., 2005), and the amygdala (McDonald et al., 2012). For instance, virtually all non-pyramidal neurons in the amygdala that have long-range projecting axons to the basal forebrain in the rat express SRIF (McDonald et al., 2012). **Figure 3** represents the projections of all long-range somatostatinergic interneurons known to date in the brain.

### SOMATOSTATIN RECEPTORS IN THE CENTRAL NERVOUS SYSTEM

Autoradiographic studies characterized initially two SRIF binding site according to their affinity for the synthetic agonist octreotide and their pattern of expression. In the early 1990s, five receptors ($sst_{1-5}$) belonging to the G-protein-coupled receptors (GPCRs) family were cloned and characterized from various species. Sequence homology is 39–57% among the five subtypes, each being highly conserved across species. They activate multiple intracellular targets (Olias et al., 2004) and display distinct internalization and dimerization properties (Csaba et al., 2012). Based on structural, pharmacological, and operational features, they are now divided into two groups displaying nanomolar affinity for both SRIF and CST: SRIF-1 ($sst_2$, $sst_3$, and $sst_5$ receptors) and SRIF-2 ($sst_1$ and $sst_4$ receptors). **Figure 2B** represents the wide expression of SRIF receptors in the CNS. In contrast to most GPCRs, $sst_{1-5}$ are unique because their gene coding sequence is devoid of introns. However, this does not preclude the generation of spliced variants such as a shorter isoform of mouse $sst_2$, named $sst_{2B}$, originating by the excision of a cryptic intronic sequence (Vanetti et al., 1992), and spliced variants of $sst_5$ in human and rodents (Córdoba-Chacón et al., 2011). While some data suggested that CST also acts through the proadrenomedullin receptor MgrX2 or the ghrelin orexigenic peptide receptors, the existence of specific CST receptors has not been demonstrated (Siehler et al., 2008). Neuronostatin does not bind to SRIF receptors, but some of its effects seem mediated through the central melanocortin system (Yosten et al., 2011). Recent findings have shown that neuronostatin is involved in regulating depressive behavior and nociception (Yang et al., 2011a,b, 2012).

The extended distribution of $sst_2$ receptors in the CNS together with studies using subtype selective SRIF analogs in both *in vivo* and *in vitro* experiments, suggested that these subtypes are the major players in the SRIF receptor family. They have broad inhibitory effects in many neuronal networks including cortex, hippocampus, limbic regions, and sensory systems (retina and olfactory system; Viollet et al., 2008; Lepousez et al., 2010a; Radojevic et al., 2011). The $sst_1$ receptor may function as an autoreceptor in basal ganglia, hypothalamus, and sensory systems (Thermos et al., 2006), and in the hippocampus (de Bundel et al., 2010). $sst_3$ receptors are localized to mature neuronal cilia in most brain regions (Stanić et al., 2008), and pharmacological or genetic blockade of $sst_3$ have marked behavioral effects (Einstein et al., 2010). $sst_4$ receptors are highly expressed in the olfactory bulb, cortex, and hippocampus, where their role remains to be clarified. In the mouse they modulate epileptic activity, whereas in the rat it seems that this effect is largely related to $sst_2$ receptors. Hippocampal $sst_4$ have also been involved in cognitive processes (Gastambide et al., 2009; Sandoval et al., 2011), functionally interacting with $sst_2$ (Dutar et al., 2002; Gastambide et al., 2010). $sst_5$ receptors mediate regulation of GH release and inhibit cell proliferation by SRIF/CST, mainly through $sst_2$/$sst_5$ receptors interaction. The detection of functional truncated forms of $sst_5$ suggests that they could interfere in and modulate those interactions (Córdoba-Chacón et al., 2011).

## SOMATOSTATINERGIC FUNCTIONS IN THE BRAIN

### NEURONAL ACTIONS OF SRIF

#### *Presynaptic mechanisms*

Somatostatin, like other neuropeptides, can modulate CNS excitability via presynaptic mechanisms (Baraban and Tallent, 2004). In rat hippocampus and cortex, SRIF induces a presynaptic inhibition of excitatory neurotransmission leading to a decrease in glutamate release and in the amplitude of evoked synaptic responses (Ishibashi and Akaike, 1995; Boehm and Betz, 1997; Tallent and Siggins, 1997; Grilli et al., 2004). The SRIF-induced decrease in glutamate release is explained by an inhibition of excitatory transmission via a G-protein of the Gi/Go family and modulation of calcium channels. Indeed, SRIF selectively inhibits N-type $Ca^{2+}$ channel via the picrotoxin-sensitive G(i)/G(o) protein. Somatostatin can also inhibit N-type $Ca^{2+}$ channels in the dentate gyrus (Baratta et al., 2002). By these inhibitory effects on excitatory synaptic transmission, SRIF, co-released with GABA on dendritic shafts of principal neurons, increases and prolongs GABA effect. This presynaptic action on $Ca^{2+}$ conductance could explain, at least in part, the inhibitory effect of SRIF on long-term potentiation in the mouse dentate gyrus (Baratta et al., 2002). Other studies suggest that presynaptic $K^+$ channels modulation may also be involved in the SRIF inhibition of excitatory transmission (Tallent and Siggins, 1997). More precisions on the mechanisms have been given by Grilli et al. (2004), demonstrating on synaptosomal preparations from mouse cerebral cortex that activation of $sst_2$ presynaptic receptors may inhibit the cAMP/PKA pathway stimulated by high potassium concentration, leading to a decrease of the evoked glutamate release. If in the hippocampus, cortex and also hypothalamus, the presynaptic effects of SRIF concern almost exclusively the excitatory transmission (Peineau et al., 2003), SRIF is also able to decrease GABA release in different brain structures, such as the rat basal forebrain (Momiyama and Zaborszky, 2006), the neostriatum (Lopez-Huerta et al., 2008), and the thalamus (Leresche et al., 2000). In the basal forebrain, SRIF presynaptically inhibits both GABA and glutamate release onto cholinergic neurons in a $Ca^{2+}$-dependent way.

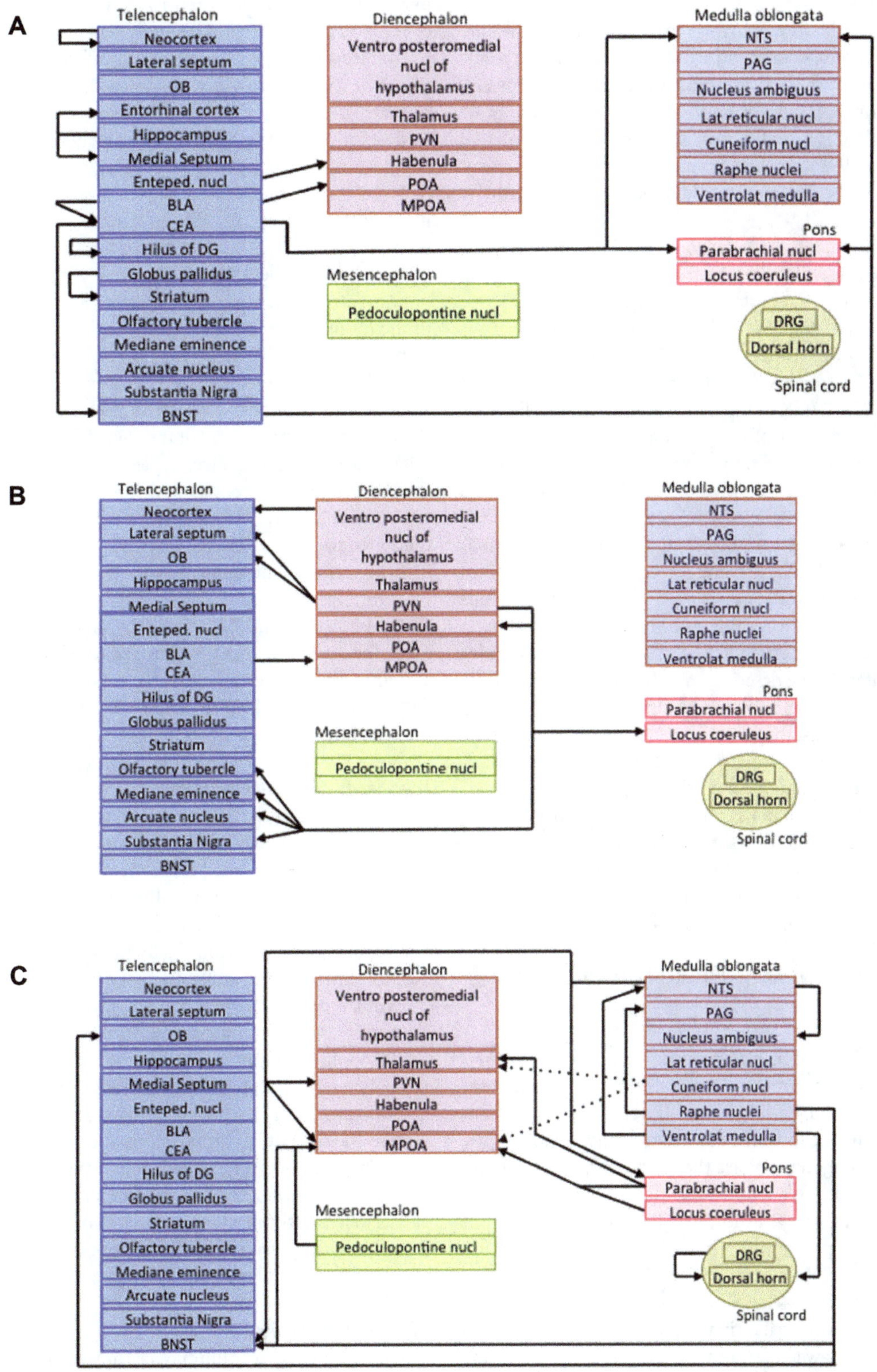


**FIGURE 3 | Schematic representations of long-range somatostatinergic interneurons in the central nervous system. (A)** Telencephalic efferent projections to the rest of the brain. **(B)** Efferent projections arising from the diencephalon and projecting to the telencephalon and the pons. **(C)** Efferent projections arising from the mesencephalon, the medulla oblongata, the pons and the spinal cord. Enteped, entopeduncular; BLA, basolateral amygdala; BNST, bed nucleus of the stria terminalis; CEA, central amygdala; DG, dentate gyrus; DRG, dorsal root ganglia; MPOA, medial preoptic area; NTS, nucleus of the solitary tract; OB, olfactory bulb; PAG, periaqueductal gray; POA, preoptic area; PVN, paraventricular nucleus.

### Postsynaptic mechanisms

Effects of SRIF on intrinsic neuronal membrane properties are well documented. Somatostatin induces a membrane hyperpolarization resulting from the activation of two distinct $K^+$ current, the voltage-sensitive $K^+$ current or M-current ($I_M$; Moore et al., 1988; Jiang et al., 2003), and a voltage-insensitive leak current (Schweitzer et al., 1998). In hippocampal CA1 pyramidal neurons, $sst_4$ seems to be the receptor subtype that couples to $I_M$ (Qiu et al., 2008).

In medium spiny neostriatal neurons, SRIF produces a qualitative change in the firing pattern from a tonic regular to an interrupted "stuttering"-like pattern (Galarraga et al., 2007). These authors demonstrated that SRIF changes the firing pattern via $sst_2$-subtype activation, which reduces the small conductance $Ca^{2+}$-activated $K^+$ currents (SK-channels) and activates large conductance $g(K)Ca^{2+}$ (GK channels). These results highlight the fact that SRIF is a regulator of cellular function in the striatum. The numerous effects of SRIF on $Ca^{2+}$ and $K^+$ channel conductance in different structures are reviewed by Cervia and Bagnoli (2007).

A huge amount of literature has tried to define the pharmacological nature of SRIF effects, using agonists and antagonists of SRIF receptors or mice invalidated for receptor subtypes. Results are often controversial and are different in mice and rats (Aourz et al., 2011). Therefore, the classification of SRIF effects is complex and it is accentuated by the description of functional cooperation between different receptor subtypes $sst_2/sst_3$, $sst_2/sst_4$, $sst_3/sst_4$ (Moneta et al., 2002; Gastambide et al., 2010; Aourz et al., 2011). Recent publications suggest that $sst_3$ and $sst_4$ (but not $sst_1$; de Bundel et al., 2010) have potent anticonvulsive properties (Aourz et al., 2011), and that $sst_2$, the major receptor subtype involved in the anticonvulsant effect of SRIF in the hippocampus exerts a functional cooperation with $sst_3/sst_4$. In hippocampus, $sst_1$ activation inhibits both NMDA- and AMPA-mediated responses but did not affect the inhibitory transmission (Cammalleri et al., 2009).

## SRIF-CONTAINING NEURONS ARE INVOLVED IN PHYSIOLOGICAL FUNCTIONS

### Interneurons

A large diversity of inhibitory interneurons is able to exert inhibition on specific compartments of principal cells. Among these populations is the dendrite-targeting SRIF-expressing interneuron located in oriens-lacunosum moleculare of the hippocampus. These SRIF-containing neurons are the only subtype of interneuron that reliably follows synaptic stimulation of the alveus in the theta frequency range via activation of their kainate receptors, suggesting that they play an important role in theta band frequency oscillations (Goldin et al., 2007). Spontaneous activities of inhibitory interneurons have been characterized and SRIF-containing neurons are described in the cortex and piriform cortex as regular-spiking (Kawaguchi and Kubota, 1998; Suzuki and Bekkers, 2010) or low-threshold spiking neurons (Goldberg et al., 2004), often opposed to the fast spiking PV-containing neurons. In the hippocampus, SRIF neurons are locked to the ascending phase of the theta cycle. However, using an optogenetic inhibition of different populations of interneurons, it was recently demonstrated that silencing SRIF interneurons increases burst firing of pyramidal cells without altering the theta phase of spikes (Royer et al., 2012). Applying optogenetic technique to animals trained to run head-fixed on a treadmill belt rich with visual-tactile stimuli, these authors provided evidence that the dendritic (but not somatic) inhibition of pyramidal neurons by SRIF interneurons is critical for controlling spike burst firing during active exploration. They concluded that perisomatic PV-targeting interneurons control the spikes' theta phase while the dendrite-targeting SRIF interneurons control the rate of discharge. This is in agreement with the fact that dendritic but not somatic GABAergic inhibition is decreased in experimental epilepsy (Cossart et al., 2001). Combining optogenetic stimulation with *in vivo* two-photon imaging in the mouse visual cortex, Wilson et al. (2012) demonstrate that soma-targeting PV neurons regulate the gain of cortical response, while dendritic-targeting SRIF neurons shift response level and alter stimulus selectivity, leaving response gain unaffected.

Another demonstration of the role of SRIF interneurons in cellular function has been given recently (Gentet et al., 2012). In this study, SRIF neurons recorded in the barrel cortex of awake mice were tonically active during quiet wakefulness but they decreased their firing during whisker sensorimotor processing. This decrease in firing relieves the dendrites of excitatory pyramidal neurons from inhibition.

It is known that inhibitory neurons have diverse roles in physiological and synaptic function, based on their connectivity patterns and intrinsic properties. All the experiments described above demonstrated that SRIF interneurons have a prominent role in the regulation of distal dendrites excitability.

### Long-range projecting neurons

The long-range projecting somatostatinergic non-pyramidal cells found in the hippocampus target the medial septum and the medial entorhinal cortex (Viollet et al., 2008; Melzer et al., 2012) and more specifically form inhibitory synapses on GABAergic interneurons of these areas. They coordinate activity between distant brain regions, contributing to the generation and the synchronization of rhythmic oscillatory activity in the hippocampus and entorhinal cortex (Melzer et al., 2012). They are therefore involved in spatial and temporal coding. Interestingly, early-generated GABA-containing hub neurons, dendrite-targeting interneurons, express preferentially SRIF and give long-range projecting neurons (Picardo et al., 2011). These superconnected hub cells are present early in the developing hippocampus. They develop a widespread axonal arborization and remain into adulthood. They play a key role in the control of the hippocampal giant depolarizing potentials as well as in the modulation of network dynamics. In the other brain areas, the precise contribution of these long-projecting SRIF neurons in the oscillatory activity still needs to be addressed.

### Hypophysiotropic neurons

Somatotropin release inhibiting factor was initially discovered as a neurohormone that inhibits GH secretion from anterior pituitary somatotroph cells. This function is exerted by hypophysiotropic neurons, located in the anterior periventricular hypothalamic nucleus, which project to the median eminence and release the peptide in the fenestrated capillaries of the hypothalamo–hypophyseal portal vessels; thus directly connecting the brain to the anterior pituitary. SRIF is also a potent inhibitor of many hormonal and exocrine secretions as well as an antiproliferative agent in normal and tumoral tissue (Epelbaum, 1986). SRIF analogs (octreotide and lanreotide) have potent inhibitory effects on hypersecretion, thereby alleviating the symptoms associated with neuroendocrine tumors. Furthermore, the antitumor potential of octreotide is now well documented. Pasireotide, a long-acting SRIF analog, has the advantage of targeting a wider range of SRIF receptors (subtypes 1, 2, 3, and 5) than the analogs previously used in clinical practice (which preferentially target subtype 2) and has a broader spectrum of activity (for review, see Bousquet et al., 2012).

## INVOLVEMENT OF SRIF SYSTEMS IN SENSORY, MOTOR, AND COGNITIVE FUNCTIONS

Since SRIF systems are widely expressed in CNS, they are involved in numerous functions including nociceptive and vasoconstrictor properties. Here, we will present recent advances about the role of SRIF systems in autonomic responses (digestion, cardiac rate, and respiration) and motor functions as well as cognitive functions such as learning and memory and emotion (for review, see Viollet et al., 2008).

### Somatostatinergic involvement in sensory functions

***Somatostatin and visual information.*** Somatostatinergic system is expressed in mammalian retina (for review, see Thermos, 2003; Casini et al., 2005; Cervia et al., 2008), where it is suspected to exert multiple actions on neurons and on retinal physiology. SRIF acts as a positive factor in the retina by regulating homeostasis and protecting neurons against damage. Both $sst_2$ and $sst_5$ somatostatinergic receptors are involved. Indeed, activation of $sst_2$ protects the retina from ischemic insults *ex vivo* (Mastrodimou et al., 2005) and $sst_2$ as well as $sst_5$ receptor activation protect from excitotoxicity *in vivo* (Kiagiadaki and Thermos, 2008; Kiagiadaki et al., 2010; Kokona et al., 2012). The severity of angiogenic responses to hypoxia is correlated to the $sst_2$ expression level in the retina (Dal Monte et al., 2007). Moreover, the $sst_2$-preferring agonist octreotide prevents hypoxia-induced VEGF up-regulation (Dal Monte et al., 2009).

***Somatostatinergic modulation of olfactory discrimination.*** Recent studies have shown that SRIF modulates olfactory processing in mice (Lepousez et al., 2010a,b). In mouse main olfactory bulb, SRIF is mainly concentrated in local GABAergic interneurons synaptically connected to the mitral cells by reciprocal dendrodendritic synapses. When activated by an odor, mitral cells synchronize and generate gamma oscillations of the local field potentials that are involved in olfactory processing. Pharmacological or genetic blockade of $sst_2$ transmission in the olfactory bulb of awake animal selectively decreased the gamma oscillations power while pharmacological activation of $sst_2$ had opposite effects. These treatments were respectively correlated to either impairment or improvement of odor discrimination performances of the pharmacologically injected animals. Thus, bulbar endogenous SRIF, presumably released from external plexiform layer interneurons, affects gamma oscillations through the dendrodendritic reciprocal synapse and contributes to olfactory processing.

### Involvement of SRIF in learning and memory

It has been reported for decades that SRIF plays a role in learning and memory at different stages of information processing. The first studies investigating its role in cognition showed that intracerebroventricular administrations of SRIF improved learning in active avoidance tasks (Bollok et al., 1983; Vecsei et al., 1983; Vecsei and Widerlov, 1988) and prevented electroshock-induced amnesia in passive avoidance paradigms (Vecsei et al., 1983, 1984). Conversely, the depletion of SRIF in the brain by cysteamine (which depletes SRIF levels; Szabo and Reichlin, 1981) produced major memory deficits in passive avoidance (Bakhit and Swerdlow, 1986; Schettini et al., 1988; DeNoble et al., 1989). These studies revealed that SRIF is involved in the acquisition of information but other studies showed that cysteamine produced memory deficits not only when given before the training session but also within a critical time window (0–4 h) after acquisition, suggesting that SRIF plays a critical role in memory consolidation processing (Haroutunian et al., 1987, 1989; Schettini et al., 1988; Vecsei et al., 1990).

The hippocampus is an essential structure in learning and memory (Jeneson and Squire, 2012), and is also a chosen site to study the effects of SRIF on learning and memory since injection of cysteamine impairs tasks requiring its integrity (DeNoble et al., 1989; Guillou et al., 1998). Surprisingly in the rodent hippocampus, both activation of SRIF receptors as well as depletion of SRIF contents generate hippocampal memory impairments. Indeed, microinjections of cysteamine, SRIF or CST directly into the hippocampus impaired hippocampal-dependent spatial learning (Guillou et al., 1993; Sanchez-Alavez et al., 2000; Lamirault et al., 2001; Mendez-Diaz et al., 2005; Gastambide et al., 2009). Consistent with these pharmacological results, transgenic mice overexpressing CST display a profound impairment of spatial learning (Tallent et al., 2005). Studies that investigated which SRIF receptor mediates SRIF memory effect showed that intra-hippocampal injections of the $sst_4$ agonist, but not $sst_1$, $sst_2$, or $sst_3$ agonists, dramatically impaired spatial memory formation (Gastambide et al., 2009). Importantly, these authors found that concomitantly to the impairment of spatial memory, an $sst_4$ agonist also enhanced the use of striatum-dependent memory. Therefore, it was hypothesized that hippocampal $sst_4$ controls the use of cognitive strategies by switching from hippocampus-based multiple associations to simple striatum-based behavioral response through a functional interaction with $sst_2$ receptor (Gastambide et al., 2010). The precise cellular and molecular mechanisms involved in this functional interaction between $sst_2$ and $sst_4$ are not fully understood but some studies showed that $sst_4$ mediates increases in glutamatergic excitability and bursting frequency, which were blocked by $sst_2$ agonists or antagonists and were lacking in $sst_2$ knockout (KO) mice (Moneta et al., 2002; Cammalleri et al., 2006). Therefore, $sst_4$ is not the unique SRIF receptor in the hippocampus mediating SRIF memory effects as $sst_2$ also modulates memory as previously suggested by Dutar et al. (2002).

### Involvement of SRIF in the control of emotion

Somatostatin and its receptors are strongly expressed in the different nuclei of the amygdala (Hannon et al., 2002), a key brain structure involved in the emotional assessment of the environment (Schumann et al., 2011). Despite the extensive expression of SRIF systems in this area, the effects of SRIF on emotions have not yet been studied extensively. Nevertheless, some studies reported an involvement of SRIF systems in the control of emotion and anxiety. Indeed, a very recent work revealed that the pattern of activation of SRIF-positive interneurons was specific to the nuclei of the amygdala considered and also to the kind of stressor used (Butler et al., 2012). Moreover, SRIF has anxiolytic- and antidepressant-like effects (Engin et al., 2008b) that are associated with the suppression of the frequency of hippocampal theta activity, a neurophysiological signature common to most classes of anxiolytic drugs (i.e., benzodiazepines, selective 5-HT reuptake inhibitors, 5-HT1A agonists). These effects seem to be mediated by $sst_2$ receptor since both intra-septal and intra-amygdala SRIF microinfusions induced anxiolytic effects that were completely reversed by selective $sst_2$ receptor antagonist injection in these brain areas (Yeung and Treit, 2012). Additional evidence for a specific role of $sst_2$ receptor came from the observation that a stressful experience is associated with an increase of $sst_2$ mRNA levels within the amygdala (Nanda et al., 2008) and that mice lacking $sst_2$ receptor display increased anxiety-like behaviors associated with increased pituitary ACTH levels, a main regulator of the stress response (Viollet et al., 2000).

#### *Involvement of SRIF in locomotion*

An involvement for SRIF was also reported in motor functions. Increased motor activity was shown in rats receiving intracerebroventricular administration of SRIF (Havlicek et al., 1976) as well as in mice receiving unilateral striatal infusions of the peptide by retrodialysis (Hathway et al., 2004) and in animals receiving direct injections of SRIF in the nucleus accumbens (Raynor et al., 1993). Tashev et al. (2001) showed that SRIF modulated locomotor activity in biphasic manner. Indeed, shortly after SRIF striatal injection a decrease of locomotor activity is observed whereas later, the locomotor behavior is increased. Similar effects have been found after striatal injection of $sst_2$ and $sst_4$ agonists. On the other hand, genetic invalidation of $sst_2$ receptor in two different strains of mice as well as SRIF null mice showed an impairment of motor functions (Viollet et al., 2000; Zeyda et al., 2001; Allen et al., 2003). But the role of SRIF in locomotion seems to be limited to fine motor control since these different lines of transgenic mice only develop impaired motor coordination in tasks that require a fine motor control and display normal levels of motor activity and coordination in undemanding tasks (Viollet et al., 2000; Zeyda et al., 2001; Allen et al., 2003).

#### *Autonomic responses*

Somatotropin release inhibiting factor and its receptors are found in several medulla oblongata nuclei that control autonomic functions such as digestion, cardiac rate, and respiration (Llona and Eugenín, 2005; Spary et al., 2008; Viollet et al., 2008). In the preBötzinger complex (preBötC), a critical component of the respiratory rhythm generator that underlies mammalian breathing, SRIF is expressed in a subpopulation of glutamatergic neurokinin 1 receptor-positive neurons, a kind of neuron rhythmically active (Stornetta et al., 2003). Originating from the homeogene Dbx1 lineage, these cells are mandatory for breathing, since invalidation of the Dbx1 gene impaired their differentiation and disrupted respiratory rhythm generation in the preBötC (Bouvier et al., 2010; Gray et al., 2010). Acute silencing of somatostatinergic preBötC neurons increased respiratory rhythm, leading to persistent apnea (Tan et al., 2008). Similar effects were found *in vitro* after pharmacological blockade of $sst_2$ transmission, while exogenous SRIF application decreased rhythms generation (Pantaleo et al., 2011; Ramírez-Jarquín et al., 2012). This demonstrated that the peptide exerts a tonic inhibitory control on the rythmogenic neurons in order to avoid deleterious overactivity, probably through cellular subdomain-specific inhibitory and excitatory synaptic contacts (Wei et al., 2012). The existence of long-range somatostatinergic projections to either contralateral PreBötC (Stornetta et al., 2003) or downstream premotor neurons (Tan et al., 2010) favors a neuromodulatory role for PreBötC SRIF (Llona and Eugenín, 2005), whose developmental impairment may be involved in human pathologies (Schwarzacher et al., 2011) such as the sudden infant death syndrome (Lavezzi and Matturri, 2008).

## SOMATOSTATINERGIC NETWORKS IN PATHOLOGICAL CONDITIONS

In animals, an alteration of SRIF systems is observed during normal aging (Stanley et al., 2012) and pathological models of aging. In human a similar specific dysregulation is observed in normal pathological disorders such as some neurodegenerative and psychiatric diseases (Glorioso et al., 2011; Gleichmann et al., 2012).

### ALZHEIMER'S DISEASE

Somatostatin has been involved in Alzheimer's disease (AD) pathology for a number of years. Indeed, since the early 1980s, it is known that SRIF levels in cortex and hippocampus are decreased in AD patients (Davies et al., 1980). Later, it was demonstrated that the decline in SRIF concentrations in the CSF (Tamminga et al., 1987) or in the middle frontal gyrus (Dournaud et al., 1995) correlates with cognitive deficits. Using quantitative real-time PCR, a recent study confirmed this decrease of SRIF in the inferior, medial, and superior temporal lobe of AD patients (Gahete et al., 2010). Interestingly, SRIF concentrations were reported to be significantly lower in Alzheimer patients carrying the epsilon 4 allele of APOE (Grouselle et al., 1998), the main genetic risk factor described to date for late-onset AD (Genin et al., 2011). In addition, two different studies found in Finnish and Chinese patients that polymorphisms in the SST gene are associated with the risk of developing AD (Vepsalainen et al., 2007; Xue et al., 2009).

Regarding SRIF receptors, data are limited and controversial. Although all studies agreed on a decrease of SRIF receptors in AD, controversies appeared about the proportion, the localization, and receptor subtype specificity of this decrease. SRIF receptor quantification using quantitative real-time PCR in AD temporal lobe showed a decrease of $sst_1$, $sst_3$, and $sst_4$ receptors whereas $sst_2$ and $sst_5$ receptors were unchanged (Gahete et al., 2010). Previously, an immunohistochemistry study reported a similar decrease of $sst_4$ but showed a reduction in neuronal $sst_5$ – and a modest decrease in $sst_2$ –like immunoreactivity without any changes in $sst_1$ immunoreactive neurons (Kumar, 2005). Surprisingly, in the same study, an increase of $sst_3$ subtype was observed in AD cortex. A radioligand binding and functional study showed a general receptor decrease in AD brain (Beal et al., 1985). More specifically, receptors levels in the frontal and temporal cortex were reduced by approximately 50% of control values in AD patients while a 40% reduction was reported in the hippocampus and no significant changes were found in the cingulate cortex, postcentral gyrus, temporal pole, and superior temporal gyrus. Another radioligand binding study revealed that while the maximal binding capacity of the SRIF-1 receptor subtype (primarily $sst_2$, and possibly $sst_5$) is altered in frontal and temporal cortices, other putative cortical SRIF receptor classes (SRIF-2 sites, i.e., $sst_1$ and $sst_4$) are not as broadly affected (Krantic et al., 1992). Finally, a last study showed a significant decrease only in the frontal cortex, but not in other brain regions (Bergstrom et al., 1991). Because of the cholinergic hypothesis regarding AD etiology, it was concluded that the pattern of change of SRIF binding in AD cortex might be secondary to the degeneration of SRIF receptor-bearing cholinergic afferents arising from the nucleus basalis. In line with this idea, experiments in the literature demonstrate that the selective destruction of cholinergic neurons of the basal forebrain with intracerebroventricular injection of 192-IgG saporin produces an irreversible loss of SRIF-immunoreactive neurons in the hilus of the hippocampus (Jolkkonen et al., 1997) and in the cortex (Zhang et al., 1998). This last study shows a correlation between the intensity of acetylcholinesterase in the cortex and the number of remaining SRIF cells. These data highlight a trophic dependence of SRIF neurons on cholinergic inputs and are consistent with observations in AD and aging.

Although SRIF deficit is not correlated with the amyloid load in AD brain patients (Dournaud et al., 1995), SRIF was identified as a modulator that increases brain neprilysin activity, one of the main enzymes involved in Aβ degradation (Saito et al., 2005). Recently, it has been shown that neuropeptide pituitary adenylate cyclase-activating polypeptide slows down AD-like pathology and improves cognition in a transgenic mouse model of AD through the activation of SRIF-neprilysin cascade (Rat et al., 2011). In mouse primary embryonic neurons, SRIF concomitantly increased neprilysin activity and decreased Aβ42 in the culture medium and these effects were blocked by an $sst_5$ antagonist (but also an agonist at $sst_1$ and $sst_3$ receptors; for review, see Epelbaum et al., 2009). Moreover, neprilysin activity was decreased by 50% and Aβ42 increased by a similar extent in SRIF KO mice (Saito et al., 2005). Such findings may have important implications for understanding the cellular mechanisms leading to AD and suggest that SRIF and its receptors are potential pharmacological targets for AD. Indeed, FK962, which promotes SRIF production in the brain, co-administrated with donepezil, an acetylcholinesterase inhibitor widely used to treat patients, enhances cognition in rat and has been proposed as an add-on therapy for AD (McCarthy et al., 2011). In addition, Rubio et al. (2012) recently suggested that SRIF and CST act as a protective agent against Aβ toxicity. However, in APP transgenic mouse models, data concerning SRIF-containing interneurons are contradictory. In the triple-transgenic model of AD, 3×Tg-AD, inhibitory neurotransmission is unchanged in the cerebral cortex and hippocampus (Gleichmann et al., 2012). In a APP/PS1 mouse model of AD, as soon as 6 months of age, a decrease in the number of oriens-lacunosum moleculare hilar perforant path-associated SRIF-positive interneurons was evidenced in the hippocampus, when no change was demonstrated for 21 additional mRNA markers tested (Ramos et al., 2006). In the APPswe/PS1dE9 mouse model, Aβ deposition disrupted cognitive circuits when the cholinergic and somatostatinergic systems remained relatively intact (Savonenko et al., 2005). Another study on this last model even found that, in most brain regions tested, SRIF concentrations were increased rather than decreased relative to controls (Horgan et al., 2007). Thus, the validity of a direct and major role for SRIF in the regulation of Aβ42 degradation remains to be further confirmed (Iwata et al., 2005). More recent studies, focusing on olfaction, an early-altered function in AD (Wilson et al., 2009), account for evidence of a relationship between Aβ pathology and SRIF alterations in the disease. Indeed, SRIF interneurons and receptors are selectively reduced by approximately 50% in the anterior olfactory nucleus of AD patients (Saiz-Sanchez et al., 2010). These authors suggested that SRIF decreases in AD might be linked with Aβ. Moreover, an increase in the levels of aggregated Aβ peptide is observed with aging in olfactory cortices of APP/PS1 transgenic mouse model of AD, and it is accompanied by a fall in numbers of SRIF-positive interneurons (Saiz-Sanchez et al., 2012).

Experiments from our laboratory demonstrated that intrahippocampal injections of Aβ in rats induced aberrant inhibitory septo-hippocampal network activity associated with an impairment of hippocampal memory processes (Villette et al., 2010). This effect can be explained by the selective loss of long-range hippocampo-septal projecting neurons population containing calbindin and SRIF (Villette et al., 2012). This population of SRIF neurons could be a favored target for Aβ, explaining the early decrease of SRIF observed in AD.

Somatotropin release inhibiting factor is not only interacting with Aβ42 in AD, it has also an effect on Tau phosphorylation. Rubio et al. (2008) indicated that in mouse cortex SRIF and CST induce Tau phosphorylation at Ser262, a site modified in AD (Wang et al., 2007), although with different kinetics. An $sst_2/sst_4$ interaction seems implicated in this process but the types of phosphatases that are involved remain to be determined. Moreover, in human apoE4 knock-in mice where Tau phosphorylation and intracellular neurofibrillary tangle-like deposits are detected (Huang et al., 2001; Harris et al., 2003; Brecht et al., 2004), Huang's group showed that the number of SRIF-positive interneurons correlated inversely with the performance of these mice in a spatial memory task (Andrews-Zwilling et al., 2010).

## PARKINSON'S DISEASE

Alteration of SRIF levels is also observed in other neurodegenerative diseases. Indeed, decrease in SRIF levels has been described in demented Parkinson's disease patients (Epelbaum et al., 1989) as well as in a unilateral 6-OHDA experimental mouse model of Parkinson's disease (Nilsson et al., 2009). Recent data obtained in a rat model of Parkinsonism showed that an alteration of presynaptic modulation by SRIF after dopamine deprivation. This observation may underlie a homeostatic mechanism trying to compensate for the excitability imbalance between direct and indirect basal ganglia pathways found during Parkinson's disease (Lopez-Huerta et al., 2012).

## MAJOR DEPRESSIVE DISORDER

Evidence in major depressive disorder (MDD) suggests an impaired excitation/inhibition balance that is potentially mediated by decreased GABA content (Levinson et al., 2010). More specifically, Sibille et al. (2011) reported a down-regulation of SRIF in the dorsolateral prefrontal cortex (PFC), the subgenual cingulate cortices (Tripp et al., 2011), and the amygdala (Guilloux et al., 2011) of MDD patients. Engin et al. (2008a) and Engin and Treit (2009) revealed an antidepressant effect of SRIF mediated by either $sst_2$ or $sst_3$ receptor and suggested that while SRIF itself is not appropriate for clinical use because of its short half-life and diverse range of effects (Pinter et al., 2006), a closely related SRIF derivative may have some potential for the pharmacological treatment of depression.

## SCHIZOPHRENIA

One of the most consistent findings in schizophrenia neuropathology is deficits in cortical inhibitory interneurons across multiple cortical regions (Hashimoto et al., 2008). It has been known for years that cerebral cortical concentrations of SRIF are reduced in schizophrenics (Roberts et al., 1983) as well as hippocampal concentration (Ferrier et al., 1983; Konradi et al., 2011). Moreover, Hashimoto et al. (2008) found that subjects with schizophrenia exhibited deficits in SRIF expression in the PFC, and this was further confirmed after global analysis from six previously published microarray studies (Perez-Santiago et al., 2012). A recent study suggested that this decrease of SRIF-positive inhibitory interneurons in the PFC may be related to changes in an inflammatory response pathway that are often observed in schizophrenics (Fillman et al., 2012). In addition, Beneyto et al. (2012) showed that SRIF neurotransmission in the PFC of subjects with schizophrenia is also altered at the postsynaptic level in a receptor subtype-, layer-, and cell type-specific manner. The expression of $sst_2$, but not $sst_1$, mRNA is preferentially lower in layers 5–6, and in larger, putative pyramidal neurons in those layers. These authors suggested converging pre- and postsynaptic mechanisms to reduce inhibitory neurotransmission in pyramidal neurons in the PFC, which could alter the synchronization of low frequency oscillations and disturb working memory performance in subjects with schizophrenia.

## EPILEPSY

Somatostatin is highly expressed in brain regions associated with seizures and has been implicated as playing a prominent role in epilepsy (Vezzani and Hoyer, 1999) based on the observation of an activity-dependent release of SRIF during seizures, the modulation of SRIF mRNA expression, peptide and receptors levels by seizures and the effect of SRIF and its analogs on seizures (Tallent and Qiu, 2008; Zafar et al., 2012). Temporal lobe epilepsy (TLE) is characterized by hippocampal sclerosis together with profound phenotypic changes of different classes of interneurons. Hilar SRIF interneurons undergo extensive degeneration in patients with hippocampal sclerosis (de Lanerolle et al., 1989; Robbins et al., 1991). Recently, this selective neurodegeneration has been linked to the specific enrichment of somatostatinergic neurons in striatum-enriched phosphatase, an enzyme that counteracts the MAPK neuroprotective pathway (Choi et al., 2007; Florio et al., 2008). SRIF receptors may represent potential therapeutic targets for TLE. Indeed, SRIF is released in characteristic conditions of seizures and SRIF and its analogs affect seizures (Vezzani and Hoyer, 1999; Buckmaster et al., 2002). However, information on the precise contribution of each SRIF receptor on the SRIF-induced inhibition of epileptiform activity is still limited. Although the $sst_2$ receptor is likely to mediate the anticonvulsant effects of SRIF in rat hippocampus (Vezzani and Hoyer, 1999), observations in the mouse support a central role for $sst_4$ (Moneta et al., 2002) and/or $sst_1$ receptors (Cammalleri et al., 2004, 2006) in mediating SRIF inhibition of epileptiform activity. In a rodent model of cortical focal ischemia, $sst_2$ is also activated while the infarct size is significantly reduced in $sst_2$ KO mice (Stumm et al., 2004). However, recent data in rats showed that $sst_1$ receptors do not appear to mediate the *in vivo* anticonvulsive effect of SRIF (de Bundel et al., 2010), whereas $sst_3$ and $sst_4$ mediate this effect through a functional interaction with $sst_2$ receptor (Aourz et al., 2011).

## CONCLUSION

Somatostatin systems are widely expressed in the different brain regions and are involved in numerous processes from sensory to cognitive functions, suggesting that they play major roles in brain functioning. These key roles are illustrated by the decrease of SRIF concentrations observed in neurodegenerative diseases such as AD and Parkinson's disease but also in psychiatric diseases such as schizophrenia and MDD. From this perspective, SRIF systems represent a potential and challenging therapeutic target. Further studies need to be carried on to unravel the role of SRIF systems in all functions they have been implicated in.

## ACKNOWLEDGMENTS

Supported by NeRF post-doctoral fellowship (to Guillaume Martel), ANR-10-MALZ-003-01 SOMADOLF and Fondation Recherche Plan Alzheimer.

## REFERENCES

Allen, J. P., Hathway, G. J., Clarke, N. J., Jowett, M. I., Topps, S., Kendrick, K. M., et al. (2003). Somatostatin receptor 2 knockout/lacZ knockin mice show impaired motor coordination and reveal sites of somatostatin action within the striatum. *Eur. J. Neurosci.* 17, 1881–1895.

Andrews-Zwilling, Y., Bien-Ly, N., Xu, Q., Li, G., Bernardo, A., Yoon, S. Y., et al. (2010). Apolipoprotein E4 causes age- and Tau-dependent impairment of GABAergic interneurons, leading to learning and memory deficits in mice. *J. Neurosci.* 30, 13707–13717.

Aourz, N., De Bundel, D., Stragier, B., Clinckers, R., Portelli, J., Michotte, Y., et al. (2011). Rat hippocampal somatostatin $sst_3$ and $sst_4$ receptors mediate anticonvulsive effects *in vivo*: indications of functional interactions with $sst_2$ receptors. *Neuropharmacology* 61, 1327–1333.

Bakhit, C., and Swerdlow, N. (1986). Behavioral changes following central injection of cysteamine in rats. *Brain Res.* 365, 159–163.

Baraban, S. C., and Tallent, M. K. (2004). Interneuron Diversity Series: interneuronal neuropeptides – endogenous regulators of neuronal excitability. *Trends Neurosci.* 27, 135–142.

Baratta, M. V., Lamp, T., and Tallent, M. K. (2002). Somatostatin depresses long-term potentiation and $Ca^{2+}$ signaling in mouse dentate gyrus. *J. Neurophysiol.* 88, 3078–3086.

Beal, M. F., Mazurek, M. F., Tran, V. T., Chattha, G., Bird, E. D., and Martin, J. B. (1985). Reduced numbers of somatostatin receptors in the cerebral cortex in Alzheimer's disease. *Science* 229, 289–291.

Beneyto, M., Morris, H. M., Rovensky, K. C., and Lewis, D. A. (2012). Lamina- and cell-specific alterations in cortical somatostatin receptor 2 mRNA expression in schizophrenia. *Neuropharmacology* 62, 1598–1605.

Bergstrom, L., Garlind, A., Nilsson, L., Alafuzoff, I., Fowler, C. J., Winblad, B., et al. (1991). Regional distribution of somatostatin receptor binding and modulation of adenylyl cyclase activity in Alzheimer's disease brain. *J. Neurol. Sci.* 105, 225–233.

Boehm, S., and Betz, H. (1997). Somatostatin inhibits excitatory transmission at rat hippocampal synapses via presynaptic receptors. *J. Neurosci.* 17, 4066–4075.

Bollok, I., Vecsei, L., and Telegdy, G. (1983). The effects of interaction between propranolol and somatostatin on the active avoidance behavior, open-field activity and electroconvulsive shock-induced amnesia of rats. *Neuropeptides* 3, 263–270.

Bousquet, C., Lasfargues, C., Chalabi, M., Billah, S. M., Susini, C., Vezzosi, D., et al. (2012). Clinical review: current scientific rationale for the use of somatostatin analogs and mTOR inhibitors in neuroendocrine tumor therapy. *J. Clin. Endocrinol. Metab.* 97, 727–737.

Bouvier, J., Thoby-Brisson, M., Renier, N., Dubreuil, V., Ericson, J., Champagnat, J., et al. (2010). Hindbrain interneurons and axon guidance signaling critical for breathing. *Nat. Neurosci.* 13, 1066–1074.

Brazeau, P., Vale, W., Burgus, R., Ling, N., Butcher, M., Rivier, J., et al. (1973). Hypothalamic polypeptide that inhibits the secretion of immunoreactive pituitary growth hormone. *Science* 179, 77–79.

Brecht, W. J., Harris, F. M., Chang, S., Tesseur, I., Yu, G. Q., Xu, Q., et al. (2004). Neuron-specific apolipoprotein e4 proteolysis is associated with increased tau phosphorylation in brains of transgenic mice. *J. Neurosci.* 24, 2527–2534.

Brunjes, P. C., Kay, R. B., and Arrivillaga, J. P. (2011). The mouse olfactory peduncle. *J. Comp. Neurol.* 519, 2870–2886.

Buckmaster, P. S., Otero-Corchon, V., Rubinstein, M., and Low, M. J. (2002). Heightened seizure severity in somatostatin knockout mice. *Epilepsy Res.* 48, 43–56.

Butler, R. K., White, L. C., Frederick-Duus, D., Kaigler, K. F., Fadel, J. R., and Wilson, M. A. (2012). Comparison of the activation of somatostatin- and neuropeptide Y-containing neuronal populations of the rat amygdala following two different anxiogenic stressors. *Exp. Neurol.* 238, 52–63.

Cammalleri, M., Cervia, D., Dal Monte, M., Martini, D., Langenegger, D., Fehlmann, D., et al. (2006). Compensatory changes in the hippocampus of somatostatin knockout mice: upregulation of somatostatin receptor 2 and its function in the control of bursting activity and synaptic transmission. *Eur. J. Neurosci.* 23, 2404–2422.

Cammalleri, M., Cervia, D., Langenegger, D., Liu, Y., Dal Monte, M., Hoyer, D., et al. (2004). Somatostatin receptors differentially affect spontaneous epileptiform activity in mouse hippocampal slices. *Eur. J. Neurosci.* 20, 2711–2721.

Cammalleri, M., Martini, D., Timperio, A. M., and Bagnoli, P. (2009). Functional effects of somatostatin receptor 1 activation on synaptic transmission in the mouse hippocampus. *J. Neurochem.* 111, 1466–1477.

Casini, G., Catalani, E., Dal Monte, M., and Bagnoli, P. (2005). Functional aspects of the somatostatinergic system in the retina and the potential therapeutic role of somatostatin in retinal disease. *Histol. Histopathol.* 20, 615–632.

Cervia, D., and Bagnoli, P. (2007). An update on somatostatin receptor signaling in native systems and new insights on their pathophysiology. *Pharmacol. Ther.* 116, 322–341.

Cervia, D., Casini, G., and Bagnoli, P. (2008). Physiology and pathology of somatostatin in the mammalian retina: a current view. *Mol. Cell. Endocrinol.* 286, 112–122.

Choi, Y. S., Lin, S. L., Lee, B., Kurup, P., Cho, H. Y., Naegele, J. R., et al. (2007). Status epilepticus-induced somatostatinergic hilar interneuron degeneration is regulated by striatal enriched protein tyrosine phosphatase. *J. Neurosci.* 27, 2999–3009.

Córdoba-Chacón, J., Gahete, M. D., Durán-Prado, M., Luque, R. M., and Castaño, J. P. (2011). Truncated somatostatin receptors as new players in somatostatin-cortistatin pathophysiology. *Ann. N. Y. Acad. Sci.* 1220, 6–15.

Cossart, R., Dinocourt, C., Hirsch, J. C., Merchan-Perez, A., De Felipe, J., Ben-Ari, Y., et al. (2001). Dendritic but not somatic GABAergic inhibition is decreased in experimental epilepsy. *Nat. Neurosci.* 4, 52–62.

Csaba, Z., Peineau, S., and Dournaud, P. (2012). Molecular mechanisms of somatostatin receptor trafficking. *J. Mol. Endocrinol.* 48, R1–R12.

Dal Monte, M., Cammalleri, M., Martini, D., Casini, G., and Bagnoli, P. (2007). Antiangiogenic role of somatostatin receptor 2 in a model of hypoxia-induced neovascularization in the retina: results from transgenic mice. *Invest. Ophthalmol. Vis. Sci.* 48, 3480–3489.

Dal Monte, M., Ristori, C., Cammalleri, M., and Bagnoli, P. (2009). Effects of somatostatin analogues on retinal angiogenesis in a mouse model of oxygen-induced retinopathy: involvement of the somatostatin receptor subtype 2. *Invest. Ophthalmol. Vis. Sci.* 50, 3596–3606.

Davies, P., Katzman, R., and Terry, R. D. (1980). Reduced somatostatin-like immunoreactivity in cerebral cortex from cases of Alzheimer disease and Alzheimer senile dementa. *Nature* 288, 279–280.

de Bundel, D., Aourz, N., Kiagiadaki, F., Clinckers, R., Hoyer, D., Kastellakis, A., et al. (2010). Hippocampal sst(1) receptors are autoreceptors and do not affect seizures in rats. *Neuroreport* 21, 254–258.

de Lanerolle, N. C., Kim, J. H., Robbins, R. J., and Spencer, D. D. (1989). Hippocampal interneuron loss and plasticity in human temporal lobe epilepsy. *Brain Res.* 495, 387–395.

de Lecea, L. (2008). Cortistatin – functions in the central nervous system. *Mol. Cell. Endocrinol.* 286, 88–95.

De Lecea, L., Criado, J. R., Prospero-Garcia, O., Gautvik, K. M., Schweitzer, P., Danielson, P. E., et al. (1996). A cortical neuropeptide with neuronal depressant and sleep-modulating properties. *Nature* 381, 242–245.

DeNoble, V. J., Hepler, D. J., and Barto, R. A. (1989). Cysteamine-induced depletion of somatostatin produces differential cognitive deficits in rats. *Brain Res.* 482, 42–48.

Dournaud, P., Delaere, P., Hauw, J. J., and Epelbaum, J. (1995). Differential correlation between neurochemical deficits, neuropathology, and cognitive status in Alzheimer's disease. *Neurobiol. Aging* 16, 817–823.

Dutar, P., Vaillend, C., Viollet, C., Billard, J. M., Potier, B., Carlo, A. S., et al. (2002). Spatial learning and synaptic hippocampal plasticity in type 2 somatostatin receptor knock-out mice. *Neuroscience* 112, 455–466.

Einstein, E. B., Patterson, C. A., Hon, B. J., Regan, K. A., Reddi, J., Melnikoff, D. E., et al. (2010). Somatostatin signaling in neuronal cilia is critical for object recognition memory. *J. Neurosci.* 30, 4306–4314.

Engin, E., Stellbrink, J., Treit, D., and Dickson, C. (2008a). Anxiolytic and antidepressant effects of intracerebroventricularly administered somatostatin: behavioral and neurophysiological evidence. *Neuroscience* 157, 666–676.

Engin, E., Stellbrink, J., Treit, D., and Dickson, C. T. (2008b). Anxiolytic and antidepressant effects of intracerebroventricularly administered somatostatin: behavioral and neurophysiological evidence. *Neuroscience* 157, 666–676.

Engin, E., and Treit, D. (2009). Anxiolytic and antidepressant actions of somatostatin: the role of sst2 and sst3 receptors. *Psychopharmacology (Berl.)* 206, 281–289.

Epelbaum, J. (1986). Somatostatin in the central nervous system: physiology and pathological modifications. *Prog. Neurobiol.* 27, 63–100.

Epelbaum, J., Agid, F., Agid, Y., Beaudet, A., Bertrand, P., Enjalbert, A., et al. (1989). Somatostatin receptors in brain and pituitary. *Horm. Res.* 31, 45–50.

Epelbaum, J., Guillou, J. L., Gastambide, F., Hoyer, D., Duron, E., and Viollet, C. (2009). Somatostatin, Alzheimer's disease and cognition: an old story coming of age? *Prog. Neurobiol.* 89, 153–161.

Eyre, M. D., Kerti, K., and Nusser, Z. (2009). Molecular diversity of deep short-axon cells of the rat main olfactory bulb. *Eur. J. Neurosci.* 29, 1397–1407.

Ferrier, I. N., Roberts, G. W., Crow, T. J., Johnstone, E. C., Owens, D. G., Lee, Y. C., et al. (1983). Reduced cholecystokinin-like and somatostatin-like immunoreactivity in limbic lobe is associated with negative symptoms in schizophrenia. *Life Sci.* 33, 475–482.

Fillman, S. G., Cloonan, N., Catts, V. S., Miller, L. C., Wong, J., Mccrossin, T., et al. (2012). Increased inflammatory markers identified in the dorsolateral prefrontal cortex of individuals with schizophrenia. *Mol. Psychiatry.* doi: 10.1038/mp.2012.110 [Epub ahead of print].

Fino, E., and Yuste, R. (2011). Dense inhibitory connectivity in neocortex. *Neuron* 69, 1188–1203.

Florio, P., Abella, R., Marinoni, E., Di Iorio, R., Letizia, C., Meli, M., et al. (2008). Adrenomedullin blood concentrations in infants subjected to cardiopulmonary bypass: correlation with monitoring parameters and prediction of poor neurological outcome. *Clin. Chem.* 54, 202–206.

Gahete, M. D., Rubio, A., Duran-Prado, M., Avila, J., Luque, R. M., and Castano, J. P. (2010). Expression of Somatostatin, cortistatin, and their receptors, as well as dopamine receptors, but not of neprilysin, are reduced in the temporal lobe of Alzheimer's disease patients. *J. Alzheimers Dis.* 20, 465–475.

Galarraga, E., Vilchis, C., Tkatch, T., Salgado, H., Tecuapetla, F., Perez-Rosello, T., et al. (2007). Somatostatinergic modulation of firing pattern and calcium-activated potassium currents in medium spiny neostriatal neurons. *Neuroscience* 146, 537–554.

Gastambide, F., Lepousez, G., Viollet, C., Loudes, C., Epelbaum, J., and Guillou, J. L. (2010). Cooperation between hippocampal somatostatin receptor subtypes 4 and 2: functional relevance in interactive memory systems. *Hippocampus* 20, 745–757.

Gastambide, F., Viollet, C., Lepousez, G., Epelbaum, J., and Guillou, J. L. (2009). Hippocampal SSTR4 somatostatin receptors control the selection of memory strategies. *Psychopharmacology (Berl.)* 202, 153–163.

Genin, E., Hannequin, D., Wallon, D., Sleegers, K., Hiltunen, M., Combarros, O., et al. (2011). APOE and Alzheimer disease: a major gene with semi-dominant inheritance. *Mol. Psychiatry* 16, 903–907.

Gentet, L. J., Kremer, Y., Taniguchi, H., Huang, Z. J., Staiger, J. F., and Petersen, C. C. (2012). Unique functional properties of somatostatin-expressing GABAergic neurons in mouse barrel cortex. *Nat. Neurosci.* 15, 607–612.

Gleichmann, M., Zhang, Y., Wood, W. H. III, Becker, K. G., Mughal, M. R., Pazin, M. J., et al. (2012). Molecular changes in brain aging and Alzheimer's disease are mirrored in experimentally silenced cortical neuron networks. *Neurobiol. Aging* 33, 205.e201–205.e218.

Glorioso, C., Oh, S., Douillard, G. G., and Sibille, E. (2011). Brain molecular aging, promotion of neurological disease and modulation by sirtuin 5 longevity gene polymorphism. *Neurobiol. Dis.* 41, 279–290.

Goldberg, J. H., Lacefield, C. O., and Yuste, R. (2004). Global dendritic calcium spikes in mouse layer 5 low threshold spiking interneurones: implications for control of pyramidal cell bursting. *J. Physiol.* 558, 465–478.

Goldin, M., Epsztein, J., Jorquera, I., Represa, A., Ben-Ari, Y., Crepel, V., et al. (2007). Synaptic kainate receptors tune oriens-lacunosum moleculare interneurons to operate at theta frequency. *J. Neurosci.* 27, 9560–9572.

Gonchar, Y., Wang, Q., and Burkhalter, A. (2007). Multiple distinct subtypes of GABAergic neurons in mouse visual cortex identified by triple immunostaining. *Front. Neuroanat.* 1, 1–11.

Gray, P. A., Hayes, J. A., Ling, G. Y., Llona, I., Tupal, S., Picardo, M. C. D., et al. (2010). Developmental origin of preBötzinger complex respiratory neurons. *J. Neurosci.* 30, 14883–14895.

Grilli, M., Raiteri, L., and Pittaluga, A. (2004). Somatostatin inhibits glutamate release from mouse cerebrocortical nerve endings through presynaptic sst2 receptors linked to the adenylyl cyclase-protein kinase A pathway. *Neuropharmacology* 46, 388–396.

Grouselle, D., Winsky-Sommerer, R., David, J. P., Delacourte, A., Dournaud, P., and Epelbaum, J. (1998). Loss of somatostatin-like immunoreactivity in the frontal cortex of Alzheimer patients carrying the apolipoprotein epsilon 4 allele. *Neurosci. Lett.* 255, 21–24.

Guillou, J. L., Micheau, J., and Jaffard, R. (1993). Effects of intrahippocampal injections of somatostatin and cysteamine on spatial discrimination learning in mice. *Psychobiology* 21, 265–271.

Guillou, J. L., Micheau, J., and Jaffard, R. (1998). The opposite effects of cysteamine on the acquisition of two different tasks in mice are associated with bidirectional testing-induced changes in hippocampal adenylyl cyclase activity. *Behav. Neurosci.* 112, 900–908.

Guilloux, J. P., Douillard-Guilloux, G., Kota, R., Wang, X., Gardier, A. M., Martinowich, K., et al. (2011). Molecular evidence for BDNF- and GABA-related dysfunctions in the amygdala of female subjects with major depression. *Mol. Psychiatry* 17, 1130–1142.

Hannon, J. P., Petrucci, C., Fehlmann, D., Viollet, C., Epelbaum, J., and Hoyer, D. (2002). Somatostatin sst2 receptor knock-out mice: localisation of sst1-5 receptor mRNA and binding in mouse brain by semi-quantitative RT-PCR, *in situ* hybridisation histochemistry and receptor autoradiography. *Neuropharmacology* 42, 396–413.

Haroutunian, V., Kanof, P. D., and Davis, K. L. (1989). Interactions of forebrain cholinergic and somatostatinergic systems in the rat. *Brain Res.* 496, 98–104.

Haroutunian, V., Mantin, R., Campbell, G. A., Tsuboyama, G. K., and Davis, K. L. (1987). Cysteamine-induced depletion of central somatostatin-like immunoactivity: effects on behavior, learning, memory and brain neurochemistry. *Brain Res.* 403, 234–242.

Harris, F. M., Brecht, W. J., Xu, Q., Tesseur, I., Kekonius, L., Wyss-Coray, T., et al. (2003). Carboxyl-terminal-truncated apolipoprotein E4 causes Alzheimer's disease-like neurodegeneration and behavioral deficits in transgenic mice. *Proc. Natl. Acad. Sci. U.S.A.* 100, 10966–10971.

Hashimoto, T., Arion, D., Unger, T., Maldonado-Aviles, J. G., Morris, H. M., Volk, D. W., et al. (2008). Alterations in GABA-related transcriptome in the dorsolateral prefrontal cortex of subjects with schizophrenia. *Mol. Psychiatry* 13, 147–161.

Hathway, G. J., Humphrey, P. P., and Kendrick, K. M. (2004). Somatostatin induces striatal dopamine release and contralateral turning behaviour in the mouse. *Neurosci. Lett.* 358, 127–131.

Havlicek, V., Rezek, M., and Friesen, H. (1976). Somatostatin and thyrotropin releasing hormone: central effect on sleep and motor system. *Pharmacol. Biochem. Behav.* 4, 455–459.

Horgan, J., Miguel-Hidalgo, J. J., Thrasher, M., and Bissette, G. (2007). Longitudinal brain corticotropin releasing factor and somatostatin in a transgenic mouse (TG2576) model of Alzheimer's disease. *J. Alzheimers Dis.* 12, 115–127.

Hu, H., Ma, Y., and Agmon, A. (2011). Submillisecond firing synchrony between different subtypes of cortical interneurons connected chemically but not electrically. *J. Neurosci.* 31, 3351–3361.

Huang, Y., Liu, X. Q., Wyss-Coray, T., Brecht, W. J., Sanan, D. A., and Mahley, R. W. (2001). Apolipoprotein E fragments present in Alzheimer's disease brains induce neurofibrillary tangle-like intracellular inclusions in neurons. *Proc. Natl. Acad. Sci. U.S.A.* 98, 8838–8843.

Hwang, I. K., Lee, J. C., Park, S.-K., An, S.-J., Lee, H. Y., Lee, Y.-B., et al. (2004). Age-related change of somatostatin-immunoreactive neurones in the main olfactory bulb of the rat. *Anat. Histol. Embryol.* 33, 59–63.

Ishibashi, H., and Akaike, N. (1995). Somatostatin modulates high-voltage-activated $Ca^{2+}$ channels in freshly dissociated rat hippocampal neurons. *J. Neurophysiol.* 74, 1028–1036.

Iwata, N., Higuchi, M., and Saido, T. C. (2005). Metabolism of amyloid-beta peptide and Alzheimer's disease. *Pharmacol. Ther.* 108, 129–148.

Jeneson, A., and Squire, L. R. (2012). Working memory, long-term memory, and medial temporal lobe function. *Learn. Mem.* 19, 15–25.

Jiang, N., Furue, H., Katafuchi, T., and Yoshimura, M. (2003). Somatostatin directly inhibits substantia gelatinosa neurons in adult rat spinal dorsal horn *in vitro*. *Neurosci. Res.* 47, 97–107.

Jinno, S., Klausberger, T., Marton, L. F., Dalezios, Y., Roberts, J. D., Fuentealba, P., et al. (2007). Neuronal diversity in GABAergic long-range projections from the hippocampus. *J. Neurosci.* 27, 8790–8804.

Jolkkonen, J., Kahkonen, K., and Pitkanen, A. (1997). Cholinergic deafferentation exacerbates seizure-induced loss of somatostatin-immunoreactive neurons in the rat hippocampus. *Neuroscience* 80, 401–411.

Kapfer, C., Glickfeld, L. L., Atallah, B. V., and Scanziani, M. (2007). Supralinear increase of recurrent inhibition during sparse activity in the somatosensory cortex. *Nat. Neurosci.* 10, 743–753.

Kawaguchi, Y., and Kubota, Y. (1998). Neurochemical features and synaptic connections of large physiologically-identified GABAergic cells in the rat frontal cortex. *Neuroscience* 85, 677–701.

Kiagiadaki, F., Savvaki, M., and Thermos, K. (2010). Activation of somatostatin receptor (sst 5) protects the rat retina from AMPA-induced neurotoxicity. *Neuropharmacology* 58, 297–303.

Kiagiadaki, F., and Thermos, K. (2008). Effect of intravitreal administration of somatostatin and sst2 analogs on AMPA-induced neurotoxicity in rat retina. *Invest. Ophthalmol. Vis. Sci.* 49, 3080–3089.

Kokona, D., Mastrodimou, N., Pediaditakis, I., Charalampopoulos, I.,

Schmid, H. A., and Thermos, K. (2012). Pasireotide (SOM230) protects the retina in animal models of ischemia induced retinopathies. *Exp. Eye Res.* 103, 90–98.

Konradi, C., Yang, C. K., Zimmerman, E. I., Lohmann, K. M., Gresch, P., Pantazopoulos, H., et al. (2011). Hippocampal interneurons are abnormal in schizophrenia. *Schizophr. Res.* 131, 165–173.

Kosaka, K., and Kosaka, T. (2007). Chemical properties of type 1 and type 2 periglomerular cells in the mouse olfactory bulb are different from those in the rat olfactory bulb. *Brain Res.* 1167, 42–55.

Krantic, S., Robitaille, Y., and Quirion, R. (1992). Deficits in the somatostatin SS1 receptor sub-type in frontal and temporal cortices in Alzheimer's disease. *Brain Res.* 573, 299–304.

Kumar, U. (2005). Expression of somatostatin receptor subtypes (SSTR1-5) in Alzheimer's disease brain: an immunohistochemical analysis. *Neuroscience* 134, 525–538.

Lahlou, H., Guillermet, J., Hortala, M., Vernejoul, F., Pyronnet, S., Bousquet, C., et al. (2004). Molecular signaling of somatostatin receptors. *Ann. N. Y. Acad. Sci.* 1014, 121–131.

Lamirault, L., Guillou, J. L., Micheau, J., and Jaffard, R. (2001). Intrahippocampal injections of somatostatin dissociate acquisition from the flexible use of place responses. *Eur. J. Neurosci.* 14, 567–570.

Lavezzi, A. M., and Matturri, L. (2008). Functional neuroanatomy of the human pre-Bötzinger complex with particular reference to sudden unexplained perinatal and infant death. *Neuropathology* 28, 10–16.

Lepousez, G., Csaba, Z., Bernard, V., Loudes, C., Videau, C., Lacombe, J., et al. (2010a). Somatostatin interneurons delineate the inner part of the external plexiform layer in the mouse main olfactory bulb. *J. Comp. Neurol.* 518, 1976–1994.

Lepousez, G., Mouret, A., Loudes, C., Epelbaum, J., and Viollet, C. (2010b). Somatostatin contributes to *in vivo* gamma oscillation modulation and odor discrimination in the olfactory bulb. *J. Neurosci.* 30, 870–875.

Leresche, N., Asprodini, E., Emri, Z., Cope, D. W., and Crunelli, V. (2000). Somatostatin inhibits GABAergic transmission in the sensory thalamus via presynaptic receptors. *Neuroscience* 98, 513–522.

Levinson, A. J., Fitzgerald, P. B., Favalli, G., Blumberger, D. M., Daigle, M., and Daskalakis, Z. J. (2010). Evidence of cortical inhibitory deficits in major depressive disorder. *Biol. Psychiatry* 67, 458–464.

Llona, I., and Eugenín, J. (2005). Central actions of somatostatin in the generation and control of breathing. *Biol. Res.* 38, 347–352.

Lopez-Huerta, V. G., Blanco-Hernandez, E., Bargas, J., and Galarraga, E. (2012). Presynaptic modulation by somatostatin in the rat neostriatum is altered in a model of Parkinsonism. *J. Neurophysiol.* 108, 1032–1043.

Lopez-Huerta, V. G., Tecuapetla, F., Guzman, J. N., Bargas, J., and Galarraga, E. (2008). Presynaptic modulation by somatostatin in the neostriatum. *Neurochem. Res.* 33, 1452–1458.

Ma, Y., Hu, H., Berrebi, A. S., Mathers, P. H., and Agmon, A. (2006). Distinct subtypes of somatostatin-containing neocortical interneurons revealed in transgenic mice. *J. Neurosci.* 26, 5069–5082.

Mastrodimou, N., Lambrou, G. N., and Thermos, K. (2005). Effect of somatostatin analogues on chemically induced ischaemia in the rat retina. *Naunyn Schmiedebergs Arch. Pharmacol.* 371, 44–53.

McCarthy, A. D., Owens, I. J., Bansal, A. T., Mctighe, S. M., Bussey, T. J., and Saksida, L. M. (2011). FK962 and donepezil act synergistically to improve cognition in rats: potential as an add-on therapy for Alzheimer's disease. *Pharmacol. Biochem. Behav.* 98, 76–80.

McDonald, A. J., Mascagni, F., and Zaric, V. (2012). Subpopulations of somatostatin-immunoreactive non-pyramidal neurons in the amygdala and adjacent external capsule project to the basal forebrain: evidence for the existence of GABAergic projection neurons in the cortical nuclei and basolateral nuclear complex. *Front. Neural Circuits* 6:46. doi: 10.3389/fncir.2012.00046

McGarry, L. M., Packer, A. M., Fino, E., Nikolenko, V., Sippy, T., and Yuste, R. (2010). Quantitative classification of somatostatin-positive neocortical interneurons identifies three interneuron subtypes. *Front. Neural Circuits* 4:12. doi: 10.3389/fncir.2011.00012

Melzer, S., Michael, M., Caputi, A., Eliava, M., Fuchs, E. C., Whittington, M. A., et al. (2012). Long-range-projecting GABAergic neurons modulate inhibition in hippocampus and entorhinal cortex. *Science* 335, 1506–1510.

Mendez-Diaz, M., Irwin, L., Gomez-Chavarin, M., Jimenez-Anguiano, A., Cabeza, R., Murillo-Rodriguez, E., et al. (2005). Cortistatin modulates memory evocation in rats. *Eur. J. Pharmacol.* 507, 21–28.

Momiyama, T., and Zaborszky, L. (2006). Somatostatin presynaptically inhibits both GABA and glutamate release onto rat basal forebrain cholinergic neurons. *J. Neurophysiol.* 96, 686–694.

Moneta, D., Richichi, C., Aliprandi, M., Dournaud, P., Dutar, P., Billard, J. M., et al. (2002). Somatostatin receptor subtypes 2 and 4 affect seizure susceptibility and hippocampal excitatory neurotransmission in mice. *Eur. J. Neurosci.* 16, 843–849.

Moore, S. D., Madamba, S. G., Joels, M., and Siggins, G. R. (1988). Somatostatin augments the M-current in hippocampal neurons. *Science* 239, 278–280.

Nanda, S. A., Qi, C., Roseboom, P. H., and Kalin, N. H. (2008). Predator stress induces behavioral inhibition and amygdala somatostatin receptor 2 gene expression. *Genes Brain Behav.* 7, 639–648.

Nilsson, A., Falth, M., Zhang, X., Kultima, K., Skold, K., Svenningsson, P., et al. (2009). Striatal alterations of secretogranin-1, somatostatin, prodynorphin, and cholecystokinin peptides in an experimental mouse model of Parkinson disease. *Mol. Cell. Proteomics* 8, 1094–1104.

Olias, G., Viollet, C., Kusserow, H., Epelbaum, J., and Meyerhof, W. (2004). Regulation and function of somatostatin receptors. *J. Neurochem.* 89, 1057–1091.

Oliva, A. A. Jr., Jiang, M., Lam, T., Smith, K. L., and Swann, J. W. (2000). Novel hippocampal interneuronal subtypes identified using transgenic mice that express green fluorescent protein in GABAergic interneurons. *J. Neurosci.* 20, 3354–3368.

Pantaleo, T., Mutolo, D., Cinelli, E., and Bongianni, F. (2011). Respiratory responses to somatostatin microinjections into the Bötzinger complex and the pre-Bötzinger complex of the rabbit. *Neurosci. Lett.* 498, 26–30.

Peineau, S., Potier, B., Petit, F., Dournaud, P., Epelbaum, J., and Gardette, R. (2003). AMPA-sst2 somatostatin receptor interaction in rat hypothalamus requires activation of NMDA and/or metabotropic glutamate receptors and depends on intracellular calcium. *J. Physiol.* 546, 101–117.

Perez-Santiago, J., Diez-Alarcia, R., Callado, L. F., Zhang, J. X., Chana, G., White, C. H., et al. (2012). A combined analysis of microarray gene expression studies of the human prefrontal cortex identifies genes implicated in schizophrenia. *J. Psychiatr. Res.* 46, 1464–1474.

Perrenoud, Q., Rossier, J., Geoffroy, H., Vitalis, T., and Gallopin, T. (2012). Diversity of GABAergic interneurons in layer VIa and VIb of mouse barrel cortex. *Cereb. Cortex.* doi: 10.1093/cercor/bhs032 [Epub ahead of print].

Picardo, M. A., Guigue, P., Bonifazi, P., Batista-Brito, R., Allene, C., Ribas, A., et al. (2011). Pioneer GABA cells comprise a subpopulation of hub neurons in the developing hippocampus. *Neuron* 71, 695–709.

Pinter, E., Helyes, Z., and Szolcsanyi, J. (2006). Inhibitory effect of somatostatin on inflammation and nociception. *Pharmacol. Ther.* 112, 440–456.

Qiu, C., Zeyda, T., Johnson, B., Hochgeschwender, U., De Lecea, L., and Tallent, M. K. (2008). Somatostatin receptor subtype 4 couples to the M-current to regulate seizures. *J. Neurosci.* 28, 3567–3576.

Radojevic, V., Hanusek, C., Setz, C., Brand, Y., Kapfhammer, J. P., and Bodmer, D. (2011). The somatostatinergic system in the mammalian cochlea. *BMC Neurosci.* 12:89. doi: 10.1186/1471-2202-12-89

Ramírez-Jarquín, J. O., Lara-Hernández, S., López-Guerrero, J. J., Aguileta, M. A., Rivera-Angulo, A. J., Sampieri, A., et al. (2012). Somatostatin modulates generation of inspiratory rhythms and determines asphyxia survival. *Peptides* 34, 360–372.

Ramos, B., Baglietto-Vargas, D., Del Rio, J. C., Moreno-Gonzalez, I., Santa-Maria, C., Jimenez, S., et al. (2006). Early neuropathology of somatostatin/NPY GABAergic cells in the hippocampus of a PS1xAPP transgenic model of Alzheimer's disease. *Neurobiol. Aging* 27, 1658–1672.

Rat, D., Schmitt, U., Tippmann, F., Dewachter, I., Theunis, C., Wieczerzak, E., et al. (2011). Neuropeptide pituitary adenylate cyclase-activating polypeptide (PACAP) slows down Alzheimer's disease-like pathology in amyloid precursor protein-transgenic mice. *FASEB J.* 25, 3208–3218.

Raynor, K., Lucki, I., and Reisine, T. (1993). Somatostatin receptors in the nucleus accumbens selectively mediate the stimulatory effect of somatostatin on locomotor activity in rats. *J. Pharmacol. Exp. Ther.* 265, 67–73.

Robbins, R. J., Brines, M. L., Kim, J. H., Adrian, T., De Lanerolle, N., Welsh, S., et al. (1991). A selective loss of somatostatin in the hippocampus of patients with temporal lobe epilepsy. *Ann. Neurol.* 29, 325–332.

Roberts, G. W., Ferrier, I. N., Lee, Y., Crow, T. J., Johnstone, E. C., Owens, D. G., et al. (1983). Peptides, the limbic lobe and schizophrenia. *Brain Res.* 288, 199–211.

Royer, S., Zemelman, B. V., Losonczy, A., Kim, J., Chance, F., Magee, J. C., et al. (2012). Control of timing, rate and bursts of hippocampal place cells by dendritic and somatic inhibition. *Nat. Neurosci.* 15, 769–775.

Rubio, A., Perez, M., De Lecea, L., and Avila, J. (2008). Effect of cortistatin on tau phosphorylation at Ser262 site. *J. Neurosci. Res.* 86, 2462–2475.

Rubio, A., Sanchez-Mut, J. V., Garcia, E., Velasquez, Z. D., Oliver, J., Esteller, M., et al. (2012). Epigenetic control of somatostatin and cortistatin expression by beta amyloid peptide. *J. Neurosci. Res.* 90, 13–20.

Rudy, B., Fishell, G., Lee, S., and Hjerling-Leffler, J. (2011). Three groups of interneurons account for nearly 100% of neocortical GABAergic neurons. *Dev. Neurobiol.* 71, 45–61.

Saito, T., Iwata, N., Tsubuki, S., Takaki, Y., Takano, J., Huang, S. M., et al. (2005). Somatostatin regulates brain amyloid beta peptide Abeta42 through modulation of proteolytic degradation. *Nat. Med.* 11, 434–439.

Saiz-Sanchez, D., Ubeda-Banon, I., De La Rosa-Prieto, C., Argandona-Palacios, L., Garcia-Munozguren, S., Insausti, R., et al. (2010). Somatostatin, tau, and beta-amyloid within the anterior olfactory nucleus in Alzheimer disease. *Exp. Neurol.* 223, 347–350.

Saiz-Sanchez, D., Ubeda-Banon, I., De La Rosa-Prieto, C., and Martinez-Marcos, A. (2012). Differential expression of interneuron populations and correlation with amyloid-beta deposition in the olfactory cortex of an AbetaPP/PS1 transgenic mouse model of Alzheimer's disease. *J. Alzheimers Dis.* 31, 113–129.

Samson, W. K., Zhang, J. V., Avsian-Kretchmer, O., Cui, K., Yosten, G. L., Klein, C., et al. (2008). Neuronostatin encoded by the somatostatin gene regulates neuronal, cardiovascular, and metabolic functions. *J. Biol. Chem.* 283, 31949–31959.

Sanchez-Alavez, M., Gomez-Chavarin, M., Navarro, L., Jimenez-Anguiano, A., Murillo-Rodriguez, E., Prado-Alcala, R. A., et al. (2000). Cortistatin modulates memory processes in rats. *Brain Res.* 858, 78–83.

Sandoval, K. E., Farr, S. A., Banks, W. A., Niehoff, M. L., Morley, J. E., Crider, A. M., et al. (2011). Chronic peripheral administration of somatostatin receptor subtype-4 agonist NNC 26-9100 enhances learning and memory in SAMP8 mice. *Eur. J. Pharmacol.* 654, 53–59.

Savonenko, A., Xu, G. M., Melnikova, T., Morton, J. L., Gonzales, V., Wong, M. P., et al. (2005). Episodic-like memory deficits in the APPswe/PS1dE9 mouse model of Alzheimer's disease: relationships to beta-amyloid deposition and neurotransmitter abnormalities. *Neurobiol. Dis.* 18, 602–617.

Schettini, G., Florio, T., Magri, G., Grimaldi, M., Meucci, O., Landolfi, E., et al. (1988). Somatostatin and SMS 201-995 reverse the impairment of cognitive functions induced by cysteamine depletion of brain somatostatin. *Eur. J. Pharmacol.* 151, 399–407.

Schumann, C. M., Bauman, M. D., and Amaral, D. G. (2011). Abnormal structure or function of the amygdala is a common component of neurodevelopmental disorders. *Neuropsychologia* 49, 745–759.

Schwarzacher, S. W., Rüb, U., and Deller, T. (2011). Neuroanatomical characteristics of the human pre-Bötzinger complex and its involvement in neurodegenerative brainstem diseases. *Brain* 134, 24–35.

Schweitzer, P., Madamba, S. G., and Siggins, G. R. (1998). Somatostatin increases a voltage-insensitive K+ conductance in rat CA1 hippocampal neurons. *J. Neurophysiol.* 79, 1230–1238.

Shipley, M. T., and Ennis, M. (1996). Functional organization of olfactory system. *J. Neurobiol.* 30, 123–176.

Sibille, E., Morris, H. M., Kota, R. S., and Lewis, D. A. (2011). GABA-related transcripts in the dorsolateral prefrontal cortex in mood disorders. *Int. J. Neuropsychopharmacol.* 14, 721–734.

Siehler, S., Nunn, C., Hannon, J., Feuerbach, D., and Hoyer, D. (2008). Pharmacological profile of somatostatin and cortistatin receptors. *Mol. Cell. Endocrinol.* 286, 26–34.

Silberberg, G., and Markram, H. (2007). Disynaptic inhibition between neocortical pyramidal cells mediated by Martinotti cells. *Neuron* 53, 735–746.

Sousa, V. H., Miyoshi, G., Hjerling-Leffler, J., Karayannis, T., and Fishell, G. (2009). Characterization of Nkx6-2-derived neocortical interneuron lineages. *Cereb. Cortex* 19(Suppl. 1), i1–i10.

Spary, E. J., Maqbool, A., and Batten, T. F. C. (2008). Expression and localisation of somatostatin receptor subtypes sst1–sst5 in areas of the rat medulla oblongata involved in autonomic regulation. *J. Chem. Neuroanat.* 35, 49–66.

Stanić, D., Malmgren, H., He, H., Scott, L., Aperia, A., and Hökfelt, T. (2008). Developmental changes in frequency of the ciliary somatostatin receptor 3 protein. *Brain Res.* 1249, 101–112.

Stanley, E. M., Fadel, J. R., and Mott, D. D. (2012). Interneuron loss reduces dendritic inhibition and GABA release in hippocampus of aged rats. *Neurobiol. Aging* 33, 431.e1–13.

Stornetta, R. L., Rosin, D. L., Wang, H., Sevigny, C. P., Weston, M. C., and Guyenet, P. G. (2003). A group of glutamatergic interneurons expressing high levels of both neurokinin-1 receptors and somatostatin identifies the region of the pre-Bötzinger complex. *J. Comp. Neurol.* 455, 499–512.

Stumm, R. K., Zhou, C., Schulz, S., Endres, M., Kronenberg, G., Allen, J. P., et al. (2004). Somatostatin receptor 2 is activated in cortical neurons and contributes to neurodegeneration after focal ischemia. *J. Neurosci.* 24, 11404–11415.

Suzuki, N., and Bekkers, J. M. (2010). Distinctive classes of GABAergic interneurons provide layer-specific phasic inhibition in the anterior piriform cortex. *Cereb. Cortex* 20, 2971–2984.

Szabo, S., and Reichlin, S. (1981). Somatostatin in rat tissues is depleted by cysteamine administration. *Endocrinology* 109, 2255–2257.

Tahvildari, B., Wölfel, M., Duque, A., and Mccormick, D. A. (2012). Selective functional interactions between excitatory and inhibitory cortical neurons and differential contribution to persistent activity of the slow oscillation. *J. Neurosci.* 32, 12165–12179.

Tallent, M. K., Fabre, V., Qiu, C., Calbet, M., Lamp, T., Baratta, M. V., et al. (2005). Cortistatin overexpression in transgenic mice produces deficits in synaptic plasticity and learning. *Mol. Cell. Neurosci.* 30, 465–475.

Tallent, M. K., and Qiu, C. (2008). Somatostatin: an endogenous antiepileptic. *Mol. Cell. Endocrinol.* 286, 96–103.

Tallent, M. K., and Siggins, G. R. (1997). Somatostatin depresses excitatory but not inhibitory neurotransmission in rat CA1 hippocampus. *J. Neurophysiol.* 78, 3008–3018.

Tamminga, C. A., Foster, N. L., Fedio, P., Bird, E. D., and Chase, T. N. (1987). Alzheimer's disease: low cerebral somatostatin levels correlate with impaired cognitive function and cortical metabolism. *Neurology* 37, 161–165.

Tan, W., Janczewski, W. A., Yang, P., Shao, X. M., Callaway, E. M., and Feldman, J. L. (2008). Silencing preBötzinger Complex somatostatin-expressing neurons induces persistent apnea in awake rat. *Nat. Neurosci.* 11, 538–540.

Tan, W., Pagliardini, S., Yang, P., Janczewski, W. A., and Feldman, J. L. (2010). Projections of preBötzinger complex neurons in adult rats. *J. Comp. Neurol.* 518, 1862–1878.

Taniguchi, H., He, M., Wu, P., Kim, S., Paik, R., Sugino, K., et al. (2011). A resource of Cre driver lines for genetic targeting of GABAergic neurons in cerebral cortex. *Neuron* 71, 995–1013.

Tashev, R., Belcheva, S., Milenov, K., and Belcheva, I. (2001). Behavioral effects of somatostatin microinjected into caudate putamen. *Neuropeptides* 35, 271–275.

Thermos, K. (2003). Functional mapping of somatostatin receptors in the retina: a review. *Vision Res.* 43, 1805–1815.

Thermos, K., Bagnoli, P., Epelbaum, J., and Hoyer, D. (2006). The somatostatin sst1 receptor: an autoreceptor for somatostatin in brain and retina? *Pharmacol. Ther.* 110, 455–464.

Tomioka, R., Okamoto, K., Furuta, T., Fujiyama, F., Iwasato, T., Yanagawa, Y., et al. (2005). Demonstration of long-range GABAergic connections distributed throughout the mouse neocortex. *Eur. J. Neurosci.* 21, 1587–1600.

Tripp, A., Kota, R. S., Lewis, D. A., and Sibille, E. (2011). Reduced somatostatin in subgenual anterior cingulate cortex in major depression. *Neurobiol. Dis.* 42, 116–124.

Vanetti, M., Kouba, M., Wang, X., Vogt, G., and Höllt, V. (1992). Cloning and expression of a novel mouse somatostatin receptor (SSTR2B). *FEBS Lett.* 311, 290–294.

Vecsei, L., Alling, C., and Widerlov, E. (1990). Comparative studies of intracerebroventricularly administered cysteamine and pantethine in different behavioral tests and on brain catecholamines in rats. *Arch. Int. Pharmacodyn. Ther.* 305, 140–151.

Vecsei, L., Bollok, I., and Telegdy, G. (1983). Intracerebroventricular somatostatin attenuates electroconvulsive shock-induced amnesia in rats. *Peptides* 4, 293–295.

Vecsei, L., Kiraly, C., Bollok, I., Nagy, A., Varga, J., Penke, B., et al. (1984). Comparative studies with somatostatin and cysteamine in different behavioral tests on rats. *Pharmacol. Biochem. Behav.* 21, 833–837.

Vecsei, L., and Widerlov, E. (1988). Effects of intracerebroventricularly administered somatostatin on passive avoidance, shuttle-box behaviour and open-field activity in rats. *Neuropeptides* 12, 237–242.

Vepsalainen, S., Helisalmi, S., Koivisto, A. M., Tapaninen, T., Hiltunen, M., and Soininen, H. (2007). Somatostatin genetic variants modify the risk for Alzheimer's disease among Finnish patients. *J. Neurol.* 254, 1504–1508.

Vezzani, A., and Hoyer, D. (1999). Brain somatostatin: a candidate inhibitory role in seizures and epileptogenesis. *Eur. J. Neurosci.* 11, 3767–3776.

Villette, V., Poindessous-Jazat, F., Bellessort, B., Roullot, E., Peterschmitt, Y., Epelbaum, J., et al. (2012). A new neuronal target for beta-amyloid peptide in the rat hippocampus. *Neurobiol. Aging* 33, 1126.e1121–1114.

Villette, V., Poindessous-Jazat, F., Simon, A., Lena, C., Roullot, E., Bellessort, B., et al. (2010). Decreased rhythmic GABAergic septal activity and memory-associated theta oscillations after hippocampal amyloid-beta pathology in the rat. *J. Neurosci.* 30, 10991–11003.

Viollet, C., Lepousez, G., Loudes, C., Videau, C., Simon, A., and Epelbaum, J. (2008). Somatostatinergic systems in brain: networks and functions. *Mol. Cell. Endocrinol.* 286, 75–87.

Viollet, C., Vaillend, C., Videau, C., Bluet-Pajot, M. T., Ungerer, A., L'Heritier, A., et al. (2000). Involvement of sst2 somatostatin receptor in locomotor, exploratory activity and emotional reactivity in mice. *Eur. J. Neurosci.* 12, 3761–3770.

Wang, J. Z., Grundke-Iqbal, I., and Iqbal, K. (2007). Kinases and phosphatases and tau sites involved in Alzheimer neurofibrillary degeneration. *Eur. J. Neurosci.* 25, 59–68.

Wei, X.-Y., Zhao, Y., Wong-Riley, M. T. T., Ju, G., and Liu, Y.-Y. (2012). Synaptic relationship between somatostatin- and neurokinin-1 receptor-immunoreactive neurons in the pre-Bötzinger complex of rats. *J. Neurochem.* 122, 923–933.

Wilson, N. R., Runyan, C. A., Wang, F. L., and Sur, M. (2012). Division and subtraction by distinct cortical inhibitory networks *in vivo*. *Nature* 488, 343–348.

Wilson, R. S., Arnold, S. E., Schneider, J. A., Boyle, P. A., Buchman, A. S., and Bennett, D. A. (2009). Olfactory impairment in presymptomatic Alzheimer's disease. *Ann. N. Y. Acad. Sci.* 1170, 730–735.

Xu, X., Roby, K. D., and Callaway, E. M. (2006). Mouse cortical inhibitory neuron type that coexpresses somatostatin and calretinin. *J. Comp. Neurol.* 499, 144–160.

Xu, X., Roby, K. D., and Callaway, E. M. (2010). Immunochemical characterization of inhibitory mouse cortical neurons: three chemically distinct classes of inhibitory cells. *J. Comp. Neurol.* 518, 389–404.

Xue, S., Jia, L., and Jia, J. (2009). Association between somatostatin gene polymorphisms and sporadic Alzheimer's disease in Chinese population. *Neurosci. Lett.* 465, 181–183.

Yang, A. M., Ge, W. W., Lu, S. S., Yang, S. B., Su, S. F., Mi, Z. Y., et al. (2011a). Central administration of neuronostatin induces antinociception in mice. *Peptides* 32, 1893–1901.

Yang, A. M., Ji, Y. K., Su, S. F., Yang, S. B., Lu, S. S., Mi, Z. Y., et al. (2011b). Intracerebroventricular administration of neuronostatin induces depression-like effect in forced swim test of mice. *Peptides* 32, 1948–1952.

Yang, S. B., Yang, A. M., Su, S. F., Wang, H. H., Wang, N. B., and Chen, Q. (2012). Neuronostatin induces hyperalgesia in formalin test in mice. *Neurosci. Lett.* 506, 126–130.

Yeung, M., and Treit, D. (2012). The anxiolytic effects of somatostatin following intra-septal and intra-amygdalar microinfusions are reversed by the selective sst2 antagonist PRL2903. *Pharmacol. Biochem. Behav.* 101, 88–92.

Yosten, G. L., Pate, A. T., and Samson, W. K. (2011). Neuronostatin acts in brain to biphasically increase mean arterial pressure through sympatho-activation followed by vasopressin secretion: the role of melanocortin receptors. *Am. J. Physiol. Regul. Integr. Comp. Physiol.* 300, R1194–R1199.

Young, A., and Sun, Q.-Q. (2009). GABAergic inhibitory interneurons in the posterior piriform cortex of the GAD67-GFP mouse. *Cereb. Cortex* 19, 3011–3029.

Zafar, R., King, M. A., and Carney, P. R. (2012). Adeno associated viral vector-mediated expression of somatostatin in rat hippocampus suppresses seizure development. *Neurosci. Lett.* 509, 87–91.

Zeyda, T., Diehl, N., Paylor, R., Brennan, M. B., and Hochgeschwender, U. (2001). Impairment in motor learning of somatostatin null mutant mice. *Brain Res.* 906, 107–114.

Zhang, Z. J., Lappi, D. A., Wrenn, C. C., Milner, T. A., and Wiley, R. G. (1998). Selective lesion of the cholinergic basal forebrain causes a loss of cortical neuropeptide Y and somatostatin neurons. *Brain Res.* 800, 198–206.

14

# Role of neuropeptide FF in central cardiovascular and neuroendocrine regulation

**Jack H. Jhamandas[1]* and Valeri Goncharuk[1,2]**

[1] Division of Neurology, Department of Medicine, Centre for Neuroscience, University of Alberta, Edmonton, AB, Canada
[2] Russian Cardiology Research Center, Moscow, Russia

**Edited by:**
Hubert Vaudry, University of Rouen, France

**Reviewed by:**
Michiru Hirasawa, Memorial University, Canada
Jean-Marie Zajac, Centre National de la Recherche Scientifique, France
Guy Simonnet, Université Bordeaux Ségalen et Centre National de la Recherche Scientifique, France

***Correspondence:**
Jack H. Jhamandas, Department of Medicine (Neurology), 530 Heritage Medical Research Centre, University of Alberta, Edmonton, AB, Canada T6G 2S2.
e-mail: jack.jhamandas@ualberta.ca

Neuropeptide FF (NPFF) is an octapeptide belonging to the RFamide family of peptides that have been implicated in a wide variety of physiological functions in the brain including central cardiovascular and neuroendocrine regulation. The effects of these peptides are mediated via NPFF1 and NPFF2 receptors that are abundantly expressed in the rat and human brain. Herein, we review evidence for the role of NPFF in central regulation of blood pressure particularly within the brainstem and the hypothalamic paraventricular nucleus (PVN). At a cellular level, NPFF demonstrates distinct responses in magnocellular and parvocellular neurons of the PVN, which regulate the secretion of neurohypophyseal hormones and sympathetic outflow, respectively. Finally, the presence of NPFF system in the human brain and its alterations within the hypertensive brain are discussed.

**Keywords: RFamide, FMRFamide, NPFF1, NPFF2, hypothalamus, paraventricular nucleus, blood pressure, hypertension**

## INTRODUCTION

An understanding of the mechanisms that regulate arterial blood pressure under physiological conditions and in the context of pathophysiological situations such as hypertension represents a major challenge. Essential hypertension is the most common form of hypertension in humans, although its cause is poorly understood. However, there is substantial evidence to indicate that essential hypertension may be related to elevated levels of sympathetic nervous activity, which originate within the central nervous system (CNS). Within the CNS, neural networks governing arterial blood pressure are contained within topographically segregated but interactive cell groups represented at all levels of the neuraxis. Amongst the many neurotransmitters and neuropeptides present in these autonomic regions, emerging evidence indicates that a group of RFamide peptides play an important role in CNS regulation of cardiovascular function.

## WHAT ARE RFamide PEPTIDES?

Historically, the cardioexcitatory peptide FMRFamide from the bivalve mollusc *Macrocallista nimbosa* was the first peptide isolated and identified with an Arg-Phe-amide C-terminus (Price and Greenberg, 1977). Since then many bioactive peptides have been isolated from invertebrates and vertebrates, and the extended family of peptides terminating in a penultimate Arg and an amidated Phe residue at the C-terminus (RFamide) exists in all phyla (Yang et al., 1985). These peptides are designated as FMRFamide related peptides (FaRPs) and collectively referred to as RFamide peptides. RFamide peptides have been identified to have diverse biological functions that include pain modulation, inhibition of food intake, regulation of water balance, and potent cardiovascular actions that are mediated through the peripheral and CNSs (Raffa, 1988; Murase et al., 1996; Panula et al., 1996; Hinuma et al., 2000; Zajac and Gouarderes, 2000; Sunter et al., 2001; Fukusumi et al., 2003; Samson et al., 2003; Dockray, 2004).

The recent rapid accumulation of cDNA and genomic DNA sequence data and the development of bioinformatics have had a profound impact on the field of RFamide peptide research, especially on gene identification and analyses of RFamide peptides and their receptors. While some confusion exists on the precise nomenclature used in the literature, five genes encoding five prepropeptide precursors that yield five groups of RFamide peptides have been described in mammals (**Figure 1**). These include the prolactin-releasing peptide (PrRP) family (Hinuma et al., 1998), the family of neuropeptide FF (NPFF; and related peptides neuropeptide AF (NPAF), neuropeptide SF (NPSF), and neuropeptide VF (NPVF); Perry et al., 1997; Vilim et al., 1999; Bonini et al., 2000; Liu et al., 2001), human RFamide related peptides (hRFRPs; Hinuma et al., 2000; Fukusumi et al., 2001), metastin/kisspeptins (Ohtaki et al., 2001), and pyroglutamylated RFamide peptide (QRFP) (26RFa) family (Chartrel et al., 2003; Fukusumi et al., 2003). Of these, NPFF peptides and PrRP have been identified by our laboratory and others to play an important role in CNS regulation of cardiovascular function (Thiemermann et al., 1991; Allard et al., 1995; Jhamandas et al., 1998; Samson et al., 2000; Jhamandas and MacTavish, 2002). hRFRPs, which are encoded by a human gene, have a significant homology to the NPFF family of peptides and their receptors (Fukusumi et al., 2006). Members of the RFRP family (RFRP-1 and RFRP-3) have been recently identified as mammalian orthologs of the avian gonadotropin inhibitory hormone and administration of the selective NPFF receptor antagonist results in potent secretion of gonadotropins that is presumed to be mediated via the NPFF1

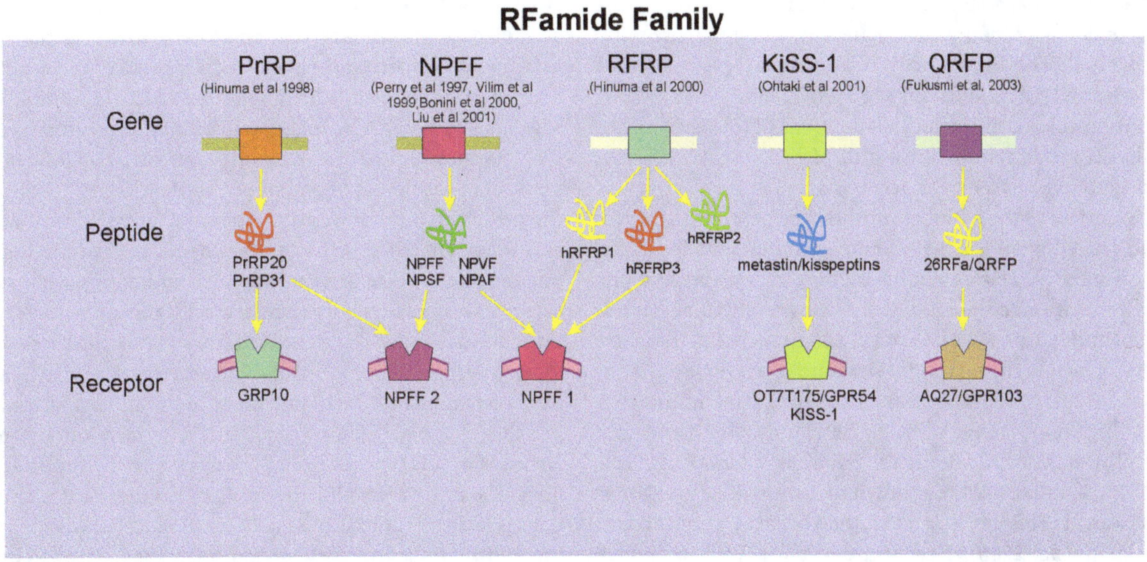


**FIGURE 1 | Members of the mammalian RFamide family.** These include the prolactin releasing peptide (PrRP) family, the family of NPFF (and related peptides NPAF, NPSF, and NPVF), human RFamide related peptides (hRFRPs), metastin/kisspeptins, and QRFP family. Specific receptors for each family of peptides have been identified, although in a number of instances cross-talk amongst these peptides and their receptors exists (denoted by arrows).

receptor (Pineda et al., 2010), Metastatin/kisspeptins have been shown to have anti-migratory effects *in vitro*, metastasis-inhibiting effects *in vivo* (Muir et al., 2001; Ohtaki et al., 2001), and identified to play an important role in regulation of puberty and reproduction via gonadotropin release (Richard et al., 2009). QRFPs are the most recently discovered members of the RFamide family and postulated to play a role in food intake and increased locomotor activity (Chartrel et al., 2003; Fukusumi et al., 2006; Bruzzone et al., 2007).

## NEUROPEPTIDE FF

### CHARACTERISTICS AND TISSUE DISTRIBUTION

Neuropeptide FF (Phe-Leu-Phe-Gln-Pro-Gln-Arg-Phe-$NH_2$) is an important member of the RFamide peptide family that is present in the CNS and in the periphery of several mammalian species including humans (for review see Panula et al., 1996). Initial interest in NPFF stemmed from its ability to modulate the antinociceptive effects of opioids (Yang et al., 1985; Chen et al., 2006; Mouledous et al., 2010), however, emerging studies have shown that the neuropeptide may play an equally important role in the central processing of visceral autonomic signals related to feeding, generation of central cardiovascular responses, stress, and neuroendocrine regulation (Panula et al., 1996; Jhamandas and MacTavish, 2003; Simonin et al., 2006). NPFF was the first RFamide peptide to be identified in mammals (Yang et al., 1985). The gene for NPFF has been cloned from human, bovine, rat, and mouse tissue and is highly conserved amongst these species (Yang et al., 1985; Vilim et al., 1999; Hinuma et al., 2000). The precursor mRNA encodes for NPFF and other related peptides (NPAF, NPSF, and NPVF) and distribution of the NPFF mRNA in the brain matches that of NPFF immunoreactivity (Kivipelto et al., 1989; Vilim et al., 1999; Liu et al., 2001). Immunocytochemical and receptor autoradiographic studies reveal that brain regions involved in pain transmission, autonomic and endocrine regulation are enriched in NPFF and its binding sites (Kivipelto et al., 1989; Allard et al., 1992). Concentrations of NPFF and its receptors in the hypothalamus are amongst the highest in the brain (Bonini et al., 2000; Zajac and Gouarderes, 2000; Liu et al., 2001).

### LIGANDS AND RECEPTORS

Two NPFF receptors, NPFF1 (also referred to as OT7TO22) and NPFF2 (also known as HLWAR77), have been cloned and characterized (Bonini et al., 2000; Elshourbagy et al., 2000; Zajac and Gouarderes, 2000). Both receptors are $G_{i/o}$ protein-coupled when expressed in Chinese hamster ovary cells or human embryonic kidney 293 cells (Kotani et al., 2001). These receptors demonstrate some of the highest levels of expression within the rat and human brain and spinal cord but data on distribution of specific NPFF receptor subtypes in these regions is controversial (Bonini et al., 2000; Zajac and Gouarderes, 2000). The emerging picture, based on autoradiographic binding, immunohistochemical and *in situ* hybridization studies, is that NPFF1 receptors are predominantly localized in the hypothalamus and the forebrain, whereas NPFF2 receptors are mainly within the spinal cord, the brainstem visceral autonomic sensory nuclei, and the hypothalamus (Bonini et al., 2000; Gouarderes et al., 2002; Zeng et al., 2003; Goncharuk and Jhamandas, 2004).

NPFF1 receptor has a high affinity for the avian peptide LPLRFamide and is the candidate receptor for NPVF, NPSF as well as hRPRF1 and hRPRF2 peptides (Bonini et al., 2000; Elshourbagy et al., 2000; Liu et al., 2001). NPFF2, on the other hand, binds NPFF and NPAF (Liu et al., 2001; Fukusumi et al., 2006). Interestingly, PrRP, for which GPR10 has been identified as the endogenous receptor (**Figure 1**), has a relatively high affinity for the NPFF2 receptor and may even have a higher efficacy at the NPFF2 receptor than NPFF (Engström et al., 2003). When administered intracerebroventricular (icv), PrRP has been observed to produce elevations in arterial blood pressure and heart rate that are strikingly similar to those evoked by icv NPFF and in fact can be blocked with the selective NPFF antagonist, RF9 (Ma et al., 2009). Thus, many of the postulated physiological functions of the newer members of the RFamide family, PrRP and hRFRPs, may in fact be mediated via NPFF1 and NPFF2 receptors.

In the past few years, with the synthesis of peptide analogs of NPFF and related peptides, the essential requirements for ligand recognition at the NPFF receptor have emerged (Vyas et al., 2006). However, a major impediment to delineating a physiological role for NPFF peptides has been a lack of suitable antagonists that show selectivity for each of the receptors. DesaminoYLFQPQRa was the first analog to attenuate morphine abstinence signs induced by NPFF (Malin et al., 1995; Prokai et al., 2001) but suffers from poor bioavailability and/or low affinity for NPFF receptors (Fang et al., 2005). PFR(Tic)amide has been shown to demonstrate antagonist activity toward NPFF effect *in vitro*, but behaves as an agonist *in vivo* (Chen et al., 2006). Neuropeptide Y (NPY) ligands such as BIBP 3226 have been reported to interact with NPFF receptors, likely on the basis of structural similarities between these receptors and the C-terminal end of NPY peptides (Mollereau et al., 2002; Fang et al., 2006). Unfortunately, BIBP 3226 and its derivatives that were most potent at the NPFF1 receptor were also able to displace NPY $Y_1$ binding (Fang et al., 2005). The discovery of RF9, a *selective* antagonist at the NPFF receptor (Simonin et al., 2006) has represented a significant advance in dissecting the role of NPFF in a variety of physiological functions. This compound potently and selectively binds to NPFF receptors and indeed blocks the acute cardiovascular effects induced by icv NPFF. In addition, its chronic administration blocks delayed and long-lasting opioid-induced hyperalgesia.

## NPFF AND CENTRAL CARDIOVASCULAR AND NEUROENDOCRINE REGULATION

Experimental evidence supporting a key role for NPFF in cardiovascular regulation first became apparent in the mid-1980s when Roth et al. (1987) reported that two NPFF analogs could produce significant pressor effects when administered systemically. Subsequently, focal injections of NPFF into the brainstem nucleus of tractus solitarius, which is the first terminus for cardiovascular inputs originating from the periphery, resulted in an increase in blood pressure and bradycardia that could be attenuated with adrenergic antagonists (Laguzzi et al., 1996). NPFF-synthesizing neurons in the same brainstem nucleus were shown to be activated in response to hemorrhage and to a lesser extent acute drug-induced hypertension (Jhamandas et al., 1998). These NPFF neurons in turn project to more rostral brainstem and hypothalamic cardiovascular centers. Intrathecal and icv administration of NPFF has been demonstrated to evoke dose-dependent elevations in arterial blood pressure and heart rate (Jhamandas and MacTavish, 2002, 2003; Fang et al., 2010). Identity of neural circuits that participate in centrally generated NPFF responses have been best studied in the hypothalamus, where icv NPFF evokes activation of specific sets of chemically defined paraventricular nucleus (PVN) neurons, that control CNS humoral and autonomic outflow to the periphery (Jhamandas and MacTavish, 2003).

### WHOLE ANIMAL OBSERVATIONS

The PVN is viewed as a key site for homeostasis and a model nucleus for understanding the central regulation of autonomic and neuroendocrine function in the brain (Cunningham and Sawchenko, 1991). The magnocellular neurosecretory cells of the PVN synthesize either vasopressin or oxytocin and following stimulation, release these hormones from their axonal projections to the posterior pituitary into the systemic circulation (Sawchenko and Swanson, 1982). On the other hand, the parvocellular component of the PVN is more complex and consists of two broad categories of cells, neurosecretory cells and non-neurosecretory (autonomic) cells. The neurosecretory parvocellular neurons are located within the dorsal medial and periventricular PVN and their axons terminate on median eminence portal capillaries to facilitate the release of "factors" regulating anterior pituitary secretion. Neurons of this type for example express corticotrophin-releasing hormone or thyrotrophin-releasing hormone. Parvocellular non-neurosecretory (autonomic) neurons are located within the dorsal cap and ventral medial PVN and project their axons to the brainstem and the spinal cord. Some of the chemical messengers expressed in these types of cells include tyrosine hydroxylase, oxytocin, and somatostatin (Roland and Sawchenko, 1993; Dawson et al., 1998). Central administration of NPFF results in a preferential activation of oxytocin-synthesizing parvocellular PVN neurons that project to the brainstem. Oxytocinergic projections to the solitary-vagal complex have previously been shown to modulate baroreflex control of heart rate and other aspects of circulatory control (Higa et al., 2002; Vela et al., 2010). On the other hand, icv NPFF does not activate the magnocellular vasopressin-secreting PVN neurons as measured by Fos immunohistochemistry suggesting that the effects of NPFF on these subset of PVN neurons are inhibitory (Jhamandas et al., 2006). The latter posit being supported by observation from electrophysiological studies where NPFF inhibits activity of magnocellular vasopressin neurons (see below).

### CELLULAR ACTIONS OF NPFF

Work from whole animal experiments described above suggests that the differential activation of subsets of hypothalamic PVN neurons may result from distinct effects of NPFF on synaptic activation of magno- and parvocellular neurons of this nucleus. Indeed, cellular electrophysiological recordings from hypothalamic brain slices reveal that NPFF increases the inhibitory synaptic drive to magnocellular PVN neurons through a GABA-synthesizing network of interneurons located within the sub-PVN region (Roland and Sawchenko, 1993; Jhamandas et al., 2006; **Figure 2**). This observation of NPFF augmenting an inhibition of magnocellular vasopressin-secreting PVN cells fits well with the *in vivo* hormone release data, which shows that hypovolemia-induced vasopressin release from the pituitary is blunted by centrally administered NPFF (Arima et al., 1996). On the other hand, NPFF presynaptically *disinhibits* the GABAergic input to the parvocellular PVN, thereby increasing the net excitability of these neurons (**Figure 2**). NPFF also exerts a distinct depolarizing [tetrodotoxin (TTX)-independent] postsynaptic effect on parvocellular PVN neurons (Jhamandas et al., 2007). NPFF-induced excitation of parvocellular PVN neurons

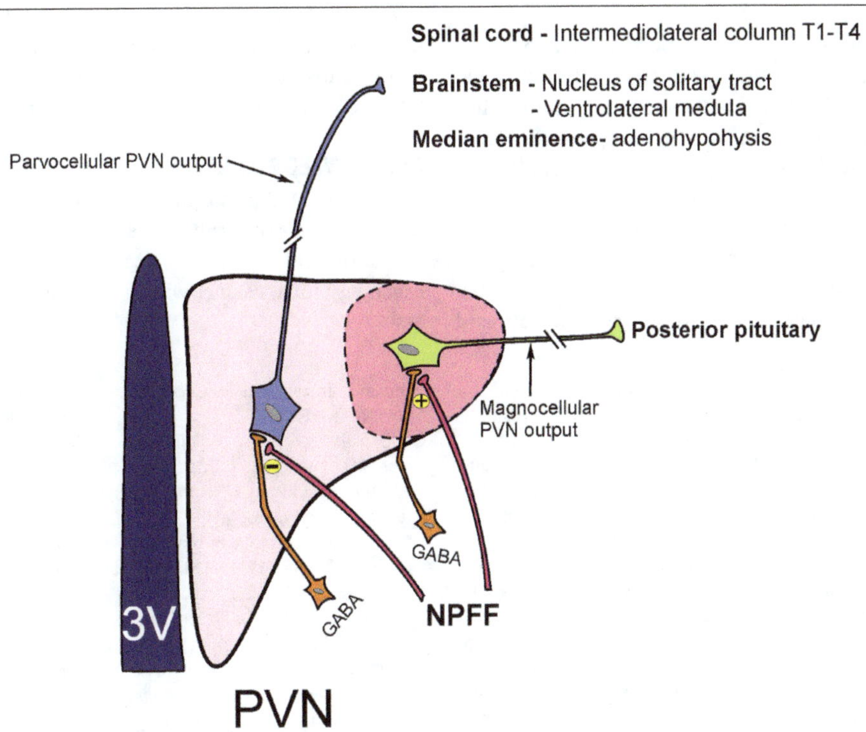


**FIGURE 2 | Schematic depicting parvocellular and magnocellular components of the hypothalamic paraventricular nucleus (PVN) and their projection sites.** NPFF differentially modulates GABAergic input (originating from the adjacent subPVN region) to parvocellular and magnocellular neurons of the PVN. NPFF inhibits activity of GABAergic terminals that project to the parvocellular PVN neurons resulting in a disinhibition of these neurons. On the other hand, NPFF augments GABA synaptic input to magnocellular PVN neurons.

would be expected to result in an increase in autonomic outflow and sympathetic activation which is precisely what is observed with acute infusions of icv NPFF in the conscious animal. At present the lack of selective antagonists acting at NPFF1 versus NPFF2 receptors makes it difficult to determine whether the differential effects of NPFF are in fact mediated via distinct NPFF receptor subtypes. However, PrRP, which binds to NPFF2 receptors, shows a similar profile of electrophysiological effects on parvocellular PVN neurons as NPFF. Moreover RF9, a selective NPFF receptor antagonist, blocks PrRP actions on these neurons suggesting that both the PrRP and the NPFF effects in the parvocellular PVN are likely NPFF2 receptor mediated (Ma et al., 2009).

## NPFF AND HUMAN HYPERTENSION

There is currently a paucity of knowledge on the role of NPFF, and RFamide peptides in general, in human pathophysiological states such as essential hypertension. All of our current knowledge on the role of NPFF in the regulation of arterial blood pressure is derived from paradigms that rely on studying acute effects of this peptide in experimental animal models, which do not recapitulate the chronic human hypertensive condition. Nonetheless, anatomical relationships between NPFF and its receptors within autonomic centers in the human brain may provide important clues as to the role of this peptide in diverse biological functions. In this regard, immunohistochemical data from our laboratory over several years has identified striking similarities in the distribution of NPFF and its receptors, NPFF1 and NPFF2, in the normal human brain compared to the rat, a species in which much of the behavioral and physiological studies have been done to date(Goncharuk and Jhamandas, 2004, 2008; Goncharuk et al., 2006). In these studies, we have identified significant numbers of NPFF fibers, NPFF1, and NPFF2 receptors in the human parvocellular PVN. The relative preponderance of NPFF (and its receptors) and its intimate anatomical relationship to important cardiovascular regulatory peptides such as corticotropin releasing hormone (CRH) in human hypothalamus suggests an important role for this peptide in hypertension. Interestingly, an up-regulation of CRH-secreting cells in the human hypothalamic PVN of patients who suffered from essential hypertension has been reported (Goncharuk et al., 2001, 2002). Recent immunohistochemical observations from post-mortem brain tissue of hypertensive individuals and age-matched controls indicate a marked reduction of NPFF in discrete cardiovascular brainstem and hypothalamic nuclei of hypertensives (Goncharuk et al., 2011, 2012). In these studies, NPFF immunoreactivity was severely reduced in a subnuclear zone adjacent to the hypothalamic PVN and supraoptic nucleus, a site where dense networks of GABAergic neurons reside. These GABAergic neurons have been identified to mediate arterial baroreceptor inputs that control the release of the pressor hormone vasopressin from the neurohypophysis (Jhamandas et al., 1989). Thus loss of NPFF input to GABaergic cells has the potential to dysregulate cardiovascular reflexes and control of arterial blood pressure.

## CONCLUSION

Emerging evidence indicates that structure of RFamide peptides including NPFF is remarkably conserved during evolution. What makes these peptides attractive as therapeutic targets is that they are involved in essential functions such as pain, appetite and feeding, stress, and cardiovascular regulation. Anatomical, molecular, and physiological studies indicate that NPFF plays an important role in brain control of neurohormones and sympathetic outflow. Advances in identification and pharmacology of NPFF receptors and the availability of new and specific antagonists such as RF9 provide a unique opportunity to identify the specific role and relevance of these receptors in physiological function and in pathophysiological states such as hypertension. NPFF receptor based compounds could serve as potential therapeutic agents in the treatment of hypertension and other autonomic disorders.

## ACKNOWLEDGMENTS

Research contributions of the author were supported by the Canadian Institutes of Health Research and the Institute of Diabetes, Nutrition and Metabolism (MOP 111426). We thank Mr. David Mactavish for assistance with graphics and Ms. C. Krys for editorial assistance.

## REFERENCES

Allard, M., Labrouche, S., Nosjean, A., and Laguzzi, R. (1995). Mechanisms underlying the cardiovascular responses to peripheral administration of NPFF in the rat. *J. Pharmacol. Exp. Ther.* 274, 577–583.

Allard, M., Zajac, J.-M., and Simonnet, G. (1992). Autoradiographic distribution of receptors to FLFQPQRFamide, a morphine-modulating peptide in rat central nervous system. *Neuroscience* 49, 101–116.

Arima, H., Murase, T., Kondo, K., Iwasaki, Y., and Oiso, Y. (1996). Centrally administered neuropeptide FF inhibits arginine vasopressin release in conscious rats. *Endocrinology* 137, 1523–1529.

Bonini, J. A., Jones, K. A., Adham, N., Forray, C., Artymyshyn, R., Durkin, M. M., et al. (2000). Identification and characterization of two G protein-coupled receptors for neuropeptide FF. *J. Biol. Chem.* 275, 39324–39331.

Bruzzone, F., Lectz, B., Alexandre, D., Jegou, S., Mounien, L., Tollemer, H., et al. (2007). Distribution of 26RFa binding sites and GPR103 mRNA in the central nervous system of the rat. *J. Comp. Neurol.* 503, 573–591.

Chartrel, N., Dujardin, C., Anouar, Y., Leprince, J., Decker, A., Clerens, S., et al. (2003). Identification of 26RFa, a hypothalamic neuropeptide of the RFamide peptide family with orexigenic activity. *Proc. Natl. Acad. Sci. U.S.A.* 100, 15247–15252.

Chen, J.-C., Lee, W.-H., Chen, P.-C., Tseng, C.-P., and Huang, E. Y.-K. (2006). Rat $NPFF_1$ receptor-mediated signalling: functional comparison of neuropeptides FF (NPFF), FMRFamide and PFR(Tic)amide. *Peptides* 27, 1005–1014.

Cunningham, E. T., and Sawchenko, P. E. (1991). Reflex control of magnocellular vasopressin and oxytocin secretion. *Trends Neurosci.* 14, 406–411.

Dawson, C. A., Jhamandas, J. H., and Krukoff, T. L. (1998). Activation by systemic Angiotensin II of neurochemically identified neurones in rat hypothalamic paraventricular nucleus. *J. Neuroendocrinol.* 10, 453–459.

Dockray, G. J. (2004). The expanding family of -Rfamide peptides and their effects on feeding behaviour. *Exp. Physiol.* 89, 229–235.

Elshourbagy, N. A., Ames, R. S., Fitzgerald, L. R., Foley, J. J., Chambers, J. K., Szekeres, P. G., et al. (2000). Receptor for the pain modulatory neuropeptides NPFF and NPAF is an orphan G-protein-coupled receptor. *J. Biol. Chem.* 275, 25965–25971.

Engström, M., Brandt, A., Wurster, S., Savola, J.-M., and Panula, P. (2003). Prolactin releasing peptide has high affinity and efficacy at Neuropeptide FF2 receptors. *J. Pharmacol. Exp. Ther.* 305, 825–832.

Fang, Q., Guo, J., Peng, Y. L., Chang, M., He, F., Chen, Q., et al. (2005). In vitro and in vivo studies of dansylated compounds, the putative agonists and antagonists on Neuropeptide FF receptors. *Peptides* 27, 1297–1304.

Fang, Q., Guo, J., He, F., Peng, Y. L., Chang, M., and Wang, R. (2006). In vivo inhibition of neuropeptides FF agonism by BIBP3226, an NPY Y1 receptor antagonist. *Peptides* 27, 2207–2213.

Fang, Q., Li, N., Jiang, T. N., Liu, Q., Li, Y. L., and Wang, R. (2010). Pressor and tachycardic responses to intrathecal administration of neuropeptide FF in anesthetized rats. *Peptides* 31, 683–688.

Fukusumi, S., Fujii, R., and Hinuma, S. (2006). Recent advances in mammalian RFamide peptides: the discovery and functional analyses of PrRP, RFRPs and QRFP. *Peptides* 27, 1073–1086.

Fukusumi, S., Habata, Y., Yoshida, H., Iijima, N., Kawamata, Y., Hosoya, M., et al. (2001). Characteristics and distribution of endogenous RFamide-related peptide-1. *Biochim. Biophys. Acta* 1540, 221–232.

Fukusumi, S., Yoshida, H., Fujii, R., Maruyama, M., Komatsu, H., Habata, Y., et al. (2003). A new peptide ligand and its receptor regulating adrenal function in rats. *J. Biol. Chem.* 278, 46387–46395.

Goncharuk, V., Buijs, R., Jhamandas, J. H., and Swaab, D. F. (2011). Vasopressin (VP) and Neuropeptide FF (NPFF) systems in the normal and hypertensive human brainstem. *J. Comp. Neurol.* 519, 93–124.

Goncharuk, V., Buijs, R. M., Swaab, D. F., and Jhamandas, J. H. (2012). The hypothalamic Neuropeptide FF (NPFF) system is impaired in hypertensive patients. *Soc. Neurosci. Abstr.* (New Orleans, LA, USA. 387.12).

Goncharuk, V., and Jhamandas, J. H. (2004). The distribution of the Neuropeptide FF1 (FF1) in the human hypothalamus and surrounding basal forebrain structures: an immunocytochemical study. *J. Comp. Neurol.* 474, 487–503.

Goncharuk, V., and Jhamandas, J. H. (2008). Neuropeptide FF2 receptor distribution in the human brain: an immunohistochemical study. *Peptides* 29, 1544–1553.

Goncharuk, V. D., Buijs, R. M., MacTavish, D., and Jhamandas, J. H. (2006). Neuropeptide FF distribution in the human and rat forebrain: a comparative immunohistochemical study. *J. Comp. Neurol.* 496, 572–593.

Goncharuk, V. D., van Heerikhuize, J., Dai, J. P., Swaab, D. F., and Buijs, R. M. (2001). Neuropeptide changes in the suprachiasmatic nucleus in primary hypertension indicate functional impairment of the biological clock. *J. Comp. Neurol.* 431, 320–330.

Goncharuk, V. D., van Heerikhuize, J., Swaab, D. F., and Buijs, R. M. (2002). Paraventricular nucleus of the human hypothalamus in primary hypertension: activation of corticotropin-releasing hormone neurons. *J. Comp. Neurol.* 443, 321–331.

Gouarderes, C., Quelven, I., Mollereau, C., Mazarguil, H., Rice, S. Q. J., and Zajac, J. M. (2002). Quantitative autoradiographic distribution of NPFF1 Neuropeptide FF receptor in the rat brain and comparison with NPFF2 receptor by using [125]YVP and [125I]EYF as selective radioligands. *Neuroscience* 115, 349–361.

Higa, K. T., Mori, E., Vianna, F. F., Morris, M., and Michelini, L. C. (2002). Baroreflex control of heart rate by oxytocin in the solitary-vagal complex. *Am. J. Physiol. Regul. Integr. Comp. Physiol.* 282, R537–R545.

Hinuma, S., Habata, Y., Fujii, R., Kawamata, Y., Hosoya, M., Fukusumi, S., et al. (1998). A prolectin-releasing peptide in the brain. *Nature* 393, 272–276.

Hinuma, S., Shitani, Y., Fukusumi, S., Iijima, N., Matsumoto, Y., Hosoya, M., et al. (2000). New neuropeptides containing carboxy-terminal RFamide and their receptor in mammals. *Nat. Cell Biol.* 2, 703–708.

Jhamandas, J. H., Raby, W., Rogers, J., Buijs, R. M., and Renaud, L. P. (1989). Diagonal band projection towards the hypothalamic supraoptic nucleus: light and electron microscopic observations in the rat. *J. Comp. Neurol.* 282, 15–23.

Jhamandas, J. H., Harris, K. H., Petrov, T., Yang, H.-Y. T., and Jhamandas, K. H. (1998). Activation patterns of Neuropeptide FF (NPFF) neurons within the brainstem nucleus tractus solitarius following autonomic stimulation. *J. Comp. Neurol.* 402, 210–221.

Jhamandas, J. H., and MacTavish, D. (2002). Central administration of Neuropeptide FF (NPFF) causes increased neuronal activation and upregulation of NPFF gene expression in the rat brainstem. *J. Comp. Neurol.* 447, 300–307.

Jhamandas, J. H., and MacTavish, D. (2003). Central administration of Neuropeptide FF (NPFF) causes activation of oxytocin paraventricular hypothalamic neurones that project to the brainstem. *J. Neuroendocrinol.* 15, 24–32.

Jhamandas, J. H., MacTavish, D., and Harris, K. H. (2006). Neuropeptide FF (NPFF) control of magnocellular neurosecretory cells of the rat hypothalamic paraventricular nucleus (PVN). *Peptides* 27, 973–979.

Jhamandas, J. H., Simonin, F., Bourguignon, J.-J., and Harris, K. H. (2007). Neuropeptide FF and Neuropeptide VF inhibit GABAergic neurotransmission in parvocellular neurons of the rat hypothalamic paraventricular nucleus. *Am. J. Physiol.* 292, R1872–R1880.

Kivipelto, L., Majane, E. A., Yang, H.-Y. T., and Panula, P. (1989). Immunohistochemical distribution and partial characterization of FLFQPQRF amide like peptides in the central nervous system of rats. *J. Comp. Neurol.* 286, 269–287.

Kotani, M., Mollereau, C., Detheux, M., Le Poul, E., Brezillon, S., Vakili, J., et al. (2001). Functional characterization of a human receptor for neuropeptide FF and related peptides. *Br. J. Pharmacol.* 133, 138–144.

Laguzzi, R., Nosjean, A., Mazarguil, H., and Allard, M. (1996). Cardiovascular effects induced by the stimulation of neuropeptide FF receptors in the dorsal vagal complex: an autoradiographic and pharmacological study in the rat. *Brain Res.* 711, 193–202.

Liu, Q., Guan, X. M., Martin, W. J., McDonald, T. P., Clemens, M. K., Jiang, Q., et al. (2001). Identification and characterization of novel mammalian neuropeptide FF-like peptides that attenuate morphine-induced antinociception. *J. Biol. Chem.* 276, 36961–36969.

Ma, L., MacTavish, D., Simonin, F., Bourguignon, J.-J., and Jhamandas, J. H. (2009). Prolactin releasing peptide (PrRP) effects in the rat brain are mediated through the Neuropeptide FF (NPFF) receptor. *Eur. J. Neurosci.* 30, 1585–1593.

Malin, D. H., Lake, J. R., Smith, D. A., Jones, J. A., Morel, J., Claunch, A. E., et al. (1995). Subcutaneous injection of an analog of neuropeptides FF prevents naloxone-precipitated morphine abstinence syndrome. *Drug Alcohol Depend.* 40, 37–42.

Mollereau, C., Mazarguil, H., Marcus, D., Quelven, I., Kotani, M., Lanoy, V., et al. (2002). Pharmacological characterization of human $NPFF_1$ and NPFF receptors expressed in CHO cells by using NPY $Y_1$ receptor antagonists. *Eur. J. Pharmacol.* 451, 245–256.

Mouledous, L., Mollereau, C., and Zajac J.-M. (2010). Opioid modulating properties of the neuropeptide FF system. *Biofactors* 36, 423–429.

Muir, A. I., Chamberlain, L., Elshourbagy, N. A., Michalovich, D., Moore, D. J., Calamari, A., et al. (2001). AXOR12, a novel human G protein-coupled receptor, activated by the peptide KiSS-1. *J. Biol. Chem.* 276, 28969–28975.

Murase, T., Arima, H., Kondo, K., and Oiso, Y. (1996). Neuropeptide FF reduces food intake in rats. *Peptides* 17, 353–354.

Ohtaki, T., Shintani, Y., Honda, S., Matsumoto, H., Hori, A., Kanehashi, K., et al. (2001). Metastasis suppressor gene KiSS-1 encodes peptide ligand of a G-protein-coupled receptor. *Nature (Lond.)* 411, 613–617.

Panula, P., Aarnisalo, A. A., and Wasowicz, K. (1996). Neuropeptide FF, a mammalian neuropeptide with multiple functions. *Prog. Neurobiol.* 48, 461–487.

Perry, S. J., Huang, E. Y., Cronk, D., Bagust, J., Sharma, R., Walker, R. J., et al. (1997). A human gene encoding morphine modulating peptides related to NPFF and FMRFamide. *FEBS Lett.* 409, 426–430.

Pineda, R., Garcia-Galiano, D., Sanchez-Garrido, M. A., Romero, M., Ruiz-Pino, F., Aguilar, E., et al. (2010). Characterization of the potent gonadotropin-releasing activity of RF9, a selective antagonist of RF-amide-related peptides and neuropeptide FF receptors: physiological and pharmacological implications. *Endocrinology* 151, 1902–1913.

Price, D. A., and Greenberg, M. J. (1977). Structure of a molluscan cardioexcitatory neuropeptide. *Science* 197, 670–671.

Prokai, L., Prokai-Tatrai, K., Zharikova, A., Li, X., and Rocca, J. R. (2001). Combinatorial optimization of a neuropeptide FF antagonist. *J. Med. Chem.* 44, 1623–1626.

Roth, B. L., Disimone, J., Majane, E. A., and Yang, H. Y. (1987). Elevation of arterial pressure in rats by two new vertebrate peptides FLFQPQRF-NH2 and AGEGLSSPFWSLAAPQRF-NH2 which are immunoreactive to FMRF-NH2 antiserum. *Neuropeptides* 10, 37–42.

Raffa, R. B. (1988). The action of FMRFamide (Phe-Met-Arg-Phe-$NH_2$) and related peptides on mammals. *Peptides* 9, 915–922.

Richard, N., Corvaisier, S., Camacho, E., and Kottler, M. L. (2009). KiSS-1 and GPR54 at the pituitary level: overview and recent insights. *Peptides* 30, 123–129.

Roland, B. L., and Sawchenko, P. E. (1993). Local origins of some GABAergic projections to the paraventricular and supraoptic nuclei of the hypothalamus in the rat. *J. Comp. Neurol.* 332, 123–143.

Samson, W. K., Resch, Z. T., and Murphy, T. C. (2000). A novel action of the newly described prolactin-releasing peptides: cardiovascular regulation. *Brain Res.* 858, 19–25.

Samson, W. K., Taylor, M. M., and Baker, J. R. (2003). Prolactin-releasing peptides. *Regul. Pept.* 114, 1–5.

Sawchenko, P. E., and Swanson, L. W. (1982). Immunohistochemical identification of neurons in the paraventricular nucleus of the hypothalamus that project to the medulla or to the spinal cord in the rat. *J. Comp. Neurol.* 205, 260–272.

Simonin, F., Schmitt, M., Laulin, J. P., Laboureyras, E., Jhamandas, J. H., MacTavish, D., et al. (2006). RF9, a potent and selective neuropeptides FF receptor antagonist, prevents opioid-induced tolerance associated with hyperalgesia. *Proc. Natl. Acad. Sci. U.S.A.* 103, 466–471.

Sunter, D., Hewson, A. K., Lynam, S., and Dickson, S. L. (2001). Intracerebroventricular injection of neuropeptide FF, an opioid modulating neuropeptide, acutely reduces food intake and stimulates water intake in the rat. *Neurosci. Lett.* 313, 145–148.

Thiemermann, C., Al-Damluji, S., Hecker, M., and Vane, J. R. (1991). FMRF-amide and L-Arg-L-Phe increase blood pressure and heart rate in the anesthetized rat by central stimulation of the sympathetic nervous system. *Biochem. Biophys. Res. Commun.* 175, 318–324.

Vela, C., Diaz-Cabiale, Z., Parrado, C., Narvaez, M., Covenas, R., and Narvaez, J. A. (2010). Involvement of oxytocin in the nucleus tractus solitarii on central cardiovascular control: interactions with glutamate. *J. Physiol. Pharmacol.* 61, 59–65.

Vilim, F. S., Aarnisalo, A. A., Nieminen, M.-L., Lintunen, M., Karlstedt, K., Kontinen, V. K., et al. (1999). Gene for pain modulatory neuropeptide NPFF: induction in spinal cord by noxious stimuli. *Mol. Pharmacol.* 55, 804–811.

Vyas, N., Mollereau, C, Cheve, G., and McCurdy, C. R. (2006). Structure-activity relationships of neuropeptides FF and related peptidic and non-peptidic derivatives. *Peptides* 27, 990–996.

Yang, H.-Y. T., Fratta, W., Majane, E. A., and Costa, E. (1985). Isolation, sequencing, syntheses and pharmacological characterization of two neuropeptides that modulate the action of morphine. *Proc. Natl. Acad. Sci. U.S.A.* 82, 7757–7761.

Zajac, J. M., and Gouarderes, C. (2000). "Neuropeptide FF receptors," in *Handbook of Chemical Neuroanatomy*, Vol. 16, eds R. Quirion, A. Bjorklund, and T. Hokfelt (Amsterdam: Elsevier), 163–193.

Zeng, Z., McDonald, T. P., Wang, R., Liu, Q., and Austin, C. P. (2003). Neuropeptide FF receptor 2 (NPFF2) is localized to pain-processing regions in the primate spinal cord and the lower level of the medulla oblongata. *J. Chem. Neuroanat.* 25, 269–278.

# 15

# Different distribution of neuromedin S and its mRNA in the rat brain: NMS peptide is present not only in the hypothalamus as the mRNA, but also in the brainstem

***Miwa Mori*[1†], *Kenji Mori*[1†], *Takanori Ida*[2], *Takahiro Sato*[3], *Masayasu Kojima*[3], *Mikiya Miyazato*[1]* and *Kenji Kangawa*[1]**

[1] *Department of Biochemistry, National Cerebral and Cardiovascular Center Research Institute, Osaka, Japan*
[2] *Interdisciplinary Research Organization, University of Miyazaki, Miyazaki, Japan*
[3] *Molecular Genetics, Institute of Life Sciences, Kurume University, Fukuoka, Japan*

***Edited by:***
*Hubert Vaudry, University of Rouen, France*

***Reviewed by:***
*Etienne Challet, Centre National de la Recherche Scientifique, France*
*Manuel Tena-Sempere, University of Cordoba, Spain*

***Correspondence:**
*Mikiya Miyazato, Department of Biochemistry, National Cerebral and Cardiovascular Center Research Institute, 5-7-1 Fujishirodai, Suita, Osaka 565-8565, Japan.*
*e-mail: miyazato@ri.ncvc.go.jp*

*†Miwa Mori and Kenji Mori have contributed equally to this work.*

Neuromedin S (NMS) is a neuropeptide identified as another endogenous ligand for two orphan G protein-coupled receptors, FM-3/GPR66 and FM-4/TGR-1, which have also been identified as types 1 and 2 receptors for neuromedin U structurally related to NMS. Although expression of NMS mRNA is found mainly in the brain, spleen, and testis, the distribution of its peptide has not yet been investigated. Using a newly prepared antiserum, we developed a highly sensitive radioimmunoassay for rat NMS. NMS peptide was clearly detected in the rat brain at a concentration of $68.3 \pm 3.4$ fmol/g wet weight, but it was hardly detected in the spleen and testis. A high content of NMS peptide was found in the hypothalamus, midbrain, and pons–medulla oblongata, whereas abundant expression of NMS mRNA was detected only in the hypothalamus. These differing distributions of the mRNA and peptide suggest that nerve fibers originating from hypothalamic NMS neurons project into the midbrain, pons, or medulla oblongata. In addition, abundant expression of type 2 receptor mRNA was detected not only in the hypothalamus, but also in the midbrain and pons–medulla oblongata. These results suggest novel, unknown physiological roles of NMS within the brainstem.

**Keywords: neuromedin S, neuropeptide, radioimmunoassay, peptide distribution, brain, brainstem**

## INTRODUCTION

Neuromedin S (NMS) is a neuropeptide originally isolated by our group from the rat brain as an additional endogenous ligand for neuromedin U (NMU) receptors types 1 (NMUR1) and 2 (NMUR2), which were previously identified as the orphan G protein-coupled receptors FM-3/GPR66 and FM-4/TGR-1, respectively (Mori et al., 2005). In rats, NMS and NMU are structurally related peptides composed respectively of 36 and 23 amino-acid residues (Brighton et al., 2004; Mori et al., 2005). They have an identical C-terminal amidated seven-residue sequence that is essential for their agonist activity. NMS and NMU precursors are encoded by separate genes mapped to human chromosomes 2q11.2 and 4q12, respectively (Mori et al., 2005). Because these genes are under different transcriptional control, the mRNAs of NMS and NMU have different patterns of distribution (Brighton et al., 2004; Mori et al., 2005), indicating that they have different physiological roles despite having the same agonist effect on their receptors. Expression of NMS mRNA is observed mainly in the brain, spleen, and testis, and the highest level of expression is found in the hypothalamus (Mori et al., 2005). In the rat brain, NMS mRNA is expressed predominantly in the suprachiasmatic nucleus (SCN) of the hypothalamus, although low-level expression of NMS mRNA is also found in other hypothalamic nuclei, such as the arcuate nucleus (ARC), paraventricular nucleus (PVN), and supraoptic nucleus (SON; Mori et al., 2005). In contrast to the mRNA distribution, the distribution of the NMS peptide in the brain has not yet been elucidated.

Because of the high level expression of NMS mRNA in the hypothalamus, there has been a focus on the role of NMS in the brain. The functions of NMS in the brain have been validated by intracerebroventricular (ICV) administration of the peptide to rats: ICV-administered NMS causes a phase shift in circadian rhythm (Mori et al., 2005), suppresses food intake (Ida et al., 2005), reduces urine volume (Sakamoto et al., 2007), increases milk secretion (Sakamoto et al., 2008), and elevates plasma levels of luteinizing hormone (Vigo et al., 2007). The activity of NMS is approximately 10 times as great as that of NMU in the brain, although ICV-administered NMU induces the same responses (Nakahara et al., 2004; Ida et al., 2005; Mori et al., 2005; Sakamoto et al., 2007, 2008). These findings suggest that NMS plays important roles in the brain. However, it is not certain whether these actions described above are the physiological roles of NMS. Interesting results have been obtained by ICV administration of anti-NMS antibody to rats to neutralize the activity of endogenous NMS. In contrast to the actions induced by NMS administration, ICV pretreatment with anti-NMS IgG, but not anti-NMU IgG, blocks the suppression of food intake induced by both ICV and intraperitoneally administered leptin in rats (Nakahara et al., 2010), and ICV administration of anti-NMS antiserum suppresses suckling-induced milk ejection in lactating rats

(Sakamoto et al., 2008), suggesting that endogenous NMS plays physiological roles in the regulation of food intake and milk ejection. However, there is no anatomical evidence supporting these roles in the brain: NMS mRNA expression levels are low in the ARC, PVN, and SON in the hypothalamus (Mori et al., 2005), even though these nuclei are involved in the control of feeding behavior and release of oxytocin, a hormone important for milk ejection. Therefore, to understand completely the physiological role of NMS, it is necessary to elucidate the neural circuits formed by NMS-producing neurons in the brain.

Here, to clarify the physiological significance of NMS, we analyzed the regional distribution of NMS in the rat brain at the peptide level. We established a highly sensitive radioimmunoassay (RIA) specific for rat NMS by using a newly prepared antiserum. We then characterized NMS-immunoreactive molecules separated by reversed-phase high performance liquid chromatography (RP-HPLC) and determined the NMS content of the brain and other tissues. An examination of both NMS content and NMS mRNA expression in the various regions of the brain suggested that NMS neurons project directly from the hypothalamus to the brainstem.

## MATERIALS AND METHODS

### PREPARATION OF ANTI-RAT NMS ANTISERA

[$Cys^{21}$]-rat NMS[1-20], a C-terminally Cys-extended rat NMS fragment (positions 1–20), was synthesized and then conjugated to maleimide-activated mariculture keyhole limpet hemocyanin. Anti-rat-NMS serum (batch OB1321-1) was obtained from a Japanese white rabbit after 10 weekly subcutaneous injections of conjugate with adjuvant; a second batch (OB1321-2) was obtained from another rabbit in the same way. The titers of the antisera were determined by RIA.

### RADIOIODINATION OF TRACER LIGAND

A tracer ligand, [$Tyr^{21}$]-rat NMS[1-20], was synthesized and then radioiodinated by using the lactoperoxidase method (Washimine et al., 1994). After radioiodination, monoiodinated tracer was purified by RP-HPLC on a COSMOSIL $5C_{18}$-AR-II column (4.6 × 150 mm; Nacalai Tesque, Japan). The purified tracer was stored at −30°C after the addition of bovine serum albumin at a concentration of 0.1%.

### RIA FOR RAT NMS

The RIA for rat NMS was performed by using the method used for ghrelin, with minor modifications (Hosoda et al., 2000). Each RIA incubation mixture was composed of 100 μl of standard rat NMS or unknown sample in RIA buffer (50 mM $Na_2HPO_4$, 80 mM NaCl, 25 mM EDTA, 0.5% Triton X-100, 0.5% bovine serum albumin, 0.05% $NaN_3$, pH 7.4) and 100 μl antiserum diluted with RIA buffer containing 3.1% dextran T40. OB1321-2 anti-rat-NMS antiserum was used at a final dilution of 1/295,000. After a 24-h incubation, 18,000 cpm of [$^{125}I$-$Tyr^{21}$]-rat NMS[1-20] in 100 μl of RIA buffer containing 3.1% dextran T40 was added. Bound and free tracers were separated by precipitation with polyethylene glycol (PEG). After an additional 24-h incubation, 100 μl of 1% γ-globulin in precipitation buffer [50 mM phosphate buffer (pH 7.4) containing 80 mM NaCl and 0.05% $NaN_3$] and 500 μl of 16% PEG-6000 in precipitation buffer were added. The solution was then mixed vigorously and incubated for 15 min. The bound tracer was precipitated by centrifugation at 1500 *g* for 20 min, and then the free tracer was removed by aspiration. All procedures described above were performed at 4°C. The radioactivity in the precipitation was counted with a γ-counter ARC-600 (Aloka, Japan).

### PREPARATION OF TISSUE EXTRACTS FOR RIA

All procedures using animal experiments were performed in accordance with the Japanese Physiological Society's guidelines for animal care and the National Cerebral and Cardiovascular Center Research Institute Guide for the Care and Use of Experimental Animals. Ten-week-old male Wistar rats were maintained under 12 h light/dark cycles (light on from 7:00 to 19:00). Food and water were provided *ad libitum* except during the fasting experiments. The brains were sampled during the light period at ZT6 (Zeitgeber time, ZT; ZT0 is lights on and ZT12 is lights off) from free-fed and 48 h-fasted rats, and during the dark period at ZT18 from free-fed rats. Immediately after decapitation of rats, the brain, spleen, and testis were resected. The brain was dissected into the cerebral cortex, cerebellum, hippocampus–thalamus–striatum, hypothalamus, midbrain, and pons–medulla oblongata by using the method of Glowinski and Iversen (1966). After being weighed, each tissue was minced and then boiled for 5 min in 5× volumes of water. After being cooled, acetic acid was added to make a final concentration of 1 M, and then the boiled tissue was homogenized with a Polytron homogenizer (Kinematica, Switzerland). The supernatant of the extract, obtained after a 10-min centrifugation for at 14,000 g, was concentrated by evaporation and then subjected to precipitation with acetone at a concentration of 66% acetone. After removal of precipitates, the supernatant was evaporated to remove the acetone, and then loaded onto a Sep-Pak C18 cartridge (Waters, USA) equilibrated with 0.1% trifluoroacetic acid (TFA). After the cartridge had been washed with 10% acetonitrile ($CH_3CN$) in 0.1% TFA, the absorbed material was eluted with 60% $CH_3CN$ in 0.1% TFA, lyophilized, and dissolved in RIA buffer. Portions of samples, equivalent to 20–300 mg wet weight, were subjected to RIA.

The cerebrospinal fluid was collected from three anesthetized 12-week-old male Wistar rats, and then subjected to Sep-Pak purification.

### CHROMATOGRAPHIC CHARACTERIZATION OF IMMUNOREACTIVE NMS IN RAT BRAINS

Immediately after peptide extraction, a portion of sample equivalent to 1.2 g wet weight of whole brain was separated by RP-HPLC on a Symmetry 300 C18 column (3.9 × 150 mm; Waters, USA), with a linear gradient from 10 to 60% of $CH_3CN$ in 0.1% TFA for 40 min at a flow rate 1 ml/min. The purified cerebrospinal fluid was also subjected to RP-HPLC under the same conditions. The eluates were collected every minute, evaporated, and then lyophilized. The portions of eluate equivalent to 0.5 g wet weight of tissue and 130 μl of cerebrospinal fluid were subjected to RIA for rat NMS. Synthetic rat NMS was also applied to the same RP-HPLC system to compare the retention time with that of immunoreactive (ir)-NMS.

### QUANTITATIVE REVERSE TRANSCRIPTION–POLYMERASE CHAIN REACTION

The brains were sampled from 10-week-old male Wistar rats and various brain regions were dissected as described above. RNA was isolated by using TRIzol reagent (Ambion, USA). Reverse transcription was performed with a QuantiTect reverse transcription kit (Qiagen, USA). Quantitative PCR was conducted with a LightCycler system (Roche, USA) using a SYBR Premix Ex Taq kit (TaKaRa, Japan). The primer set used for rat NMS was 5′-CTCATCTGTGGTCTGCAAAGAG-3′ and 5′-GCATACAGAAGCAGTAGATGAC-3′, and for rat NMUR1 was 5′-CTCAGTCCACTCTATGTACC-3′ and 5′-AGAAGAGCAGTATGGTCGTC-3′, and for rat NMUR2 was 5′-ACTTGAACAGCACAGAGGAG-3′ and 5′-TTCAAAGTCTGATGTCGGAC-3′. Known amounts of rat NMS, NMUR1, and NMUR2 cDNA were used to obtain a standard curve. The data were normalized against total RNA quantity, wet weight of tissues, or 36B4 level.

## RESULTS

### RIA FOR RAT NMS

To generate specific antibodies, the N-terminal fragment (positions 1–20) of rat NMS was used as antigen, because this region has no sequence homology to other known peptides including rat NMU, a structurally related peptide (**Figure 1A**). Two types of antisera were obtained; antiserum OB1321-2 exhibited a titer against [$^{125}$I-Tyr$^{21}$]-rat NMS[1-20] approximately 17 times higher than OB1321-1 (**Figure 1B**). Therefore, the OB1321-2 antiserum was used in the subsequent experiments. On the standard RIA curve, the half-maximum inhibition of [$^{125}$I-Tyr$^{21}$]-rat NMS[1-20] binding to antibody by rat NMS was 6.2 fmol/tube, and the peptide was detectable at a low level of 0.25 fmol/tube (**Figure 1C**). The intra- and inter-assay variations were 3.1 and 3.8%, respectively. This antiserum had no cross-reactivity with rat NMU (**Figure 1C**) as well as neuropeptide Y, somatostatin, pituitary adenylate cyclase activating polypeptide, vasoactive intestinal polypeptide, calcitonin gene-related peptide, adrenocorticotropic hormone, α-melanocyte-stimulating hormone, and orexin-A, which are abundantly present in the hypothalamus (data not shown).

In rats, apparent expression of NMS mRNA is found in the brain, spleen, and testis (Mori et al., 2005). Therefore, we quantified NMS peptide in these tissues. The dilution curve generated from whole-brain extract paralleled the standard curve (**Figure 1C**), and the concentration of NMS in rat whole brain was 68.3 ± 3.4 fmol/g wet weight (mean ± SEM, $n = 3$). A small amount of ir-NMS was detected in the cerebrospinal fluid of rats. However, its concentration was not determined, because the value was outside of the range of the standard curve. On the other hand, specific ir-NMS was hard to detect in the spleen and testis (data not shown).

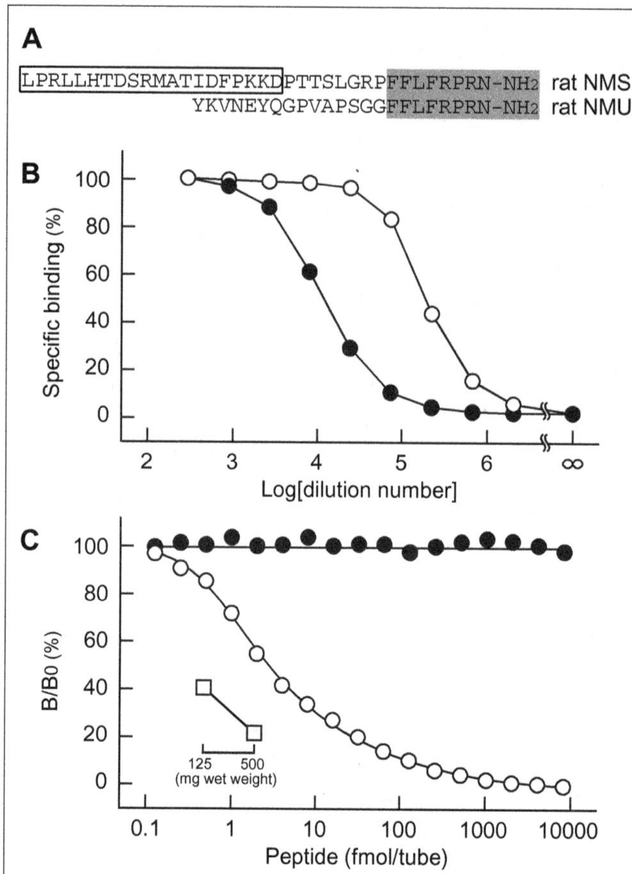


**FIGURE 1 | Characterization of antisera for rat neuromedin S (NMS).** **(A)** Structural comparison of rat NMS and rat neuromedin U (NMU). Structure conserved in the two peptides is shaded. The box indicates the sequence used as antigen peptide to obtain antisera specific for rat NMS. **(B)** Specific binding curves of antisera. [$^{125}$I-Tyr$^{21}$]-rat NMS[1-20] was incubated with serially diluted OB1321-1 (closed circles) and OB1321-2 (open circles) antisera, and then co-precipitated with antibody in a concentration-dependent manner. **(C)** Standard curve of radioimmunoassay for rat NMS using antiserum OB1321-2. [$^{125}$I-Tyr$^{21}$]-rat NMS[1-20] binding to antibody was displaced by increasing concentrations of rat NMS (open circles) but not rat NMU (closed circles). B/B0 means tracer bound/tracer bound in zero standards. Inset shows the inhibition of tracer ligand binding to antibody by diluted rat brain extract (open squares).

### CHROMATOGRAPHIC CHARACTERIZATION OF ir-NMS IN RAT WHOLE BRAIN

The molecular forms of ir-NMS found in the extract of rat whole brain were characterized by RIA coupled with RP-HPLC. More than 90% of ir-NMS was eluted as a single peak, with a retention time (20–21 min) identical to that of synthetic rat NMS (**Figure 2**). A very minor ir-NMS was also detected at a retention time of 18–20 min; this corresponded to that observed for oxidized NMS (data not shown). Non-specific immunoreactivity was not observed in any other eluted fractions.

On the other hand, ir-NMS in the cerebrospinal fluid was also eluted at a retention time identical to that of synthetic rat NMS (data not shown).

### REGIONAL DISTRIBUTION OF ir-NMS AND NMS mRNA IN RAT BRAIN

The rat brain was dissected into six parts, and both the NMS contents and the NMS mRNA expression levels in these regions were then determined. The highest concentration of ir-NMS was observed in the midbrain (286.5 ± 26.6 fmol/g wet weight, mean ± SEM), followed by the pons–medulla oblongata

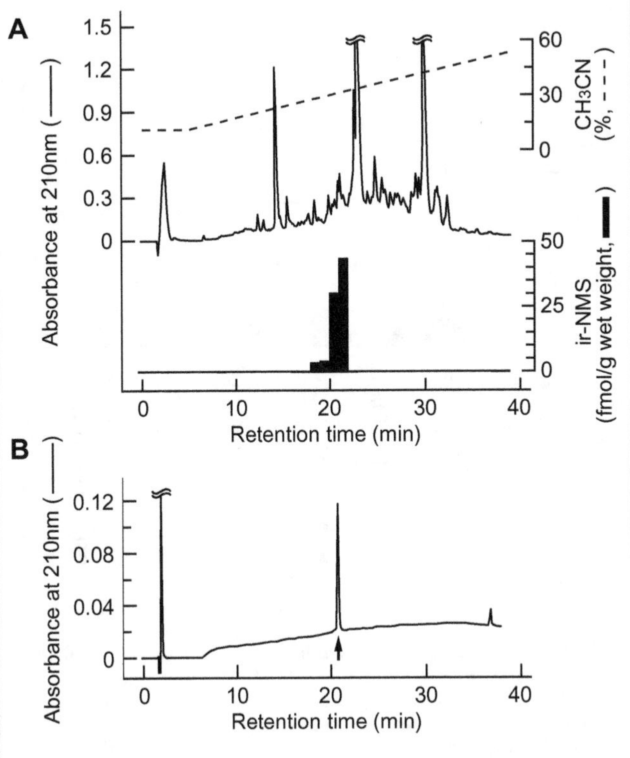


**FIGURE 2 | Representative reversed-phase high performance liquid chromatography (RP-HPLC) profile of neuromedin S (NMS) immunoreactivity in rat brain.** Peptide extract (equivalent to 1.2 g wet weight) from rat whole brain **(A)** and synthetic rat NMS **(B)** were applied to RP-HPLC under the same conditions. Black bars indicate immunoreactive NMS detected by radioimmunoassay **(A)**. Elution position of rat NMS is indicated by the arrow **(B)**.

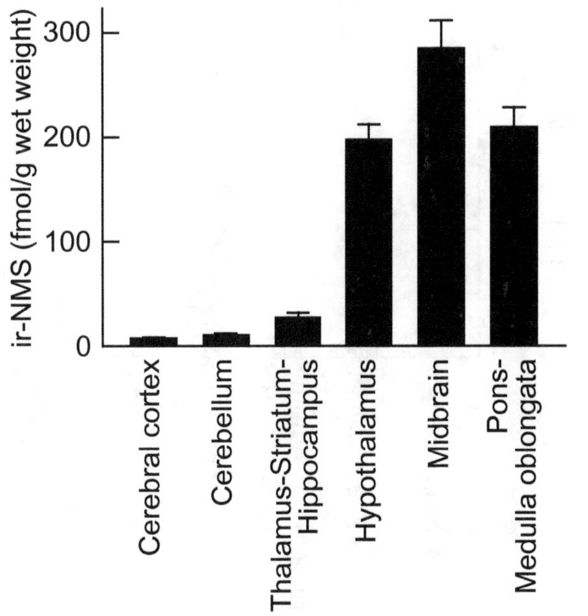


**FIGURE 3 | Regional distribution of immunoreactive neuromedin S (ir-NMS) in rat brain.** Concentrations of ir-NMS in various brain areas were quantified by radioimmunoassay. The brains were sampled during the light period. Data represent means ± SEM of three rats.

(208.8 ± 18.7 fmol/g wet weight) and hypothalamus (196.2 ± 15.2 fmol/g wet weight; **Figure 3**). Non-specific immunoreactivity was not found in these brain regions by RIA coupled with RP-HPLC (data not shown). Low levels of ir-NMS were detected in the other brain regions.

Abundant expression of NMS mRNA was found only in the hypothalamus (4.69 ± 0.52 copies/ng total RNA, mean ± SEM); low levels of mRNA expression were observed in the other regions (**Figure 4**). Normalization of the mRNA levels against the wet weight of tissues or 36B4 expression did not change this mRNA expression profile in the rat brain (data not shown).

### REGIONAL DISTRIBUTION OF NMUR1 AND NMUR2 mRNA IN RAT BRAIN

To elucidate the regional distribution of NMS receptor in rat brain, the mRNA expression level of NMUR1 and NMUR2 was analyzed by quantitative PCR (**Figure 5**). NMUR1 mRNA was widely distributed throughout the brain with low level of expression (approximately 0.8 copies/ng total RNA). On the other hand, abundant expression of NMUR2 mRNA was observed not only in the hypothalamus (7.27 ± 0.81 copies/ng total RNA, mean ± SEM), but also in the thalamus–striatum–hippocampus (3.72 ± 1.11 copies/ng total RNA), midbrain (4.20 ± 0.16 copies/ng total RNA), and pons–medulla oblongata (4.76 ± 0.40 copies/ng total RNA).

### LEVELS OF NMS PEPTIDE IN THE BRAIN OF RATS MAINTAINED UNDER LIGHT/DARK CYCLING, AND OF FASTED RATS

Most abundant expression of NMS mRNA is found in the SCN within the brain, and its expression level fluctuates under light/dark cycling (Mori et al., 2005). Therefore, we measured the levels of NMS peptide in the hypothalamus, midbrain, and pons–medulla oblongata of rats during both light and dark periods. The brains were sampled during the light period at ZT6 and the dark period at ZT18. In these brain regions, there is no significant difference in peptide levels between groups of rats at ZT6 and ZT18 (**Figures 6A–C**).

On the other hand, because ICV-administered NMS suppresses the food intake (Ida et al., 2005), we examined the effect of fasting on the levels of NMS peptide in the hypothalamus, midbrain, and pons–medulla oblongata. The peptide levels in the brain regions tested did not significantly differ between groups of free-fed and 48-h fasted rats (**Figures 6D–F**).

## DISCUSSION

We developed a highly sensitive RIA for rat NMS; the lowest detection limit was 0.25 fmol/tube (equivalent to 10.6 pg/ml). We evaluated the specificity of the assay by using a peptide extract of rat whole brain, because NMS was originally isolated from this tissue (Mori et al., 2005). The dilution curve for rat brain extract paralleled the standard curve. Moreover, no immunoreactivity other than that originating from native (major) and oxidized (minor) NMS was detected in any of the fractions of extracts

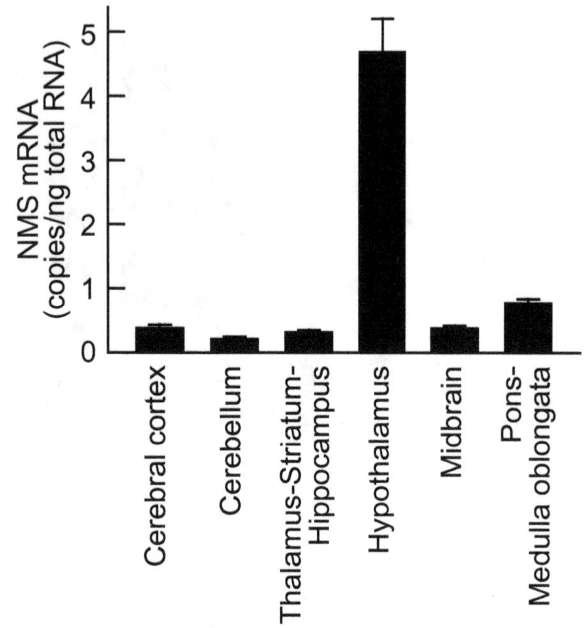


**FIGURE 4 | Expression of neuromedin S (NMS) mRNA in rat brain.** Rat NMS mRNA was quantified by quantitative reverse transcription–polymerase chain reaction analysis. The brains were sampled during the light period. Data represent means ± SEM of three rats.

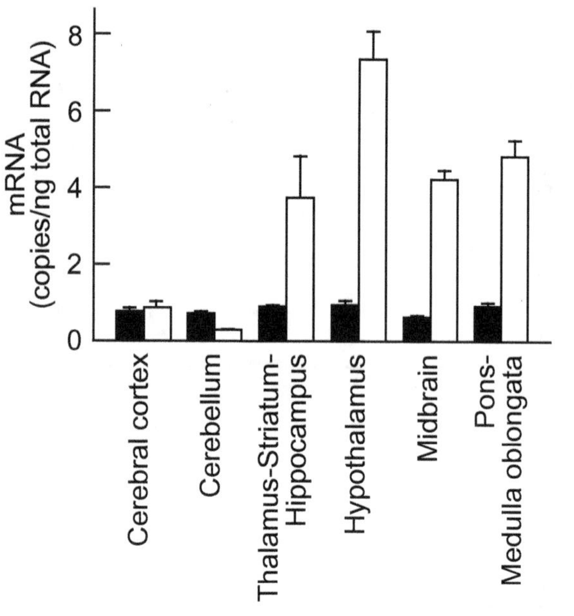


**FIGURE 5 | Expression of neuromedin U receptors types 1 (NMUR1) and 2 (NMUR2) mRNA in rat brain.** Rat NMUR1 (closed bars) and NMUR2 (open bars) mRNA were quantified by quantitative reverse transcription–polymerase chain reaction analysis. Data represent means ± SEM of three rats.

separated by RP-HPLC, suggesting that the OB1321-2 antiserum is not cross-reactive to other neuropeptides that are abundantly expressed in the brain. This is no doubt because NMS shows no sequence homology with any other known neuropeptide except for NMU, a structurally related peptide. In addition, this RIA is unable to detect rat NMU. These data indicate that the assay was highly specific.

Within the rat brain, the distribution profile of ir-NMS was different from that of NMS mRNA. It was interpreted that we clearly detected NMS peptide in the hypothalamus, because its mRNA was abundantly expressed in this region. However, we also detected NMS peptide in the midbrain and pons–medulla oblongata at levels comparable to those in the hypothalamus, whereas the mRNA levels in these regions were much lower than in the hypothalamus. Differences in the distributions of the orexin peptide and its mRNA have also been observed. Expression of orexin mRNA is restricted to the lateral hypothalamic area (LHA) and posterior hypothalamus (PH; Sakurai et al., 1998), whereas orexin peptides are distributed in various areas of the brain (Mondal et al., 1999). Furthermore, immunohistochemical mapping has shown that orexin-containing nerve fibers are abundant in various brain areas, including the olfactory bulb, cerebral cortex, thalamus, hypothalamus, and brainstem (Date et al., 1999). These data indicate that orexin neurons in the LHA or PH send projections widely across the brain (Date et al., 1999). The predominant expression of NMS mRNA only in the hypothalamus thus indicates that the cell bodies of the NMS neurons are located mainly in this region. In addition, NMS-containing nerve fibers are likely to be present in the midbrain and pons–medulla oblongata, because NMS peptide was abundant in these regions despite the low levels of expression of NMS mRNA. On the other hand, it is likely that there are fewer NMS-producing cells in the spinal cord than in the hypothalamus, because NMS mRNA expression levels are low in the spinal cord, as they are in the brainstem (Mori et al., 2005). Therefore, it is likely that nerve fibers originating from hypothalamic NMS neurons project to the brainstem, which consists of midbrain, pons, and medulla oblongata.

In our previous study, quantitative RT-PCR and *in situ* hybridization analyses showed that NMS mRNA was predominantly expressed in the SCN of the hypothalamus (Mori et al., 2005), indicating that, within the hypothalamus, most NMS neurons are located in this nucleus. Together with this situation, in view of the larger distribution in the brain of NMS peptide compared to NMS mRNA, we speculated the existence of neural circuits from NMS neurons located in the SCN to the brainstem. Little is known that the nerve fibers originating from SCN neurons project directly to the brainstem, although it is reported that the SCN indirectly projects to the locus coeruleus of pons (Aston-Jones et al., 2001) and the ventral tegmental area of midbrain (Luo and Aston-Jones, 2009). The results we described here may lead to the discovery of novel neural circuits. On the other hand, another possibility is that NMS peptide in the brainstem comes from hypothalamic nuclei other than the SCN, such as the PVN that are known to project to various targets in the brainstem (Geerling et al., 2010), whereas the levels of NMS mRNA in the PVN and other hypothalamic nuclei are extremely low compared with that in the SCN (Mori et al., 2005). To clarify these possibilities, immunohistochemical analysis of NMS in the brain is needed, and further investigation is continued in this regard.

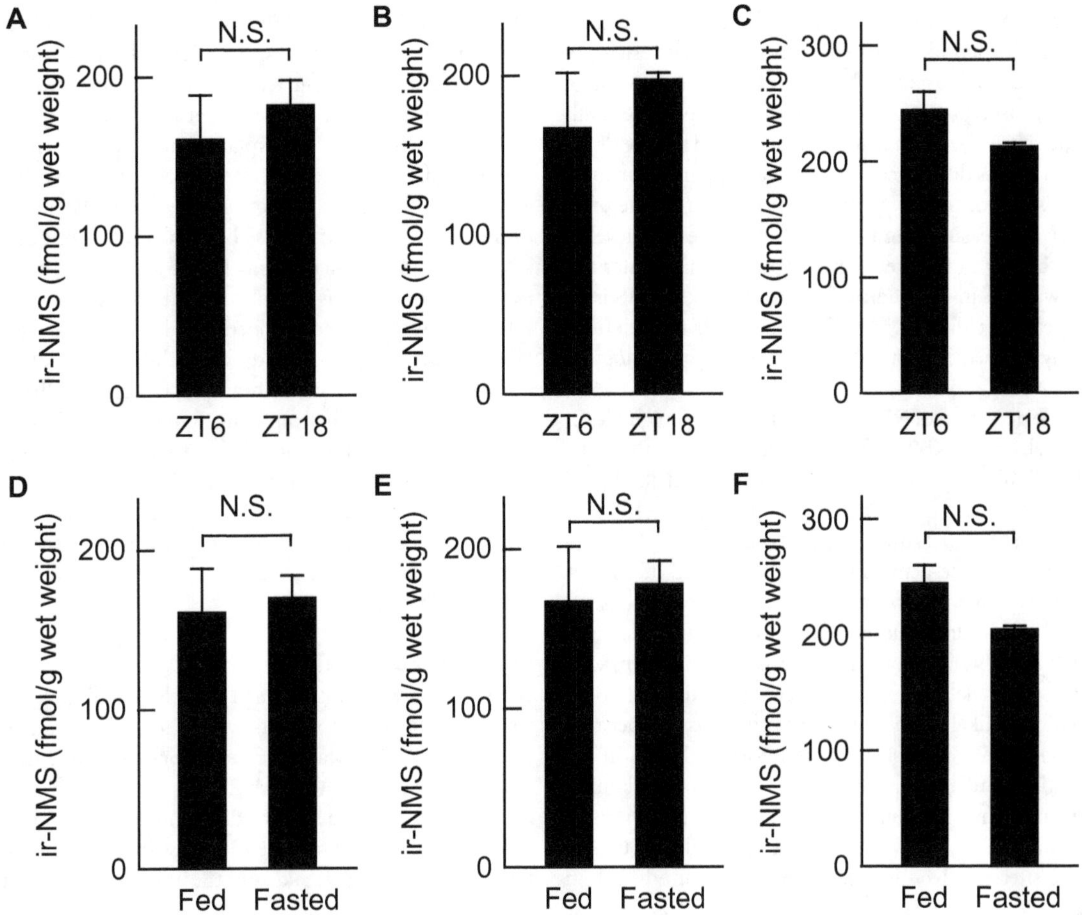


**FIGURE 6 | Levels of immunoreactive neuromedin S (ir-NMS) in the brain of rats maintained under light/dark cycling, and of fasted rats. (A–C)** Concentrations of ir-NMS were quantified in the hypothalamus **(A)**, midbrain **(B)**, and pons–medulla oblongata **(C)** of rats under the light at ZT6 and dark at ZT18. **(D–F)** Concentrations of ir-NMS were quantified in the hypothalamus **(D)**, midbrain **(E)**, and pons–medulla oblongata **(F)** of free-fed and 48 h-fasted rats. Data represent means ± SEM of three rats. Data were analyzed statistically by Student's *t*-test.

There are two kinds of receptors for NMS, NMUR1 and NMUR2 (Brighton et al., 2004; Mori et al., 2005), and their expression patterns are unique. Expression of NMUR1 is widely distributed throughout various tissues, and high levels of expression are found in peripheral tissues (Fujii et al., 2000). In contrast, NMUR2 mRNA is mainly expressed in the central nervous system (Hosoya et al., 2000), and its expression is clearly detected in the PVN, the wall of the third ventricle in the hypothalamus, and the CA1 region of the hippocampus (Howard et al., 2000). In addition, regional distribution of these receptors in rat brain was investigated in this study. Quantitative RT-PCR showed the apparent expression of NMUR2 mRNA in the midbrain and pons–medulla oblongata as well as in the hypothalamus. These data suggest the functional possibility of NMS within the brainstem.

We and another group have demonstrated that ICV administration of NMS induces a phase shift in the circadian rhythm (Mori et al., 2005), suppression of food intake (Ida et al., 2005), reduction of urine volume (Sakamoto et al., 2007), increased in milk ejection (Sakamoto et al., 2008), and release of luteinizing hormone (Vigo et al., 2007). All of actions are induced as a result of the direct effects of NMS on hypothalamic nuclei such as the SCN, ARC, PVN, and SON (Ida et al., 2005; Mori et al., 2005; Sakamoto et al., 2007, 2008; Vigo et al., 2007). On the other hand, NMS peptide and NMUR2 mRNA are present in the brainstem, suggesting the physiological role of NMS system in this region. However, the function of NMS by direct action on the brainstem remains to be clarified. The brainstem is important for basic bodily functions (especially regulation of the cardiovascular and respiratory systems). Therefore, regulation of these systems may be a major role of NMS within the brainstem, although it is not yet certain whether this action is a result of a direct effect of NMS in this region. On the other hand, our group recently reported that, in mice, NMS regulates the heart rate through the sympathetic nervous system (Sakamoto et al., 2011).

In the rat brain, NMS mRNA is predominantly expressed in the SCN, with weak expression in other nuclei of hypothalamus, and its expression fluctuates within the SCN under light/dark cycling: the largest decrease occurs during the dark period, followed by a gradual increase until the late light period (Mori et al., 2005). In contrast, there is no difference in hypothalamic content of NMS peptide between groups of rats during the light and dark periods. In general, the neuropeptide is stored in the secretory vesicles of neuron, and released in response to relevant stimuli. In view of this mechanism, discrepancy between mRNA and peptide levels of NMS may be caused by mechanism of storage and release of the neuropeptide as well as differences in mRNA and peptide turnover rates, because tissue content of peptide is modulated by the presence or absence of releasing stimuli, even if the expression level of mRNA is constant. On the other hand, hypothalamic content of NMS peptide was not influenced by fasting, although NMS is an anorexigenic peptide (Ida et al., 2005). To consider the relationship between hypothalamic content of peptide and physiology of NMS, further investigation is needed.

The negligible detection of NMS peptide in the spleen and testis was unexpected, because NMS gene expression levels in these tissues are higher than that in the whole brain (Mori et al., 2005). Several neuropeptides are produced in the spleen and testis. For example, somatostatin and its mRNA are detected in the spleen and pituitary adenylate cyclase-activating polypeptide and its mRNA are detected in the testis, indicating that both neuropeptides are synthesized and stored until release in these tissues (Aquila et al., 1991; Shioda et al., 1994). In contrast, because only NMS mRNA – not its peptide – was detected in the spleen and testis, NMS peptide accumulation is likely to be difficult in these tissues because NMS may be secreted *via* constitutive secretory pathways in the spleen and testis, similar to the way in which adrenomedullin is secreted from both endothelial and vascular smooth muscle cells (Sugo et al., 1994a,b). This may occur because the sequences of the cleavage sites involved in post-translational modification of the NMS precursor coincide with those of the consensus motifs (Arg-X-Lys/Arg-Arg and Arg-X-Arg-X-X-Arg) for proteolytic processing by furin and/or furin-like proteases (proprotein convertases functioning within constitutive secretory pathways; Seidah and Chrétien, 1999; Mori et al., 2005). On the other hand, there is another possible explanation as follows: if NMS mRNA is highly expressed in a discrete cell population within the spleen and testis, the peptide gets massively diluted when whole organ is homogenized. To verify these hypotheses, it is important to identify the NMS-producing cells in the spleen and testis by *in situ* hybridization analysis and immunohistochemistry.

In conclusion, we developed a highly sensitive and highly specific RIA for rat NMS. The different distribution of NMS peptide and its mRNA within the brain suggested the direct projection of nerve fibers originating from hypothalamic NMS neurons to the brainstem. In addition, the gene expression of NMS receptor, NMUR2, was clearly detected in the brainstem. Because the functions of NMS within the brainstem have not yet been identified, our findings provide a foundation on which further research can build to provide novel insights into the physiological roles of NMS in the brain.

## ACKNOWLEDGMENTS

We thank Dr. Kazuhiko Harada for helpful support. This work was supported in part by Grants-in-Aid for Scientific Research from the Ministry of Education, Science, Sports, and Culture of Japan, the Improvement of Research Environment for Young Researchers Program of the Ministry of Education, Science, Sports, and Culture of Japan, a grant for Scientific Research on Priority Areas from the University of Miyazaki, and the Takeda Science Foundation.

## REFERENCES

Aquila, M. C., Dees, W. L., Haensly, W. E., and McCann, S. M. (1991). Evidence that somatostatin is localized and synthesized in lymphoid organs. *Proc. Natl. Acad. Sci. U.S.A.* 88, 11485–11489.

Aston-Jones, G., Chen, S., Zhu, Y., and Oshinsky, M. L. (2001). A neural circuit for circadian regulation of arousal. *Nat. Neurosci.* 4, 732–738.

Brighton, P. J., Szekeres, P. G., and Willars, G. B. (2004). Neuromedin U and its receptors: structure, function, and physiological roles. *Pharmacol. Rev.* 56, 231–248.

Date, Y., Ueta, Y., Yamashita, H., Yamaguchi, H., Matsukura, S., Kangawa, K., et al. (1999). Orexins, orexigenic hypothalamic peptides, interact with autonomic, neuroendocrine and neuroregulatory systems. *Proc. Natl. Acad. Sci. U.S.A.* 96, 748–753.

Fujii, R., Hosoya, M., Fukusumi, S., Kawamata, Y., Habata, Y., Hinuma, S., et al. (2000). Identification of neuromedin U as the cognate ligand of the orphan G protein-coupled receptor FM-3. *J. Biol. Chem.* 275, 21068–21074.

Geerling, J. C., Shin, J. W., Chimenti, P. C., and Loewy, A. D. (2010). Paraventricular hypothalamic nucleus: axonal projections to the brainstem. *J. Comp. Neurol.* 518, 1460–1499.

Glowinski, J., and Iversen, L. L. (1966). Regional studies of catecholamines in the rat brain-I: the disposition of [3H]norepinephrine, [3H]dopamine and [3H]dopa in various regions of the brain. *J. Neurochem.* 13, 655–669.

Hosoda, H., Kojima, M., Matsuo, H., and Kangawa, K. (2000). Ghrelin and des-acyl ghrelin: two major forms of rat ghrelin peptide in gastrointestinal tissue. *Biochem. Biophys. Res. Commun.* 279, 909–913.

Hosoya, M., Moriya, T., Kawamata, Y., Ohkubo, S., Fujii, R., Matsui, H., et al. (2000). Identification and functional characterization of a novel subtype of neuromedin U receptor. *J. Biol. Chem.* 275, 29528–29532.

Howard, A. D., Wang, R., Pong, S. S., Mellin, T. N., Strack, A., Guan, X. M., et al. (2000). Identification of receptors for neuromedin U and its role in feeding. *Nature* 406, 70–74.

Ida, T., Mori, K., Miyazato, M., Egi, Y., Abe, S., Nakahara, K., et al. (2005). Neuromedin S is a novel anorexigenic hormone. *Endocrinology* 146, 4217–4223.

Luo, A. H., and Aston-Jones, G. (2009). Circuit projection from suprachiasmatic nucleus to ventral tegmental area: a novel circadian output pathway. *Eur. J. Neurosci.* 20, 748–760.

Mondal, M. S., Nakazato, M., Date, Y., Murakami, N., Yanagisawa, M., and Matsukura, S. (1999). Widespread distribution of orexin in rat brain and its regulation upon fasting. *Biochem. Biophys. Res. Commun.* 256, 495–499.

Mori, K., Miyazato, M., Ida, T., Murakami, N., Serino, R., Ueta, Y., et al. (2005). Identification of neuromedin S and its possible role in the mammalian circadian oscillator system. *EMBO J.* 24, 325–335.

Nakahara, K., Hanada, R., Murakami, N., Teranishi, H., Ohgusu, H., Fukushima, N., et al. (2004). The gut-brain peptide neuromedin U is involved in the mammalian circadian oscillator system. *Biochem. Biophys. Res. Commun.* 318, 156–161.

Nakahara, K., Katayama, T., Maruyama, K., Ida, T., Mori, K., Miyazato, M., et al. (2010). Comparison of feeding suppression by the anorexigenic hormones neuromedin U and neuromedin S in rats. *J. Endocrinol.* 207, 185–193.

Sakamoto, T., Mori, K., Nakahara, K., Miyazato, M., Kangawa, K., Sameshima, H., et al. (2007). Neuromedin S exerts an antidiuretic action in rats. *Biochem. Biophys. Res. Commun.* 361, 457–461.

Sakamoto, T., Mori, K., Miyazato, M., Kangawa, K., Sameshima, H., Nakahara, K., et al. (2008). Involvement of neuromedin S in the oxytocin release response to suckling stimulus. *Biochem. Biophys. Res. Commun.* 375, 49–53.

Sakamoto, T., Nakahara, K., Maruyama, K., Katayama, T., Mori, K., Miyazato, M., et al. (2011). Neuromedin S regulates cardiovascular function through the sympathetic nervous system in mice. *Peptides* 32, 1020–1026.

Sakurai, T., Amemiya, A., Ishii, M., Matsuzaki, I., Chemelli, R. M., Tanaka, H., et al. (1998). Orexins and orexin receptors: a family of hypothalamic neuropeptides and G protein-coupled receptors that regulate feeding behavior. *Cell* 92, 573–585.

Seidah, N. G., and Chrétien, M. (1999). Proprotein and prohormone convertases: a family of subtilases generating diverse bioactive polypeptides. *Brain Res.* 848, 45–62.

Shioda, S., Leqradi, G., Leung, W. C., Nakajo, S., Nakaya, K., and Arimura, A. (1994). Localization of pituitary adenylate cyclase-activating polypeptide and its messenger ribonucleic acid in the rat testis by light and electron microscopic immunocytochemistry and *in situ* hybridization. *Endocrinology* 135, 818–825.

Sugo, S., Minamno, N., Kangawa, K., Miyamoto, K., Kitamura, K., Sakata, J., et al. (1994a). Endothelial cells actively synthesize and secrete adrenomedullin. *Biochem. Biophys. Res. Commun.* 201, 1160–1166.

Sugo, S., Minamino, N., Shoji, H., Kangawa, K., Kitamura, K., Eto, T., et al. (1994b). Production and secretion of adrenomedullin from vascular smooth muscle cells: augmented production by tumor necrosis factor-α. *Biochem. Biophys. Res. Commun.* 203, 719–726.

Vigo, E., Roa, J., López, M., Castellano, J. M., Fernandez-Fernandez, R., Navarro, V. M., et al. (2007). Neuromedin S as novel putative regulator of luteinizing hormone secretion. *Endocrinology* 148, 813–823.

Washimine, H., Kitamura, K., Ichiki, Y., Yamamoto, Y., Kangawa, K., Matsuo, H., et al. (1994). Immunoreactive proadrenomedullin N-terminal 20 peptide in human tissue, plasma and urine. *Biochem. Biophys. Res. Commun.* 202, 1081–1087.

16

# NPBWR1 and NPBWR2: implications in energy homeostasis, pain, and emotion

***Takeshi Sakurai****

*Kanazawa University, Kanazawa, Japan*

***Edited by:***
*Hubert Vaudry, University of Rouen, France*

***Reviewed by:***
*Kazuhiro Nakamura, Kyoto University, Japan*
*Olivier Civelli, University of California, Irvine, USA*

****Correspondence:***
*Takeshi Sakurai, Kanazawa University, 13-1 Takara-machi, Kanazawa 920-8640, Japan.*
*e-mail: takeshi.sakurai@gmail.com*

Neuropeptide B/W receptor-1 (NPBWR1) and NPBWR2 had been known as orphan receptors GPR7 and 8, respectively. Endogenous peptide ligands of these receptors, neuropeptide B (NPB) and neuropeptide W (NPW), were identified in 2002 and 2003 (Fujii et al., 2002; Brezillon et al., 2003; Tanaka et al., 2003). These peptides have been implicated in regulation of feeding behavior, energy homeostasis, neuroendocrine function, and modulating inflammatory pain. In addition, strong and discrete expression of their receptors in the extended amygdala and bed nucleus of the stria terminalis suggests a potential role in regulating stress responses, emotion, anxiety, and fear. Recent studies of NPB/NPW using both pharmacological and phenotypic analyses of genetically engineered mice as well as a human study support this hypothesis.

**Keywords: neuropeptide B, neuropeptide W, hypothalamus, limbic system, amygdala, pain, emotions**

## INTRODUCTION

Receptors for neuropeptide B (NPB)/neuropeptide W (NPW) were originally identified as orphan receptors GPR7 and GPR8, which share 70% nucleotide identity and 64% amino acid identity with each other. They have relatively high similarities with opioid and somatostatin receptors. GPR8 was not found in the rodent genomes, while GPR7 was highly conserved in both human and rodents (O'Dowd et al., 1995). This suggests the GPR8 gene was relatively recently generated through gene duplication.

In 2002–2003, two endogenous peptide ligands for these receptors were identified and named NPB/NPW (Fujii et al., 2002; Shimomura et al., 2002; Brezillon et al., 2003; Tanaka et al., 2003). Following the deorphaning of these receptors, GPR7 and GPR8 were reclassified by IUPHAR as NPB/W receptor-1 (NPBWR1) and NPB/W receptor-2 (NPBWR2), respectively (Davenport and Singh, 2005).

In rodents, *Npbwr1* mRNA is localized in some discrete brain regions, including the hypothalamus (dorsomedial hypothalamus and suprachiasmatic nucleus), hippocampus, ventral tegmental area (VTA), and extended amygdala (CeA and bed nucleus of the stria terminalis; BNST) (Lee et al., 1999; Tanaka et al., 2003), suggesting this receptor is involved in regulatory mechanisms of homeostasis, reward system, and emotion.

This review discusses recent findings concerning the pharmacology, histology, and phenotypic analysis of genetically engineered mice of the NPB/NPW system.

## IDENTIFICATION OF NPB AND NPW

In 2002–2003, three groups independently identified endogenous peptide ligands for GPR7 and GPR8 by so-called "reverse pharmacology" in combination with bioinformatics approaches. To identify the cognate endogenous ligands for GPR7 (NPBWR1) and GPR8 (NPBWR2), Shimomura et al. (2002) expressed these receptors in Chinese Hamster Ovary (CHO) cells and measured the decrease in forskolin-induced cAMP production in these cells as the read-out for receptor activation. While screening the bovine hypothalamic extract fractions, they detected activities that specifically inhibit cAMP production in those cells, and purified the activities. During their purification process, they identified two forms of NPW with different peptide lengths of 23 and 30 amino acid residues, and named them NPW23 and NPW30, respectively.

In a similar manner, three groups (Fujii et al., 2002; Brezillon et al., 2003; Tanaka et al., 2003) independently purified and identified an additional endogenous ligand for NPBW1 and NPBW2. Fujii et al. first screened the Celera database to identify novel secretory peptides and then expressed the cDNAs of the putative secretory peptides to find novel peptide ligands. Subsequent pharmacological studies and purification of the peptide from bovine hypothalamic extracts led to identification of the second ligand for GPR7 and GPR8, which was named NPB due to the unique modification, namely, bromination of the first tryptophan residue. Brezillon et al. (2003) also identified human NPB mRNA using a bioinformatics approach by searching the EST database using the NPW sequence as a query.

Tanaka et al. used a unique melanin-pigment aggregation assay in *Xenopus* melanophore cells expressing GPR7 as the assay system to purify NPB from bovine hypothalamus. Through EST database searches they also identified NPW as a putative paralogous peptide (Tanaka et al., 2003).

## STRUCTURES OF NPW AND NPB

Neuropeptide W and NPB do not display any significant sequence similarity to members of other known peptide families, while sharing a high degree of sequence similarity with each other, constituting a distinct family of peptides (**Figure 1A**) (Fujii et al., 2002; Shimomura et al., 2002; Brezillon et al., 2003; Tanaka et al., 2003).

As mentioned earlier, sequence analysis of purified peptides showed that NPW has two isoforms with lengths of 23 and 30 amino acid residues, i.e., neuropeptide W23 (NPW23) and

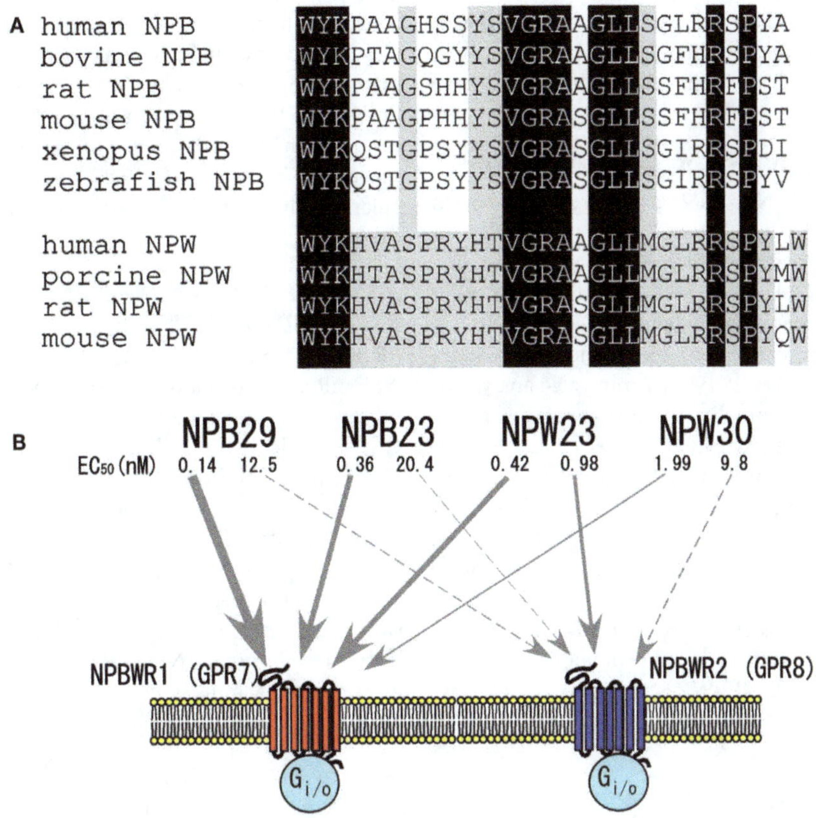


**FIGURE 1 | The NPB/NPW system. (A)** Amino acid sequences of NPB and NPW. Dark shadow shows amino acid identity between NPB and NPW. Light shadow shows conserved amino acids within NPB or NPW. **(B)** NPB/W and their receptors. $EC_{50}$ values were determined by assay of inhibition of cAMP production in CHO cells expressing each receptor (Brezillon et al., 2003). Modified from Hondo et al. (2008).

neuropeptide W30 (NPW30), respectively. NPW23 is produced as a result of proteolytic processing at a pair of arginine residues in the 24th and 25th positions in NPW30 (Fujii et al., 2002; Brezillon et al., 2003; Tanaka et al., 2003). *In vitro* experiments using cells expressing these receptors showed that synthetic NPW23 activates and binds to both NPBWR1 and NPBWR2 at similar effective doses, while NPW30 shows slightly lower affinity to both receptors as compared with NPW23 (**Figure 1B**) (Brezillon et al., 2003; Tanaka et al., 2003).

As mentioned earlier, NPB has a unique modification at the N-terminus tryptophan residue, C-6-bromination (Fujii et al., 2002; Tanaka et al., 2003). While this represents the first evidence of bromination of the protein in mammals, the biological significance of this modification is unclear, as it has been demonstrated that des-bromo-NPB is equipotent to brominated NPB in *in vitro* cAMP inhibition assays (Tanaka et al., 2003). By analogy with NPW, Brezillon et al. (2003) predicted that two isoforms of NPB, NPB23 and NPB29, could be produced from the processing of a 125-amino acid human precursor through the alternative usage of a dibasic amino acid pair. However, the dibasic motif, Arg24–Arg25, which is seen in human NPB, does not exist in NPB of other mammalian species including bovine, rat, and mouse. Therefore, it is unlikely that the NPB23 isoform exists as a mature peptide in non-human species. Consistently, both Fujii et al. and Tanaka et al. were only able to isolate NPB29 from bovine hypothalamus extracts during their purification procedures.

In *X. laevis* melanophore pigment aggregation assay, NPB29 binds and activates human NPBWR1 or NPBWR2 with median effective concentrations ($EC_{50}$) of 0.23 and 15.8 nM, respectively (Tanaka et al., 2003), suggesting that NPB is a relatively selective agonist for NPBWR1 (**Figure 1B**).

The preferred conformations of des-bromo-NPB and -NPW have been determined by a combination of $^{1}H$ NMR, CD, and molecular modeling (Lucyk and Miskolzie, 2005).

## STRUCTURE-ACTIVITY RELATIONSHIPS OF NPW AND NPB

The rank order of potency of NPB and NPW isoforms has been determined in cell lines expressing NPBWR1 and NPBWR2. Both NPW and NPB bind and activate NPBWR1 and NPBWR2 receptors with varying degrees of affinity. NPBWR1 has slightly higher affinity for NPB as compared with both forms of NPW, whereas NPBWR2 shows a potency rank order of NPW23 > NPW30 > NPB (**Figure 1B**) (Fujii et al., 2002; Shimomura et al., 2002; Brezillon et al., 2003; Tanaka et al., 2003). NPB23 and NPB29 have similar affinity for both receptors. NPW23 and NPW30 bind to both receptors almost equally, while NPB acts as a relatively selective agonist for NPBWR1.

Tanaka et al. (2003) showed that deletion of Trp-1 from NPB or NPW markedly decreased their activity, suggesting that the N-terminus is involved in receptor binding. This is consistent with the fact that NPB and NPW have similarity in their sequences in the N-terminal region.

## STRUCTURES AND FUNCTIONS OF NPBWR1 AND NPBWR2

The human NPBWR1 and NPBWR2 genes are localized on chromosome 10q11.2–121.1 and 20q13.3, respectively. Human NPBWR1 and NPBWR2 have 328 and 333 amino acid residues, respectively, and share 64% sequence homology with each other (**Figure 2**). Among other family members of GPCRs, NPBW1 and NPBW2 are most closely related to opioid and somatostatin receptors (**Figure 2**) (O'Dowd et al., 1995). Amino acid analysis of NPBW1 orthologs in other mammalian species has revealed a high degree of conservation throughout evolution (Lee et al., 1999). In contrast, while the gene encoding NPBWR2 has been discovered in several mammalian species such as monkey, lemur, bat, shrew, and rabbit, it has not been found in rodent genomes (Lee et al., 1999), suggesting that these two receptors were produced by relatively phylogenetically recent gene duplication (Lee et al., 1999).

As suggested by the assay systems used during their purification process and structural similarities to somatostatin/opioid receptors, both NPBWR1 and NPBWR2 couple to the Gi-class of G-proteins (Tanaka et al., 2003). This suggests that these neuropeptides have inhibitory properties on neurons via activation of GIRK (Kir3) channels. NPB and NPW were also shown to stimulate Erk p42/p44 activity in human adrenocortical carcinoma-derived NCI-H295 cells (Andreis et al., 2005). This activation is probably mediated by beta/gamma subunits released from Gi-proteins (Tim van et al., 1995). Recently, a synthetic low molecular weight antagonist for NPBWR1 has been reported (Anthony Romero et al., 2012).

## DISTRIBUTION OF NPB/NPW AND NPBWR1/NPBWR2 IN BRAIN AND OTHER TISSUE

### NEUROPEPTIDE B

*Npb* mRNA was found in several specific regions in the mouse brain such as the paraventricular hypothalamic nucleus (PVN), CA1–CA3 fields of the hippocampus, and several nuclei in the midbrain and brainstem, including the Edinger–Westphal (EW) nucleus, the sensory and motor nuclei of the trigeminal nerve, locus coeruleus (LC), inferior olive, and lateral parabrachial nucleus (**Figure 3**) (Tanaka et al., 2003; Jackson et al., 2006).

Schulz et al. reported that NPB-immunoreactive cell bodies were observed in many regions within the hypothalamus. High levels of *Npbwr1* and *Npb* mRNA expression were also observed in the hypothalamus, including the ventromedial hypothalamic

```
GPR7                                                            MD-NASFSEP-WPANASGPDP   19
GPR8                                                   MQAAGHPEPLDSRGSFSLPTMGANVS-QD-   28
SOMATOSTATIN RECEPTOR SSTR3                                 MDMLHPSSVSTTSEPENASSAWPPD-   25
DELTA OPIOID RECEPTOR                        MEPAPSAGAELQPPLFANASDAYPSAFPSAG---ANASGP-P   38
KAPPA OPIOID RECEPTOR               MDSPIQIFRGEPGPTCAPSACLPPNSSAWFPGWAEPDSNGSAG-SEDAQ   48
M1 OPIOID RECEPTOR           MDSSAAPTNASNCTDALAYSSCSPAPSPGSWVNLSHLDGNLSDPCGP-NRTN---   51

                              TRANSMEMBRANE 1                TRANSMEMBRANE 2
GPR7     ALSCSNASTLAPLPAP-LAVAVPVVYAVICAVGLAGNSAVLYVLLRAPRMKTVTNLFILNLAIADELFTLVLPINIADFLLRQWPFGELMC   109
GPR8     NGTGHNATFSEPLPF--LYVLLPAVYSGICAVGLTGNTAVILVILRAPKMKTVTNVFILNLAVADGLFTLVLPVNIAEHLLQYWPFGELLC   117
SSTR3    ATLGNVSAGPSPAGLAVSGVLIPLVYLVVCVVGLLGNSLVIYVVLRHTASPSVTNVYILNLALADELFMLGLPFLAAQNALSYWPFGSLMC   116
DELTA    -GARS-AS------SLALAIAITALYSAVCAVGLLGNVLVMFGIVRYTKMKTATNIYIFNLALADALATSTLPFQSAKYLMETWPFGELLC   121
KAPPA    --------LEPAHISPAIPVIITAVYSVVFVVGLVGNSLVMFVIIRYTKMKTATNIYIFNLALADALVTTTMPFQSTVYLMNSWPFGDVLC   131
M1       LGGRDSLCPPTGSPSMITAITIMALYSIVCVVGLFGNFLVMYVIVRYTKMKTATNIYIFNLALADALATSTLPFQSVNYLMGTWPFGTILC   142

              TRANSMEMBRANE 3                        TRANSMEMBRANE 4
GPR7     KLIV-AIDQYNTFSSLYFLTVMSADRYLVVLATAESRRVAGRTYSAARAVSLAVWGIVTLVVLPFAVFA---RLDDEQGRRQCVLVFPQP   195
GPR8     KL-VLAVDHYNIFSSIYFLAVMSVDRYLVVLATVRSRHMPWRTYRGAKVASLCVWLGVTVLVLPFFSFAGVYSNELQVPS---CGLSFPWP   204
SSTR3    R-LVMAVDGINQFTSIFCLTVMSVDRYLAVVHPTRSARW--RTAPVARTVSAAVWVASAVVVLPVVVFSGV-PRGMST-----CHMQWPEP   196
DELTA    K-AVLSIDYYNMFTSIFTLTMMSVDRYIAVCHPVKALDF--RTPAKAKLINICIWVLASGVGVPIMVMAVTRPR-DGAVV---CMLQFPSP   205
KAPPA    K-IVISIDYYNMFTSIFTLTMMSVDRYIAVCHPVKALDF--RTPLKAKIINICIWLLSSSVGISAIVLGGTKVREDVDV--IECSLQFPDD   217
M1       K-IVISIDYYNMFTSIFTLCTMSVDRYIAVCHPVKALDF--RTPRNAKIINVCNWILSSAIGLPVMFMATTKYR----QGSIDCTLTFSHP   226

                   TRANSMEMBRANE 5                            TRANSMEMBRANE 6
GPR7     EAFWWRAS-RLYTLVLGFAIPVSTICVLYTT-LLCRLHAM--RLDSHAKALERA-KKRVTFLVVAILAVCLLCWTPYHLSTVV-ALTTDLP   280
GPR8     EQVWFKAS-RVYTLVLGFVLPVCTICVLYTD-LLRRLRAV--RLRSGAKALGKA-RRKVTVLVLVVLAVCLLCWTPFHLASVV-ALTTDLP   283
SSTR3    -AAAWRAGFIIYTAALGFFGPLLVICLCYLLIVV-KVRSAGRRVWAPSCQRRRRSERRVTRMVVAVVALFVLCWMPFYVLNIVNVVCP-LP   286
DELTA    -SWYWDTVTKICVFLFAFVVPILIITVCYGLMLL-RLRSV--RLLSGSKEKDR-SLRRITRMVLVVVGAFVVCWAPIHIFVIVWTLVDIDR   295
KAPPA    DYSWWDLFMKICVFIFAFVIPVLIIIVCYTLMIL-RLKSV--RLLSGSREKDRN-LRRITRLVLVVVAVFVVCWTPIHIFILVEALGSTSH   304
M1       -TWYWENLVKICVFIFAFIMPVLIITVCYGLMIL-RLKSV--RMLSGSKEKDRN-LRRITRMVLVVVAVFIVCWTPIHIYVIIKALVTI-P   311

                 TRANSMEMBRANE 7
GPR7     QTPLVIAISYF-ITSLTYANSCLNPFLYAFLDASFRRNLRQL-I-TC-RAAA                                       328
GPR8     QTPLVISMSYV-ITSLSYANSCLNPFLYAFLDDNFRKNFR--SILRC                                            333
SSTR3    EEPAFFG-LYFLVVALPYANSCANPILYGFLSYRFKQGFRRVLLRPSRRVRSQEPTVGPPEKTEEEDEEEEDGEESREGGKGKEMNGRVSQ   378
DELTA    RDPLVVAALHLCI-ALGYANSSLNPVLYAFLDENFKRCFRQLCRKPCGRPDPSSFSRAREATARERVTACTPSDGPGGGAAA          372
KAPPA    STAAL-SSYYFCI-ALGYTNSSLNPILYAFLDENFKRCFRDFCFPLKMRMERQSTSRVR--NTVQDPAYLRDIDGMNKPV            380
M1       ETTFQTVSWHFCI-ALGYTNSCLNPVLYAFLDENFKRCFREFCIPTSSNIEQQNSTRIRQ-NTRDHPSTANTVDRTNHQLENLEAETAPLP 400
```

**FIGURE 2 | Primary structures of NPBWR1/NPBWR2 compared to somatostatin and opioid receptors.** Conserved amino acid residues are shown in red. Each transmembrane domain is boxed. Modified from Hondo et al. (2008).

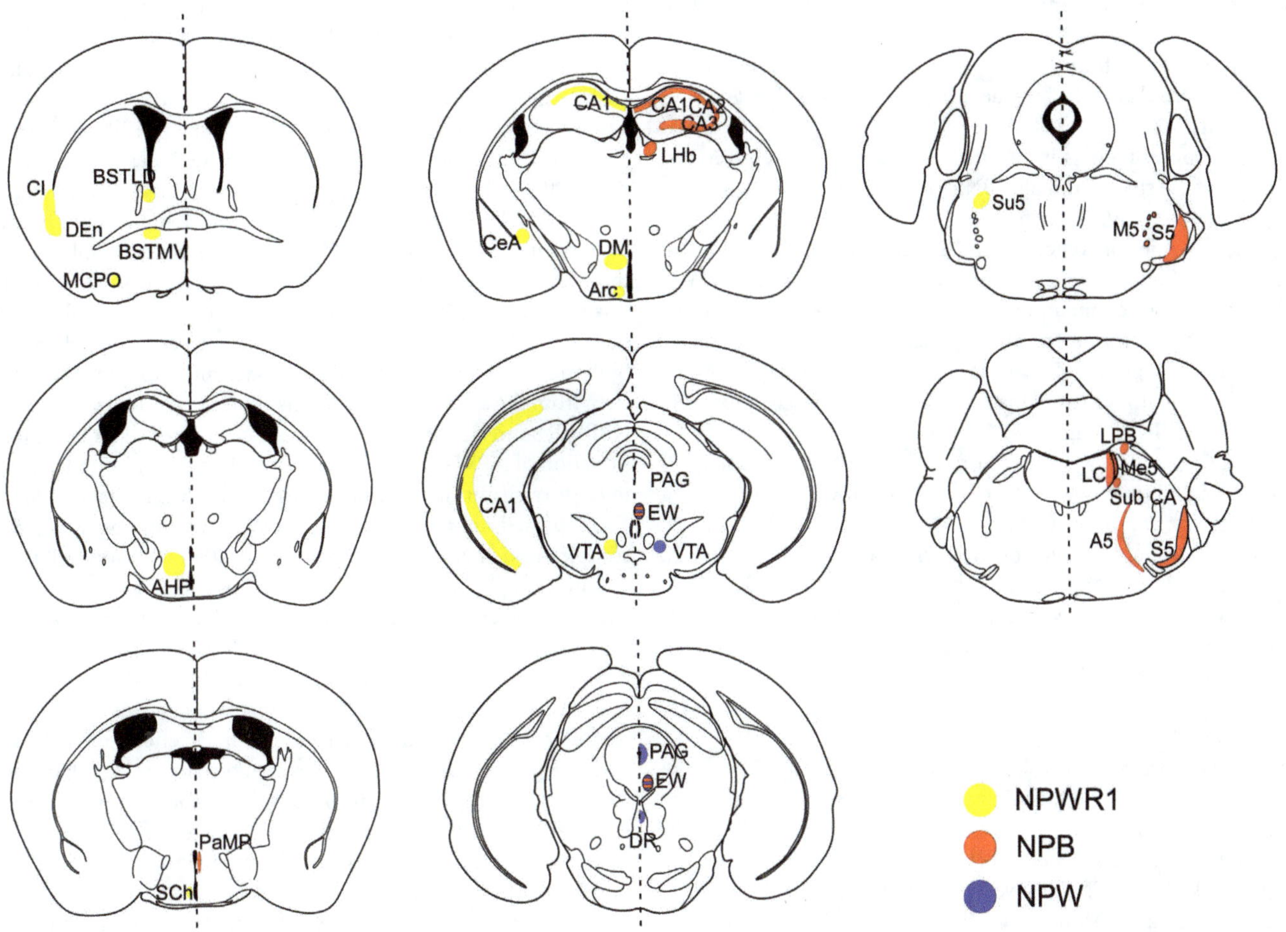


**FIGURE 3 | Schematic representation of distribution of NPB/NPW and *Npbwr1* mRNA in mouse brain coronal sections.** Receptor distribution is shown in the right hemisphere, while ligand distribution is shown in the left. *Npb* mRNA (red regions) was observed in the hippocampus (CA1, CA2, CA3), lateral habenular nucleus (LHb), paraventricular hypothalamic nucleus, medial parvicellular part (PaMP), Edinger–Westphal (EW) nucleus, motor root of the trigeminal nerve (m5), sensory root of the trigeminal nerve (s5), lateral parabrachial nucleus alpha part (Sub CA), locus coeruleus (LC), noradrenergic cell group A5 (A5), and inferior olive subnucleus B (IOB) (Tanaka et al., 2003). *Npw* mRNA (blue regions) was observed in the periaqueductal gray (PAG) matter, EW nucleus (EW), ventral tegmental area (VTA), and dorsal raphe nucleus (DR). NPBWR1 mRNA (yellow regions) was observed in the claustrum (Cl), dorsal endopiriform nucleus (DEn), bed nucleus of the stria terminals, laterodorsal part (BSTLD), bed nucleus of the stria terminalis, medioventral part (BSTMV), suprachiasmatic nucleus (Sch), magnocellular preoptic nucleus (MCPO), paraventricular hypothalamic nucleus, posterior part (PaPo), dorsomedial hypothalamic nucleus (DM), central amygdala (CeA), CA1 field, hippocampus (CA1), ventral tegmental area (VTA), sensory root trigeminal nerve (Su5), subiculum (S), anterior hypothalamic area, posterior part (AHP), and arcuate hypothalamic nucleus (Arc). Modified from Hondo et al. (2008).

nucleus, dorsomedial hypothalamic nucleus, arcuate nucleus, supraoptic retrochiasmatic nucleus, and in the area ventral to the zona incerta (Schulz et al., 2007). Although *Npb* mRNA was detected in several regions outside the hypothalamus such as the hippocampus and brain stem (Tanaka et al., 2003; Jackson et al., 2006; Schulz et al., 2007), the existence of NPB-immunoreactive neurons in these regions in the brain has not been clearly demonstrated, since no good antibody for NPB is available.

In peripheral tissues, expression of human *Npb* mRNA was detected by RT-PCR in the kidney, uterus, ovary, testis, and placenta, while murine *Npb* mRNA was detected by Northern blot at high levels in the stomach, spinal cord, and testis and at lower levels in the liver and kidney (Brezillon et al., 2003). The biological significance of this expression remains unknown.

## NEUROPEPTIDE W

The existence of NPW in the mouse brain was more confined to several nuclei in the midbrain and brainstem including the EW, VTA, periaqueductal gray (PAG), and dorsal raphe nucleus (DR) (**Figure 3**) (Tanaka et al., 2003; Kitamura et al., 2006). Most of these neurons expressed tyrosine hydroxylase (TH), suggesting that these cells are also catecholaminergic (our unpublished observation). In humans, high levels of *Npw* mRNA were detected in the substantia nigra, and moderate expression levels were detected in the amygdala and hippocampus (Fujii et al., 2002). In peripheral tissues, expression of human *Npw* mRNA was confirmed by RT-PCR in the progenital system, comprising the kidney, testis, uterus, ovary, and placenta, and also in the stomach and respiratory system, while murine *Npw* mRNA was detected by Northern blot at high levels in the lung and lower levels in the stomach (Brezillon et al., 2003).

Consistent with the mRNA distribution, NPW-immunoreactive (ir) cells were also exclusively detected in the EW, VTA, PAG, and DR in rats (Kitamura et al., 2006). NPW-ir fibers were observed in several brain regions in rats including the lateral septum, bed nucleus of the stria terminalis (BNST), dorsomedial and posterior hypothalamus, CeA, CA1 field of hippocampus, interpeduncular nucleus, inferior colliculus, lateral parabrachial nucleus, facial nucleus, and hypoglossal nucleus. Among these regions, NPW-ir fibers were most abundantly observed in the CeA and BNST, the output nuclei of the extended amygdala. These observations suggest that NPW-producing neurons are exclusively localized to the mid brain, and they project mainly to the limbic system, especially the CeA and BNST (**Figure 3**).

Some reports showed the existence of NPW-ir cell bodies in the PVN in rats and mice (Dun et al., 2003). However, the staining of NPW-like immunoreactivity-positive cells in the PVN is likely to be non-specific staining, for two main reasons (Kitamura et al., 2006). First, PVN immunoreactivity is also observed in $NPW^{-/-}$ mice using many of the commercially available antibodies. Second, *Npw* mRNA is not expressed in the PVN in either mice or rats (Kitamura et al., 2006).

### NPBWR1 (GPR7)

*In situ* hybridization study showed that the CeA and BNST express the highest levels of NPBWR1 mRNA expression in the mouse brain (**Figure 3**) (Tanaka et al., 2003; Singh et al., 2004; Jackson et al., 2006). Other nuclei with high levels of *Npbwr1* are the suprachiasmatic (SCN) and ventral tuberomammillary nuclei of the hypothalamus. Moderate levels of expression are seen in the CA1–CA3 regions of the hippocampus, dorsal endopiriform, dorsal tenia tecta, bed nucleus, and red nucleus. Low level expression of *Npbwr1* is seen in the olfactory bulb, parastrial nucleus, hypothalamus, laterodorsal tegmentum, superior colliculus, LC, and nucleus of the solitary tract.

### NPBWR2 (GPR8)

Because *Npbwr* 2 does not exist in rodent genomes, very limited information about the tissue distribution of NPBWR2 has been available thus far. RT-PCR analysis showed that *Npbwr2* mRNA is strongly expressed in the human amygdala and hippocampus. Lower levels of expression were also detected in the corpus callosum, cerebellum, substantia nigra, and caudate nucleus (Brezillon et al., 2003).

## BIOLOGICAL ACTIVITIES OF NPB AND NPW

Several papers reported pharmacological actions of NPB and NPW *in vivo* (**Table 1**). In this section, I discuss biological activities of these peptides, referring the pharmacological actions and phenotypes of genetically-modified mice on NPB/W systems (**Table 2**).

### FEEDING AND ENERGY HOMEOSTASIS

The NPB/W system was initially thought to be involved in regulation of feeding behavior (Shimomura et al., 2002; Tanaka et al., 2003), and therefore many of the currently available reports have focused on the roles of NPB/W in this function. The first physiological study on the action of NPW showed acute hyperphagia in male rats when NPW was administered intracerebroventricularly (i.c.v.) (Shimomura et al., 2002; Tanaka et al., 2003). However, Tanaka et al. (2003) showed that the effect of NPB on feeding behavior in mice is very complex. When NPB was i.c.v. injected during the light period, no significant effect of NPB on feeding was observed (Tanaka et al., 2003). In contrast, in the dark period, i.c.v. administration of 3 nmol NPB increased feeding only within the first 2 h. A higher dose of NPB suppressed food intake in this period. After 2 h, both doses of NPB decreased food intake. Because rodents only have NPBWR1 as a receptor for NPB, the biphasic, i.e., earlier orexigenic and later anorexic, effect cannot stem from the different potency rank orders of the two peptides on NPBWR1 and NPBWR2. In fact, we also observed a similar biphasic action of NPW on feeding behavior when administered i.c.v. in mice or rats (our unpublished observation). Mondal et al. (2003) also reported anorexic effects of NPW. These findings suggest a complex role of NPB and NPW in the regulation of food intake.

Interestingly, the anorexic effect of NPB was markedly enhanced when corticotrophin-releasing factor (CRF), a known anorexic peptide, was co-administered (Tanaka et al., 2003). The i.c.v. administration of these two peptides almost completely suppressed food intake over 4 h. The biphasic effects of NPB/W on feeding behavior and the synergistic anorexic effects of NPB and CRF suggest complex roles of these peptides in the regulation of feeding behavior in relation to the stress response. The synergic effect of NPB with CRF in suppression of feeding suggests that this neuropeptide is likely to be implicated in inhibition of feeding under stressful conditions.

Continuous i.c.v. infusion of NPW was reported to suppress feeding and body weight gain over the infusion period (Mondal et al., 2003). Conversely, i.c.v. administration of anti-NPW IgG stimulated feeding, suggesting that endogenous NPW plays an inhibitory role in feeding behavior (Mondal et al., 2003). However, unlike the results of continuous i.c.v. infusion of NPW, bolus intra-PVN microinjection of NPW23 at doses ranging from 0.1 to 3 nmol increased feeding for up to 4 h, and a bolus dose ranging from 0.3 to 3 nmol was reported to increase feeding for up to 24 h (Levine et al., 2005). These observations suggest that the orexigenic versus anorectic effects of NPB/W could result from different sites of action. When these peptides are injected into the lateral ventricle, they might initially act on the PVN, followed by diffusion to other regions implicated in the suppression of feeding. Alternatively, delayed inhibition of feeding by NPB/W might result from the production of other anorectic factors that are stimulated by NPB or NPW.

The i.c.v. administration of NPW also increased body temperature and heat production (Mondal et al., 2003). These effects suggest that endogenous NPB/W might increase energy expenditure, which is consistent with the late-onset obesity seen in male $NPBWR1^{-/-}$ mice and $NPB^{-/-}$ mice (Ishii et al., 2003; Kelly et al., 2005).

Male $NPBWR1^{-/-}$ mice have been shown to develop adult-onset obesity that progressively worsens with age and is greatly exacerbated when animals are fed a high-fat diet (Ishii et al., 2003). The obesity is caused by hyperphagia along with decreased

**Table 1 | *In vivo* pharmacological effects of NPB/NPW.**

| Substance | Effects | Animal | Preference |
|---|---|---|---|
| NPW (i.c.v.) | Food intake ↑<br>Body weight ↑ | Rat (male) | Shimomura et al. (2002)<br>Tanaka et al. (2003) |
| NPW (i.c.v.) | Body temperature ↑<br>Heat production ↑ | Rat | Mondal et al. (2003) |
| NPW | ACTH ↑<br>Estradiol ↑ | Rat | Hochol et al. (2007) |
| NPW30 (i.c.v.) | Arterial blood pressure (ABP) ↑<br>Heart rate (HR) ↑<br>Plasma catecholamine concentration ↑ | Rat | Yu et al. (2007) |
| NPB (i.c.v.) | Food intake (light period–dark period) ↑ | Mouse | Tanaka et al. (2003) |
| NPB (i.c.v.) | Prolactin ↑<br>Growth hormone ↑ | Rat (male) | Samson et al. (2004) |
| NPW23/NPB (i.t) | Inflammatory pain ↓ | Rat | Yamamoto et al. (2005) |
| NPW/NPB (i.c.v.) | Corticosterone in circulation ↑ | Rat (male) | Samson et al. (2004)<br>Taylor et al. (2005) |
| NPW/NPB (i.p) | (Plasma level) parathyroid hormone ↑<br>(Plasma level) corticosterone ↑<br>(Plasma level) testosterone ↑ | Rat | Hochol et al. (2007) |
| NPW/NPB (i.c.v.) | Circadian rhythm → | Rat/mouse | Our unpublished observations |

**Table 2 | Summary of behavioral phenotypes of NPBWR1 knockout mice (modified from Nagata-Kuroiwa et al., 2011).**

| Behavioral test | Parameter | Results |
|---|---|---|
| Open field test | Anxiety | Normal time spent in center of arena |
| Elevated plus maze test | Anxiety | Normal time spent and number of entries in open arms |
| Light-dark exploration test | Anxiety | Decrease in escape latency and time spent in light box |
| Porsolt forced swim test | Depression, learning helplessness | Normal time spent swimming |
| Prepulse inhibition test | Sensory motor reactivity | Normal percentage of prepulse inhibition |
| Marble burying behavior test | Compulsive behavior | Normal number of marbles buried |
| Cued and contextual fear conditioning test | Fear and memory | Decrease in time of freezing behavior during contextual testing while normal during auditory-cued testing |
| Morris water maze test | Spatial memory | Normal escape latency |
| Resident-intruder test | Social interaction | Abnormal social interaction (see text) |
| Stress-induced hyperthermia | Stress response | Exaggerated hyperthermia |
| Daily locomotor activity | Circadian rhythm | Normal in both light/dark cycle and constant dark condition. Normal entrainment by food or light |
| Sleep-wake behavior (EEG/EMG) | Sleep/wake cycle | Normal in each episode duration, times spent in each state in hourly sleep/wake analysis |

energy expenditure. *Npbwr1*$^{-/-}$ male mice showed decreased hypothalamic *neuropeptide Y* mRNA level and increased *proopiomelanocortin* mRNA level, a set of effects opposite to those evident in *ob/ob* mice. Furthermore, *ob/ob;NPBWR1*$^{-/-}$ and *Ay/a;NPBWR1*$^{-/-}$ double mutant male mice had an increased body weight compared with normal *ob/ob* or *Ay/a* male mice, suggesting that the obesity of *NPBWR1*$^{-/-}$ mice is independent of leptin and melanocortin signaling. Female mice did not show any significant weight increase or associated metabolic defects. These data suggest a potential role for NPBWR1 in regulating energy homeostasis independent of leptin and melanocortin signaling, in a sexually dimorphic manner (Ishii et al., 2003). Consistent with the phenotype of *Npbwr1*$^{-/-}$ mice, *Npb*$^{-/-}$ mice were also reported to exhibit mild adult-onset obesity (Kelly et al., 2005).

### PAIN REGULATION

Intracerebroventricular administration of NPB produces analgesia to pain induced by subcutaneous formalin injection in rats (Tanaka et al., 2003). Intrathecal (i.t.) injection of either NPW23 or NPB also decreased agitation behaviors induced by formalin injection into the paw and attenuated the level of mechanical allodynia (Yamamoto et al., 2005). The effects were not antagonized by naloxone, suggesting that this effect is not mediated through the opioid receptor system. While i.t. injection of either NPW23 or NPB did not show any effect in the hot plate test or mechanical nociceptive test, i.t. injection of either NPW23 or NPB significantly suppressed the expression of Fos-like immunoreactivity of the L4–5 spinal dorsal horn induced by formalin injection into the paw. These data suggest that spinally applied NPW/B suppressed the input of nociceptive information to the spinal dorsal horn, producing an analgesic effect on inflammatory pain, but not mechanical or thermal pain (Yamamoto et al., 2005).

Consistent with the pharmacological studies suggesting an analgesic action of NPB on inflammatory pain, *NPB*$^{-/-}$ mice exhibited hyperalgesia to inflammatory pain, while they showed normal responses to mechanical or thermal pain (Kelly et al., 2005). These observations suggest that NPB in the brain and/or spinal cord modulates pain in a modality-specific manner. These observations suggest that NPB might play a role in the pathophysiology of allodynia. Unfortunately, however there are no available data about expression of NPW, NPW, or NPBWR1 in the spinal cord or dorsal root ganglia.

A low level of NPBWR1 receptor expression was observed in Schwann cells in both normal human and rat nerves as well as in primary rat Schwann cell cultures. Peripheral nerve samples taken from patients exhibiting inflammatory/immune-mediated neuropathy showed a marked increase of NPBWR1 receptor expression restricted to myelin-forming Schwann cells. Complementary animal models of immune-inflammatory and ligation-induced nerve injury and neuropathic pain similarly exhibited increased myelin-associated expression of NPBWR1 (Zaratin et al., 2005). These observations suggest that NPBWR1 is involved in regulation of inflammatory pain at least in part by modulating Schwann cell function.

### NEUROENDOCRINE REGULATION

Central administration of NPB or NPW elevated the plasma corticosterone level in rats (Samson et al., 2004; Taylor et al., 2005). NPB also increased prolactin and decreased growth hormone levels (Samson et al., 2004). Pretreatment with a polyclonal anti-CRF antiserum or CRF antagonist completely blocked the effect of NPB or NPW to stimulate ACTH release, and significantly inhibited the effect of NPB/W on plasma corticosterone level (Samson et al., 2004; Taylor et al., 2005). These findings suggest that NPW and NPB play a role in the neuroendocrine response to stress via activation of the hypothalamus-pituitary-adrenal (HPA) axis. Consistent with these observations, whole cell patch-clamp recording from hypothalamic slice preparations showed that bath application of NPW depolarized and directly increased the spike frequency of neuroendocrine PVN neurons (Taylor et al., 2005).

A whole cell patch-clamp study showed that NPW23 exhibited effects on oxytocin, vasopressin, and thyrotrophin-releasing hormone neurons in the PVN, although both depolarizing and hyperpolarizing effects were observed in each of these cell groups (Price et al., 2009). Corticotrophin-releasing hormone cells were unaffected. Further subdivision of chemically phenotyped cell groups into magnocellular, neuroendocrine, or pre-autonomic neurons, using their electrophysiological fingerprints, revealed that neurons projecting to medullary and spinal targets were predominantly inhibited by NPW, whereas those that projected to the median eminence or neural lobe showed almost equivalent numbers of depolarizing and hyperpolarizing cells (Price et al., 2009).

The intracellular mechanisms of these electrophysiological effects of NPW have remained unclear. Since NPBWR1 primarily couples to Gi subclass of G-proteins, activation of this receptor should lead to inhibition of neurons. Depolarizing effect of NPW described in above mentioned report might be indirect effect due to inhibition of inhibitory interneurons of recorded cells.

### AUTONOMIC REGULATION

Intracerebroventricular administration of NPW to rats was reported to increase arterial blood pressure (ABP), heart rate (HR), and plasma catecholamine concentration (Yu et al., 2007). The same report showed that most of the PVN neurons were excited, while a subset of a smaller population of PVN neurons was inhibited by NPW30, although the chemical identities of these neurons were not determined. These observations suggest that NPB/W modulate PVN neuronal activities, which play an important role in regulation of the autonomic nervous system as well as the HPA axis. The expression of NPB mRNA in the PVN suggests that NPB is more likely to be involved in HPA axis regulation. However, *NPBWR1*$^{-/-}$ mice have normal blood pressure and HR in a basal state (Nagata-Kuroiwa et al., 2011). The physiological relevance of the NPB/W system in regulation of the autonomic nervous system remains unclear.

### SLEEP AND WAKEFULNESS

Neuropeptide B is reported to induce slow wave sleep in mice when injected intracerebroventricularly (Hirashima et al., 2011). However, since *NPBWR1*$^{-}$/– mice did not show any sleep abnormality, the biological relevance of this finding remains unclear.

### EMOTION AND BEHAVIOR

*Npbwr1* mRNA is abundantly expressed in discrete brain regions in rodents, including the hypothalamus (dorsomedial hypothalamus and suprachiasmatic nucleus), hippocampus, VTA, and extended amygdala (the CeA and bed nucleus of the stria terminalis; BNST) (Lee et al., 1999; Tanaka et al., 2003). These regions are implicated in mood and emotion. Especially, the particularly strong expression of *Npbwr1* in the CeA and BNST, together with the robust projections of NPW-containing axons to these regions (Kitamura et al., 2006), suggest that this receptor might be an important modulator or regulator of the output signal from the extended amygdala, which is a well-defined subcortical nuclear group that is the center of emotion including fear (Phelps and LeDoux, 2005).

A sensory stimulus associated with an aversive outcome will change neural transmission in the amygdala to produce somatic, autonomic, and endocrine signs of fear, as well as increased attention to that stimulus. Fear learning involves the lateral and basolateral amygdala (BLA), where the association between incoming sensory stimuli leads to potentiation of synaptic transmission. The BLA receives sensory information from the thalamus, hippocampus, and cortex, and then activates or modulates synaptic transmission in target areas appropriate for the reinforcement signal with which the sensory information has been associated. The BLA projects to the CeA and BSNT, whose efferents to the hypothalamus and brainstem trigger the expression of fear. Histological and electrophysiological studies have shown that NPBWR1 acts as an inhibitory regulator on a subpopulation of GABAergic neurons in the lateral division of the CeA and terminates stress responses (Nagata-Kuroiwa et al., 2011). These anatomical and functional findings suggest that the NPB/W systems might have important roles in the modulation of output from the extended amygdala.

The role of NPBWR1 in social behavior was recently investigated using *Npbwr1*$^{-/-}$ mice (Nagata-Kuroiwa et al., 2011). When presented with an intruder mouse, *Npbwr1*$^{-/-}$ mice showed impulsive contact with the strange mice, produced more intense approaches toward them, and had longer contact and chasing time along with greater and sustained elevation of HR and blood pressure compared to wild type mice. *Npbwr1*$^{-/-}$ mice also showed increased autonomic and neuroendocrine responses to various physical stresses, suggesting that NPBWR1 might play a role in coping with stress.

Another interesting phenotype of *NPBWR1*$^{-/-}$ mice is the impairment of contextual fear conditioning and inversion of "safety conditioning." In the safety conditioning paradigm, mice received unpaired presentations of a CS (tone) and a US (electrical shock). Because the shock never occurs during the CS, mice typically learn to treat the CS as a safety signal, so that fear-related behavior is inhibited during presentation of the CS. *Npbwr1*$^{-/-}$ mice show an inversion of this learning in that the safety-trained CS elicits fear rather than a reduction in fear. This observation suggests that *Npbwr1*$^{-/-}$ mice undergo trace conditioning rather than safety conditioning in this procedure, in that they associate the CS and US across a long trace interval, while the control mice treat CS and US as unpaired. These results suggest that *Npbwr1*$^{-/-}$ mice are more stimulus-bound, meaning that they preferentially attend to discrete stimuli, to the exclusion of more complex, conjunctive stimuli such as context. This hypothesis would also explain the deficit in contextual fear conditioning. To determine the neural mechanisms and the possible developmental and/or extra-amygdalar origins of the phenotype, further investigation using spatially restricted knockout mice and/or genetic rescue of the phenotype of these mice by expressing NPBWR1 in a region-specific manner is needed.

The human *NPBWR1* gene has a frequent single nucleotide polymorphism at nucleotide 404 (SNP rs33977775) in the coding region (404A >T). Importantly, this polymorphism causes an amino acid substitution (Y135F) within the highly conserved DRY motif of G-protein-coupled receptors at the junction of the third transmembrane domain and second intracellular loop, which is known to play an important role in G-protein coupling. Recently, Watanabe et al. (2012) demonstrated that this change partially impairs receptor function as measured by inhibition of cAMP production. Furthermore, this variation affects the emotional response to stimuli showing human faces with four categories of emotional expression (anger, fear, happiness, and neutral). The subject's emotional levels at seeing these faces were rated on scales of hedonic valence, emotional arousal, and dominance (V–A–D). A significant genotype difference was observed in valence evaluation; the 404AT group (position 404 in one allele is replaced by T) perceived the face as more pleasant than did the 404AA group (position 404 in both alleles of *NPBWR1* is A), regardless of the category of facial expression. The 404AT group tended to feel less submissive to an angry face than did the 404AA group. These results suggest that a single nucleotide polymorphism of NPBWR1 seems to affect human behavior in a social context. Future studies using functional brain imaging of human subjects are needed to clarify the mechanisms of the effects of the polymorphisms.

## EFFECTS ON CIRCADIAN RHYTHM

The abundant expression of NPBWR1 in the suprachiasmatic nucleus suggests the possibility that this neuropeptides/receptor system has a role in regulating circadian rhythm (Lee et al., 1999; Tanaka et al., 2003; Singh et al., 2004). However, we did not observe any effects of NPB/W on circadian activity in rats or mice when administered by i.c.v. injection. *Npbwr1*$^{-/-}$ mice displayed a normal circadian pattern of behavior in both light-dark and constant dark conditions (Uchio et al., 2009). Both light-entrainable and food-entrainable oscillation were also normal in these mice (our unpublished observations). The function of NPBWR1 in the SCN remains unclear thus far.

## PERIPHERAL ACTIONS

Expression of *Npb*, *Npw*, and *Npbwr1* mRNA in both the adrenal cortex and adrenal medulla has been reported (Andreis et al., 2005; Mazzocchi et al., 2005; Hochol et al., 2007). NPB and NPW were shown to pharmacologically stimulate adrenal glucocorticoid secretion by an ACTH-independent mechanism. It was also reported that NPW stimulates *in vitro* aldosterone secretion by enhancing the release of medullary catecholamines, which activate beta-adrenoceptors located on zona glomerulosa cells (Hochol et al., 2007).

Bolus intraperitoneal (i.p.) injection of NPB or NPW increased the plasma levels of parathyroid hormone, corticosterone, and testosterone. NPB was also reported to increase the blood concentration of thyroxine, and NPW was shown to increase ACTH and estradiol levels. These findings suggest that NPB and NPW play a role in regulation of the endocrine system (Hochol et al., 2006).

The existence of NPW in rat gastric antral cells was reported. The level of NPW in the stomach was decreased in fasted animals, while it was increased by re-feeding (Mondal et al., 2003), which is consistent with the notion that NPW may act as a suppressant of feeding. However, we did not observe any effects on feeding in mice when NPB or NPW was intravenously administered, suggesting that peripheral NPB/W has limited, if any, significant role in modulating feeding behavior (our unpublished observations).

Neuropeptide B and NPW are reported to inhibit proliferative activity of rat calvarial osteoblast-like (ROB) cells (Ziolkowska et al., 2009). However, the physiological relevance of this finding is unknown, and requires further investigation.

## CONCLUSION

Neuropeptide B and NPW are likely to be multi-tasking factors. Both $Npb^{-/-}$ and $Npbwr1^{-/-}$ mice show late-onset obesity and hyperphagia, suggesting that the endogenous NPB-NPBWR1 pathway negatively regulates feeding behavior and positively regulates energy expenditure (Ishii et al., 2003; Kelly et al., 2005). This notion is further supported by several pharmacological studies that showed that i.c.v. NPB/W increased heat production and sympathetic outflow (Yu et al., 2007). However, the biphasic (early orexigenic followed by anorexic) effects of NPB/NPW suggest complex actions of NPB and NPW in the regulation of food intake.

Many studies have also shown that the NPB/W system is involved in the modulation of inflammatory pain. Consistent with these results, $Npb^{-/-}$ mice are hypersensitive to inflammatory pain but display no significant difference in chemical or thermal pain. These data together strongly support a physiological role of central NPB in pain regulation, and agonists for NPBWR1 or NPBWR2 might be good candidates for analgesic drugs for chronic inflammatory pain.

Finally, the strong, discrete expression of NPBWR1 in the extended amygdala and abundant projections of NPW fibers in these regions suggest that this neuropeptide system has a role in the regulation of fear and anxiety. The CeA and BNST have been implicated in a variety of emotional functions including expression of fear, modulation of memory, and mediation of social communication (Davis and Shi, 1999) (**Figure 3**). Therefore, the expression of NPBWR1 in the CeA and BNST suggests modulatory roles of this receptor in these functions. Recent studies in $Npbwr1^{-/-}$ mice support this concept (**Table 2**). Furthermore, a recent report suggested that a human polymorphism in the *NPBWR1* gene might affect emotional responses to facial expressions (Watanabe et al., 2012). In daily life, people show various emotional reactions to others depending on their personalities, even in the same situation. NPBWR1 may provide part of the cause for such differences in reactions in social interactions.

## ACKNOWLEDGMENTS

This study was supported in part by a Technology (MEXT) of Japan, and the Cabinet Office, Government of Japan through its "Funding Program for Next Generation World-Leading Researchers."

## REFERENCES

Andreis, P., Rucinski, M., Neri, G., Conconi, M., Petrelli, L., Parnigotto, P., et al. (2005). Neuropeptides B and W enhance the growth of human adrenocortical carcinoma-derived NCI-H295 cells by exerting MAPK p42/p44-mediated proliferogenic and antiapoptotic effects. *Int. J. Mol. Med.* 16, 1021–1028.

Anthony Romero, F., Hastings, N. B., Moningka, R., Guo, Z., Wang, M., Di Salvo, J., et al. (2012). The discovery of potent antagonists of NPBWR1 (GPR7). *Bioorg. Med. Chem. Lett.* 22, 1014–1018.

Brezillon, S., Lannoy, V., Franssen, J. D., Le Poul, E., Dupriez, V., Lucchetti, J., et al. (2003). Identification of natural ligands for the orphan G protein-coupled receptors GPR7 and GPR8. *J. Biol. Chem.* 278, 776–783.

Davenport, A., and Singh, G. (2005). *Neuropeptide W/Neuropeptide B Receptors – NPBW1.* IUPHAR Receptor database. [doi:10.1786/080844542445].

Davis, M., and Shi, C. (1999). Extended amygdala and basal forebrain. *Ann. N. Y. Acad. Sci.* 877, 281–291.

Dun, S. L., Brailoiu, G. C., Yang, J., Chang, J. K., and Dun, N. J. (2003). Neuropeptide W-immunoreactivity in the hypothalamus and pituitary of the rat. *Neurosci. Lett.* 349, 71–74.

Fujii, R., Yoshida, H., Fukusumi, S., Habata, Y., Hosoya, M., Kawamata, Y., et al. (2002). Identification of a neuropeptide modified with bromine as an endogenous ligand for GPR7. *J. Biol. Chem.* 277, 34010–34016.

Hirashima, N., Tsunematsu, T., Ichiki, K., Tanaka, H., Kilduff, T. S., and Yamanaka, A. (2011). Neuropeptide B induces slow wave sleep in mice. *Sleep* 34, 31–37.

Hochol, A., Belloni, A., Rucinski, M., Ziolkowska, A., Di Liddo, R., Nussdorfer, G., et al. (2006). Expression of neuropeptides B and W and their receptors in endocrine glands of the rat. *Int. J. Mol. Med.* 18, 1101–1106.

Hochol, A., Tortorella, C., Ricinski, M., Ziolkowska, A., Nussdorfer, G., and Malendowicz, L. (2007). Effects of neuropeptides B and W on the rat pituitary-adrenocortical axis: in vivo and in vitro studies. *Int. J. Mol. Med.* 19, 207–211.

Hondo, M., Ishii, M., and Sakurai, T. (2008). The NPB/NPW neuropeptide system and its role in regulating energy homeostasis, pain, and emotion. *Results Probl. Cell Differ.* 46, 239–256.

Ishii, M., Fei, H., and Friedman, J. M. (2003). Targeted disruption of GPR7, the endogenous receptor for neuropeptides B and W, leads to metabolic defects and adult-onset obesity. *Proc. Natl. Acad. Sci. U.S.A.* 100, 10540–10545.

Jackson, V. R., Lin, S. H., Wang, Z., Nothacker, H. P., and Civelli, O. (2006). A study of the rat neuropeptide B/neuropeptide W system using in situ techniques. *J. Comp. Neurol.* 497, 367–383.

Kelly, M. A., Beuckmann, C. T., Williams, S. C., Sinton, C. M., Motoike, T., Richardson, J. A., et al. (2005). Neuropeptide B-deficient mice demonstrate hyperalgesia in response to inflammatory pain. *Proc. Natl. Acad. Sci. U.S.A.* 102, 9942–9947.

Kitamura, Y., Tanaka, H., Motoike, T., Ishii, M., Williams, S. C., Yanagisawa, M., et al. (2006). Distribution of neuropeptide W immunoreactivity and mRNA in adult rat brain. *Brain Res.* 1093, 123–134.

Lee, D. K., Nguyen, T., Porter, C. A., Cheng, R., George, S. R., and O'Dowd, B. F. (1999). Two related G protein-coupled receptors: the distribution of GPR7 in rat brain and the absence of GPR8 in rodents. *Brain Res. Mol. Brain Res.* 71, 96–103.

Levine, A., Winsky-Sommerer, R., Huitron-Resendiz, S., Grace, M., and de Lecea, L. (2005). Injection of neuropeptide W into paraventricular nucleus of hypothalamus increases food intake. *Am. J. Physiol. Regul. Integr. Comp. Physiol.* 288, R1727–R1732.

Lucyk, S., and Miskolzie, M. K. G. (2005). NMR conformational analyses on (des-bromo) neuropeptide B [1-23] and neuropeptide W [1-23]: the importance of alpha-helices, a cation-pi interaction and a beta-turn. *J. Biomol. Struct. Dyn.* 23, 77–90.

Mazzocchi, G., Rebuffat, P., Ziolkowska, A., Rossi, G., Malendowicz, L., and Nussdorfer, G. (2005). G protein receptors 7 and 8 are expressed in human adrenocortical cells, and their endogenous ligands neuropeptides B and w enhance cortisol secretion by activating adenylate cyclase- and phospholipase C-dependent signaling cascades. *J. Clin. Endocrinol. Metab.* 90, 3466–3471.

Mondal, M. S., Yamaguchi, H., Date, Y., Shimbara, T., Toshinai, K., Shimomura, Y., et al. (2003). A role for neuropeptide W in the regulation of feeding behavior. *Endocrinology* 144, 4729–4733.

Nagata-Kuroiwa, R., Furutani, N., Hara, J., Hondo, M., Ishii, M., Abe, T., et al. (2011). Critical role of neuropeptides B/W receptor 1 signaling in social behavior and fear memory. *PLoS ONE* 6:e16972. doi:10.1371/journal.pone.0016972

O'Dowd, B. F., Scheideler, M. A., Nguyen, T., Cheng, R., Rasmussen, J. S., Marchese, A., et al. (1995). The cloning and chromosomal mapping of two novel human opioid-somatostatin-like receptor genes, GPR7 and GPR8, expressed in discrete areas of the brain. *Genomics* 28, 84–91.

Phelps, E. A., and LeDoux, J. E. (2005). Contributions of the amygdala to emotion processing: from animal models to human behavior. *Neuron* 48, 175–187.

Price, C. J., Samson, W. K., and Ferguson, A. V. (2009). Neuropeptide W has cell phenotype-specific effects on the excitability of different subpopulations of paraventricular nucleus neurones. *J. Neuroendocrinol.* 21, 850–857.

Samson, W. K., Baker, J. R., Samson, C. K., Samson, H. W., and Taylor, M. M. (2004). Central neuropeptide B administration activates stress hormone secretion and stimulates feeding in male rats. *J. Neuroendocrinol.* 16, 842–849.

Schulz, S., Stumm, R., and Hollt, V. (2007). Immunofluorescent identification of neuropeptide B-containing nerve fibers and terminals in the rat hypothalamus. *Neurosci. Lett.* 411, 67–71.

Shimomura, Y., Harada, M., Goto, M., Sugo, T., Matsumoto, Y., Abe, M., et al. (2002). Identification of neuropeptide W as the endogenous ligand for orphan G-protein-coupled receptors GPR7 and GPR8. *J. Biol. Chem.* 277, 35826–35832.

Singh, G., Maguire, J. J., Kuc, R. E., Fidock, M., and Davenport, A. P. (2004). Identification and cellular localisation of NPW1 (GPR7) receptors for the novel neuropeptide W-23 by [125I]-NPW radioligand binding and immunocytochemistry. *Brain Res.* 1017, 222–226.

Tanaka, H., Yoshida, T., Miyamoto, N., Motoike, T., Kurosu, H., Shibata, K., et al. (2003). Characterization of a family of endogenous neuropeptide ligands for the G protein-coupled receptors GPR7 and GPR8. *Proc. Natl. Acad. Sci. U.S.A.* 100, 6251–6256.

Taylor, M., Yuill, E., Baker, J., Ferri, C., Ferguson, A., and Samson, W. (2005). Actions of neuropeptide W in paraventricular hypothalamus: implications for the control of stress hormone secretion. *Am. J. Physiol. Regul. Integr. Comp. Physiol.* 288, R270–R275.

Tim van, B., Brian, E. H., Deirdre, K. L., Kathleen, M. K., Kazushige, T., Emilio, P., et al. (1995). Receptor-tyrosine-kinase-and Gβγ-mediated MAP kinase activation by a common signalling pathway. *Nature* 376, 781–784.

Uchio, N., Doi, M., Matsuo, M., Yamazaki, F., Mizoro, Y., Hondo, M., et al. (2009). Circadian characteristics of mice depleted with GPR7. *Biomed. Res.* 30, 357–364.

Watanabe, N., Wada, M., Irukayama-Tomobe, Y., Ogata, Y., Tsujino, N., Suzuki, M., et al. (2012). A single nucleotide polymorphism of the neuropeptide B/W receptor-1 gene influences the evaluation of facial expressions. *PLoS ONE* 7:e35390. doi:10.1371/journal.pone.0035390

Yamamoto, T., Saito, O., Shono, K., and Tanabe, S. (2005). Anti-hyperalgesic effects of intrathecally administered neuropeptide W-23, and neuropeptide B, in tests of inflammatory pain in rats. *Brain Res.* 1045, 97–106.

Yu, N., Kunitake, T., Kato, K., Nakazato, M., and Kannan, H. (2007). Effects of intracerebroventricular administration of neuropeptide W30 on neurons in the hypothalamic paraventricular nucleus in the conscious rat. *Neurosci. Lett.* 15, 40–145.

Zaratin, P., Quattrini, A., Previtali, S., Comi, G., Hervieu, G., and Scheideler, M. (2005). Schwann cell overexpression of the GPR7 receptor in inflammatory and painful neuropathies. *Mol. Cell. Neurosci.* 28, 55–63.

Ziolkowska, A., Rucinski, M., Tyczewska, M., and Malendowicz, L. K. (2009). Neuropeptide B (NPB) and neuropeptide W (NPW) system in cultured rat calvarial osteoblast-like (ROB) cells: NPW and NPB inhibit proliferative activity of ROB cells. *Int. J. Mol. Med.* 24, 781–787.

# 17

# Distribution and protective function of pituitary adenylate cyclase-activating polypeptide in the retina

**Tomoya Nakamachi[1,2], Attila Matkovits[1,3], Tamotsu Seki[1,4] and Seiji Shioda[1]***

[1] Department of Anatomy, Showa University School of Medicine, Tokyo, Japan
[2] Center for Biotechnology, Showa University, Tokyo, Japan
[3] Department of Anatomy, University of Pécs, Pécs, Hungary
[4] Department of Ophthalmology, Showa University School of Medicine, Tokyo, Japan

**Edited by:**
Hubert Vaudry, University of Rouen, France

**Reviewed by:**
Dora Reglodi, University of Pécs, Hungary
Illana Gozes, Tel Aviv University, Israel

***Correspondence:**
Seiji Shioda, Department of Anatomy, Showa University School of Medicine, 1-5-8 Hatanodai, Shinagawa-ku, Tokyo 142-8555, Japan.
e-mail: shioda@med.showa-u.ac.jp

Pituitary adenylate cyclase-activating polypeptide (PACAP), which is found in 27- or 38-amino acid forms, belongs to the VIP/glucagon/secretin family. PACAP and its three receptor subtypes are expressed in neural tissues, with PACAP known to exert a protective effect against several types of neural damage. The retina is considered to be part of the central nervous system, and retinopathy is a common cause of profound and intractable loss of vision. This review will examine the expression and morphological distribution of PACAP and its receptors in the retina, and will summarize the current state of knowledge regarding the protective effect of PACAP against different kinds of retinal damage, such as that identified in association with diabetes, ultraviolet light, hypoxia, optic nerve transection, and toxins. This article will also address PACAP-mediated protective pathways involving retinal glial cells.

**Keywords: PACAP, PACAP receptor, retina, distribution, protection, rodent, review, knockout mouse**

## INTRODUCTION

Pituitary adenylate cyclase-activating polypeptide (PACAP) is a neuropeptide which was originally isolated from ovine hypothalamus on the basis of its capacity to stimulate adenylate cyclase activity in pituitary cells (Miyata et al., 1989). PACAP exists in two forms containing 27 and 38 amino acid residues, respectively, with PACAP27 sharing 68% sequence homology with that of vasoactive intestinal polypeptide (VIP). PACAP belongs to the VIP/secretin/glucagon family of peptides (Arimura and Shioda, 1995). PACAP38 is the predominantly expressed form in mammals (Arimura et al., 1991). The amino acid sequence of PACAP has been well conserved in vertebrates, implying that PACAP may act as an important neuropeptide (Sherwood et al., 2000). The receptors for PACAP, of which there are three main types, belong to the G protein-coupled receptor family with seven transmembrane domains. The PAC1 receptor (PAC1R) binds PACAP with high affinity and VIP with a much lower affinity, while the VPAC1 and VPAC2 receptors (VPAC1R, VPAC2R) bind VIP and PACAP with similar affinities (Harmar et al., 2012). PACAP is a pleiotropic biological peptide which regulates vasodilation, activates intestinal motility, increases insulin and histamine secretion, and modulates immune responses in peripheral tissues (Vaudry et al., 2009). In the central nervous system (CNS), PACAP acts as a neurotransmitter, neuromodulator, and/or neurotrophic factor (Arimura, 1998; Nakamachi et al., 2011). One of the most important functions of PACAP is that of neuroprotection. In this way, PACAP suppresses neuronal damage against acute brain injuries such as brain ischemia, traumatic brain injury, and spinal cord injury (Farkas et al., 2004; Ohtaki et al., 2008; Tsuchikawa et al., 2012). Moreover, PACAP protects the brain against neurodegenerative disease (Reglodi et al., 2011), reducing the level of neuronal damage. The retina is considered as a specialized neuronal tissue containing different types of neurons and glial cells. Therefore, to reveal any functions of PACAP in this tissue, it is necessary to understand which cell types in the retina express PACAP and PACAP receptors. The purpose of this review is to provide an overview of the distribution of PACAP and its receptors in the retina, and to summarize current knowledge of the protective functions of PACAP in animal models of retinopathy.

## EXPRESSION OF PACAP AND ITS RECEPTORS IN RETINAL TISSUE

### PACAP DISTRIBUTION

From a morphological perspective, light microscopy immunohistochemistry studies have shown PACAP-like immunoreactivity (-LI) exists in a population of sensory neurons in the rat uvea (Moller et al., 1993; Mulder et al., 1994) and in rabbit trigeminal ganglion cells (Onali and Olianas, 1994). Nerve fibers with PACAP-LI have also been found in the uvea of the rat eye (Moller et al., 1993; Mulder et al., 1994). PACAP-LI in the eye was studied by radio-immunoassay and the highest concentrations were found in the iris sphincter and ciliary body (Onali and Olianas, 1994; Wang et al., 1995). Furthermore, immunohistochemical studies revealed that PACAP-positive nerve fibers were present in the nerve fiber layer (NFL), the ganglion cell layer (GCL), and the inner plexiform layer (IPL). PACAP-positive neuronal cell bodies were also found in amacrine and horizontal cells in the inner nuclear layer (INL). No PACAP-LI was found in photoreceptors in the outer nuclear layer (ONL) or retinal pigmented epithelium (Seki et al., 1997, 1998; Izumi et al., 2000).

At the ultrastructural level, PACAP-LI was found in some amacrine and horizontal cells in the INL. PACAP-LI was detected in the plasma membrane and rough endoplasmic reticulum, and diffusible immunoreactive products were detected in the cytoplasmic matrix of amacrine cells and horizontal cells. Intense PACAP-LI was detected in cell processes of the IPL, GCL, and NFL. In the IPL, PACAP-positive amacrine cell processes make synaptic contacts with retinal ganglion cell (RGC) terminals, as well as amacrine and bipolar cell processes. PACAP-positive amacrine cell processes have also been identified to make synaptic contacts with each other. In the IPL, PACAP-positive presynaptic axon terminals were found to contain several dense granular vesicles (80–100 nm in diameter) and many small clear synaptic vesicles (30–50 nm in diameter). However, precise ultrastructural localization of PACAP-LI in the axon terminals is very difficult to determine with the pre-embedding immunostaining method. Electron microscopy observations of the IPL revealed non-specific immunoreactive products associated with post-synaptic membranes, the outer mitochondrial membrane, and the cytoplasmic matrix of axon terminals (Seki et al., 2000b). PACAP-LI is also expressed in the cell bodies of some amacrine and horizontal cells in the INL and their processes in the IPL, GCL, and NFL in the rat retina, as shown by both light and electron microscopic immunocytochemistry. PACAP-positive axon terminals make synaptic contact with RGC, bipolar cells, amacrine cells, and horizontal cells in the GCL, NFL, and IPL. On the other hand, VIP-positive cells have also been found in the GCL and INL, and their fibers have been found in the IPL (Loren et al., 1980). Both PACAP- and VIP-positive cells and fibers are found in the rat retina but their distributions are quite different from each other. These studies strongly suggest that PACAP and VIP function as neurotransmitters and/or neuromodulators, but the functions of PACAP may be different from those of VIP.

### PACAP RECEPTOR DISTRIBUTION

Receptor binding sites for PACAP and VIP, positively coupled to adenylate cyclase, have been previously described in the retina of different mammalian species (D'Agata and Cavallaro, 1998). As to the localization of PAC1R in the rat retina (Nilsson et al., 1994), we have described the distribution and localization of PAC1R and its mRNA in the rat retina by immunohistochemistry and *in situ* hybridization histochemistry (Seki et al., 1997, 2000a). PAC1R-LI was found in the cell bodies and processes of RGC and amacrine cells. No PAC1R-LI was observed in photoreceptors. At the ultrastructural level, PAC1R-LI was detected in the plasma membrane, rough endoplasmic reticulum, and the cytoplasmic matrix of RGCs and amacrine cells in the INL. There are certain areas in which the localization of PACAP does not match that of PAC1R. For example, in the rat brain, PAC1R has been found at very high levels in the olfactory bulb, hippocampus, and cerebellar cortex, where few PACAP-containing neurons are identified (Seki et al., 1997). Reports also suggest that PACAP is a transmitter and/or modulator which regulates RGCs and amacrine cells in the rat retina. Müller cells were difficult to identify in histological observations, but PAC1R-LI was observed in rat primary cultures of Müller cells (Seki et al., 2006a). PACAP and PAC1R distributions in the rodent retina are summarized in **Figure 1**.

## PACAP AND NEUROPROTECTION

Protective effect of PACAP on retina and retinal cells against various types of retinopathy animal models and toxic reagent showing below was summarized in **Table 1**.

### PACAP AND DIABETES (DIABETIC RETINOPATHY)

It is well known that diabetes causes numerous health complications in the human body, with one of the most serious consequences of this disease being diabetic retinopathy. The reason for the retinal degeneration is that the retina is unable to adapt to the metabolic changes caused by hyperglycemia. This situation leads to chronic inflammation and microvascular angiopathy (Liu et al., 2008). One of the most important consequences of diabetes is the changes to enzyme activities and altered expression patterns of growth and transcription factors (Seki et al., 2004). Another reason for the degeneration of the retina is related to oxidative stress (Kowluru and Abbas, 2003). Increased production of reactive oxygen species (ROS) may play an important role in the development of diabetic complications as it has been shown that ROS levels are elevated in the diabetic rat retina and in retinal cells incubated in high glucose media (Kowluru and Abbas, 2003; Cui et al., 2006) due to the hyperglycemia-induced impairment of antioxidant defense systems (Kowluru et al., 1996). The progression of diabetic retinopathy is slow, and leads to a decrease in a number of cell types in the retina such as amacrine cells, RGCs, and both types of photoreceptors (rod and cone cells; Holopigian et al., 1997; Gastinger et al., 2006). Müller cells and retinal astrocytes are also affected, becoming reactive within 3 months of the onset of diabetes (Lieth et al., 1998). Increased glial fibrillary acidic protein (GFAP) expression has been reported, particularly in the early phase of the disease (Lieth et al., 1998), which is closely associated with the activation of Müller cells.

Some studies have shown that PACAP treatment could protect the retina against the harmful effects of diabetes. In streptozotocin-treated rats, PACAP (100 pmol in 5 $\mu$l saline) administered into the vitreous body three times over the course of a week was able to attenuate the decrease of the cell number in the GCL (Szabadfi et al., 2012b). The PACAP treatment was also effective with respect to Müller cells in that the streptozotocin injection increased GFAP immunoreactivity in the retina due to Müller cell activation, but the PACAP treatment was able to significantly decrease the number of GFAP-positive Müller cells compared with untreated animals (Szabadfi et al., 2012b).

The PACAP treatment also increased the expression pattern of PAC1R in the diabetic retina, particularly in tyrosine-hydroxylase (TH)-positive cells (Szabadfi et al., 2012b). The most important TH-positive cells in the retina are the amacrine cells. The morphological or functional degeneration of dopaminergic amacrine cells was observed during the early stage of STZ-induced diabetes (Seki et al., 2004), and it was recently confirmed immunohistochemically that intravitreally injected PACAP is able to protect the amacrine cells from such degeneration (Atlasz et al., 2010b). Diabetes also causes changes in the expression of several apoptotic factors. Three weeks after streptozotocin injection, B-cell lymphoma 2 (Bcl-2) expression was decreased and p53 expression was increased, both of which indicate an elevated level of apoptosis

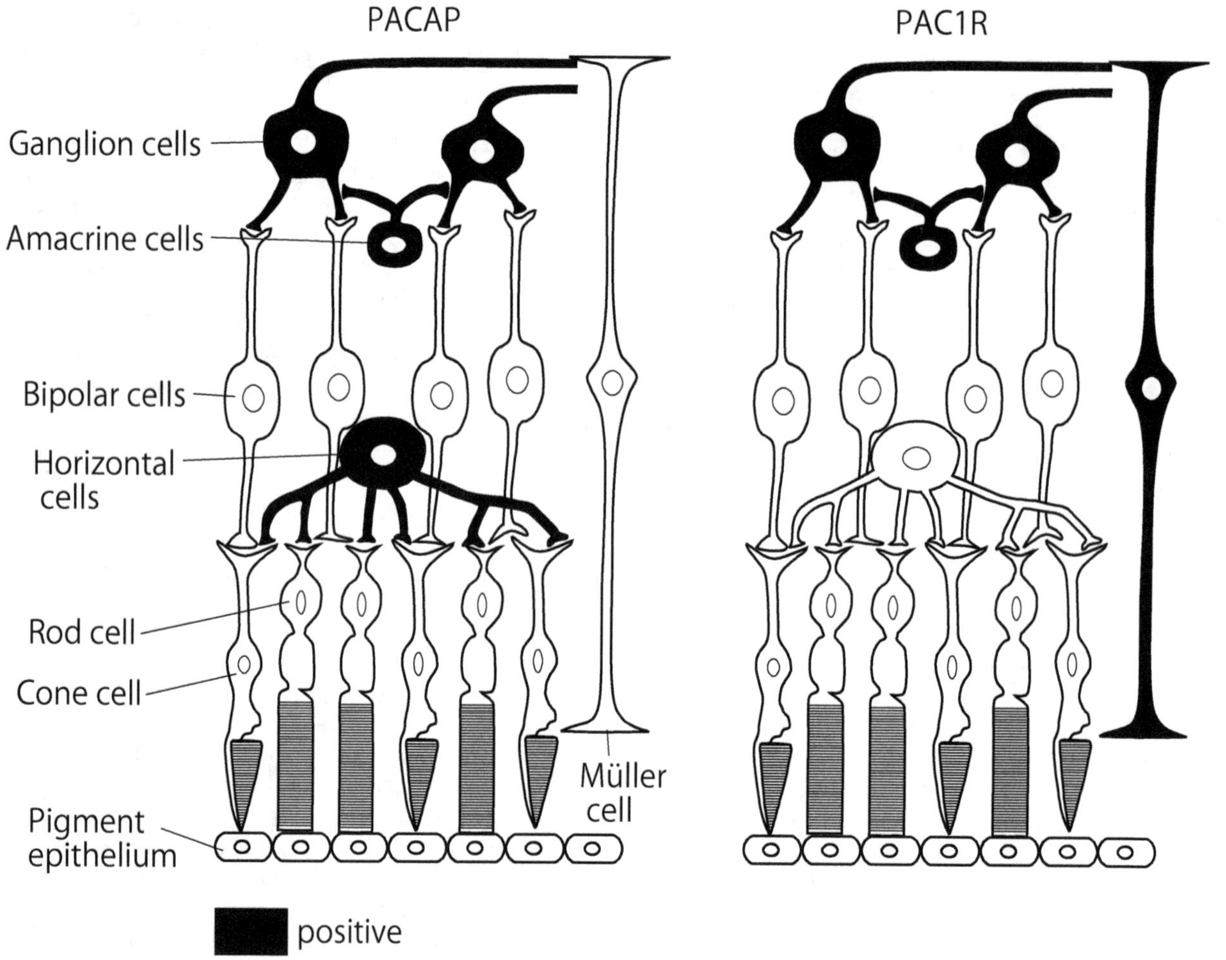


**FIGURE 1 | Schematic diagram of PACAP and PAC1R distributions in the rodent retina.** Black color indicates PACAP or PAC1R-expressing cells according to previous reports.

of the retinal cells. The intravitreal injection of PACAP (100 μmol in 5 μl of saline) was able to block these changes and restore the Bcl-2 and p53 levels to near control (Giunta et al., 2012). These results suggest that PACAP is able to up-regulate anti-apoptotic pathways and down-regulate pro-apoptotic pathways.

#### PACAP AND ULTRAVIOLET-A LIGHT-INDUCED RETINOPATHY

Only one paper has been published concerning the capacity of PACAP to protect against ultraviolet (UV) light-induced retinopathy. Exposure of animals for 45 min to diffuse UV-A irradiation caused cell death especially in the ONL and INL of the retina, and the thickness of the retina decreased in line with the duration of the UV-A treatment. One day after the UV-A treatment the GCL was not affected, but following a second day after illumination a significant decrease of the number of RGCs was observed. The intravitreal administration of PACAP (100 pmol in 5 μl saline) immediately after the irradiation was able to protect the ONL and INL of the retina which are seriously affected by the UV-A light, and the number of the cells in INL, ONL, and GCL was significantly increased as a consequence of the PACAP treatment (Atlasz et al., 2011). This effect of PACAP may have been via a reduction in the level and toxicity of free radicals generated as a consequence of the exposure to the UV-A. PACAP may thus reduce UV-A radiation-induced retinal damage and edema in a manner similar to that in which it reduces ischemia-induced cerebral damage and edema (Ohtaki et al., 2008; Nakamachi et al., 2010).

#### PACAP AND HYPOXIA

The retina has an elevated oxygen uptake compared to other tissues, making it one of the most sensitive tissues in the human body to hypoxia. Several diseases can cause retinal ischemia, the most common of which are cardiovascular disorders such as carotid artery stenosis, retinal artery occlusion, diabetic retinopathy, or high intraocular pressure, which can compress the blood vessels of the retina and cause hypoperfusion (Seki et al., 2011). An optimal way to model retinal ischemia in rats is the bilateral common carotid artery occlusion (BCCAO) technique; however the outcome of the operation may depend on the rat strain and technique used (Block et al., 1992; Szabadfi et al., 2010). The permanent ligation of both common carotid arteries leads to a reduction

**Table 1 | Summary of current knowledge on the effects of PACAP in retinal cells.**

| Toxin/model | Treatment of PACAP | | | Reference |
|---|---|---|---|---|
| | Tissue/cells | Dose | Effect | |
| ***In vitro*** | | | | |
| Glutamate (1 mM) | Retinal tissue culture from rat pups | PACAP27 or 38 (10 nM to 1 μM) | Protect neuronal cells (maximum effect at 1 μM) | Shoge et al. (1999) |
| Thapsigargin (10 nM) | Retinal tissue culture from rat pups | PACAP38 (1 nM) | Protect photoreceptor cell | Silveira et al. (2002) |
| Anisomycin (1 μg/ml) | Retinal tissue culture from rat pups | PACAP38 (100 fM to 10 nM) | Protect neuroblastic layer (maximum effect at 1 nM) | Silveira et al. (2002) |
| Anoxic condition | Turtle eyecup preparation | PACAP38 (0.165 μM) | Protect horizontal cells | Rabl et al. (2002) |
| | Primary culture of rat Müller cell | PACAP38 (1 pM to 1 μM) | Increase IL-6 levels | Nakatani et al. (2006) |
| $H_2O_2$ (0.2–0.3 mM) | ARPE19 human retinal pigment epithelium | PACAP38 (10 pM to 1 μM) | Increase the number of surviving cells (maximum effect at 100 nM) | Mester et al. (2011) |
| ***In vivo*** | | | | |
| MSG (2 mg/g, SC, three times) | Rat retina (PD21) | PACAP27 or 38 (100 pmol, IVI) | Protect INL, IPL, and GCL | Tamas et al. (2004)<br>Babai et al. (2005, 2006) |
| Kainic acid (5 nmol, IVI) | Rat retina (adult) | PACAP38 (100 pmol, IVI) | Protect GCL | Seki et al. (2006a) |
| BCCAO (permanent occlusion) | Rat retina (adult) | PACAP38 (100 pmol, IVI) | Protect GCL, OPL, and INL | Atlasz et al. (2007) |
| Optic nerve transection | Rat retina (adult) | PACAP38 (1 pM to 1 nM, 3 μl) | Protect GCL (maximum effect at 10 and 100 pM) | Seki et al. (2008) |
| UV-A irradiation | Rat retina (adult) | PACAP38 (100 pmol, IVI) | Protect ONL and GCL | Atlasz et al. (2011) |
| High intraocular pressure | Rat retina (adult) | PACAP38 (1 fM to 1 nM, 3 μl IVI) | Protect GCL (bimodal effect at 10 fM and 10 pM) | Seki et al. (2011) |
| NMDA (40 nmol, IVI) | $PACAP^{+/-}$ and $PACAP^{+/+}$ mice retina (adult) | PACAP38 (10 fM to 10 nM, 2 μl IVI) | Protect GCL (maximum effect at 100 pmol) | Endo et al. (2011) |
| MSG (2 mg/g, SC, three times) | Rat retina (PD21) | PACAP38 (100 pmol, IVI) | Retinal damage in $PACAP^{-/-}$ mice was more severe in GCL | Kiss et al. (2011)<br>Varga et al. (2011) |
| BCCAO (10 min occlusion) | $PACAP^{-/-}$ and $PACAP^{+/+}$ mice retina (adult) | PACAP38 (100 pmol, IVI) | Protect all layers of the retina, and improve ERG response | Szabadfi et al. (2012a) |
| Streptozotocin (70 mg/kg i.p.) | Rat retina (adult) | PACAP38 (100 pmol, IVI) | Retinal damage in $PACAP^{-/-}$ mice was more severe in all layers | Szabadfi et al. (2012b) |

*BCCAO, bilateral common carotid artery occlusion; ERG, electroretinography; GCL, ganglion cell layer; INL, inner nuclear layer; IPL, inner plexiform layer; IVI, intravitreal injection; MSG, monosodium glutamate; NMDA, N-methyl-D-aspartate; ONL, outer nuclear layer; OPL, outer plexiform layer; PD, postnatal day; SC, subcutaneous injection; UV, ultraviolet.*

in the cerebral blood flow in rats (Farkas et al., 2005; Lavinsky et al., 2006), which can cause severe retinal damage. All layers of the retina can be affected, with the reduction of the blood flow usually leading to a decrease of the thickness of the retina, especially with respect to the inner and outer plexiform layers (Atlasz et al., 2007; Atlasz et al., 2010b). The photoreceptors can also be damaged, with their outer segments becoming shorter, and alterations to their structure appearing after the BCCAO (Atlasz et al., 2010b).

In recent years, several studies have been published concerning retinoprotective strategies and agents developed to combat retinal ischemia. Because decreased perfusion leads to a range of changes in the retina, such as an altered metabolism of glutamate, increased levels of ROS, mitochondrial failure, and activation of inflammatory mediators, several possibilities to reduce the harmful effects of ischemia have been proposed (Szabadfi et al., 2010). For example, numerous retinoprotective agents or methods have been tested in the last few years against the harmful effects of retinal ischemia; these include VIP, poly ADP-ribose polymerase (PARP) inhibitors, brain-derived neurotrophic factor (BDNF), antioxidants, flavonoids, pre- or post-conditioning, etc. (Atlasz et al., 2010a; Szabadfi et al., 2010). Both *in vitro* and *in vivo* studies have shown PACAP to be one of the best candidates to protect retinal cells and to reduce the effects of ischemia. In an early report, turtle retina fragments were maintained in non-oxygenated Ringer solution for 46 h, with added PACAP38 (0.165 μM) able to protect the horizontal cells against ischemia; after 42 and 46 h, the light response of the cells was significantly higher than responses obtained from control group fragments (Rabl et al., 2002).

Several papers were published thereafter concerning the retinoprotective action of PACAP against the effects of hypoxia. PACAP possibly acts via PAC1R, which is detectable in all layers of the retina and is strongly expressed in the GCL, INL, NFL, and more weakly in the IPL, OPL, and ONL (Seki et al., 1997, 2000a). PACAP (10 pmol in 5 μl saline) intravitreally administered immediately after the BCCAO operation significantly reduced the harmful effects of ischemia compared to sham-operated animals. This protective effect was significantly attenuated by the PACAP38 antagonist, PACAP6-38 (Atlasz et al., 2007). Several cell types in the retina can be damaged by ischemia. A decrease of vesicular glutamate transporter 1 (VGLUT1) transporters causes damage to photoreceptors, bipolar cells, and calcium binding proteins, giving rise to the degeneration of different types of neurons. Moreover, increased GFAP expression is a sign of Müller cell and astrocyte activation. These effects were attenuated by PACAP treatment after the BCCAO (Atlasz et al., 2010b), suggesting that PACAP has a general cytoprotective effect in the retina against hypoxic conditions.

This effect of PACAP38 was confirmed in another study on wild-type and PACAP-null CD1 mice exposed to transient (10 min) BCCAO. Directly after the operation PACAP38 (100 pmol in 3 μl saline) was administered into the vitreous body. The results of the operation and treatment were tested 2 weeks later. The 10-min BCCAO resulted in a thinner retina, with significantly greater damage evident in the PACAP-null animals. In this group all the retinal layers were affected, while in the wild-type animal abnormalities were only evident in the INL. Intravitreal PACAP38 treatment significantly attenuated the deleterious effects of BCCAO in both groups. These results suggest that the retina in PACAP-null animals is more sensitive to ischemia compared to that in wild-type mice, and that PACAP treatment is effective against retinal ischemia in both wild-type and PACAP-null animals (Szabadfi et al., 2012a).

Another technique to transiently decrease retinal blood flow is to artificially elicit intraocular hypertension. This is a glaucoma model, where a thin needle is inserted into the anterior chamber of the eye of adult rats and 0.9% saline is injected to temporarily increase the intraocular pressure up to 100 mmHg for 60 min. The result of this procedure is similar to that achieved with BCCAO, in that under these experimental conditions the intraocular pressure is greater than the blood pressure in the vessels of the retina, thereby causing a hypoxic state in the retina. This treatment leads to a decrease in the number of RGCs and in the thickness of the retina, especially the IPL (Seki et al., 2011). PACAP38 treatment was also effective in combating this situation given that, compared with untreated eyeballs; the number of the RGCs was higher in animals treated with PACAP38. The effect of the PACAP was significantly stronger compared to the vehicle-treated animals when 3 μl of PACAP38 solution at concentrations of 10 fM, 10 or 100 pM was administered. This result suggests that the PACAP has a bimodal effect with peaks at 10 fM and 10–100 pM, even though the mechanism accounting for these effects was not the same. In the case of the 10 fM PACAP administration, the mitogen-activated protein kinase (MAPK) inhibitor PD-98059 significantly reduced the protective effect of PACAP, but there was no significant difference observed at the other PACAP concentrations tested. Meanwhile, the cAMP antagonist Rp-cAMP significantly decreased the effect of PACAP at all the concentrations tested (Seki et al., 2011). These results suggest that pathways involving MAPK and cAMP play key roles in the protective effect of PACAP against hypoxia. A recent study revealed additional information concerning this phenomenon. Adult rat retinas were examined 5, 30, and 60 min after BCCAO accompanied by injections of 100 nmol/3 μl of PACAP. The results showed that in the absence of any harmful stimulus, the PACAP did not cause any changes compared with the control group. Ischemia itself caused several changes, such as increases in the phosphorylation of Akt, ERK 1/2, JNK, or p38MAPK, particularly at the 30 and 60 min time points following the operation. PACAP treatment caused a significant increase in the phosphorylation of Akt and ERK 1/2 at all time points, and decreased the activity of JNK and p38MAPK (Szabo et al., 2012). Several results were published previously concerning the effect of PACAP on these signal transduction pathways in the retina and other tissues (Dohi et al., 2002; Ohtaki et al., 2006; Racz et al., 2006; Shioda et al., 2006). PACAP has important, but variable, effects on the expression of interleukins and cytokines. The expression of several interleukins such as inter interleukin (IL)-1, intercellular adhesion molecule (ICAM), L-selectin, regulated and normal T cell expressed and secreted (RANTES) etc, was decreased by PACAP, while levels of others such as IL-2, IL-6, IL-10, and tumor necrosis factor (TNF)-α were not changed. In contrast, the levels of vascular endothelial growth factor (VEGF) and thymus chemokine were increased (Szabo et al., 2012).

Not only ischemia, but also hyperoxia cause oxidative stress which could be harmful for cells in the retina. Oxidative stress is one of the most important apoptosis-inducing factors in the human body, especially in the CNS and sensory organs (Vaudry et al., 2002; Racz et al., 2010). Retinal pigment epithelial cells are sensitive to oxidative stress, with hydrogen peroxide- or aldehyde-induced oxidative stress leading to apoptosis of these cells *in vitro* (Kalariya et al., 2008; Kook et al., 2008). Given that retinal pigment epithelial cells express PAC1R and VPAC receptors (Zhang et al., 2005), PACAP could have a cytoprotective effect on these cells. When retinal pigment epithelial cells were treated with 0.25 mM $H_2O_2$ and 10 nM PACAP38 for 3 h, the survival of these cells was significantly ameliorated compared with control cells not treated with PACAP. An MAPK inhibitor in this case had no influence on the effect of PACAP38, but inhibition of the phosphoinositide 3-kinase (PI3K)/Akt pathway and PACAP6-38 treatment were able to antagonize this cytoprotective effect (Mester et al., 2011). The p38MAPK, c-Jun N-terminal kinase (JNK), extracellular signal-regulated kinase (ERK) 1/2, and Akt pathways were also activated in response to $H_2O_2$ treatment, while PACAP38 decreased the level of p38MAPK and pJNK, and increased the activity of the ERK 1/2 and Akt pathways. Other cytokine and signal transduction pathways are modified by $H_2O_2$ and PACAP38 treatment. Oxidative stress induced the expression of several apoptosis-inducing factors such as Bad, Bax, Trail, Fas-associated protein with death domain (FADD), Fas, second mitochondrial-derived activator of caspase (SMAC), and several heat-shock proteins (HSP32, HMOX2, and HSP27), as well as p53. Co-treatment with both 100 and 10 nM PACAP38 decreased the activation all of these factors (Fabian et al., 2012).

## PACAP AND OPTIC NERVE TRANSECTION

Optic nerve injury caused by trauma, glaucoma, or neurodegenerative disease can cause apoptotic RGCs death (Quigley et al., 1995), for which, based on the above findings, PACAP could be a good candidate to protect injured RGCs against apoptosis. In one recent study, different concentrations of PACAP38 were administered into the vitreous body of adult rats, and immediately after the injection, the optic nerve was transected (Seki et al., 2008). Fourteen days later the number of the RGCs was found to be significantly decreased in the control (untreated) and PACAP-treated groups due to apoptosis. The PACAP38 treated groups, however, showed increased RGC survival compared with control, particularly with regard to the groups receiving injections of 3 $\mu$l of saline containing 10 and 100 pM PACAP.

## PACAP AND TOXINS

Many toxic agents have been identified which can cause severe retinal injury. Some of them, like glutamate, are found in the retinal cells and are necessary in small concentrations for the normal functioning of the retina. Others, like anisomycin and thapsigargin, are not endogenous to the retina and are commonly used in *in vivo* studies to induce retinal injury by direct administration into the vitreous body.

### Anisomycin

The capacity of PACAP to prevent the deleterious effects of this drug was examined on *in vitro* preparations of the retinal neuroblastic layer from newborn rats. This drug inhibits protein synthesis and causes cell death in the neuroblastic layer. It was previously found that increased cAMP levels protect retinal cells against retinal damage induced by protein synthesis inhibition (Rehen et al., 1996). In this way, 1 nM PACAP38 or PACAP27 administered in parallel with anisomycin had a protective effect on the neuroblastic layer (Silveira et al., 2002). PACAP38 exerts its action via the PAC1 receptor, which is expressed in all layers of the neonatal retina, and activates the cAMP/protein kinase A (PKA) pathway, which is essential for this effect. The activation of other PAC1R-activated signal transduction pathways, such as the phospholipase C (PLC) or PI3K pathways, is not necessary for the protective effect of PACAP against anisomycin (Silveira et al., 2002). On the other hand, PACAP6-38 and Maxadilan (a specific PAC1R antagonist) inhibit this neuroprotective effect of PACAP38 (Silveira et al., 2002).

### Thapsigargin

Thapsigargin is a non-competitive inhibitor of the endoplasmic reticulum $Ca^{2+}$-ATPase. This drug inhibits autophagia, which leads to cell death. In the case of retinal explants of newborn rats, thapsigargin causes apoptosis of the photoreceptors in the ONL (Chiarini et al., 2000). PACAP38 treatment was also effective against thapsigargin-induced damage, with 1 nM PACAP38 administered simultaneously with 10 nM thapsigargin effectively preventing damage to the photoreceptors of the ONL (Silveira et al., 2002).

### Kainic acid

Kainic acid is a glutamate receptor agonist which is able to cause dose-dependent excitotoxicity-related injury to the retina. The intraocular injection of a low dose (6–20 nmol/retina) of this drug causes damage to the amacrine cells, with a 60 nmol/retina dose sufficient to cause degeneration of the bipolar and horizontal cells. Higher doses of kainic acid lead to the disappearance of the inner and outer plexiform layers in the chicken retina, while the photoreceptors and RGCs survived the treatment across the range of doses employed (Morgan and Ingham, 1981). The intravitreal administration of this drug in rats causes excitotoxic injury and cell death in the retina, especially in the INL, IPL, and CGL. PACAP (10 pmol) administered into the vitreous body 2 days before the kainic acid treatment resulted in a significantly lower incidence of cell death in the mentioned layers; however the co-administration of PACAP and kainic acid did not provide any protective effect in the retina (Seki et al., 2006b).

### N-methyl-D-aspartate

*N*-methyl-D-aspartate (NMDA) is a selective glutamate receptor agonist, which is able to mimic the effect of glutamate. It is however specific to its NMDA receptor only, and it has no effect on other glutamate receptors such as the AMPA or kainite receptors. NMDA treatment induces an excitatory effect on several cell types in the CNS (Parsons et al., 1998; Watkins and Jane, 2006). In the retina, NMDA receptors are expressed by RGCs and amacrine cells (Fletcher et al., 2000), with the overstimulation of NMDA receptors causing retinal excitotoxicity which leads to neuronal cell death in the retina (Sucher et al., 1991), particularly in the

GCL. NMDA is a drug commonly used to artificially create normotensive glaucoma models, and for testing anti-glaucoma drugs (Yamashita et al., 2011). PACAP could be a good candidate to combat NMDA-induced retinal injury because it is able to reduce the harmful effects associated with the intravitreal injection of NMDA. The effect of NMDA treatment was more severe in PACAP-null mice than in wild-type animals, with the decrease in the number of RGCs significantly greater on the first, third, and seventh days after the injection of 40 nmol NMDA in 2 μl saline (Endo et al., 2011). In this way, endogenous PACAP production can be seen to play an important role in the protection of retinal cells against NMDA-induced damage (Endo et al., 2011). PACAP38 co-injected with NMDA significantly increased the survival of RGCs both in wild-type and PACAP-null animals. The most effective concentration of PACAP38 in the case of treatment of the retina of wild-type mice was 100 pM (Endo et al., 2011).

#### *Monosodium glutamate*

Under normal conditions, the amino acid derivate glutamate is one of the most important excitatory neurotransmitters in the CNS. This molecule and its receptors are also present in the retina where they have an essential function. However, glutamate also plays a key role in neurological and retinal diseases, as well as in pathological conditions of the eye (Sucher et al., 1991; Danysz and Parsons, 2002). Monosodium glutamate (MSG) is one of the most commonly used drugs to induce retinal injury in different animal models or *in vitro* studies. In recent years, many papers have been published concerning MSG-induced retinal cytotoxicity, and treatments that are able to protect retinal cells against the harmful effects of increased glutamate levels. Several studies suggest that drugs such as glutamate receptor blockers, hormones, neuropeptides, or pre- and post-conditioning could be effective in treating pathological conditions where the glutamate level is increased (Lombardi and Moroni, 1994; Russo et al., 2008; Fernandez et al., 2009). PACAP could also be an interesting candidate for this given that it has been shown to be retinoprotective in several retinal degeneration models, as mentioned above, and is known to exert a protective effect against glutamate toxicity.

Newborn rat retinal cell primary cultures were exposed for 10 min to 1 mM glutamate which caused a significant decrease in their viability (Shoge et al., 1999). Treatment of the cells with either PACAP38 or PACAP27 was protective in a dose-dependent manner (1 nM to 1 μM) against this glutamate-induced damage, with a maximum protective effect observed at a concentration of 100 nM. After a 10-min treatment with PACAP, the level of PKA and the MAPK activity of the cells were elevated. PACAP6-38 and H-89 (a selective PKA inhibitor) were able to attenuate the positive effects of PACAP27 and PACAP38.

In addition to these in vitro results, some *in vivo* studies have suggested that PACAP is effective against glutamate toxicity. The intravitreal treatment with MSG of newborn rats causes severe degeneration in many layers of the retina. The average thickness of the retina was decreased, the IPL almost disappeared, and the INL and CGL layers seemed to fuse with each other (Tamas et al., 2004; Babai et al., 2005; Atlasz et al., 2009). Simultaneously administered PACAP38 and PACAP27 (100 pmol in 5 μl saline) were able to significantly attenuate the MSG-induced damage to the retina. Although the retina was thinner than that in untreated controls, damage to the affected layers of the retina was not so severe (Tamas et al., 2004; Babai et al., 2006; Atlasz et al., 2007). However, if more than one MSG injection was given into the vitreous body, one PACAP treatment was not enough to provide protection against the repetitive excitotoxic stimuli. The PACAP treatment was successful only in the case where PACAP (100 pmol) was administered at least two times in parallel with the MSG injection (Babai et al., 2005).

An important question concerns the combined and additive effects of different treatments against the excitotoxic effect of the glutamate. An interesting study published in 2010 addressed the effect of enriched environments to combat the effects of MSG. MSG was injected into the vitreous body of newborn rat pups and it was found that animals maintained in a bigger cage with colorful objects exhibited reduced glutamate damage compared with controls maintained under standard conditions. A similar or enhanced result was seen in cases where pups maintained under standard conditions were treated with PACAP (100 pmol diluted in 5 μl saline). However, the protective effect of the enriched environment and PACAP co-injection was not additive (Kiss et al., 2011).

Most studies published in the last few years examined the cytoprotective effect of PACAP from a morphological perspective, but no information is usually given about improvements in retinal function following the treatment of glutamate-induced damage. Until now, only one paper has been published in which the functional effects of MSG and PACAP treatments were measured by electroretinogram (ERG). Newborn rats were treated with MSG (2 mg/g bodyweight) administered subcutaneously on the first, fifth, and ninth days postnatal. PACAP (100 pmol diluted in 5 μl saline) was administered into the vitreous body in half of the pups on the same days. The ERG examination was performed 2 months later, with results showing that the subcutaneous MSG injection attenuated the ERG wave amplitude, and that PACAP treatment was able to significantly improve the functional performance of the damaged retina (Varga et al., 2011).

### DIRECT AND INDIRECT PATHWAYS

Pituitary adenylate cyclase-activating polypeptide suppresses neuronal activity in the CNS via direct and indirect pathways (Shioda et al., 2006). The direct pathway infers that PACAP affects target neurons expressing the PACAP receptor. As shown above, PAC1R was detected in GCLs and amacrine cells in the retina (**Figure 1**), suggesting that PACAP affects these kinds of neurons directly. On the other hand, PACAP is also expressed by RGCs and amacrine cells (**Figure 1**). It is known that endogenous PACAP has neuroprotective functions in the CNS (Ohtaki et al., 2006; Nakamachi et al., 2010; Reglodi et al., 2012). Indeed, PACAP knockout mouse deteriorate retinal damage in some retinopathy animal models (Endo et al., 2011; Szabadfi et al., 2012a), which implies that endogenous PACAP protects retinal neurons via auto- or paracrine mechanisms. Signaling pathways involving the protective function of PACAP on neurons have been elegantly summarized by Atlasz et al. (2010a).

In the case of indirect pathways, PACAP is known to stimulate the secretion of neuroprotective factors in the CNS (Somogyvari-Vigh and Reglodi, 2004), although little is known about PACAP's indirect mode of action in the retina. IL-6 is recognized as a proinflammatory cytokine, but it acts as a neuroprotectant in the CNS (Loddick et al., 1998; Moidunny et al., 2010), and has been considered as a possible player in PACAP's indirect neuroprotective pathway. PACAP administration significantly increases IL-6 mRNA and protein expression levels in the murine brain, with neurons and astrocytes identified as the source of PACAP-induced IL-6 secretion (Tatsuno et al., 1996; Ohtaki et al., 2006; Nakamachi et al., 2012). In the mouse brain, PACAP-induced neuroprotection is absent in the IL-6 knockout mouse, suggesting that PACAP suppresses neuronal damage via an IL-6-mediated pathway (Ohtaki et al., 2006). PACAP also has the potential to stimulate IL-6 secretion in the retina. The addition of PACAP to primary cultures of rat Müller cells significantly augmented IL-6 levels in the culture medium in a manner that was inhibited by PACAP6-38 treatment (Nakatani et al., 2006; Seki et al., 2006a). Indeed, PAC1R protein was detected in rat primary cultures of Müller cells (Kubrusly et al., 2005). These data suggest that IL-6 released from Müller cells may mediate PACAP-induced retinal protection. Recent reports suggest that Müller cells secrete many types of neurotrophic factors, growth factors, and cytokines, such as BDNF and neurotrophin-3, glial cell-line derived neurotrophic factor (GDNF), neurturin, ciliary neurotrophic factor (CNTF), endothelin-2, leukemia inhibitory factor (LIF), basic fibroblast growth factor (bFGF), and prostaglandin E2 (Bringmann et al., 2009). These factors may be related to the neuroprotective effect of PACAP as well as IL-6. Furthermore, microglial cells exist in the retina, and infiltrating macrophages were identified in the retina after injury (Chen et al., 2002; Davies et al., 2006). This microglia/macrophage system has been considered as a regulator of immunity and inflammation after retinal damage (Wraith and Nicholson, 2012). Further study focusing on retinal glial cells in the mechanism of PACAP neuroprotection will provide new insights of the protective network involving PACAP.

## CONCLUSION AND FUTURE PERSPECTIVES

In the clinical setting, retinal neuropathies are a major cause of visual impairment that are yet to have a definitive cure. Alternative therapeutic strategies for addressing optic neuropathies are therefore required. Neurotrophic factors such as BDNF, ciliary neurotrophic factor, and glial cell line-derived neurotrophic factor have been shown to ameliorate RGC damage in an animal model of retinopathy (Johnson et al., 2011). However, the actions of these growth factors have not yet been well elucidated to enable them to be considered as target candidates of neuroprotective drugs to treat retinal neuropathies. In this review, we have shown that PACAP consistently exerts a potent protective effect against neural damage in a broad range of retinal diseases. As future studies involving PACAP will likely shift to obtaining a fuller understanding of the mechanisms underlying such protective functions, an important aspect of this will be to examine pathways involving glial cells. These insights will help in the development of new neuroprotective strategies to treat retinal neuropathies.

## ACKNOWLEDGMENTS

This work was supported by Grants-in Aid for Scientific Research (KAKENHI: 23249079, 24592681, 24592680), and by the MEXT-Support Program for the Strategic Research Foundation at Showa University (2008–2012, 2012–16).

## REFERENCES

Arimura, A. (1998). Perspectives on pituitary adenylate cyclase activating polypeptide (PACAP) in the neuroendocrine, endocrine, and nervous systems. *Jpn. J. Physiol.* 48, 301–331.

Arimura, A., and Shioda, S. (1995). Pituitary adenylate cyclase activating polypeptide (PACAP) and its receptors: neuroendocrine and endocrine interaction. *Front. Neuroendocrinol.* 16, 53–88.

Arimura, A., Somogyvari-Vigh, A., Miyata, A., Mizuno, K., Coy, D. H., and Kitada, C. (1991). Tissue distribution of PACAP as determined by RIA: highly abundant in the rat brain and testes. *Endocrinology* 129, 2787–2789.

Atlasz, T., Babai, N., Kiss, P., Reglodi, D., Tamas, A., Szabadfi, K., et al. (2007). Pituitary adenylate cyclase activating polypeptide is protective in bilateral carotid occlusion-induced retinal lesion in rats. *Gen. Comp. Endocrinol.* 153, 108–114.

Atlasz, T., Szabadfi, K., Kiss, P., Marton, Z., Griecs, M., Hamza, L., et al. (2011). Effects of PACAP in UV-A radiation-induced retinal degeneration models in rats. *J. Mol. Neurosci.* 43, 51–57.

Atlasz, T., Szabadfi, K., Kiss, P., Racz, B., Gallyas, F., Tamas, A., et al. (2010a). Pituitary adenylate cyclase activating polypeptide in the retina: focus on the retinoprotective effects. *Ann. N. Y. Acad. Sci.* 1200, 128–139.

Atlasz, T., Szabadfi, K., Kiss, P., Tamas, A., Toth, G., Reglodi, D., et al. (2010b). Evaluation of the protective effects of PACAP with cell-specific markers in ischemia-induced retinal degeneration. *Brain Res. Bull.* 81, 497–504.

Atlasz, T., Szabadfi, K., Reglodi, D., Kiss, P., Tamas, A., Toth, G., et al. (2009). Effects of pituitary adenylate cyclase activating polypeptide and its fragments on retinal degeneration induced by neonatal monosodium glutamate treatment. *Ann. N. Y. Acad. Sci.* 1163, 348–352.

Babai, N., Atlasz, T., Tamas, A., Reglodi, D., Toth, G., Kiss, P., et al. (2005). Degree of damage compensation by various PACAP treatments in monosodium glutamate-induced retinal degeneration. *Neurotox. Res.* 8, 227–233.

Babai, N., Atlasz, T., Tamas, A., Reglodi, D., Toth, G., Kiss, P., et al. (2006). Search for the optimal monosodium glutamate treatment schedule to study the neuroprotective effects of PACAP in the retina. *Ann. N. Y. Acad. Sci.* 1070, 149–155.

Block, F., Schwarz, M., and Sontag, K. H. (1992). Retinal ischemia induced by occlusion of both common carotid arteries in rats as demonstrated by electroretinography. *Neurosci. Lett.* 144, 124–126.

Bringmann, A., Iandiev, I., Pannicke, T., Wurm, A., Hollborn, M., Wiedemann, P., et al. (2009). Cellular signaling and factors involved in Muller cell gliosis: neuroprotective and detrimental effects. *Prog. Retin. Eye Res.* 28, 423–451.

Chen, L., Yang, P., and Kijlstra, A. (2002). Distribution, markers, and functions of retinal microglia. *Ocul. Immunol. Inflamm.* 10, 27–39.

Chiarini, L. B., Freitas, F. G., Petrs-Silva, H., and Linden, R. (2000). Evidence that the bifunctional redox factor$^{-/-}$AP endonuclease Ref-1 is an anti-apoptotic protein associated with differentiation in the developing retina. *Cell Death Differ.* 7, 272–281.

Cui, Y., Xu, X., Bi, H., Zhu, Q., Wu, J., Xia, X., et al. (2006). Expression modification of uncoupling proteins and MnSOD in retinal endothelial cells and pericytes induced by high glucose: the role of reactive oxygen species in diabetic retinopathy. *Exp. Eye Res.* 83, 807–816.

D'Agata, V., and Cavallaro, S. (1998). Functional and molecular expression of PACAP/VIP receptors in the rat retina. *Brain Res. Mol. Brain Res.* 54, 161–164.

Danysz, W., and Parsons, C. G. (2002). Neuroprotective potential of ionotropic glutamate receptor antagonists. *Neurotox. Res.* 4, 119–126.

Davies, M. H., Eubanks, J. P., and Powers, M. R. (2006). Microglia and macrophages are increased in response to ischemia-induced retinopathy in the mouse retina. *Mol. Vis.* 12, 467–477.

Dohi, K., Mizushima, H., Nakajo, S., Ohtaki, H., Matsunaga, S., Aruga, T., et al. (2002). Pituitary adenylate cyclase-activating polypeptide (PACAP) prevents hippocampal neurons from apoptosis by inhibiting JNK/SAPK and p38 signal transduction pathways. *Regul. Pept.* 109, 83–88.

Endo, K., Nakamachi, T., Seki, T., Kagami, N., Wada, Y., Nakamura, K., et al. (2011). Neuroprotective effect of PACAP against NMDA-induced retinal damage in the mouse. *J. Mol. Neurosci.* 43, 22–29.

Fabian, E., Reglodi, D., Mester, L., Szabo, A., Szabadfi, K., Tamas, A., et al. (2012). Effects of PACAP on intracellular signaling pathways in human retinal pigment epithelial cells exposed to oxidative stress. *J. Mol. Neurosci.* 48, 493–500.

Farkas, E., Timmer, N. M., Domoki, F., Mihaly, A., Luiten, P. G., and Bari, F. (2005). Post-ischemic administration of diazoxide attenuates long-term microglial activation in the rat brain after permanent carotid artery occlusion. *Neurosci. Lett.* 387, 168–172.

Farkas, O., Tamas, A., Zsombok, A., Reglodi, D., Pal, J., Buki, A., et al. (2004). Effects of pituitary adenylate cyclase activating polypeptide in a rat model of traumatic brain injury. *Regul. Pept.* 123, 69–75.

Fernandez, D. C., Chianelli, M. S., and Rosenstein, R. E. (2009). Involvement of glutamate in retinal protection against ischemia/reperfusion damage induced by post-conditioning. *J. Neurochem.* 111, 488–498.

Fletcher, E. L., Hack, I., Brandstatter, J. H., and Wassle, H. (2000). Synaptic localization of NMDA receptor subunits in the rat retina. *J. Comp. Neurol.* 420, 98–112.

Gastinger, M. J., Singh, R. S., and Barber, A. J. (2006). Loss of cholinergic and dopaminergic amacrine cells in streptozotocin-diabetic rat and Ins2Akita-diabetic mouse retinas. *Invest. Ophthalmol. Vis. Sci.* 47, 3143–3150.

Giunta, S., Castorina, A., Bucolo, C., Magro, G., Drago, F., and D'Agata, V. (2012). Early changes in pituitary adenylate cyclase-activating peptide, vasoactive intestinal peptide and related receptors expression in retina of streptozotocin-induced diabetic rats. *Peptides* 37, 32–39.

Harmar, A. J., Fahrenkrug, J., Gozes, I., Laburthe, M., May, V., Pisegna, J. R., et al. (2012). Pharmacology and functions of receptors for vasoactive intestinal peptide and pituitary adenylate cyclase-activating polypeptide: IUPHAR review 1. *Br. J. Pharmacol.* 166, 4–17.

Holopigian, K., Greenstein, V. C., Seiple, W., Hood, D. C., and Carr, R. E. (1997). Evidence for photoreceptor changes in patients with diabetic retinopathy. *Invest. Ophthalmol. Vis. Sci.* 38, 2355–2365.

Izumi, S., Seki, T., Shioda, S., Zhou, C. J., Arimura, A., and Koide, R. (2000). Ultrastructural localization of PACAP immunoreactivity in the rat retina. *Ann. N. Y. Acad. Sci.* 921, 317–320.

Johnson, T. V., Bull, N. D., and Martin, K. R. (2011). Neurotrophic factor delivery as a protective treatment for glaucoma. *Exp. Eye Res.* 93, 196–203.

Kalariya, N. M., Ramana, K. V., Srivastava, S. K., and Van Kuijk, F. J. (2008). Carotenoid derived aldehydes-induced oxidative stress causes apoptotic cell death in human retinal pigment epithelial cells. *Exp. Eye Res.* 86, 70–80.

Kiss, P., Atlasz, T., Szabadfi, K., Horvath, G., Griecs, M., Farkas, J., et al. (2011). Comparison between PACAP- and enriched environment-induced retinal protection in MSG-treated newborn rats. *Neurosci. Lett.* 487, 400–405.

Kook, D., Wolf, A. H., Yu, A. L., Neubauer, A. S., Priglinger, S. G., Kampik, A., et al. (2008). The protective effect of quercetin against oxidative stress in the human RPE in vitro. *Invest. Ophthalmol. Vis. Sci.* 49, 1712–1720.

Kowluru, R. A., and Abbas, S. N. (2003). Diabetes-induced mitochondrial dysfunction in the retina. *Invest. Ophthalmol. Vis. Sci.* 44, 5327–5334.

Kowluru, R. A., Kern, T. S., Engerman, R. L., and Armstrong, D. (1996). Abnormalities of retinal metabolism in diabetes or experimental galactosemia. III. Effects of antioxidants. *Diabetes* 45, 1233–1237.

Kubrusly, R. C., Da Cunha, M. C., Reis, R. A., Soares, H., Ventura, A. L., Kurtenbach, E., et al. (2005). Expression of functional receptors and transmitter enzymes in cultured Muller cells. *Brain Res.* 1038, 141–149.

Lavinsky, D., Arterni, N. S., Achaval, M., and Netto, C. A. (2006). Chronic bilateral common carotid artery occlusion: a model for ocular ischemic syndrome in the rat. *Graefes Arch. Clin. Exp. Ophthalmol.* 244, 199–204.

Lieth, E., Barber, A. J., Xu, B., Dice, C., Ratz, M. J., Tanase, D., et al. (1998). Glial reactivity and impaired glutamate metabolism in short-term experimental diabetic retinopathy. Penn State Retina Research Group. *Diabetes* 47, 815–820.

Liu, X., Mameza, M. G., Lee, Y. S., Eseonu, C. I., Yu, C. R., Kang Derwent, J. J., et al. (2008). Suppressors of cytokine-signaling proteins induce insulin resistance in the retina and promote survival of retinal cells. *Diabetes* 57, 1651–1658.

Loddick, S. A., Turnbull, A. V., and Rothwell, N. J. (1998). Cerebral interleukin-6 is neuroprotective during permanent focal cerebral ischemia in the rat. *J. Cereb. Blood Flow Metab.* 18, 176–179.

Lombardi, G., and Moroni, F. (1994). Glutamate receptor antagonists protect against ischemia-induced retinal damage. *Eur. J. Pharmacol.* 271, 489–495.

Loren, I., Tornqvist, K., and Alumets, J. (1980). VIP (vasoactive intestinal polypeptide)-immunoreactive neurons in the retina of the rat. *Cell Tissue Res.* 210, 167–170.

Mester, L., Kovacs, K., Racz, B., Solti, I., Atlasz, T., Szabadfi, K., et al. (2011). Pituitary adenylate cyclase-activating polypeptide is protective against oxidative stress in human retinal pigment epithelial cells. *J. Mol. Neurosci.* 43, 35–43.

Miyata, A., Arimura, A., Dahl, R. R., Minamino, N., Uehara, A., Jiang, L., et al. (1989). Isolation of a novel 38 residue-hypothalamic polypeptide which stimulates adenylate cyclase in pituitary cells. *Biochem. Biophys. Res. Commun.* 164, 567–574.

Moidunny, S., Dias, R. B., Wesseling, E., Sekino, Y., Boddeke, H. W., Sebastiao, A. M., et al. (2010). Interleukin-6-type cytokines in neuroprotection and neuromodulation: oncostatin M, but not leukemia inhibitory factor, requires neuronal adenosine A1 receptor function. *J. Neurochem.* 114, 1667–1677.

Moller, K., Zhang, Y. Z., Hakanson, R., Luts, A., Sjolund, B., Uddman, R., et al. (1993). Pituitary adenylate cyclase activating peptide is a sensory neuropeptide: immunocytochemical and immunochemical evidence. *Neuroscience* 57, 725–732.

Morgan, I. G., and Ingham, C. A. (1981). Kainic acid affects both plexiform layers of chicken retina. *Neurosci. Lett.* 21, 275–280.

Mulder, H., Uddman, R., Moller, K., Zhang, Y. Z., Ekblad, E., Alumets, J., et al. (1994). Pituitary adenylate cyclase activating polypeptide expression in sensory neurons. *Neuroscience* 63, 307–312.

Nakamachi, T., Farkas, J., Watanabe, J., Ohtaki, H., Dohi, K., Arata, S., et al. (2011). Role of PACAP in neural stem/progenitor cell and astrocyte - from neural development to neural repair. *Curr. Pharm. Des.* 17, 973–984.

Nakamachi, T., Ohtaki, H., Yofu, S., Dohi, K., Watanabe, J., Mori, H., et al. (2010). Endogenous pituitary adenylate cyclase activating polypeptide is involved in suppression of edema in the ischemic brain. *Acta Neurochir. Suppl.* 106, 43–46.

Nakamachi, T., Tsuchida, M., Kagami, N., Yofu, S., Wada, Y., Hori, M., et al. (2012). IL-6 and PACAP Receptor Expression and Localization after Global Brain Ischemia in Mice. *J. Mol. Neurosci.* 48, 518–525.

Nakatani, M., Seki, T., Shinohara, Y., Taki, C., Nishimura, S., Takaki, A., et al. (2006). Pituitary adenylate cyclase-activating peptide (PACAP) stimulates production of interleukin-6 in rat Muller cells. *Peptides* 27, 1871–1876.

Nilsson, S. F., De Neef, P., Robberecht, P., and Christophe, J. (1994). Characterization of ocular receptors for pituitary adenylate cyclase activating polypeptide (PACAP) and their coupling to adenylate cyclase. *Exp. Eye Res.* 58, 459–467.

Ohtaki, H., Nakamachi, T., Dohi, K., Aizawa, Y., Takaki, A., Hodoyama, K., et al. (2006). Pituitary adenylate cyclase-activating polypeptide (PACAP) decreases ischemic neuronal cell death in association with IL-6. *Proc. Natl. Acad. Sci. U.S.A.* 103, 7488–7493.

Ohtaki, H., Nakamachi, T., Dohi, K., and Shioda, S. (2008). Role of PACAP in ischemic neural death. *J. Mol. Neurosci.* 36, 16–25.

Onali, P., and Olianas, M. C. (1994). PACAP is a potent and highly effective stimulator of adenylyl cyclase activity in the retinas of different mammalian species. *Brain Res.* 641, 132–134.

Parsons, C. G., Danysz, W., and Quack, G. (1998). Glutamate in CNS disorders as a target for drug development: an update. *Drug News Perspect.* 11, 523–569.

Quigley, H. A., Nickells, R. W., Kerrigan, L. A., Pease, M. E., Thibault, D. J., and Zack, D. J. (1995). Retinal ganglion cell death in experimental glaucoma and after axotomy occurs by apoptosis. *Invest. Ophthalmol. Vis. Sci.* 36, 774–786.

Rabl, K., Reglodi, D., Banvolgyi, T., Somogyvari-Vigh, A., Lengvari, I., Gabriel, R., et al. (2002). PACAP inhibits anoxia-induced changes in physiological responses in horizontal cells in the turtle retina. *Regul. Pept.* 109, 71–74.

Racz, B., Gallyas, F. Jr., Kiss, P., Toth, G., Hegyi, O., Gasz, B., et al. (2006). The neuroprotective effects of PACAP in monosodium glutamate-induced retinal lesion involve inhibition of proapoptotic signaling pathways. *Regul. Pept.* 137, 20–26.

Racz, B., Horvath, G., Reglodi, D., Gasz, B., Kiss, P., Gallyas, F. Jr., et al. (2010). PACAP ameliorates oxidative stress in the chicken inner ear: an *in vitro* study. *Regul. Pept.* 160, 91–98.

Reglodi, D., Kiss, P., Lubics, A., and Tamas, A. (2011). Review on the protective effects of PACAP in models of neurodegenerative diseases *in vitro* and *in vivo*. *Curr. Pharm. Des.* 17, 962–972.

Reglodi, D., Kiss, P., Szabadfi, K., Atlasz, T., Gabriel, R., Horvath, G., et al. (2012). PACAP is an endogenous protective factor-insights from PACAP-deficient mice. *J. Mol. Neurosci.* 48, 482–492.

Rehen, S. K., Varella, M. H., Freitas, F. G., Moraes, M. O., and Linden, R. (1996). Contrasting effects of protein synthesis inhibition and of cyclic AMP on apoptosis in the developing retina. *Development* 122, 1439–1448.

Russo, R., Cavaliere, F., Watanabe, C., Nucci, C., Bagetta, G., Corasaniti, M. T., et al. (2008). 17Beta-estradiol prevents retinal ganglion cell loss induced by acute rise of intraocular pressure in rat. *Prog. Brain Res.* 173, 583–590.

Seki, M., Tanaka, T., Nawa, H., Usui, T., Fukuchi, T., Ikeda, K., et al. (2004). Involvement of brain-derived neurotrophic factor in early retinal neuropathy of streptozotocin-induced diabetes in rats: therapeutic potential of brain-derived neurotrophic factor for dopaminergic amacrine cells. *Diabetes* 53, 2412–2419.

Seki, T., Hinohara, Y., Taki, C., Nakatani, M., Ozawa, M., Nishimura, S., et al. (2006a). PACAP stimulates the release of interleukin-6 in cultured rat Muller cells. *Ann. N. Y. Acad. Sci.* 1070, 535–539.

Seki, T., Nakatani, M., Taki, C., Shinohara, Y., Ozawa, M., Nishimura, S., et al. (2006b). Neuroprotective effect of PACAP against kainic acid-induced neurotoxicity in rat retina. *Ann. N. Y. Acad. Sci.* 1070, 531–534.

Seki, T., Itoh, H., Nakamachi, T., Endo, K., Wada, Y., Nakamura, K., et al. (2011). Suppression of rat retinal ganglion cell death by PACAP following transient ischemia induced by high intraocular pressure. *J. Mol. Neurosci.* 43, 30–34.

Seki, T., Itoh, H., Nakamachi, T., and Shioda, S. (2008). Suppression of ganglion cell death by PACAP following optic nerve transection in the rat. *J. Mol. Neurosci.* 36, 57–60.

Seki, T., Izumi, S., Shioda, S., Zhou, C. J., Arimura, A., and Koide, R. (2000a). Gene expression for PACAP receptor mRNA in the rat retina by in situ hybridization and in situ RT-PCR. *Ann. N. Y. Acad. Sci.* 921, 366–369.

Seki, T., Shioda, S., Izumi, S., Arimura, A., and Koide, R. (2000b). Electron microscopic observation of pituitary adenylate cyclase-activating polypeptide (PACAP)-containing neurons in the rat retina. *Peptides* 21, 109–113.

Seki, T., Shioda, S., Nakai, Y., Arimura, A., and Koide, R. (1998). Distribution and ultrastructural localization of pituitary adenylate cyclase-activating polypeptide (PACAP) and its receptor in the rat retina. *Ann. N. Y. Acad. Sci.* 865, 408–411.

Seki, T., Shioda, S., Ogino, D., Nakai, Y., Arimura, A., and Koide, R. (1997). Distribution and ultrastructural localization of a receptor for pituitary adenylate cyclase activating polypeptide and its mRNA in the rat retina. *Neurosci. Lett.* 238, 127–130.

Sherwood, N. M., Krueckl, S. L., and Mcrory, J. E. (2000). The origin and function of the pituitary adenylate cyclase-activating polypeptide (PACAP)/glucagon superfamily. *Endocr. Rev.* 21, 619–670.

Shioda, S., Ohtaki, H., Nakamachi, T., Dohi, K., Watanabe, J., Nakajo, S., et al. (2006). Pleiotropic functions of PACAP in the CNS: neuroprotection and neurodevelopment. *Ann. N. Y. Acad. Sci.* 1070, 550–560.

Shoge, K., Mishima, H. K., Saitoh, T., Ishihara, K., Tamura, Y., Shiomi, H., et al. (1999). Attenuation by PACAP of glutamate-induced neurotoxicity in cultured retinal neurons. *Brain Res.* 839, 66–73.

Silveira, M. S., Costa, M. R., Bozza, M., and Linden, R. (2002). Pituitary adenylyl cyclase-activating polypeptide prevents induced cell death in retinal tissue through activation of cyclic AMP-dependent protein kinase. *J. Biol. Chem.* 277, 16075–16080.

Somogyvari-Vigh, A., and Reglodi, D. (2004). Pituitary adenylate cyclase activating polypeptide: a potential neuroprotective peptide. *Curr. Pharm. Des.* 10, 2861–2889.

Sucher, N. J., Lei, S. Z., and Lipton, S. A. (1991). Calcium channel antagonists attenuate NMDA receptor-mediated neurotoxicity of retinal ganglion cells in culture. *Brain Res.* 551, 297–302.

Szabadfi, K., Atlasz, T., Kiss, P., Danyadi, B., Tamas, A., Helyes, Z., et al. (2012a). Mice deficient in pituitary adenylate cyclase activating polypeptide (PACAP) are more susceptible to retinal ischemic injury *in vivo*. *Neurotox. Res.* 21, 41–48.

Szabadfi, K., Atlasz, T., Kiss, P., Reglodi, D., Szabo, A., Kovacs, K., et al. (2012b). Protective effects of the neuropeptide PACAP in diabetic retinopathy. *Cell Tissue Res.* 348, 37–46.

Szabadfi, K., Mester, L., Reglodi, D., Kiss, P., Babai, N., Racz, B., et al. (2010). Novel neuroprotective strategies in ischemic retinal lesions. *Int. J. Mol. Sci.* 11, 544–561.

Szabo, A., Danyadi, B., Bognar, E., Szabadfi, K., Fabian, E., Kiss, P., et al. (2012). Effect of PACAP on MAP kinases, Akt and cytokine expressions in rat retinal hypoperfusion. *Neurosci. Lett.* 523, 93–98.

Tamas, A., Gabriel, R., Racz, B., Denes, V., Kiss, P., Lubics, A., et al. (2004). Effects of pituitary adenylate cyclase activating polypeptide in retinal degeneration induced by monosodium-glutamate. *Neurosci. Lett.* 372, 110–113.

Tatsuno, I., Morio, H., Tanaka, T., Uchida, D., Hirai, A., Tamura, Y., et al. (1996). Pituitary adenylate cyclase-activating polypeptide (PACAP) is a regulator of astrocytes: PACAP stimulates proliferation and production of interleukin 6 (IL-6), but not nerve growth factor (NGF), in cultured rat astrocyte. *Ann. N. Y. Acad. Sci.* 805, 482–488.

Tsuchikawa, D., Nakamachi, T., Tsuchida, M., Wada, Y., Hori, M., Farkas, J., et al. (2012). Neuroprotective effect of endogenous pituitary adenylate cyclase-activating polypeptide on spinal cord injury. *J. Mol. Neurosci.* 48, 508–517.

Varga, B., Szabadfi, K., Kiss, P., Fabian, E., Tamas, A., Griecs, M., et al. (2011). PACAP improves functional outcome in excitotoxic retinal lesion: an electroretinographic study. *J. Mol. Neurosci.* 43, 44–50.

Vaudry, D., Falluel-Morel, A., Bourgault, S., Basille, M., Burel, D., Wurtz, O., et al. (2009). Pituitary adenylate cyclase-activating polypeptide and its receptors: 20 years after the discovery. *Pharmacol. Rev.* 61, 283–357.

Vaudry, D., Rousselle, C., Basille, M., Falluel-Morel, A., Pamantung, T. F., Fontaine, M., et al. (2002). Pituitary adenylate cyclase-activating polypeptide protects rat cerebellar granule neurons against ethanol-induced apoptotic cell death. *Proc. Natl. Acad. Sci. U.S.A.* 99, 6398–6403.

Wang, Z. Y., Alm, P., and Hakanson, R. (1995). Distribution and effects of pituitary adenylate cyclase-activating peptide in the rabbit eye. *Neuroscience* 69, 297–308.

Watkins, J. C., and Jane, D. E. (2006). The glutamate story. *Br. J. Pharmacol.* 147(Suppl. 1), S100–S108.

Wraith, D. C., and Nicholson, L. B. (2012). The adaptive immune system in diseases of the central nervous system. *J. Clin. Invest.* 122, 1172–1179.

Yamashita, H., Yamada-Nakayama, C., Sugihara, K., Tsuji, S., Sakurai, T., Ban, Y., et al. (2011). Functional and morphological effects of beta-estradiol in eyes with *N*-methyl-D-aspartate-induced retinal neurotoxicity in rats. *Exp. Eye Res.* 93, 75–81.

Zhang, X. Y., Hayasaka, S., Chi, Z. L., Cui, H. S., and Hayasaka, Y. (2005). Effect of pituitary adenylate cyclase-activating polypeptide (PACAP) on IL-6, IL-8, and MCP-1 expression in human retinal pigment epithelial cell line. *Curr. Eye Res.* 30, 1105–1111.

18

# Observations on the evolution of the melanocortin receptor gene family: distinctive features of the melanocortin-2 receptor

***Robert M. Dores****

*Department of Biological Sciences, University of Denver, Denver, CO, USA*

***Edited by:***
*Eric W. Roubos, Radboud University Nijmegen, Netherlands*

***Reviewed by:***
*Dan Larhammar, Uppsala University, Sweden*
*Li Chan, Queen Mary University of London, UK*

****Correspondence:***
*Robert M. Dores, Department of Biological Sciences, University of Denver, 2190 E. Iliff, Olin Hall 102, Denver, CO 80210, USA.*
*e-mail: rdores@du.edu*

The melanocortin receptors (MCRs) are a gene family in the rhodopsin class of G protein-coupled receptors. Based on the analysis of several metazoan genome databases it appears that the MCRs are only found in chordates. The presence of five genes in the family (i.e., *mc1r, mc2r, mc3r, mc4r, mc5r*) in representatives of the tetrapods indicates that the gene family is the result of two genome duplication events and one local gene duplication event during the evolution of the chordates. The MCRs are activated by melanocortin ligands (i.e., ACTH, α-MSH, β-MSH, γ-MSH, δ-MSH) which are all derived from the polypeptide hormone/neuropeptide precursor, POMC, and as a result the functional evolution of the MCRs is intimately associated with the co-evolution of POMC endocrine and neuronal circuits. This review will consider the origin of the MCRs, and discuss the evolutionary relationship between MC2R, MC5R, and MC4R. In addition, this review will analyze the functional evolution of the *mc2r* gene in light of the co-evolution of the *MRAP* (*Melanocortin-2 Receptor Accessory Protein*) gene family.

**Keywords: melanocortin receptors, ACTH, α-MSH, MRAP, MC2R, MC5R, constructive neutral evolution, evolutionary cell biology**

## INTRODUCTION

An analysis of tetrapod (amphibians, reptiles, birds, and mammals) genomes indicates that the melanocortin receptors (MCRs) are a family of five G protein-coupled receptors (GPCRs) genes (i.e., *mc1r, mc2r, mc3r, mc4r, mc5r*) that have been implicated in the mediation of integument pigmentation, appetite regulation, glucocorticoid synthesis, and exocrine gland secretion (Gantz and Fong, 2003; Cone, 2006). A unifying feature of this gene family is that all of the receptors can be activated by one or more of the melanocortin peptides (i.e., ACTH, α-MSH, β-MSH, γ-MSH; Cone, 2006) with varying degrees of efficacy. The melanocortin ligands are derived from the precursor protein proopiomelanocortin (POMC; Nakanishi et al., 1979), a member of the opioid/orphanin gene family (Dores et al., 2002). As a result, the functional evolution of MCRs co-evolved with the *POMC* gene. However, the functional evolution of at least some of the MCRs is also tied to the co-evolution of two other gene families; the *Melanocortin-2 Receptor Accessory Protein* (*MRAP*) gene family (Metherell et al., 2005; Hinkle and Sebag, 2009; Webb and Clark, 2010; Liang et al., 2011; Vastermark and Schiöth, 2011), and the *AGRP/ASIP* gene family (Vastermark and Schiöth, 2011). The later polypeptides function as antagonists or "inverse agonists" for several MCRs. The evolution of the *AGRP/ASIP* gene family has recently been reviewed (Vastermark and Schiöth, 2011) and will not be discussed in this review. Instead, this review will consider the origins of the MCRs and POMC, the origin of the melanocortin-2 receptor (MC2R) and the melanocortin-5 receptor (MC5R), and the co-evolution of MC2R and MRAP.

## THE PHYLOGENETIC DISTRIBUTION OF MELANOCORTIN RECEPTORS AND POMC

The MCRs are placed in the A-13 family within the rhodopsin class of GPCRs (Horn et al., 2003; Vassilatis et al., 2003). In terms of origin, the MCR gene family appears to be a relatively "recent" addition as compared to other hormone/neuropeptide-activated GPCR gene families such as the vasopressin/oxytocin receptor gene family (Mohr et al., 1996), the CRH receptor gene family (Denver, 2009), or the GnRH receptor gene family (Kah et al., 2006). A search for MCRs in the genome databases of protostomes has not revealed any orthologous genes in these phyla (Vastermark and Schiöth, 2011). In addition among the deuterostomes, it appears that MCR genes also are not present in the genomes of echinoderms, cephalochordates, or urochordates (Vastermark and Schiöth, 2011). However, the presence of *MCR*-related genes in hagfish, lamprey, cartilaginous fish, teleost, and tetrapod genomes (Vastermark and Schiöth, 2011) provides support for the assumption that the MCRs are a chordate gene family.

Coincidentally, orthologous *POMC* genes have been detected in lamprey, cartilaginous fish, teleost, and tetrapod genomes as well (Dores and Baron, 2011). As a result, the proliferation of the paralogous *mcr*-coding genes and the radiation of the paralogous genes in the opioid/orphanin gene family have been influenced by the genome duplication events which have played a critical role in the proliferation of gene families within the various classes of vertebrates (Ohno et al., 1968; Lundin, 1993; Holland et al., 1994).

## GENOME DUPLICATION EVENTS AND THE EVOLUTION OF POMC AND MELANOCORTIN RECEPTORS

The chordates can be divided into three major lineages, the protochordates represented today by the arrow worm, Amphioxus, and tunicates (superclass Cephalochordata), vertebrates lacking a true jaw such as the lampreys and hagfishes (superclass Agnatha) and the jawed vertebrates such as the cartilaginous fishes, the ray-finned fishes, lobe-finned fishes, and the tetrapods (superclass Gnathostoma). These three major lineages in chordate evolution emerged sequentially; that is the ancestral protochordate lineages are most ancient and the ancestral gnathostome lineages are most recent (Carroll, 1988). There is general agreement that during the radiation of the ancestral agnathans two genome duplication events occurred in a lineage which ultimately gave rise to the ancestral gnathostomes (Ohno et al., 1968; Lundin, 1993; Holland et al., 1994). As a result where there may have been a single copy of a particular gene in the ancestral protochordates, there was now the potential for four paralogous copies of this gene in the gnathostomes. To add to the proliferation of paralogous members within a gene family the modern ray-finned fishes (teleosts) have undergone an additional genome duplication event (Meyer and Van de Peer, 2005), and there is evidence for local gene duplication events in many gnathostome gene families. It should also be noted that gene loss has occurred in several of the gnathostome gene families.

An operating assumption of the chordate genome duplication process has been that extant agnathans are 1R, where "R" indicates replication of the entire genome, extant gnathostomes are 2R, and the teleosts are 3R. Schemes based on this operating assumption for the opioid/orphanin gene family and the melanocortin receptor gene family is presented in **Figure 1**. To date neither opioid/orphanin-related genes nor melanocortin receptor-related genes have been detected in the genome of an extant cephalochordate. However, it would be reasonable to propose that the ancestral gene for each gene family emerged in some now extinct protochordate lineage. That said both *POMC*-related genes (Heinig et al., 1995; Takahashi et al., 1995) and *Melanocortin Receptor*-related genes (Haitina et al., 2007), and have been characterized from the lamprey genome.

As shown in **Figure 1A**, there are two distinct paralogs of the *POMC* gene in the lamprey genome (*POM* and *POC* genes). These genes encode overlapping yet distinct melanocortin and opioid peptides sequences and are expressed in different regions of the lamprey pituitary (Heinig et al., 1995; Takahashi et al., 1995). Enkephalin-like peptides have also been identified in the CNS of the marine lamprey, *Petromyzon marinus* (Dores and Gorbman, 1990) which would suggest that another opioid precursor is present in the lamprey genome. In this scenario, the *Proenkephalin* and *Prodynorphin* genes are the result of the 2 R event, and these genes are found in all the extant groups of gnathostomes; whereas, the *Proorphanin* gene is viewed as the result of a local gene duplication of the *pomc* gene (Sundstrom et al., 2010) which is predicted to have occurred after the 2R event.

The characterization of two melanocortin receptor genes in the lamprey genome (**Figure 1B**) that are the orthologs of the *MC1R* gene (MCaR) and the *MC4R* gene (MCbR), respectively would be consistent with the assumption that lampreys are 1R organisms

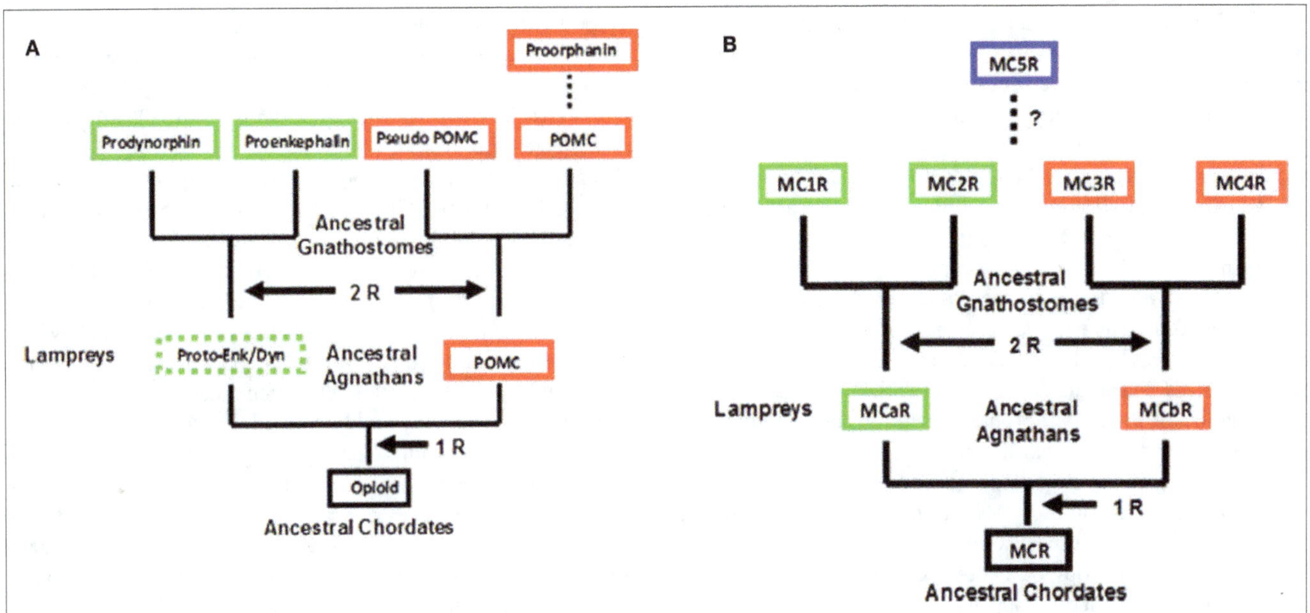


**FIGURE 1 | Scheme for the evolution of opioid/orphanin precursors and melanocortin receptors.** These evolutionary schemes assume that lampreys are 1R organisms. **(A)** Proposed evolution for the opioid/orphanin gene family. The scheme is modified from Dores and Baron (2011). **(B)** Proposed evolution of the melanocortin receptors. This scheme is modified from Baron et al. (2009). The dashed line indicates the origin of MC5R is not resolved. R, refers to the number of genome duplication events; Opioid, ancestral opioid precursor; Proto-Enk/Dyn, hypothetical proto-enkephalin/dynorphin gene; POMC, proopiomelanocortin; MCR, ancestral melanocortin receptor; MCaR, lamprey melanocortin-a receptor; MCbR, lamprey melanocortin-b receptor; MC1R, melanocortin-1 receptor; MC2R, melanocortin-2 receptor; MC3R, melanocortin-3 receptor, MC4R, melanocortin-4 receptor; MC5R, melanocortin-5 receptor.

(Haitina et al., 2007). In this scenario the second genome duplication event would result in the MC1R, MC2R, MC3R, and MC4R paralogs in the ancestral gnathostomes. At some later point it is assumed the MC5R paralog emerged as a result of a localized gene duplication of one of the other MCR paralogs. The origin of MC5R will be discussed in Section "Origin of MC5R and the Speculations on the Relationship between MC5R and MC4R." However, there are some aspects of the schemes presented in **Figure 1** which challenge the status of the lamprey as a 1R organism. For example, while plausible explanations have been made to explain the presence of three opioid coding genes in the lamprey genome, assuming that lampreys are 1R organisms (Dores et al., 2002), perhaps the status of the extant agnathan genomes needs to be reevaluated.

Although the agnathan vertebrates emerged at least 450 million years ago and at their zenith were represented by at least three subclasses and numerous orders (Carroll, 1988), today this superclass has been reduced to two extant subclasses: [Myxini (hagfishes) and Cephalaspidomorphi (lampreys; Nelson, 1994). While the lampreys have been considered a 1R group, recent analyzes of the lamprey genome database (McEwen et al., 2009) have found more members within gene families than would be predicted for a 1R organism. Collectively, these observations have led to the premise that the 2R genome duplication event may have occurred in a group of agnathans that were ancestral to both the lamprey lineage and the ancestral gnathostome lineage (Kuraku et al., 2009; Smith et al., 2013). The ramifications of this hypothesis are reflected in the revised evolutionary trees for opioid/orphanin precursors and for MCRs shown in **Figure 2**.

When considering the radiation of the opioid/orphanin gene family (**Figure 2A**), the assumption that the lampreys are 2R organisms provides a more satisfying explanation for the presence of the two *pomc* paralogous genes in the lamprey genome (i.e., *POM* and *POC*). The presence of distinct POM and POC precursor proteins synthesized in the anterior pituitary and intermediate pituitary, respectively, would appear to be the result of the second genome duplication event followed by divergence of the regulatory regions of the *POM* and *POC* genes (Takahashi and Kawauchi, 2006). This scenario also predicts that *Proenkephalin-like* and *Prodynorphin-like* genes may also be present in the lamprey genome. Since the lamprey genome project is only half completed there is likelihood that these other opioid genes may be present. This scenario also is consistent with the current view of the radiation of the opioid/orphanin genes in the gnathostomes (**Figure 2A**; Sundstrom et al., 2010).

However, regardless of whether the lamprey genome is 1R or 2R, the general organization of POMC has not been radically altered either for the lamprey or the gnathostomes (Vallarino et al., 2012). POMC encodes one copy of a core opioid sequence (YGGF; β-endorphin) and at least one copy of a core melanocortin sequence (HFRW). In the lamprey POC sequence the melanocortin ligand is a highly derived form of ACTH (Heinig et al., 1995). In the lamprey POM sequence there are two melanocortin ligands, melanotropin A and melanotropin B, that correspond to β-MSH and α-MSH, respectively (Takahashi et al., 1995). In the POMC sequences of the cartilaginous fishes there are five melanocortin sequences, ACTH, α-MSH, β-MSH, γ-MSH, and a melanocortin sequence unique to the cartilaginous fishes, δ-MSH (Amemiya et al., 1999). In teleost POMC sequences both the γ-MSH and δ-MSH are absent; whereas, among the tetrapods the γ-MSH sequence is present and there is no equivalent to a δ-MSH sequence (Dores and Lecaude, 2005; Takahashi and Kawauchi, 2006).

It should be noted that the sequence of α-MSH comprises the first 13 amino acids within the ACTH(1–39) sequence. Hence, another feature of the melanocortin network that has been rigorously retained is the differential posttranslational processing of the POMC precursor by the endoproteolytic cleavage enzymes, prohormone convertase 1 (anterior pituitary) and prohormone hormone convertase 2 (intermediate pituitary; Seidah and Chrétien, 1999).

Applying this same scenario to the evolution of the melanocortin receptor genes (**Figure 2B**), the lamprey genome may contain two additional MCRs. Hence the unique sequence motifs in the MC1R ortholog (MCaR) and the MC4R ortholog (MCbR) may be more derived features than ancestral features. Lamprey MCaR has been expressed in heterologous mammalian cells, and an unexpected observation was that this receptor is selective for ACTH-related analogs, and is much less reactive to MSH-related ligands (Haitina et al., 2007). At present the pharmacology of the lamprey MCbR has not been investigated.

Regardless of whether the lamprey genome is 1R or 2R, the genome of the ancestral gnathostomes should have had at least four paralogous melanocortin receptor genes (i.e., *MC1R, MC2R, MC3R,* and *MC4R*; **Figure 2B**), and this feature should be evident in the extant members of this subclass (i.e., the cartilaginous fishes, the bony fishes, and the lobe-finned fishes and tetrapods). To date, all five *MCR* paralogs have been found in the several tetrapod genomes that have been analyzed. However, in teleost genomes some deviations from this scheme have been observed. For example the fugu genomes (*Takifugu rubripes* and *Tetraodon nigroviridis*) lack a *MC3R* gene (Klovins et al., 2004a), and the zebrafish genome has an additional *MC5R* paralog (Ringholm et al., 2002). Finally, with respect to the cartilaginous fishes, while three MCR paralogs (*MC1R, MC2R, MC3r)* have been found in the genome of the holocephalan, *Callorhynchus milii* (Vastermark and Schiöth, 2011), and three MCR paralogs (*MC3R, MC4R, MC5R*) have been cloned from the genome of the elasmobranch, *Squalus acanthias*; Ringholm et al., 2003; Klovins et al., 2004b). However, to date all five paralogs have not been characterized from a single cartilaginous fish species. While gene loss could account for the later observation, it should be noted that the *C. milii* genome project has not been completed, and the apparent absence of *mc1r* and *mc2r* from the *S. acanthias* genome may only require a new cloning strategy that takes advantage of the sequence data on the MCR paralogs from the *C. milii* genome project. At this stage it would be reasonable to propose that the ancestral gnathostomes had a minimum of four MCR paralogs (i.e., *MC1R, MC2R, MC3R, MC4R*), which then begs the question of the origin of the *mc5r* gene.

## ORIGIN OF MC5R AND THE SPECULATIONS ON THE RELATIONSHIP BETWEEN MC5R AND MC4R

When genomes duplicate, paralogous genes will initially be located on distinct homologous chromosomes (Holland et al., 1994).

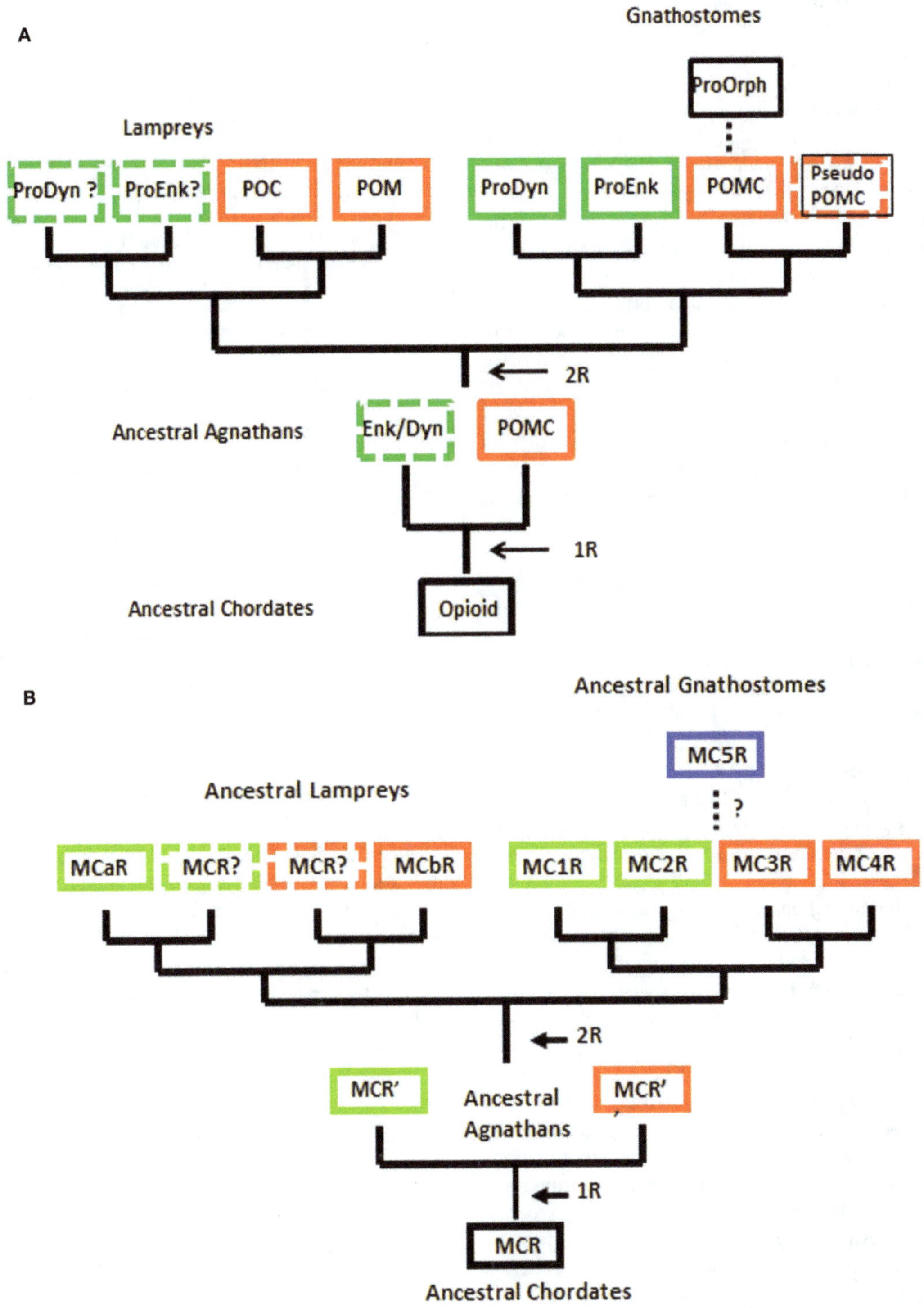


**FIGURE 2 | Alternative schemes for the evolution of opioid/orphanin precursors and melanocortin receptors (MCRs).** These evolutionary schemes assume that lampreys are 2R organisms. **(A)** Proposed evolution of the opioid/orphanin gene family. **(B)** Proposed evolution of the MCRs. The dashed line indicates the origin of MC5R is not resolved. R, refers to the number of genome duplication events; Opioid, ancestral opioid precursor; Prodyn, prodynorphin; Proenk, proenkephalin, Proorph, proorphanin; Enk/Dyn, hypothetical proto-enkephalin/dynorphin gene; POMC, proopiomelanocortin; POC, proopiocortin; POM, proopiomelanotropin; MCR, ancestral melanocortin receptor; MCaR, lamprey melanocortin-a receptor; MCbR, lamprey melanocortin-b receptor; MC1R, melanocortin-1 receptor; MC2R, melanocortin-2 receptor; MC3R, melanocortin-3 receptor, MC4R, melanocortin-4 receptor; MC5R, melanocortin-5 receptor.

However, it is appreciated that one or both of the paralogs could be subsequently lost, or that non-homologous chromosomes could fuse resulting in two paralogs on the same chromosome. However, the distribution of paralogous genes on distinct chromosomes has been considered a clear indication that a genome duplication event has occurred (Ohno et al., 1968; Lundin, 1993). For example, an analysis of the human, mouse, chicken, fugu (*Takifugu rubripes*), and zebrafish (*Danio rerio*) genomes revealed that the *MC1R* gene, the *MC2R* gene, the *MC3R* gene, and the *MC4R* gene are all located on different chromosomes (Schiöth et al., 2003; Klovins et al., 2004a). In addition, in all six genomes the *MC5R* gene was located on the same chromosome as the *MC2R* in relatively close proximity. These observations provide support for the hypothesis that the *MC5R* gene was the result of a local duplication of the *MC2R* gene (Klovins et al., 2004a). In this scenario ancestral gnathostomes are viewed as having a *MC5R/MC2R* proto-gene, which gave rise to a distinct *mc2r* gene and a distinct *mc5r* gene on the same chromosome as a result of the local gene duplication event (Baron et al., 2009).

Recently these conclusions on the relationship between the *MC2R* and the *MC5R* gene have been called into question (Vastermark and Schiöth, 2011). The issue is that a comparison of the amino acid sequences of MC2R and MC5R indicate that these two MCRs vary considerably in amino acid identity. However, when the amino acid sequences of MC4R and MC5R are compared, these two receptors share a number of identical residues. Furthermore, in a phylogenetic analysis of human and cartilaginous fish MCRs sequences, the MC4R and the MC5R sequences formed a clade (Vastermark and Schiöth, 2011). Based on these observations, Vastermark and Schiöth (2011) predicted that it is more likely that the *MC5R* gene was the result of a local duplication of the *MC4R* gene.

Are these two interpretations for the origin of the *MC5R* gene mutually exclusive? The *MC4R/MC5R* duplication could have occurred at an ancestral gnathostome locus prior to the divergence of the ancestral cartilaginous fishes and the ancestral bony fishes. In this scenario the *MC5R* locus could have moved to the chromosome carrying the *MC2R* locus in a common ancestor prior to the divergence of the ancestral cartilaginous fishes and the ancestral bony fishes. However, when genes duplicate, either as a result of a local duplication event or as a result of a genome duplication event, the new copies of the ancestral gene will accumulate mutations independent of each other. Furthermore based on selection pressures, these independently evolving genes could retain separate functions of the ancestral gene (subfunctionalization) or become adapted for some new function (neofunctionalization; Force et al., 1998).

**Figure 3** provides an alternative interpretation for the origin of *MC5R* gene that combines the major aspects of the two primary studies (Schiöth et al., 2003; Vastermark and Schiöth, 2011). **Figure 3** is based on the assumption that the *MC4R* gene was the ancestral melanocortin gene. A corollary to this assumption is that MCR paralogs would contain a "MC4R" signature; that is, sets of amino acid motifs derived from the proposed ancestral *MC4R* gene. In this scenario a *MC2R/MC5R* gene in the ancestral gnathostomes could have undergone a local gene duplication event. This assumption would be consistent with the synteny studies (Schiöth et al., 2003). Following the duplication event, selection pressures may have favored the *MC5R* duplicate gene maintaining the sequence features found in MC4R, while the *MC2R* duplicate gene apparently accumulated mutations and as a result evolved new functional properties not found in any of the other MCR paralogs.

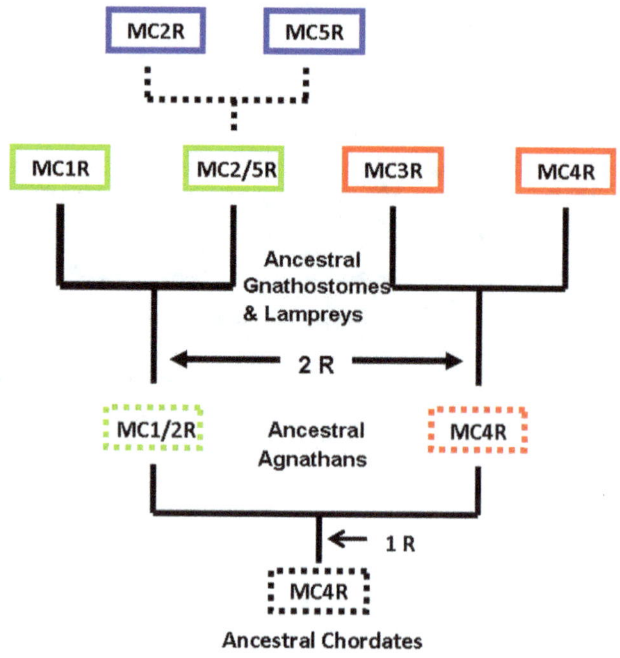


**FIGURE 3 | Revised scheme for the evolution of the melanocortin receptors.** This evolutionary scheme assumes that the melanocortin-4 receptor was the ancestral melanocortin receptor. The dashed box around a receptor indicates that the receptor is predicted but has not been identified. The dashed lines represent the hypothesis that the *MC2R* gene and the *MC5R* gene were the result of a local duplication of the proposed *MC2R/MC5R* gene.

A quick test of the preceding hypothesis would be to take a set of MCR sequences from the same group of organisms, and identify the consensus sequence common to these receptor. In **Figure A1A** in Appendix, the amino acid sequences of five cartilaginous fish MCRs were aligned, and common residues that are found at each position are identified in red. The consensus residues at 287 positions were identified. Interesting, 88% of these residues were present in the MC4R sequence. A pair-wise comparison (**Figure A1B** in Appendix) indicated that the MC4R sequence had the highest sequence identity for the MC5R sequence and the MC3R sequence, respectively. A maximum parsimony analysis of the sequences in **Figure A1** in Appendix indicated that the MC4R, the consensus sequence, and the MC3R and MC5R sequences formed a clade (**Figure A2** in Appendix). While this correlation analysis is suggestive, an analysis of the hagfish genome may be more useful for testing the validity of the hypothesis presented in **Figure 3**.

**Table 1 | Human melanocortin ligands.**

| | |
|---|---|
| ACTH | SYSMEHFRWGKPVGKKRRPVKVYPNGADDESAEAFPLEF |
| α-MSH | NAc-SYSMEHFRWGKPV-NH2 |
| β-MSH | DEGPYRMEHFRWGSPPKD |
| γ-MSH | KYVMGHFRWDRF-NH2 |

*The human melanocortin ligand sequences were derived from the sequence of human POMC (accession # CAG46625.1). The HFRW motif highlighted in red is required for the activation of all melanocortin receptor. The KKRRP motif highlighted in blue is required for the activation of the melanocortin-2 receptor (Schwyzer, 1977).*

## EVOLUTION OF MC2R LIGAND SELECTIVITY

As noted in the Introduction, the ligands for the MCRs are the melanocortins, ACTH, α-MSH, β-MSH, γ-MSH (Gantz and Fong, 2003), and for cartilaginous fishes, δ-MSH (Takahashi and Kawauchi, 2006). The sequences of the melanocortins derived from human POMC are presented in **Table 1**. The proposed origin and the primary sequence variability of vertebrate melanocortins have been reviewed recently (Dores and Baron, 2011). In brief, α-MSH is derived from the first 13 amino acids in the sequence of ACTH via posttranslational processing mechanisms (Eipper and Mains, 1980). It would appear that the γ-MSH and β-MSH are the result of duplications and reinsertions of the α-MSH sequence within the *POMC* gene (Dores et al., 2003); whereas, the δ-MSH sequence appears to be derived from a duplication and reinsertion of the β-MSH sequence in the *POMC* gene of cartilaginous fishes (Amemiya et al., 1999).

Several studies on mammalian MCRs [reviewed by Gantz and Fong (2003)], as well as a study on bird MCRs (Ling et al., 2004), and studies on teleosts (Ringholm et al., 2002; Klovins et al., 2004a) and cartilaginous fish MCRs (Ringholm et al., 2003; Klovins et al., 2004b; Reinick et al., 2012a) indicate that MC1R, MC3R, MC4R, and MC5R can be activated by ACTH or any of the MSH-sized ligands with varying degrees of efficacy. As indicated in **Table 1**, all of the melanocortin ligands have the HFRW motif which is required for activation of all MCRs (Schwyzer, 1977; Mountjoy et al., 1992; Gantz and Fong, 2003). From the perspective of the receptors, Pogozheva et al. (2005) identified critical amino acid positions in transmembrane regions 2, 3, 6, and 7 of human MC4R which are required for activation of that receptor by α-MSH. These residues are conserved in other mammalian MCRs (Pogozheva et al., 2005) and have been found in the sequences of MCRs of non-mammalian tetrapods, amphibian MCRs, teleost MCRs, and lamprey MCRs (Baron et al., 2009; Dores, 2009).

That said, none of the MSH-sized ligands in **Table 1** can activate either teleost or tetrapod MC2R (Schwyzer, 1977; Mountjoy et al., 1992; Gantz and Fong, 2003; Agulleiro et al., 2010; Liang et al., 2011). Since teleost and tetrapod MC2Rs have retained many of the residues associated with the HFRW binding site in MC1R, MC3R, MC4R, and MC5R, it would appear that the HFRW binding site in teleost and tetrapod MC2Rs is masked in some manner. The apparent key to unmasking the HFRW binding site appears to reside in the KKRRP motif in the sequence of ACTH (**Table 1**; Schwyzer, 1977; Costa et al., 2004; Liang et al., 2013a). The KKRRP motif is not present in any of the MSH-sized ligands. In addition, either deletions (Schwyzer, 1977) of this motif, or alanine substitutions (Liang et al., 2013a) within this motif will greatly decrease the potency of the ligand. All of these observations point to a KKRRP binding site in teleost and tetrapod MC2Rs, and raise the question of when MC2R orthologs became exclusively selective for ACTH.

Studies on a MC2R ortholog in the genome of the holocephalan cartilaginous fish, *Callorhynchus milii*, have provided an opportunity to address the latter question (Reinick et al., 2012b). Expression of the *C. milii MC2R* ortholog in CHO cells indicated that this receptor could be activated by either human ACTH(1–24) or NDP-MSH. In addition, stimulation of *C. milii MC2R* transiently transfected CHO cells with spiny dogfish (*Squalus acanthias*) ACTH(1–25), α-MSH, β-MSH, γ-MSH or δ-MSH yielded dose response curves with varying degrees of efficacy (Reinick et al., 2012b). Although the sample size is small, it is possible that other cartilaginous fish MC2R orthologs have similar ligand selectivity properties. If so, then the summary presented in **Figure 4A** would indicate a dichotomy in MC2R ligand selectivity between the cartilaginous fishes and the teleosts and tetrapods. In this scenario it is assumed that the MC2R ortholog in the ancestral gnathostomes could also be activated by ACTH or the MSH-related peptides. Hence, the exclusive selectivity for ACTH would appear to have evolved after the divergence of the ancestral cartilaginous fishes and the ancestral bony fishes.

## CO-EVOLUTION OF MC2R AND MRAP; AN EXAMPLE OF CONSTRUCTIVE NEUTRAL EVOLUTION

Another feature of teleost and tetrapod MC1Rs, MC3Rs, MC4Rs, and MC5Rs is that these receptors can be functionally expressed in heterologous mammalian cell lines such has HEK-293 cells, CHO cells, or COS cells (Rachel et al., 2005; Schiöth et al., 2005). These observations are in sharp contrast to teleost and tetrapod MC2Rs which cannot be functionally expressed in those cells lines unless the cells are co-transfected with accessory protein *MRAP1* cDNA (Hinkle and Sebag, 2009; Agulleiro et al., 2010; Webb and Clark, 2010; Liang et al., 2011). Melanocortin-2 Receptor Accessory Protein 1 (MRAP1) is a transmembrane protein with a single transmembrane domain (Metherell et al., 2005). The features of this accessory protein are discussed in another chapter in this book (Clark and Chan, 2013). For the purposes of this review, the salient features of MRAPs include: (a) there are two *MRAP* paralogous genes (*MRAP1* and *MRAP2*) in the vertebrate genome; (b) MRAP1 and MRAP2 form antiparallel homodimers; and (c) MRAP1 is required for the trafficking of MC2R from the ER to the plasma membrane, and for the functional activation of MC2R at the plasma membrane following the binding of ACTH; and (d) MRAP2 can only facilitate the trafficking of MC2R to the plasma membrane, but has a very weak effect on the functional activation of the receptor at the plasma membrane (Hinkle and Sebag, 2009; Webb and Clark, 2010; Gorrigan et al., 2011). In terms of the phylogeny of the *MRAP* genes, it appears that these genes may be restricted to the lamprey genome and the genomes of gnathostomes (Vastermark and Schiöth, 2011). In addition, the two *MRAP* paralogs are not uniformly distributed in these organisms. As summarized in **Figure 5**, to date only an *MRAP2* gene has been detected in the genome databases for the marine lamprey (*Petromzyon marinus*) and the cartilaginous fish, *Callorhynchus*

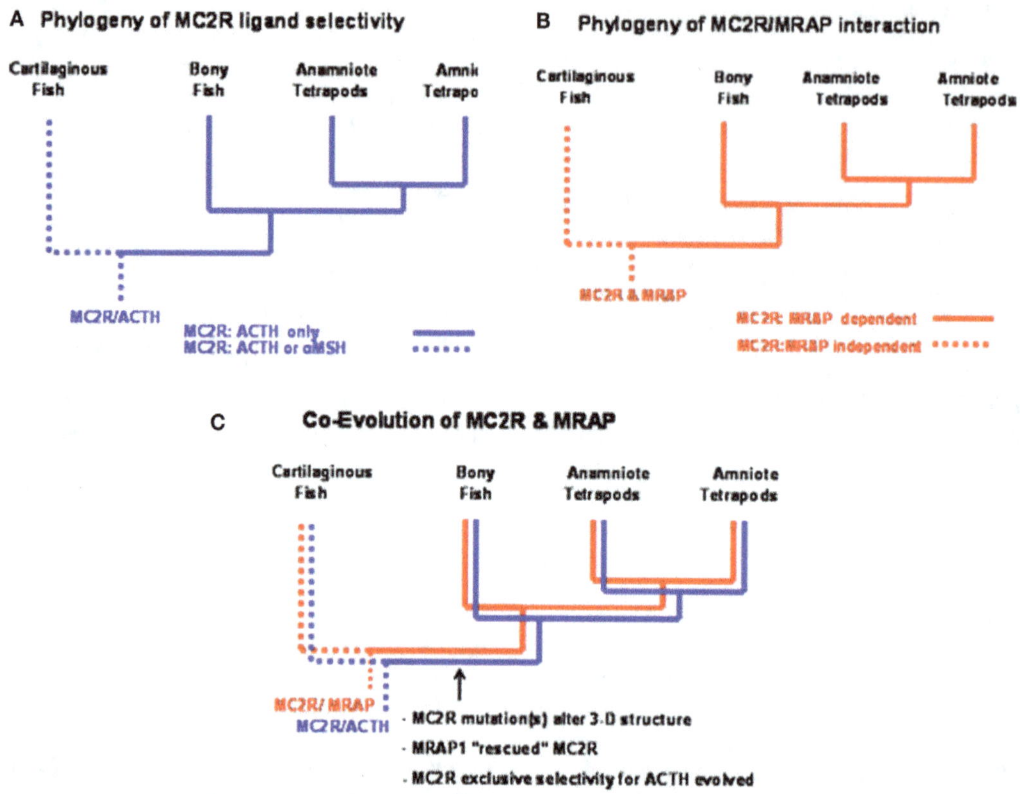


**FIGURE 4 | Functional evolution of the melanocortin-2 receptor. (A)** This summary of ligand selectivity of melanocortin-2 receptor orthologs indicates that teleost and tetrapod melanocortin-2 receptors can only be activated by ACTH, but not by any of the MSH-sized melanocortin ligands. The melanocortin-2 receptor ortholog of the cartilaginous fish, *Callorhynchus milii* can be activated by either ACTH or MSH-sized ligands (Reinick et al., 2012b). **(B)** This summary of the melanocortin-2 receptor interaction with MRAP1 indicates that teleost and tetrapod MC2R orthologs are dependent on MRAP1 for trafficking to the plasma membrane and for functional activation at the plasma membrane. The trafficking to the plasma membrane and the functional activation of the MC2R ortholog of the cartilaginous fish, *C. milii* is MRAP1 independent. **(C)** Following the divergence of the cartilaginous fishes and the bony fishes, an interaction developed between MC2R and MRAP1. As mutations occurred in the melanocortin-2 receptor, the receptor was rescued by MRAP1. In extant teleosts and tetrapods, the functional expression of MC2R is dependent on forming a complex with MRAP1.

*milii*; whereas, *MRAP1* and *MRAP2* genes have been detected in the genomes of several species of teleost fishes, the chicken (*Gallus gallus*) genome, and the genomes of several mammals (Agulleiro et al., 2010; Liang et al., 2011; Vastermark and Schiöth, 2011). It would appear that a duplication of the *MRAP* gene occurred during the radiation of the ancestral bony fishes (**Figure 5**) resulting in distinct *MRAP1* and *MRAP2* genes. In addition, it is now clear that the functional expression of teleost and tetrapod MC2Rs is dependent on interaction with MRAP1 beginning right after synthesis of MC2R at the rough endoplasmic reticulum (Sebag and Hinkle, 2007).

A *Mc2r* ortholog has been detected in genome of the cartilaginous fish, *C. milli* (Vastermark and Schiöth, 2011). When this *MC2R* ortholog was transiently transfected in CHO cells the receptor could be activated by either ACTH or MSH-sized ligand. Hence, the functional expression of the *C. milli* MC2R ortholog is MRAP1 independent (Reinick et al., 2012b). In addition, the functional expression of the *C. milii* MC2R was not affected, either in a positive or negative manner, following co-expression with either mouse MRAP1, zebrafish MRAP1, or *C. milii* MRAP2. Once again the sample size is small, but as summarized in **Figure 4B**, the MC2Rs of teleosts and tetrapods are MRAP1 dependent; whereas, the MC2R of at least one species of cartilaginous fish is MRAP independent. This conclusion would suggest that the MC2R ortholog of ancestral gnathostomes was also MRAP1 independent.

Collectively, these observations point to a number of changes and serendipitous events that have occurred during the evolution of the *MC2R* gene. To understand the functional evolution of the *MC2R* gene it may be easiest to start with the current status of this gene in mammals. In all mammals, MC2R serves as the "ACTH" receptor on cells of the adrenal cortex, and is a critical component of the hypothalamus/pituitary/adrenal axis (HPA; Clark and Cammas, 1996). Activation of MC2R results in the synthesis and release of the glucocorticoid, cortisol, a steroid that influences the normal function of many cell types, and facilitates the body's response to chronic stressors (Engelmann et al., 2004). In humans, mutations in the *MC2R* gene that either effect the trafficking of MC2R from the ER to the plasma membrane or inhibit residues on the receptor responsible for binding ACTH will result in Type 1 Familial Glucocorticoid Deficiency (FGD; Chung et al., 2008). However, the functionality of mammalian MC2Rs is totally dependent on the interaction with MRAPα, one of two splice variants of the

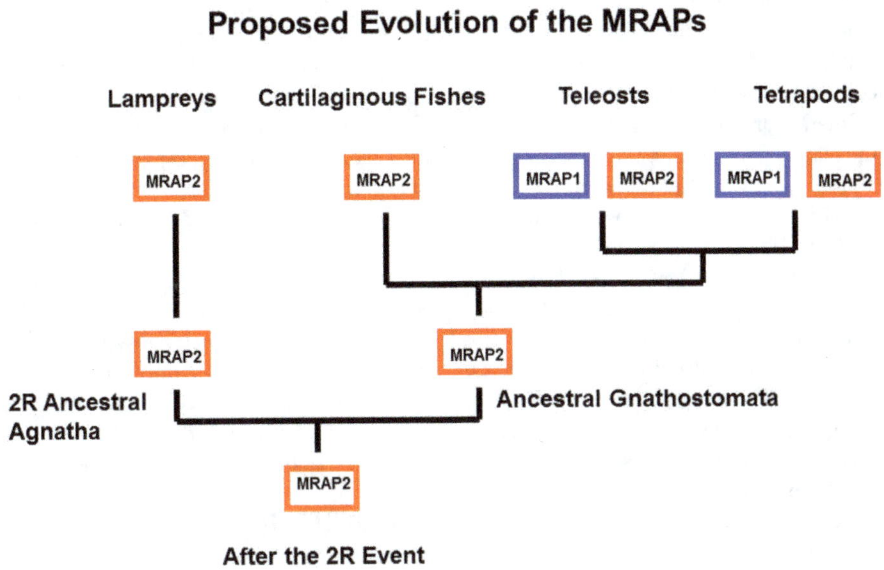


**FIGURE 5 | Proposed Evolution of MRAP1 and MRAP2.** It appears that MRAP2 may be the ancestral paralog in the MRAP gene family. This evolutionary scheme assumes that the *MRAP2* gene was in the genome of the ancestral 2R vertebrates. This gene has been retained in the lamprey genome (Vastermark and Schiöth, 2011). In this scenario only a *MRAP2* gene was present in the genome of the ancestral gnathostomes. Following the divergence of the cartilaginous fishes and the bony fishes, the *MRAP2* gene duplicated in the bony fish lineage, and as a result *MRAP2* and *MRAP1* paralogs are present in the genomes of teleosts and tetrapods.

human *MRAP1* gene (Metherell et al., 2005). Hence, mutations to critical regions in the human *MRAP1* gene will result in Type 2 Familial Glucocorticoid Deficiency (Metherell et al., 2005). In the absence of a functional MRAP1, *in vitro* experiments indicate that the MC2R is misfolded (Sebag and Hinkle, 2007) and is tagged for degradation by the ER protein quality control system. For either Type 1 or Type 2 FGD, the congenital defect is potentially life threatening if not treated.

Projecting the preceding observations to the functional activation of non-mammalian tetrapod and teleost MC2Rs, *in vitro* experiments have demonstrated that an amphibian MC2R ortholog (Liang et al., 2011) and teleost MC2R orthologs (Klovins et al., 2004a; Agulleiro et al., 2010; Liang et al., 2011) cannot be functionally expressed unless the MC2R ortholog is expressed in cells derived from a mammalian adrenal cell line (that presumably is expressing an endogenous *MRAP1* gene), or in the case of HEK-293 or CHO cells, the *MC2R* ortholog is co-expressed with a *MRAP1* cDNA. Given these observations, it would be reasonable to predict that either functional mutations in the *MC2R* gene, or mutations to the *MRAP1* gene will have a negative effect on the fitness of non-mammalian tetrapods and teleosts.

Hence, the detection of an MRAP1 independent *MC2R* ortholog in the *C. milii* genome that can be activated by either ACTH or MSH-sized ligands would suggest that the *MC2R* gene present in the ancestral gnathostomes after the 2R genome duplication event (**Figure 3**) was also MRAP independent and perhaps capable of being activated by either ACTH or MSH-sized ligands. This ancestral gene could have been the MC2R/MC5R proto-gene proposed in **Figure 3.** In any event, as shown in **Figure 4C**, following the divergence of the ancestral cartilaginous fishes and the ancestral bony fishes, an interaction between MRAP1 and MC2R in the ancestral bony fish linage must have occurred. Initially this interaction could have been neutral (no apparent advantage for the function of either transmembrane protein). However, as mutations altered the trafficking features of MC2R and the ligand selectivity of MC2R, the pre-adaptation for MC2R and MRAP1 to form a complex at the ER rescued this GPCR that if expressed alone could not function properly. Since both teleost and tetrapod MC2Rs are dependent on the interaction with MRAP1 for functional expression, the interaction must have developed in a common ancestor to both the teleosts and the tetrapods. In this scenario, the interaction between MC2R and MRAP1 would have transitioned over time from a neutral interaction to a functionally dependent interaction with respect to MC2R functionality, and serves as an example of constructive neutral evolution (Stolzfus, 1999).

## CONCLUSION

The evolution of the MCRs is intertwined with the co-evolution of the ligand-encoding *POMC* gene, the accessory protein *MRAP* genes, and the inverse agonist *AGRP/ASIP* genes. The presence of five *Melanocortin Receptor* genes in the genomes of tetrapods indicates that the gene family has been shaped by two genome duplication events and one local gene duplication event. Based on these observations, the origin of this gene family may have occurred over 500 MYA prior to the emergence of jawless vertebrates. Synteny studies provide support for the conclusions that the local gene duplication involved the *MC2R* gene and the *MC5R* gene (Schiöth et al., 2003; Klovins et al., 2004a).

Studies on the functional activation of cartilaginous fish MCRs may provide some insights into the properties of the melanocortin receptor genes in the ancestral gnathostomes (Ringholm et al.,

2003; Klovins et al., 2004b; Reinick et al., 2012a,b; Liang et al., 2013a). Current studies indicate that orthologs of MC2R, MC3R, MC4R, and MC5R can all be stimulated by ACTH or MSH-sized ligands with varying degrees of efficacy, and none of these receptors apparently requires interaction with an accessory protein to facilitate trafficking to the plasma membrane or activation once at the plasma membrane following a ligand binding event.

Among the descendents of the ancestral bony vertebrates (e.g., teleost and tetrapods) MC1R, MC3R, MC4R, and MC5R have retained the proclivity for stimulation by ACTH or the MSH-sized ligands, and none of these receptors requires an interaction with an accessory protein to facilitate trafficking to the plasma membrane. The exception to this generalization is MC2R. These features evolved in this receptor which made the receptor exclusively selective for ACTH, but also dependent on MRAP1 not only for trafficking to the plasma membrane but also for functional activation following an ACTH binding event.

The interaction between MC2R/MRAP1 in teleosts and tetrapods insures the strict signaling selectivity of the hypothalamus/pituitary/adrenal (HPA) axis and the hypothalamus/pituitary/interrenal (HPI) axis. As noted in the Introduction, MCRs are also involved in integument pigmentation, appetite regulation, glucocorticoid synthesis, and exocrine gland secretion (Gantz and Fong, 2003; Cone, 2006). The role of MCRs in these physiological processes have been extensively analyzed in mammals. For non-mammalian vertebrates it is now time to rectify the pharmacology on MCRs with the physiology of these processes in non-mammalian vertebrates. As just one example, do the cartilaginous fishes have a true HPI axis if all cartilaginous fish MCRs can be activated by either ACTH or MSH-sized ligands (Liang et al., 2013b)? What role does receptor dimerization, homo-, or hetero-play in the functionality of MCRs? Is MRAP2 an evolutionary anachronism, or does this accessory protein have a role to play in some melanocortin physiological processes? Although MCRs were characterized nearly 20 years ago, there are still many questions about this gene family that are waiting to be resolved.

## ACKNOWLEDGMENTS

This work was supported by funds provided by the University of Denver.

## REFERENCES


Agulleiro, M. J., Roy, S., Sanchez, E., Puchol, S, Gallo-Payet, N., and Cerda-Reverter, J. M. (2010). Role of melanocortin receptor accessory proteins in the function of zebrafish melanocortin receptor type 2. *Mol. Cell. Endocrinol.* 320, 145–152.

Amemiya, Y., Takahashi, A., Suzuki, N., Sasayama, Y., and Kawauchi, H. (1999). A newly characterized melanotropin in proopiomelanocortin in pituitaries of an elasmobranch, *Squalus acanthias. Gen. Comp. Endocrinol.* 114, 387–395.

Baron, A., Veo, K., Angleson, J., and Dores, R. M. (2009). Modeling the Evolution of the MC2R and MC5R genes: studies on the cartilaginous fish, *Heterondotus francisci. Gen. Comp. Endocrinol.* 161, 13–19.

Carroll, R. L. (1988). *Vertebrate Paleontology and Evolution.* New York: Freeman Press.

Chung, T. T., Webb, T. R., Chan, L. F., Cooray, S. N., Metherell, L. A., King, P. J., et al. (2008). The majority of ACTH receptor (MC2R) mutations found in familial glucocorticoid deficiency type 1 lead to defective trafficking of the receptor to the cell surface. *J. Clin. Endocrinol. Metab.* 93, 4948–4954.

Clark, A. J. L., and Cammas, F. (1996). The ACTH receptor. *Baillieres Clin. Endocrinol. Metab.* 10, 29–47.

Clark, A. J. L., and Chan, J. L. (2013). Melanocortin receptors and their accessory proteins. *Front. Endocrinol.* 4:9. doi:10.3389/fendo.2013.00009

Cone, R. D. (2006). Studies on the physiological functions of the melanocortin system. *Endocr. Rev.* 27, 736–749.

Costa, J. L., Bui, S., Reed, P., Dores, R. M., Hochgeschwender, U., and Brennan, M. B. (2004). Mutational analysis of evolutionarily conserved ACTH residues. *Gen. Comp. Endocrinol.* 136, 12–16.

Denver, R. J. (2009). Structural and functional evolution of vertebrate neuroendocrine stress systems. *Ann. N. Y. Acad. Sci.* 1163, 1–16.

Dores, R. M. (2009). ACTH, the MSHs and the Melanocortin Receptors: Revisiting the work of Robert Schwyzer – a 30 Year Retrospective. *Ann. N. Y. Acad. Sci.* 1163, 93–100.

Dores, R. M., and Baron, A. J. (2011). Evolution of POMC: origin, phylogeny, posttranslational processing, and the melanocortins. *Ann. N. Y. Acad. Sci.* 1220, 34–48.

Dores, R. M., Cameron, E., Lecaude, S., and Danielson, P. B. (2003). Presence of the δ-MSH sequence in a proopiomelanocortin cDNA cloned from the pituitary of the galeoid shark, *Heterodontus portusjacksoni. Gen. Comp. Endocrinol.* 133, 71–79.

Dores, R. M., and Gorbman, A. (1990). Detection of Met-enkephalin and Leu-enkephalin in the brain of the hagfish, *Eptatretus stouti,* and the lamprey, *Petromyzon marinus. Gen. Comp. Endocrinol.* 77, 489–500.

Dores, R. M., and Lecaude, S. (2005). Trends in the evolution of the proopiomelanocortin gene. *Gen. Comp. Endocrinol.* 142, 81–93.

Dores, R. M., Lecaude, S., Bauer, D., and Danielson, P. B. (2002). Analyzing the evolution of the opioid/orphanin gene family. *Mass. Spectrom. Rev.* 21, 220–243.

Eipper, B. A., and Mains, R. E. (1980). Structure and biosynthesis of pro-adrenocorticotropin/endorphin and related peptides. *Endocr. Rev.* 1, 1–27.

Engelmann, M., Landgraf, R., and Wotjak, C. (2004). The hypothalamic-neurohypophysial system regulates the hypothalamic-pituitary-adrenal axis under stress: an old concept revisited. *Front. Neuroendocrinol.* 25, 132–149.

Force, A., Lynch, M., Pickett, F. B., Amores, A., Yan, Y.-L., and Postlethwait, J. (1998). Preservation of duplicate genes by complementary, degenerative mutations. *Genetics* 151, 1531–1545.

Gantz, I., and Fong, T. M. (2003). The melanocortin system. *Am. J. Physiol. Endocrinol. Metab.* 284, E468–E474.

Gorrigan, R. J., Guasti, L., King, P., Clark, A. J., and Chan, L. F. (2011). Localization of the melanocortin-2-receptor accessory protein and its accessory protein in the developing and adult adrenal gland. *J. Mol. Endcrinol.* 46, 227–232.

Haitina, T., Klovins, J., Takahashi, A., Löwgren, M., Ringholm, A., Enberg, J., et al. (2007). Functional characterization of two melanocortin (MC) receptors in lamprey showing orthology to the MC1 and MC4 receptor subtypes. *BMC Evol. Biol.* 7:101. doi:10.1186/1471-2148-7-101

Heinig, J. A., Keeley, F. W., Robson, P., Sower, S. A., and Youson, J. H. (1995). The appearance of proopiomelanocortin early in vertebrate evolution: cloning and sequencing of POMC from a lamprey pituitary cDNA library. *Gen. Comp. Endocrinol.* 99, 137–144.

Hinkle, P. M., and Sebag, J. A. (2009). Structure and function of the melanocortin 2 receptor accessory protein. *Mol. Cell. Endocrinol.* 300, 25–31.

Holland, P. W., Garcia-Fernandez, J., Williams, N. A., and Sidow, A. (1994). Gene duplications and the origins of vertebrate development. *Dev. Suppl.* 125–133.

Horn, F., Bettler, E., Oliveira, L., Campagne, F., Cohen, F. E., and Vriend, G. (2003). GPCRDB information system for G protein-coupled receptors. *Nucleic Acids Res.* 31, 294–297.

Kah, O., Lethimonier, C., Somoza, G., Guilgur, L. G., Vaillant, C., and Lareyre, J. J. (2006). GnRH and GnRh receptors in metazoan: a historical, comparative, and evolutive perspective. *Gen. Comp. Endocrinol.* 153, 346–364.

Klovins, J., Haitina, T., Fridmanis, D., Kilianova, Z., Kapa, K., Fredriksson, R., et al. (2004a). The melanocortin system in fugu: determination of POMC/AGRP/MCR gene repertoire and synteny, as well as pharmacology and anatomical distribution of the MCRs. *Mol. Biol. Evol.* 21, 563–579.

Klovins, J., Haitina, T., Ringholm, A., Lowgren, M., Fridmanis, D., Slaidina, M., et al. (2004b). Cloning of two melanocortin (MC) receptors in spiny dogfish. *Eur. J. Biochem.* 271, 4320–4331.

Kuraku, S., Meyer, A., and Kuratani, S. (2009). Timing of genome duplications relative to the origin of the vertebrates: did cyclostomes diverge before, or after? *Mol. Biol. Evol.* 26, 47–59.

Liang, L., Angleson, J. K., and Dores, R. M. (2013a). Review: using the human melanocortin-2 receptor as a model for analyzing hormone/receptor interactions between a mammalian MC2 receptor and ACTH(1-24). *Gen. Comp. Endocrinol.* 181, 203–210.

Liang, L., Reinick, C., Angleson, J. E., and Dores, R. M. (2013b). Mini-review: evolution of melanocortin receptors in cartilaginous fish: melanocortin receptors and the stress axis in elasmobranches. *Gen. Comp. Endocrinol.* 181, 4–9.

Liang, L., Sebag, J. A., Eagelston, L., Serasinghe, M. N., Veo, K., Reinick, C., et al. (2011). Functional Expression of frog and rainbow trout melanocortin 2 receptors using heterologous MRAP1s. *Gen. Comp. Endocrinol.* 174, 5–14.

Ling, M. K., Hotta, E., Kilanova, Z., Haitina, T., Ringholm, A., Johansson, L., et al. (2004). The melanocortin receptor subtypes in chicken have high preference to ACTH-derived peptides. *Br. J. Pharmacol.* 143, 626–637.

Lundin, L. G. (1993). Evolution of the vertebrate genome as reflected in paralogous 827 chromosomal regions in man and the house mouse. *Genomics* 16, 1–19.

McEwen, G. K., Goode, D. K., Parker, A., Woolfe, H., Callaway, H., and Elger, G. (2009). Early evolution of conserved regulatory sequences associated with development in vertebrates. *PLoS Genet.* 5:e1000762. doi:10.1371/journal.pgen.1000762

Metherell, L. A., Chapple, J. P., Cooray, S., David, A., Becker, C., Ruschendorf, F., et al. (2005). Mutations in MRAP, encoding a new interacting partner of the ACTH receptor, cause familial glucocorticoid deficiency type 2. *Nat. Genet.* 37, 160–170.

Meyer, A., and Van de Peer, Y. (2005). From 2R to 3R: evidence for a fish-specific genome duplication (FSGD). *Bioessays* 27, 937–945.

Mohr, E., Meyerhof, W., and Richter, D. (1996). Vasopressin and oxytocin molecular biology and evolution of the peptide hormones and their receptors. *Vitam. Horm.* 51, 235–266.

Mountjoy, K. G., Robbins, L. S., Mortrud, M. T., and Cone, R. D. (1992). The cloning of a family of genes that encode the melanocortin receptors. *Science* 257, 1248–1251.

Nakanishi, S., Inoue, A., Kita, T., Nakamura, M., Chung, A. C. Y., Cohen, S. N., et al. (1979). Nucleotide sequence of cloned cDNA for bovine corticotropin-beta-lipotropin precursor. *Nature* 278, 423–427.

Nelson, J. S. (1994). *Fishes of the World*, 3rd Edn. New York: John Wiley and Sons, Inc.

Ohno, S., Wolf, U., and Atkins, N. B. (1968). Evolution from fish to mammals by gene duplication. *Herediatas* 59, 169–187.

Pogozheva, I. D., Chai, B.-X., Lomize, A. L., Fong, T. M., Weinberg, D. H., Nargund, R. P., et al. (2005). Interactions of human melanocortin 4 receptors with nonpeptide and peptide agonists. *Biochemistry* 44, 11329–11341.

Rachel, M., El Mourabit, H., Buronfosse, A., Blondet, A., Naville, D., Begeot, M., et al. (2005). Expression of the human melanocortin-2 receptor in different eukaryotic cells. *Peptides* 26, 1842–1847.

Reinick, C. L., Liang, L., Angleson, J. K., and Dores, R. M. (2012a). Functional expression of *Squalus acanthias* Melanocortin 5 Receptor in CHO Cells, ligand selectivity and interaction with MRAP. *Eur. J. Pharm.* 680, 1–7.

Reinick, C. L., Liang, L., Angleson, J. K., and Dores, R. M. (2012b). Identification of an MRAP-independent melanocortin-2 receptor: functional expression of the cartilaginous fish, *Callorhinchus milii*, melanocortin-2 receptor in CHO cells. *Endocrinology* 153, 4757–4765.

Ringholm, A., Fredriksson, R., Poliakova, N., Yan, Y. L., Postlethwait, J. H., Larhammar, D., et al. (2002). One melanocortin 4 and two melanocortin 5 receptors from zebrafish show remarkable conservation in structure and pharmacology. *J. Neurochem.* 82, 6–18.

Ringholm, A., Klovins, J., Fredriksson, R., Poliakova, N., Larson, E. T., Kukkonen, J. P., et al. (2003). Presence of melanocortin (MC4) receptor in spiny dogfish suggests an ancient vertebrate origin of central melanocortin system. *Eur. J. Biochem.* 270, 213–221.

Schiöth, H. B., Haitina, T., Ling, M. K., Ringholm, A., Fredriksson, R., Cerda-Reverter, J. M., et al. (2005). Evolutionary conservation of the structural, pharmacological, and genomic characteristics of the melanocortin receptor subtypes. *Peptides* 26, 1886–1900.

Schiöth, H. B., Raudsepp, T., Ringholm, A., Fredriksson, R., Takeuchi, S., Larhammar, D., et al. (2003). Remarkable synteny conservation of melanocortin receptors in chicken, human, and other vertebrates. *Genomics* 81, 504–509.

Schwyzer, R. (1977). ACTH: a short introductory review. *Ann. N. Y. Acad. Sci.* 297, 3–26.

Sebag, J. A., and Hinkle, P. M. (2007). Melanocortin-2 receptor accessory protein MRAP forms antiparallel homodimers. *Proc. Natl. Acad. Sci. U.S.A.* 104, 20244–20249.

Seidah, N. G., and Chrétien, M. (1999). Proprotein and prohormone convertases: a family of subtilases generating diverse bioactive polypeptides. *Brain Res.* 848, 45–62.

Smith, J. J., Kuraku, S., Holt, C., Sauka-Spengler, T., Jiang, N., Campbell, M. S., et al. (2013). Sequencing of the sea lamprey (Petromyzon marinus) genome provides insights into vertebrate evolution. *Nat. Genet.* doi:10.1038/ng.2568

Stolzfus, A. (1999). On the possibility of constructive neutral evolution. *J. Mol. Evol.* 49, 169–181.

Sundstrom, G., Dreborg, S., and Larhammar, D. (2010). Concomitant duplication of the 888 opioid peptide and receptor genes before the origin of jawed vertebrates. *PLoS ONE* 5:e10512. doi:10.1371/journal.pone.0010512

Takahashi, A., Amemiya, Y., Sarashi, M., Sower, S. A., and Kawauchi, H. (1995). Melanotropin and corticotropin are encoded on two distinct genes in the lamprey, the earliest evolved extant vertebrate. *Biochem. Biophys. Res. Commun.* 213, 490–496.

Takahashi, A., and Kawauchi, H. (2006). Evolution of melanocortin systems in fish. *Gen. Comp. Endocrinol.* 148, 85–94.

Vallarino, M., d'Amora, M., and Dores, R. M. (2012). New insights into the neuroanatomical distribution and phylogeny of opioids and POMC-derived peptides in fish." *Gen. Comp. Endocrinol.* 177, 338–347.

Vassilatis, D. K., Hohmann, J. G., Zeng, H., Li, F., Ranchalis, J. E., Mortrud, M. T., et al. (2003). The G protein-coupled receptor repertoires of human and mouse. *Proc. Natl. Acad. Sci. U.S.A.* 100, 4903–4908.

Vastermark, A., and Schiöth, H. B. (2011). The early origin of melanocortin receptors, agouti-related peptide, agouti signaling peptide, and melanocortin receptor-accessory proteins, with emphasis on pufferfishes, elephant shark, lampreys, and amphioxus. *Eur. J. Pharmacol.* 660, 61–69.

Webb, T. R., and Clark, A. J. (2010). Mini-review: the melanocortin 2 receptor accessory proteins. *Mol. Endocrinol.* 24, 475–484.

## APPENDIX

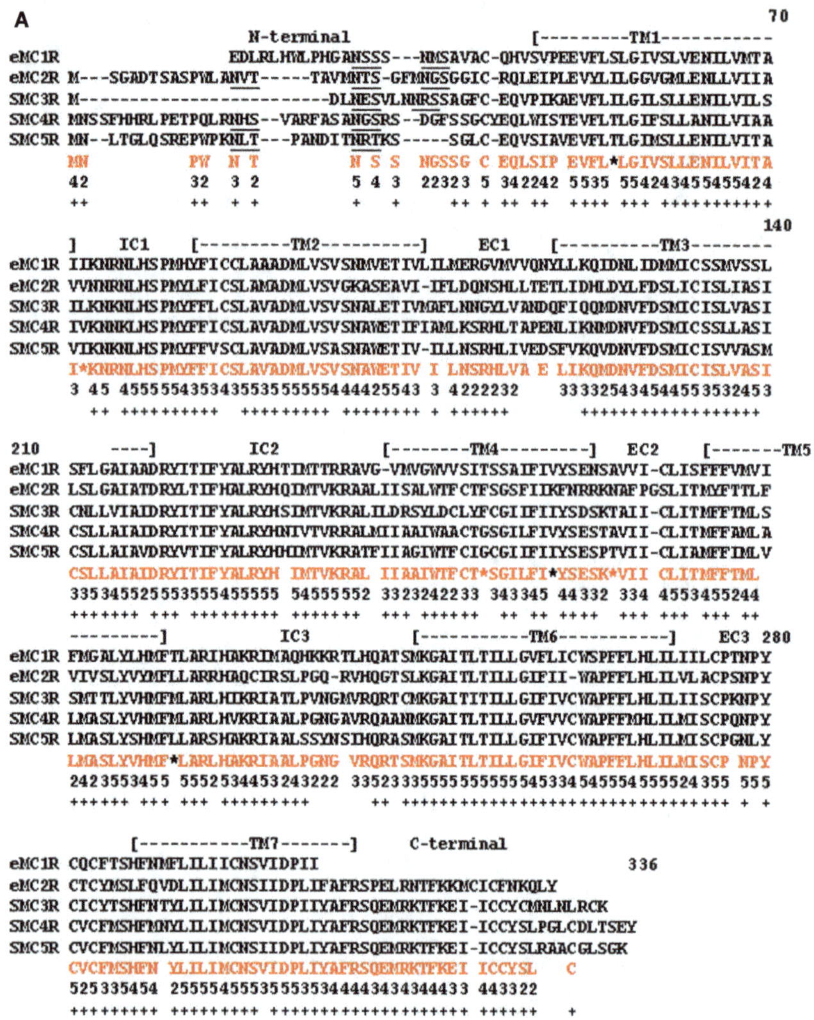

**B**

### Pair-wise Comparison of Amino Acid Identity

| | eMC1R | eMC2R | sMC3R | sMC5R | sMC4R |
|---|---|---|---|---|---|
| eMC1R | - | 47% | 55% | 57% | 55% |
| eMC2R | | - | 48% | 50% | 49% |
| SMC3R | | | - | 67% | 67% |
| sMC5R | | | | - | 70% |
| sMC4R | | | | | - |

**FIGURE A1 | Alignment of cartilaginous fish melanocortin receptors.** **(A)** The amino acid sequences of the elephant shark (*C. milii*) MC1R (AAVX01456471.1; http://esharkgenome.lmcb.a-star.edu.sg), elephant shark MC2R (accession number: FAA704.1), dogfish (*Squalus acanthias*) MC3R (accession number: AAS66720.1), dogfish MC4R (accession number: AA039833.1), and dogfish MC5R (accession number: AA867890.1) were aligned as described in Liang et al. (2011). In amino acids in red are the consensus amino acids for each position. Consensus was defined as two or more of the same amino acid at that position. Number below each consensus amino acid indicates the number of times that amino acid is present at the position. Positions marked by ∗ there were two pairs of amino acids. These positions were not used in the analysis presented in **Figure A2**. Positions in which there was no consensus were left blank. The underlined amino acids indicate a N-linked glycosylation site. **(B)** A pair-wise comparison of sequence identity for these receptors is included.

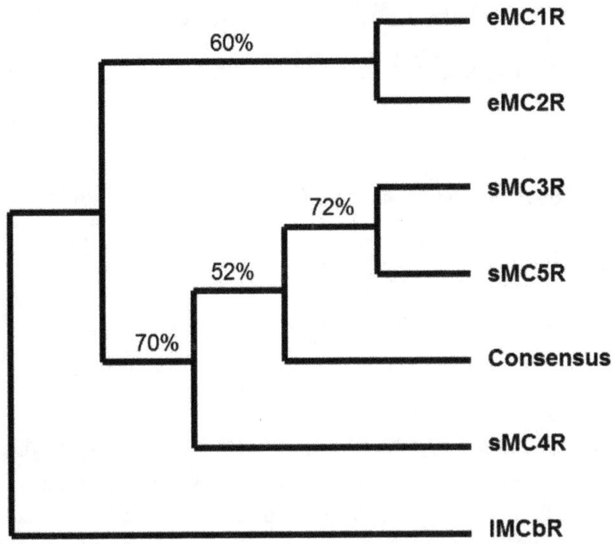


**FIGURE A2 | Maximum parsimony analysis of cartilaginous fish melanocortin receptors.** The sequences presented in **Figure A1** including the consensus sequence were analyzed by maximum parsimony using the heuristic program in PAUP. The analysis yield a single tree and the jackknife values for 100 repetitions are included. The outgroup for the rooted tree was the lamprey MCb receptor (accession number: DQ213060) sequence. eMC1R, elephant shark MC1R; eMC2R, elephant shark MC2R; sMC3R, dogfish MC3R; sMC4R, dogfish MC4R; sMC5R, dogfish MC5R.

# 19

# Comparative evolutionary histories of kisspeptins and kisspeptin receptors in vertebrates reveal both parallel and divergent features

***Jérémy Pasquier*[1]*, Anne-Gaëlle Lafont*[1]*, Hervé Tostivint*[2]*, Hubert Vaudry*[3]*, Karine Rousseau*[1] *and Sylvie Dufour*[1]****

*[1] Research Unit BOREA, Biology of Aquatic Organisms and Ecosystems, Centre National de la Recherche Scientifique 7208, Institut de Recherche pour le Développement 207, Université Pierre et Marie Curie, Muséum National d'Histoire Naturelle, Paris, France*

*[2] UMR 7221 CNRS/MNHN Evolution des Régulations Endocriniennes, Muséum National d'Histoire Naturelle, Paris, France*

*[3] Laboratory of Cellular and Molecular Neuroendocrinology, INSERM U982, European Institute for Peptide Research (IFRMP 23), University of Rouen, Mont-Saint-Aignan, France*

***Edited by:***
*Jae Young Seong, Korea University, South Korea*

***Reviewed by:***
*Kazuyoshi Tsutsui, Waseda University, Japan*
*Robert Dores, University of Minnesota, USA*

****Correspondence:***
*Sylvie Dufour, Muséum National d'Histoire Naturelle – UMR BOREA, 7 rue Cuvier, CP32, 75231 Paris Cedex 05, France.*
*e-mail: sylvie.dufour@mnhn.fr*

During the past decade, the kisspeptin system has been identified in various vertebrates, leading to the discovery of multiple genes encoding both peptides (Kiss) and receptors (Kissr). The investigation of recently published genomes from species of phylogenetic interest, such as a chondrichthyan, the elephant shark, an early sarcopterygian, the coelacanth, a non-teleost actinopterygian, the spotted gar, and an early teleost, the European eel, allowed us to get new insights into the molecular diversity and evolution of both *Kiss* and *Kissr* families. We identified four *Kissr* in the spotted gar and coelacanth genomes, providing the first evidence of four *Kissr* genes in vertebrates. We also found three *Kiss* in the coelacanth and elephant shark genomes revealing two new species, in addition to *Xenopus*, presenting three *Kiss* genes. Considering the increasing diversity of kisspeptin system, phylogenetic, and synteny analyses enabled us to clarify both *Kiss* and *Kissr* classifications. We also could trace back the evolution of both gene families from the early steps of vertebrate history. Four *Kissr* and four *Kiss* paralogs may have arisen *via* the two whole genome duplication rounds (1R and 2R) in early vertebrates. This would have been followed by multiple independent *Kiss* and *Kissr* gene losses in the sarcopterygian and actinopterygian lineages. In particular, no impact of the teleost-specific 3R could be recorded on the numbers of teleost *Kissr* or *Kiss* paralogs. The origin of their diversity *via* 1R and 2R, as well as the subsequent occurrence of multiple gene losses, represent common features of the evolutionary histories of *Kiss* and *Kissr* families in vertebrates. In contrast, comparisons also revealed un-matching numbers of *Kiss* and *Kissr* genes in some species, as well as a large variability of *Kiss/Kissr* couples according to species. These discrepancies support independent features of the *Kiss* and *Kissr* evolutionary histories across vertebrate radiation.

**Keywords: kisspeptin, kisspeptin receptor, phylogeny, synteny, evolutionary history, spotted gar, coelacanth, European eel**

## INTRODUCTION

As increasing vertebrate genomes have been explored, the understanding of their structure and evolution has progressed in parallel. Indeed, the comparison of their gene organization shed light on various large-scale genomic events that occurred along vertebrate radiation. Among those events, in the early stages of their history, vertebrates experienced two rounds of whole genome duplication (1R and 2R), resulting in fourfold-replicated genomes (Dehal and Boore, 2005; Van de Peer et al., 2010). These two events can be traced through the study of gene families currently presenting up to four paralogs. In addition, the comparison of teleost genomes with other vertebrate genomes revealed a teleost-specific third round of whole genome duplication (3R), resulting in up to eight paralogs in the same gene family in this lineage (Amores et al., 1998; Meyer and Van de Peer, 2005; Kasahara et al., 2007).

In 1996, kisspeptin was first discovered as an anti-metastatic peptide in human carcinoma (Lee et al., 1996). In 2001, the orphan receptor GPR54 was identified as the cognate receptor of kisspeptin (Kotani et al., 2001; Muir et al., 2001). Two years later, both kisspeptin (Kiss) and its receptor (Kissr) were demonstrated as key players of the reproductive function in mammals (de Roux et al., 2003; Funes et al., 2003; Seminara et al., 2003). They act upstream in the gonadotropic axis mediating gonadotropin releasing hormone (GnRH) and steroid effects on gonadotropin secretion, and are considered as major puberty gatekeepers and reproduction regulators (Pinilla et al., 2012). To date, the kisspeptin system has been identified in various vertebrate species, leading to the discovery of multiple genes encoding Kiss as well as multiple genes encoding Kissr (Biran et al., 2008; Felip et al., 2009; Kitahashi et al., 2009; Lee et al., 2009).

Concerning *Kiss* and *Kissr* diversity, contrasting situations are found in the different vertebrate phyla. Indeed, in eutherian species, one single gene, named *Kiss1r*, encodes the kisspeptin receptor and one single gene, named *Kiss1*, encodes kisspeptin. In prototherians, such as platypus (*Ornithorhynchus anatinus*), two *Kiss*, and two *Kissr* are present (Lee et al., 2009). To date, in teleosts, two situations have been reported. One *Kiss* gene and one *Kissr* gene are present in some species such as fugu (*Takifugu niphobles*), tetraodon (*Tetraodon nigroviridis*), and stickleback (*Gasterosteus aculeatus*). In contrast, a second *Kiss* as well as a second *Kissr* genes have been characterized in some species including zebrafish (*Danio rerio*; Biran et al., 2008), goldfish (*Carassius auratus*; Li et al., 2009), medaka (*Oryzias latipes*; Lee et al., 2009), and striped bass (*Morone saxatilis*; Zmora et al., 2012). Until recently the maximum number of *Kiss* and *Kissr* genes was found in an amphibian species, the *Xenopus* (*Xenopus tropicalis*), with three paralogs of each gene. On the opposite, in birds (chicken, *Gallus gallus*, zebra finch, *Taeniopygia guttata*, and turkey, *Meleagris gallopavo*) neither *Kiss* nor *Kissr* have been found. So far, in all these cases, a matching number of *Kiss* and *Kissr* genes had been reported, leading to the suggestion of the occurrence of "paired Kiss/Kissr" systems in vertebrates (Kim et al., 2012).

The recent publications of genomes from representative species of key phylogenetic positions makes it possible to revisit the diversity, the origin and the evolution of *Kiss* and *Kissr* in vertebrates. These genomes include a chondrichthyan, the elephant shark (*Callorhinchus milii*; Venkatesh et al., 2007), a representative of early sarcopterygian, the coelacanth (*Latimeria chalumnae*, coelacanth genome project, Broad Institute), a non-teleost actinopterygian, the spotted gar (*Lepisosteus oculatus*; Amores et al., 2011), and an early teleost (elopomorphe), the European eel (*Anguilla anguilla*; Henkel et al., 2012). Gene characterization, phylogenetic, and syntenic analyses allowed us to provide new insights on the respective evolutionary histories of *Kiss* and *Kissr* families. Furthermore, the comparison of proposed *Kiss* and *Kissr* phylogenetic histories highlighted common processes as well as divergent events leading to discuss the existence of conserved Kiss/Kissr couples among the various vertebrate lineages.

## MATERIALS AND METHODS

### GENOMIC DATABASES

The following genomic databases were investigated:

- the chicken genome[1],
- the coelacanth genome[2],
- the elephant shark genome[3],
- the European eel genome[4],
- the human genome[5],
- the lizard genome[6],
- the platypus genome[7],
- the sea lamprey genome[8],
- the spotted gar genome[9],
- the stickleback genome[10],
- the *Xenopus* genome[11],
- the zebrafish genome[12].

### TBLASTN SEARCH

The TBLASTN algorithm of the CLC DNA Workbench software (CLC bio, Aarhus, Denmark) was used on the European eel genome database and the elephant shark genome database. The TBLASTN algorithm (search sensitivity: near exact matches) of the *e*!ENSEMBL website[13] was used on the coelacanth and spotted gar genomic databases.

### GENE PREDICTIONS

Considering that *Kissr* gene structure as well as coding sequences (CDS) are well conserved among vertebrate species, it was possible to predict the exon and intron sequences for new *Kissr* genes (Pasquier et al., 2012). The splicing junctions were predicted using the empirical nucleotidic splicing signatures, i.e., intron begins with "GT" and ends with "AG." Concerning *Kiss* structures, the fact that their CDS are split on two exons (**Figure 1**), appear to be conserved across vertebrates (for review: Tena-Sempere et al., 2012). However, they are highly variable among species, except for the sequence encoding the Kp(10) localized on the final exon (**Figure 1**). Therefore, only this Kp(10) conserved sequence can be predicted when investigating new genomes. This small sequence was used to identify the open reading frame (ORF) encompassing a part of the putative *Kiss* final exon and a part of the putative intron sequence (**Figure 1**). We therefore focused on this ORF encompassing the sequence encoding Kp(10), in the various genomes. The ORFs of the European eel, the coelacanth, the spotted gar, and the elephant shark, were determined using ORF finder tool of the CLC DNA Workbench software.

### SYNTENIC ANALYSES

The synteny analyses of the eel genomic regions were manually performed using CLC DNA Workbench 6 software and the European eel genome database. The analyses of the spotted gar genomic regions were performed using the preliminary gene annotation of the genome assembly LepOcul generated by Ensembl release 67. Synteny maps of the conserved genomic regions in human, platypus, lizard (*Anolis carolinensis*), *Xenopus*, zebrafish, medaka, stickleback, tetraodon, and coelacanth, as well as of the corresponding region in chicken, *G. gallus*, were performed using the PhyloView of Genomicus v67.01 web site[14] (Muffato et al., 2010).

---

[1] http://www.ensembl.org/Gallus_gallus/Info/Index/
[2] http://www.ensembl.org/Latimeria_chalumnae/Info/Index/
[3] http://esharkgenome.imcb.a-star.edu.sg/resources.html
[4] http://www.zfgenomics.org/sub/eel
[5] http://www.ensembl.org/Homo_sapiens/Info/Index/
[6] http://www.ensembl.org/Anolis_carolinensis/Info/Index/
[7] http://www.ensembl.org/Ornithorhynchus_anatinus/Info/Index/
[8] http://www.ensembl.org/Petromyzon_marinus/Info/Index/
[9] http://pre.ensembl.org/Lepisosteus_oculatus/Info/Index
[10] http://www.ensembl.org/Gasterosteus_aculeatus/Info/Index/
[11] http://www.ensembl.org/Xenopus_tropicalis/Info/Index/
[12] http://www.ensembl.org/Danio_rerio/Info/Index/
[13] http://www.ensembl.org/index.html
[14] http://www.dyogen.ens.fr/genomicus-67.01/cgi-bin/search.pl

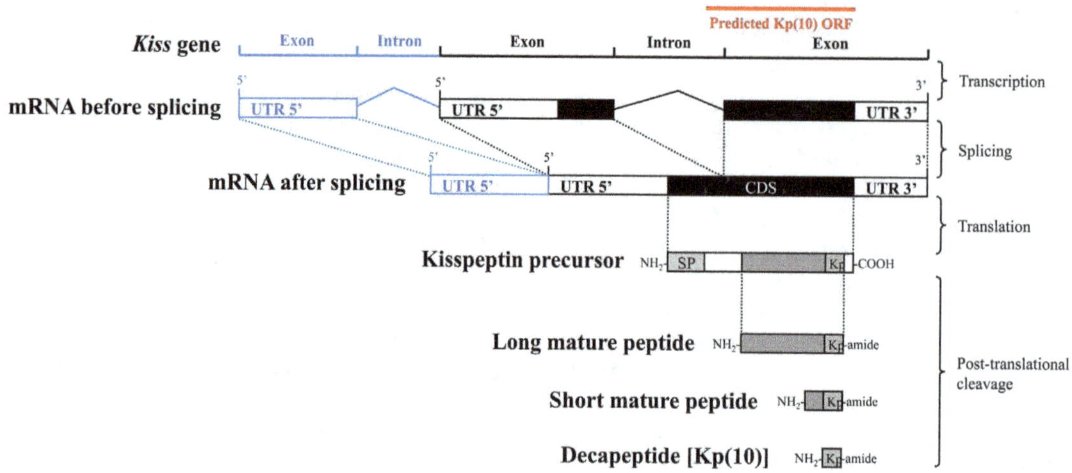


**FIGURE 1 | Main steps leading from the *Kiss* gene to the Kp(10) peptide.** ORF, open reading frame; UTR, un-translated region; CDS, coding sequence; SP, signal peptide; Kp, mature kisspeptin. Predicted ORF sequence containing Kp(10) is represented as a red line. The intron and exon represented in blue have been observed in some mammalian *Kiss1* genes including human *Kiss1*, pig *Kiss1*, and mouse *Kiss1*.

## RESULTS AND DISCUSSION

As one of the aims of this study was to compare the *Kiss* and *Kissr* histories, we first propose to make a short overview of our recent findings concerning the diversity, classification, and origin of *Kissr* gene family. Then, we will expose and discuss our new findings concerning *Kiss* family. Finally, we will compare and discuss the *Kiss* and *Kissr* evolutionary histories in order to get a better understanding of the kisspeptin system evolution.

### DIVERSITY AND EVOLUTIONARY HISTORY OF *Kissr* IN VERTEBRATES

#### Diversity and classification of Kissr

***New advances in Kissr gene characterization.*** Recently, we described three *Kissr* genes in the genome of a basal teleost, the European eel, providing the first evidence of the existence of three *Kissr* genes in a teleost species (Pasquier et al., 2012). Furthermore, we described four *Kissr* in the genome of a non-teleost actinopterygian, the spotted gar, as well as in the genome of a basal sarcopterygian, the coelacanth (Pasquier et al., 2012). This provided the first evidence for four *Kissr* genes in vertebrate species and revealed a larger diversity of *Kissr* than previously described.

So far, no *Kissr* sequence has been reported in chondrichthyans. Our search in the elephant shark genome has only led to the identification of multiple partial sequences, corresponding at least to two *Kissr* (unpublished data). Ongoing sequencing of other chondrichthyan genomes, such as dogfish (*Scyliorhinus canicula*), may provide more insights into the *Kissr* diversity in the sister group of osteichthyans.

#### Phylogeny, synteny, and classification of Kissr

Phylogenetic analysis of 51 peptidic Kissr sequences clustered the osteichthyan Kissr into four clades, each one encompassing a coelacanth and spotted gar Kissr (Pasquier et al., 2012). Clade-1 mainly encompassed mammalian Kissr including human Kiss1r, as well as *Xenopus* Kissr-1a, European eel Kissr-1, spotted gar Kissr-1, and coelacanth Kissr-1. Clade-2 mainly encompassed teleost Kissr including European eel Kissr-2, as well as amphibian, spotted gar, and coelacanth Kissr-2. Clade-3 encompassed a few teleost Kissr including European eel Kissr-3 as well as *Xenopus* Kissr1b, spotted gar, and coelacanth Kissr-3. Clade-4 encompassed two early osteichthyan (spotted gar and coelacanth) Kissr-4 and two tetrapod Kissr (lizard and platypus; Pasquier et al., 2012).

Synteny analysis of *Kissr* neighboring genes, performed on 11 representative vertebrate species including the European eel, coelacanth, and spotted gar, fully supported the phylogenetic repartition of Kissr in four clades. Based on this classification, we proposed a new nomenclature of the *Kissr* family (*Kissr-1*, *Kissr-2*, *Kissr-3*, and *Kissr-4*; Pasquier et al., 2012).

### EVOLUTIONARY HISTORY OF *Kissr*

#### Origin of Kissr diversity via 1R and 2R

Synteny analysis revealed that the four *Kissr* neighboring genomic regions were highly conserved, each presenting paralogs from eight gene families, i.e., *PALM*, *PTBP*, *GRIN3*, *GADD45*, *DIRAS*, *ZCCHC*, *LPAR*, *ZNF644/WIZ* (Pasquier et al., 2012). The hypothesis of the potential existence of four *Kissr* paralogons in vertebrates had been previously raised by Lee et al. (2009) and Kim et al. (2012), although only a maximum of three *Kissr* genes had been discovered at that time. Our finding of four *Kissr* genes, located on four paralogous genomic regions, in coelacanth and spotted gar, provides direct evidence validating this former hypothesis. These four *Kissr* paralogons likely resulted from the two successive genomic duplications (1R and 2R) of a single ancestral genomic region (**Figure 2**).

The currently available data led to a polytomy of the four Kissr clades. This polytomy did not allow to fully solve the homology relationships between the four *Kissr* resulting from the 2R (Pasquier et al., 2012). A recent study proposed the phylogenetic reconstruction of the *PALM* family (Hultqvist et al., 2012). The study of these genes, located in the vicinity of *Kissr* genes, allows us to infer further relationships between the four *Kissr*. We can

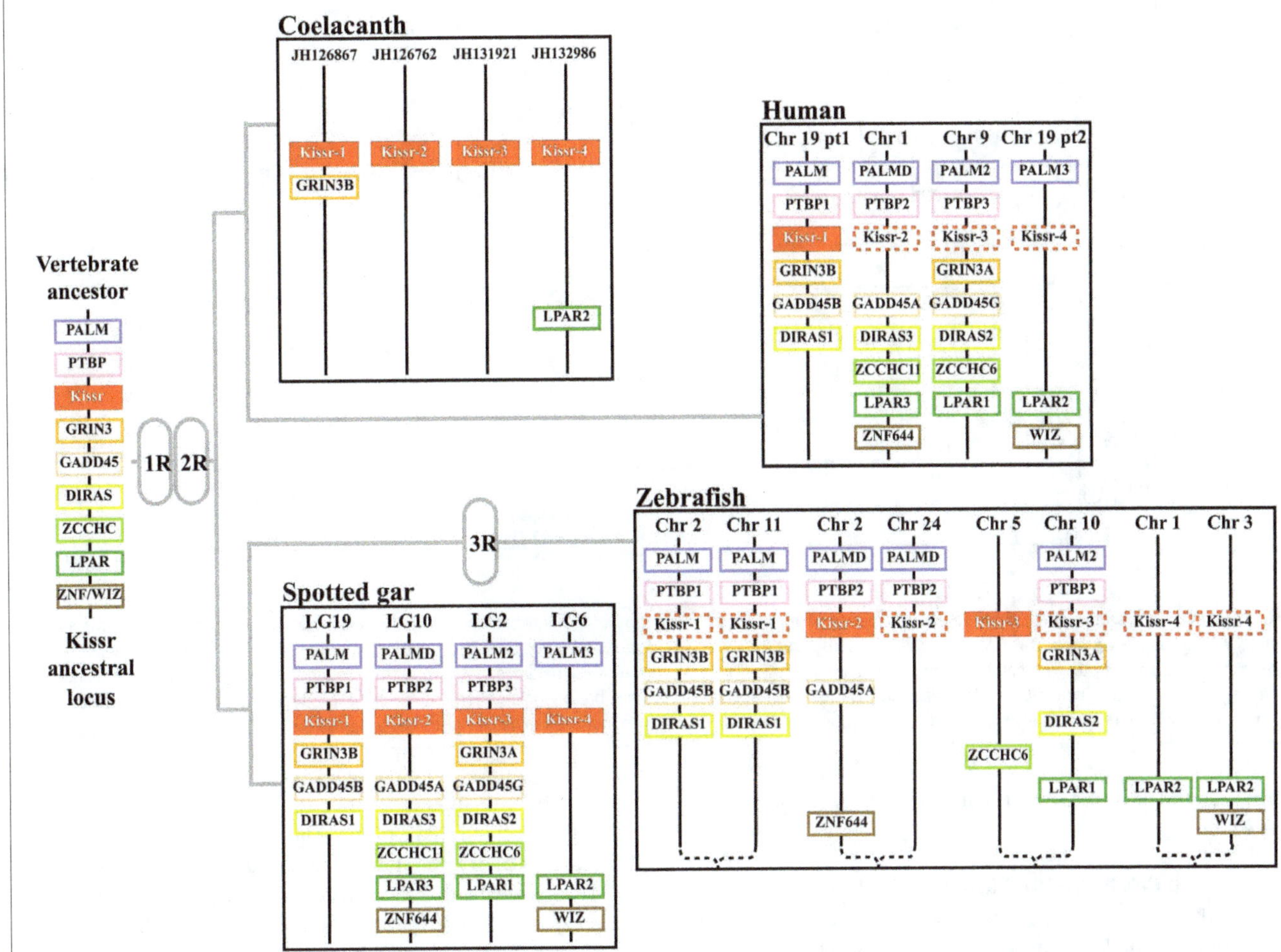


**FIGURE 2 | Proposed origin of osteichthyan *Kissr* tetra-paralogons.** The paralogous genes of each of the eight identified families delineate four paralogons in the spotted gar, coelacanth, and human genomes and a duplicated tetra-paralogon in the zebrafish genome. This suggests a common origin of the four *Kissr* before the two whole genome duplication rounds (1R and 2R) which occurred in the early vertebrate history. This also suggests no impact of the teleost-specific 3R on *Kissr* number in current teleosts. Chr, chromosome; LG, linkage group.

thus hypothesize that *Kissr-1* and *Kissr-3*, on one side, and *Kissr-2* and *Kissr-4*, on the other side, could be sister genes resulting from the 2R.

Recently, one study proposed the reconstruction of 10 proto-chromosomes of the ancestral vertebrate karyotype and their linkage to the corresponding tetra-paralogons in the human genome (Nakatani et al., 2007). Considering our localization of the four *Kissr* syntenic regions in the human genome, we can hypothesize that the corresponding tetra-paralogons resulted from the duplications of one single region localized on the proto-chromosome-A of the vertebrate ancestor (Pasquier et al., 2012).

### *A subsequent history of Kissr losses*

Since the spotted gar and the coelacanth are the only two vertebrate species in which we discovered four paralogous *Kissr*, we can hypothesize multiple *Kissr* loss events to explain the status of this receptor in current vertebrates (**Figure 3A**). In the sarcopterygian lineage, *Kissr-4* may have been lost in amphibians, while *Kissr-1* and *Kissr-2* would have been lost in early amniotes. Subsequent additional losses may have led to the presence of only *Kissr-1* in eutherian mammals and to the absence of any *Kissr* in birds.

Considering the presence of four *Kissr* in a non-teleost actinopterygian, the spotted gar, the teleost-specific 3R could have resulted in the potential existence of up to eight *Kissr* genes. However, we only found three *Kissr* in the European eel, representing the current maximum number of this gene in teleosts. Furthermore, each eel *Kissr* is orthologous to a different tetrapod *Kissr*, supporting the absence of any teleost-specific *Kissr*. Synteny analysis demonstrated that each of the four *Kissr* paralogous genomic regions, present in the spotted gar, was duplicated in zebrafish, in agreement with the 3R. This analysis also indicated that all 3R-copies of *Kissr* were lacking in the corresponding duplicated regions (**Figure 2**). This suggests an early loss of duplicated *Kissr* genes, which would have suppressed the impact of the 3R on the number of *Kissr* in teleosts (**Figure 3A**). Additional successive deletions may have led to the presence of three *Kissr* in a basal teleost (the eel), two *Kissr* in a cypriniform

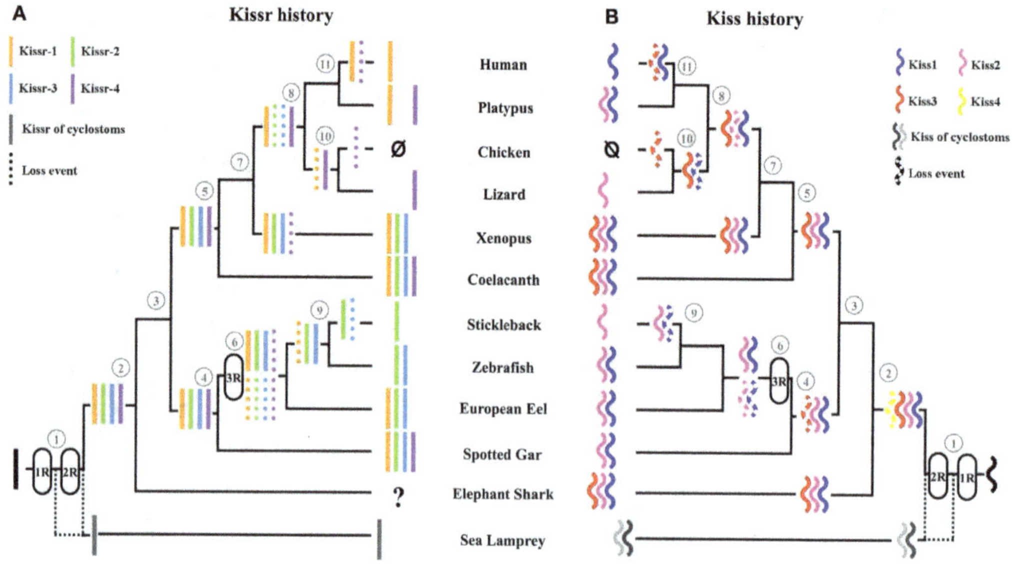


**FIGURE 3 | Current status and proposed evolutionary history of *Kissr* genes (A) versus *Kiss* genes (B).** (1) Vertebrates, (2) gnathostomes, (3) osteichthyans, (4) actinopterygians, (5) sarcopterygians, (6) teleosts, (7) tetrapods, (8) amniotes, (9) euteleosts, (10) diapsides, (11) mammals. The names of the current representative species of each phylum are given at the end of the final branches, together with the symbol of the *Kiss* and *Kissr* genes they possess. These hypotheses assume the presence of four *Kiss* and four *Kissr* paralogs in the vertebrate lineage resulting from the two rounds of vertebrate whole genome duplication. Multiple subsequent gene loss events are indicated in the various lineages.

(zebrafish), and only one Kissr in a more recent teleost (stickleback; **Figure 3A**).

## DIVERSITY AND EVOLUTIONARY HISTORY OF *Kiss* IN VERTEBRATES

In contrast to the receptor proteins which present several conserved domains, the *Kiss* genes encode precursors which are highly variable among vertebrates, except for the short sequence of the mature decapeptide [Kp(10)]. This makes it difficult to obtain *Kiss* mRNA sequences by classical molecular strategies. Genomic database analyses thus represent the best approach to characterize the *Kiss* set for a given species. However, the small characteristic sequence of *Kiss*, encoding Kp(10), could be missing in genomic databases due to sequencing or assembly limitations.

All previously investigated osteichthyan species possessed the same number of *Kiss* and *Kissr* genes: one in eutherian mammals, two in prototherians, three in *Xenopus*, none in birds, and one or two in teleosts (Lee et al., 2009). In cyclostomes, two *Kiss* genes have been reported (Lee et al., 2009), while only one *Kissr* could be predicted until now (Pasquier et al., 2011).

### *Diversity and classification of Kiss*

***New advances in Kiss gene characterization.*** To further assess the *Kiss* diversity in vertebrates, we re-investigated the presence of these genes in the genome of the elephant shark, the coelacanth, the spotted gar, and the European eel, representative species from four groups of relevant phylogenetical positions. Most of the vertebrate *Kiss* genes are made of two exons except for some mammalian *Kiss1*, including human *Kiss1*, pig (*Sus scrofa*) *Kiss1*, and mouse *Kiss1*, that are made of three exons (**Figure 1**). However, the CDS of all the *Kiss* described so far are split on two exons (**Figure 1**). In fact the first of those two exons encodes the signal peptide while the final exon encodes mainly the mature peptides including the conserved Kp(10) (**Figures 1** and **4**; Tomikawa et al., 2010, 2012; Cartwright and Williams, 2012; Tena-Sempere et al., 2012). Considering that the *Kiss* gene sequences are highly variable among species except for the sequence encoding the Kp(10), we focused our prediction on the ORF containing this sequence. We performed TBLASTN in the four genomes, resulting in the identification of several ORF containing conserved sequences encoding for Kp(10).

*Two Kiss genes in the European eel genome.* The two ORFs containing the sequences encoding Kp(10) are 296 and 327 bp long, respectively (**Figure A1** in Appendix). Once translated, each of them leads to a peptidic sequence encompassing a putative Kp(10): YNWNSFGLRY [European eel Kp1(10)] and FNRNPFGLRF [European eel Kp2(10)], respectively (**Figure 4**). The C-terminal end of the Kp1(10) sequence is followed by a GK-Stop motif, while the Kp2(10) sequence is followed by a GKR motif (**Figure A1** in Appendix). The sequences "X-G-Basic-Basic" or "X-G-Basic" are characteristic of the conserved proteolytic cleavage and alpha-amidation sites of neuropeptides (Eipper et al., 1992).

*Two Kiss genes in the spotted gar genome.* The two ORFs containing the sequences encoding Kp(10) are 348 and 300 bp long, respectively (**Figure A2** in Appendix). Once translated, each of them leads to a peptidic sequence presenting a putative Kp(10): YNWNSFGLRY [spotted gar Kp1(10)] and FNFNPFGLRF [spotted gar Kp2(10)], respectively (**Figure 4**). The C-terminal ends of these two sequences are followed by a GKR motif (**Figure A2** in Appendix).

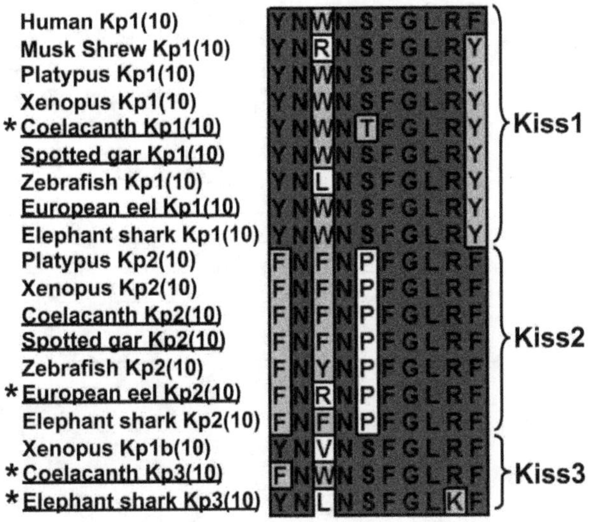


**FIGURE 4 | Sequence alignment of vertebrate Kp(10).** At each position, identical amino-acids are shaded in dark gray and similar amino-acids in light gray. Newly identified sequences are underlined and unique sequences are marked by an asterisk.

*Three Kiss genes in the coelacanth genome.* The three ORFs containing the sequences encoding Kp(10) are 363, 396, and 81 bp long, respectively (**Figure A3** in Appendix). Once translated, each of them leads to a peptidic sequence encompassing a putative Kp(10): YNWNTFGLRY [coelacanth Kp1(10)], FNFNPFGLRF [coelacanth Kp2(10)], and FNWNSFGLRF [coelacanth Kp3(10)], respectively (**Figure 4**). The C-terminal ends of the Kp1(10) and the Kp2(10) sequences are followed by a GKR motif, while the Kp3(10) is followed by a GKK motif (**Figure A3** in Appendix). Seven amino-acids up-stream the sequence of the Kp3(10), a stop codon appears (**Figure A3** in Appendix) suggesting that coelacanth *Kiss3* gene could have a different intro-exon structure compared to what has been described so far or it can suggest that this gene is no longer expressed.

*A third Kiss gene in the elephant shark genome.* While two *Kiss* (*Kiss1* and *Kiss2*) were previously identified in the elephant shark genome (Lee et al., 2009), we were able to localize a new ORF of 315 bp containing a third sequence encoding a Kp(10) (**Figure A4** in Appendix). Once translated, it leads to a peptidic sequence encompassing a putative Kp(10): YNLNSFGLKF [elephant shark Kp3(10)] (**Figure 4**). The C-terminal end of this peptide is followed by a GKR motif (**Figure A4** in Appendix).

***Kiss sequence alignment and comparisons.*** The alignment of 56 kisspeptin precursors revealed a high variability of their amino-acid sequences except for the sequences corresponding to Kp(10) and its few surrounding amino-acids which, in contrast, are highly conserved (data not shown). Such a pattern, which is representative of many other neuropeptide precursors, provides poor phylogenetic information within alignment matrix. This lack of information makes the use of phylogenetic analysis inappropriate to establish homology relationships within this kind of peptide precursor family.

***Novel Kp(10).*** Among the new Kiss genes predicted in the present study, four of them encode novel Kp(10) (**Figure 4**). The singularity of the elephant shark Kp3(10) is the presence of a lysine (K) instead of an arginine (R) at the ninth position. The coelacanth Kp1(10) provides the first case of a threonine (T) at the fifth position. The coelacanth Kp3(10) is the only one to present both a phenylalanine (F) at the first position and a serine (S) at the fifth position. The European eel Kp2(10) presents at its third position an arginine (R), which possesses different physical and chemical properties from amino-acids commonly present at this position. Up to now, only the musk shrew (*Suncus murinus*) Kp1(10) presented an arginine at the third position and it was demonstrated that its kisspeptin system was involved in the reproductive function as in other mammals (Inoue et al., 2011). Since the impacted positions by the amino-acid substitutions have not been characterized as highly critical for Kp(10) functional properties (Gutiérrez-Pascual et al., 2009; Curtis et al., 2010), those novel Kp(10) may have conserved their functionality. Since Kp(10) is considered as the smallest required sequence to specifically bind to the receptor (Kotani et al., 2001), it could be of interest to test all those peptides in future pharmacological studies in order to assess their structure/function relationships.

***Syntenic analysis and classification of Kiss genes.*** In order to classify the different *Kiss* paralogs, we performed a syntenic analysis of the *Kiss* neighboring genes. We considered the following vertebrate representatives: mammals (human), birds (chicken), squamates (lizard), amphibians (*Xenopus*), basal sarcopterygian (coelacanth), non-teleost actinopterygians (spotted gar), and teleosts (zebrafish, stickleback, and European eel). Our syntenic analysis demonstrated that the *Kiss* genes are localized in three different genomic regions.

The human *Kiss1*, *Xenopus Kiss1a*, coelacanth *Kiss1*, spotted gar *Kiss1*, and zebrafish *Kiss1* are positioned in genomic regions containing common loci, including *TEAD3*, *NAV1*, *PPP1R12B*, *PPFIA4*, *MYBPH*, *KCNC4*, *REN*, *GOLT1A*, *PLEKHA6*, *PPP1R15B*, *PIK3C2B*, and *SYT6*, thus exhibiting well conserved synteny (**Figure 5A**). This supports the orthology of these *Kiss* genes, all considered as *Kiss1* genes. Syntenic analysis suggests that the stickleback, lizard, and chicken genomes do not contain any *Kiss1* gene, although the above-mentioned neighboring genes are present in the corresponding genomic regions (**Figure 5A**). The peptidic sequence of eel Kiss1 presents many similarities to the other Kiss1, but the eel *Kiss1* gene is located on too small scaffolds to contain any other gene, preventing from any syntenic analysis.

The lizard *Kiss2*, coelacanth *Kiss2*, spotted gar *Kiss2*, zebrafish *Kiss2*, stickleback *Kiss2*, and European eel *Kiss2* genes are positioned in genomic regions containing common loci including *STRAP*, *PLEKHA5*, *GOLT1B*, *C12orf39*, *GYS2*, *LDHB*, *KCNJ8*, *ABCC9*, *CMAS*, *SYT10*, *NAV3*, *PPFIA2*, and *KCNC2*, thus exhibiting well conserved synteny (**Figure 5B**). This supports the orthology of these *Kiss* genes, all considered as *Kiss2* genes. Syntenic analysis suggests that human and chicken genomes do not contain

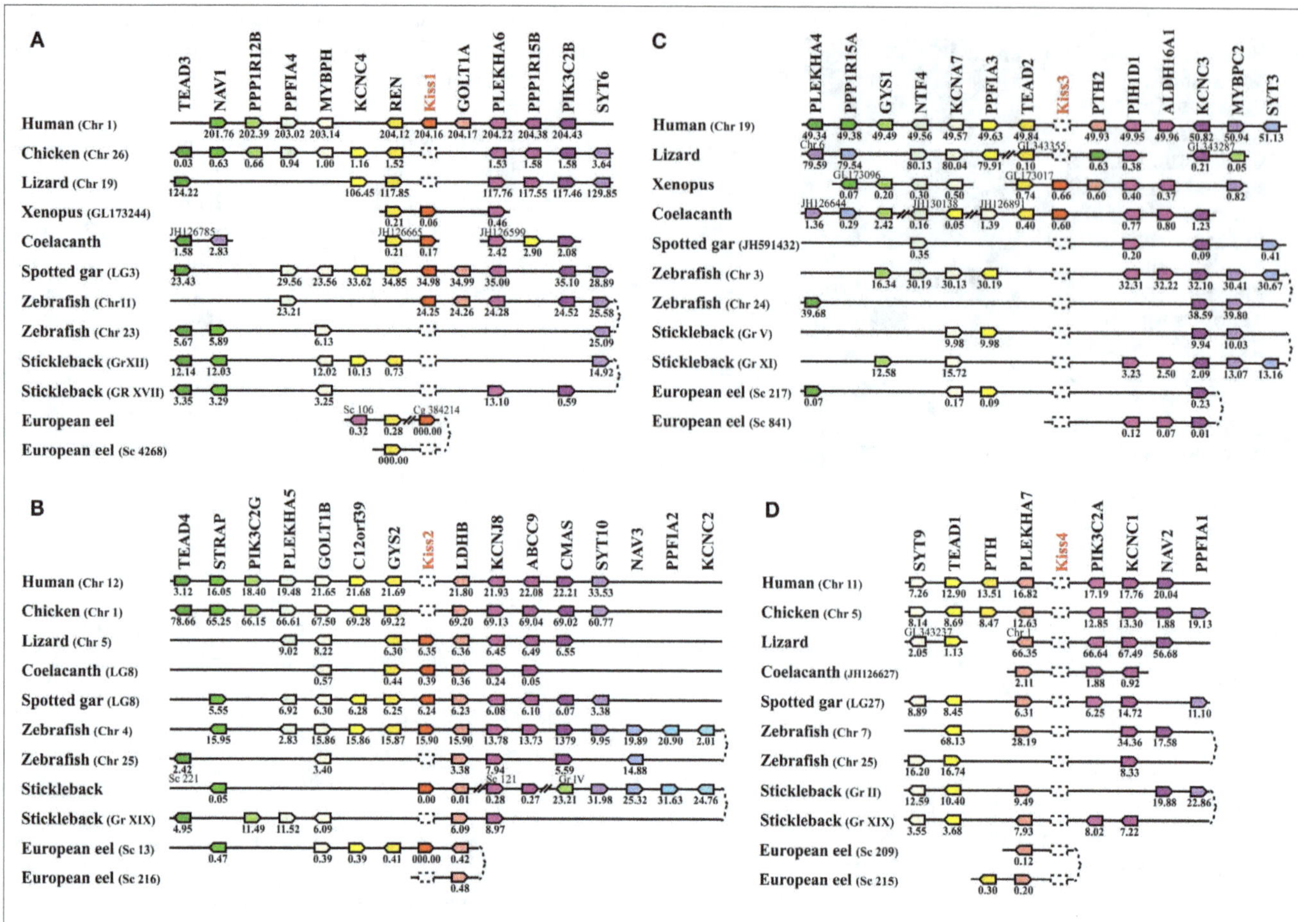


**FIGURE 5 | Conserved genomic synteny of osteichthyan *Kiss*.** Genomic synteny maps comparing the orthologs of *Kiss1* **(A)**, *Kiss2* **(B)**, *Kiss3* **(C)**, *Kiss4* **(D)**, and their neighboring genes. Analyses were performed on the genomes of human (*Homo sapiens*), platypus (*Ornithorhynchus anatinus*), lizard (*Anolis carolinensis*), chicken (*Gallus gallus*), *Xenopus* (*Xenopus tropicalis*), coelacanth (*Latimeria chalumnae*), spotted gar (*Lepisosteus oculatus*), zebrafish (*Danio rerio*), stickleback (*Gasterosteus aculeatus*), and European eel (*Anguilla anguilla*). This map was established using the PhyloView of Genomicus v67.01 web site, manual annotation of the European eel genome using CLC DNA Workbench 6 software and the gene annotation of the coelacanth and spotted gar genomic databases. *Kiss* genes are named according to our proposed nomenclature (*Kiss1* to *Kiss4*). The other genes are named after their human orthologs according to the Human Genome Naming Consortium (HGNC). Orthologs of each gene are shown in the same color. The direction of arrows indicates the gene orientation, with the position of the gene (in $10^{-6}$ base pairs) indicated below. The full gene names and detailed genomic locations are given in Table S1 in Supplementary Material. Chr, chromosome; LG, linkage group; Gr, group; Sc, scaffold; Cg, contig.

any *Kiss2* gene, although the above-mentioned neighboring genes are present in the corresponding genomic region (**Figure 5B**).

The coelacanth *Kiss3* and the *Xenopus Kiss1b* genes are positioned in genomic regions containing common loci, including *TEAD2*, *PIH1D1*, and *ALDH16A1*, thus exhibiting well conserved synteny (**Figure 5C**). This supports the orthology of these two *Kiss* genes, both considered here as *Kiss3* genes. Syntenic analysis suggests that human, lizard, spotted gar, and teleost genomes do not contain any *Kiss3* gene, although the above-mentioned neighboring genes are present in the corresponding genomic regions (**Figure 5C**). Syntenic analysis also suggests that the whole considered region is absent from the chicken genome.

### Evolutionary history of Kiss

***Origin of Kiss diversity via 1R and 2R.*** The syntenic analysis also allowed us to investigate the origin of the multiple *Kiss* genes found in vertebrates. The three conserved genomic regions, presenting *Kiss* genes, also comprise other paralogs from 11 gene families: *TEAD* (4 paralogs), *NAV* (3 paralogs), *PPFIA* (4 paralogs), *KCNC* (4 paralogs), *GOLT1* (2 paralogs), *PLEKHA* (4 paralogs), *PPP1R15* (2 paralogs), *PIK3C2* (3 paralogs), *SYT* (4 paralogs), *GYS* (2 paralogs), and *PTH* (2 paralogs) (**Figures 5A–C**). The members of those families are present among the three *Kiss* syntenic regions and they also delineate a fourth conserved region (**Figure 5D**), which does not present any *Kiss* gene in the osteichthyan representative species studied so far. The four conserved regions delineated by the 11 gene families can be considered as paralogous (tetra-paralogon).

Considering the reconstruction of the ancestral vertebrate chromosomes, their linkage to the tetra-paralogons in the human genome (Nakatani et al., 2007) and our localization of the four *Kiss* syntenic regions in the human genome (on Chromosomes 1, 11, 12, and 19), we can hypothesize that the *Kiss* tetra-paralogons resulted from the duplications of one single genomic region localized on the proto-chromosome-D of the vertebrate ancestor. Therefore, we can infer that the current three *Kiss* genes may have resulted from a single ancestral gene duplicated through 1R and 2R that occurred in early steps of vertebrate evolution (**Figure 6**).

***A subsequent history of Kiss losses.***

*Multiple loss events in sarcopterygians and actinopterygians.* The 1R and 2R events should have resulted in four different *Kiss* genes in vertebrates. Since the fourth *Kiss* gene (referred to as *Kiss4* in this study) has not been observed in any species studied so far, we can hypothesize an early loss of this gene after the 2R. As only a chondrichthyan, the elephant shark, and two sarcopterygians, the coelacanth and *Xenopus*, still present three *Kiss* genes, whereas all other species possess less than three *Kiss*, we can hypothesize multiple additional events of *Kiss* losses in vertebrates (**Figure 3B**).

Among the sarcopterygian lineage, in tetrapods, *Kiss3* would have been lost in amniotes. Further alternative losses may have occurred in this lineage, with only *Kiss1* remaining in eutherian mammals and only *Kiss2* in squamates (lizard). Finally, additional losses would have led to the complete absence of *Kiss* in birds (**Figure 3B**). Among the actinopterygian lineage, an early loss of *Kiss3* would have occurred since it is lacking in the actinopterygian species investigated so far (**Figure 3B**).

*No impact of the teleost-specific 3R on Kiss number in current species.* In the actinopterygian lineage, the teleost-specific 3R and the presence of two *Kiss* in a non-teleost actinopterygian, the spotted gar, implied the potential existence of at least four *Kiss* genes in the early teleost history. However, our study showed that so far the largest number of *Kiss* exhibited by current teleosts, including the eel, is two. Furthermore, each teleost *Kiss* is orthologous to a different tetrapod *Kiss*, indicating that no teleost-specific *Kiss* exists. Synteny analysis revealed that each of the four *Kiss* genomic regions present in the spotted gar is duplicated in teleosts in agreement with the 3R event but that duplicated *Kiss* genes are lacking (**Figures 5** and **6**). This suggests an early loss of duplicated *Kiss* genes suppressing the impact of the 3R on the number of *Kiss* in teleosts (**Figure 3B**). Additional deletion may have led to the presence of only *Kiss2* in gasterosteiforms (the stickleback; **Figure 3B**). *Kiss* evolutionary history was punctuated by numerous loss events through vertebrate radiation (**Figure 3B**).

## COMPARISON OF THE EVOLUTIONARY HISTORIES OF *Kiss* AND *Kissr* IN VERTEBRATES

These new data concerning *Kiss* and *Kissr* diversities enabled us to improve their respective classifications and evolutionary histories. A remaining challenge was to elucidate whether *Kiss* and *Kissr* families have experienced parallel histories during vertebrate radiation. The comparative study of the current status of both families in vertebrates allows a better understanding of the whole kisspeptin system.

### *Features in agreement with parallel histories*

***Origin of the Kiss and Kissr multiplicity via 1R and 2R.*** Our syntenic studies suggest that the vertebrate *Kiss* and *Kissr* families both resulted from the successive duplications of a single ancestral gene through the 1R and 2R (**Figure 3**). Thus, *Kiss* and *Kissr* experienced, in parallel, the two first genome duplication rounds resulting in four copies of each gene in the early steps of the vertebrate evolutionary history (**Figure 3**). While *Kissr* gene homologs were characterized in non-vertebrate species (*Strongylocentrotus purpuratus*, GenBank accession numbers: XP_793873.1 and XP_796286.1; *Saccoglossus kowalevskii*, GenBank accession numbers: NP_001161573.1 and NP_001161574.1), tracing back the presence of an ancestral *Kissr* in early deuterostomes, *Kiss* genes have not yet been discovered in non-vertebrate species.

***Subsequent history of gene losses.*** Both *Kiss* and *Kissr* families were composed of four genes in the early steps of the vertebrate history. However, most of the current vertebrate species investigated so far present less than four copies of *Kiss* and *Kissr* genes. The current numbers of both *Kiss* and *Kissr* genes suggest that both families underwent numerous independent loss events across vertebrate history (**Figure 3**).

***No impact of the teleost-specific 3R.*** The teleost lineage, which has experienced a third whole genome duplication round (3R), could have been expected to possess up to eight *Kiss* and *Kissr* genes. However, the analyses of the *Kiss* and *Kissr* within teleost genomes revealed a maximum of three *Kissr* and two *Kiss* genes and did not reveal any 3R-specific copies of *Kiss* or *Kissr* genes. This suggests that the teleost-specific 3R did not impact the current number of *Kiss* or *Kissr* genes, reflecting massive losses of the 3R-copies of both *Kiss* and *Kissr* genes in early teleosts (**Figure 3**).

### *Features in opposition to parallel histories: independent loss events*

***Un-matching number of Kiss and Kissr in some species.*** In the current gnathostomes, we observed a maximum of four *Kissr* but only three *Kiss* paralogs. This difference suggests that this lineage inherited the four *Kissr* copies resulting from the 1R and 2R, whereas the fourth *Kiss* may have been lost before or at an early stage of the gnathostome emergence (**Figure 3**). This situation was observed in an early sarcopterygian, the coelacanth, while an even larger difference in *Kissr* (four) and *Kiss* (two) numbers was found in the spotted gar, reflecting an additional independent loss of *Kiss* in the actinopterygian lineage. An un-matching number of *Kissr* (three) and *Kiss* (two) was also observed in an early teleost, the European eel, while additional losses may have led to equal numbers of *Kissr* and *Kiss* in more recent teleosts (two or one according to the species). These variations in *Kissr/Kiss* numbers reflect different timing of *Kiss* and *Kissr* loss events. Those hypotheses suggest that *Kiss* losses occurred independently among the different gnathostome lineages and also independently from the *Kissr* losses.

***Various Kiss/Kissr combinations across vertebrates.*** The hypothesis of independent *Kiss* and *Kissr* evolutionary histories is also strengthened by the comparison of the gene sets present in species with even matching numbers of *Kiss* and *Kissr*. For example, lizard, and stickleback both present the *Kiss2* gene, whereas they possess different *Kissr*, i.e., *Kissr-4* in the lizard and *Kissr-2* in the stickleback (**Figure 3**). The same observation can be done comparing the kisspeptin systems of platypus and zebrafish, which both present the *Kiss1* and *Kiss2* genes, whereas their sets of receptors are completely different, i.e., *Kissr-1* and *Kissr-4* in platypus versus *Kissr-2*

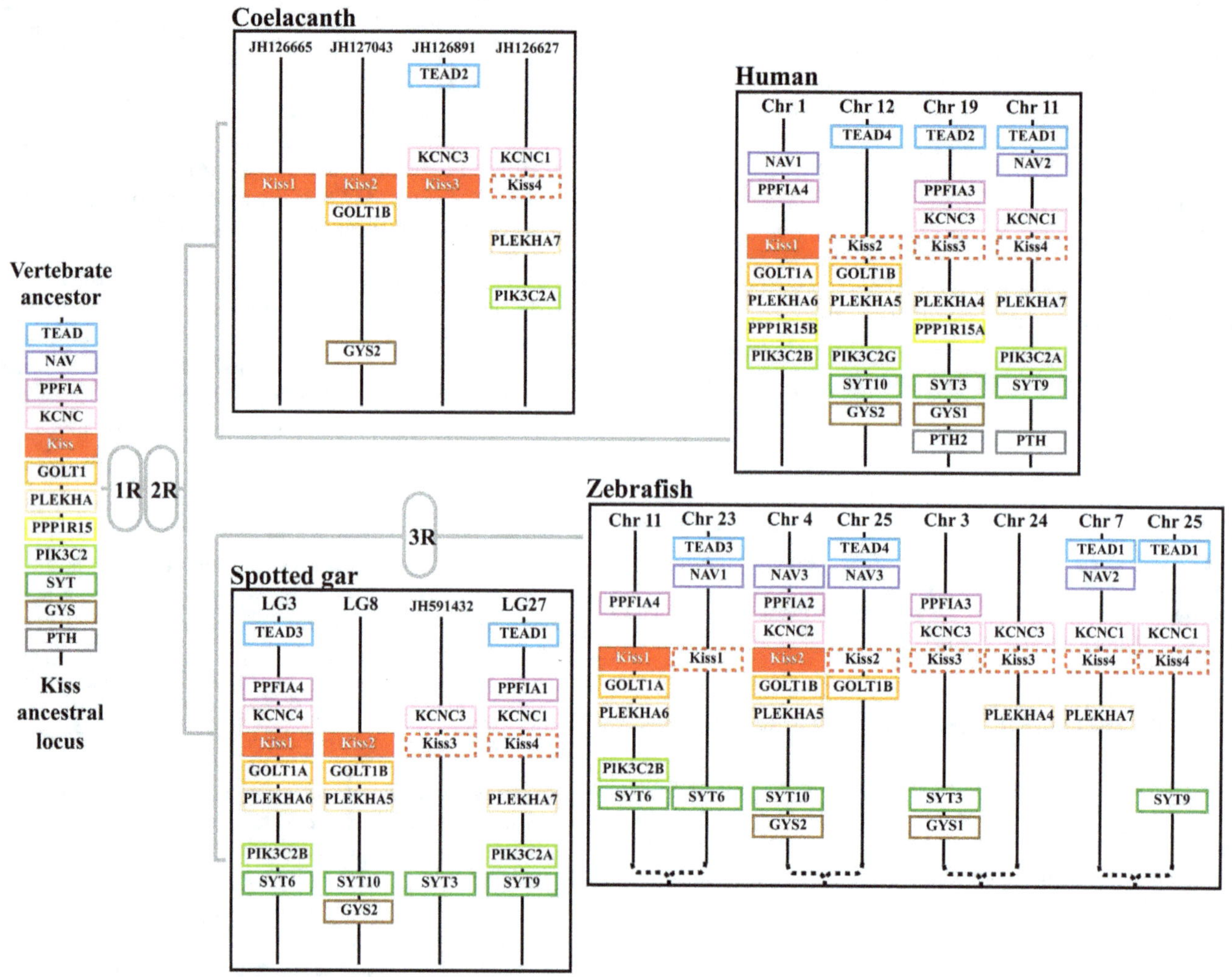


**FIGURE 6 | Proposed origin of osteichthyan *Kiss* tetra-paralogons.** The paralogous genes of each of the 11 identified families delineate four paralogons in spotted gar, coelacanth, and human genomes and a duplicated tetra-paralogon in the zebrafish genome. This suggests a common origin of the three *Kiss* before the two whole genome duplication rounds (1R and 2R) which occurred in the early vertebrate history. This also suggests no impact of the teleost-specific 3R on *Kiss* number in current teleost species. Chr, chromosome; LG, linkage group.

and *Kissr-3* in zebrafish (**Figure 3**). These observations strongly suggest a large variety of *Kiss* and *Kissr* combinations, resulting from independent loss events. These data shed new lights on the evolution of the kisspeptin system in vertebrates and challenge the former hypothesis of a conservation of *Kiss/Kissr* couples across vertebrate evolution. This diversity among vertebrates opens new research avenues for comparative physiology and endocrinology of kisspeptin system.

***What could have favored the independent evolutions of* Kiss *and* Kissr?** A few *in vitro* studies using recombinant receptors have showed cross-reactivities between various kisspeptins and kisspeptin receptors (Biran et al., 2008;Lee et al., 2009; Li et al., 2009). For instance, Lee et al. (2009) tested the specificity of recombinant human GPR54 (Kissr-1 according to our nomenclature), zebrafish GPR54-1, and -2 (Kissr-3 and Kissr-2 according to our nomenclature), and *Xenopus* GPR54-1a, -1b, and -2 (Kissr-1, Kissr-4, and Kissr-2 according to our nomenclature) toward various kisspeptins. They showed that human, zebrafish, and *Xenopus* kisspeptins were able to activate all the receptors with differential intra and inter-specific ligand selectivity. Such cross-reactivity could have promoted the independence of the *Kiss* and *Kissr* evolutionary histories. This could explain the situation of species presenting un-matching numbers of *Kiss* and *Kissr* genes, as well as the high variability of *Kiss/Kissr* gene combinations across vertebrate species. Another study, using goldfish recombinant GPR54a and GPR54b (Kissr-3 and Kissr-2 according to our nomenclature), revealed that the ligand potency strikingly differed depending on the responsive element used in the reporter gene construction (Li et al., 2009). These data showed the difficulty to define specific Kiss/Kissr couples based only on pharmacological properties.

In the case of the presence of multiple *Kiss/Kissr* genes in a given species, anatomical relationships between projections of *Kiss* neurons and target cells expressing *Kissr* may provide further cues for determining Kiss/Kissr functional couples. Thus, in zebrafish which possess two *Kiss* genes and two *Kissr* genes, *in situ* hybridization and immunocytochemical studies localized the *Kiss1* neurons in different nuclei from *Kiss2* neurons (Servili et al., 2011). Moreover, *Kiss1* neurons are projecting to *Kiss1r* (*Kissr-3* according to our nomenclature) expressing cells, while *Kiss2* neurons are projecting to *Kiss2r* (*Kissr-2* according to our nomenclature) expressing cells (Servili et al., 2011). This reveals anatomically separated kisspeptin systems and distinct specific Kiss/Kissr functional couples in zebrafish (Servili et al., 2011). In striped bass, another teleost possessing two *Kiss* genes and two *Kissr* genes, *in situ* hybridization and laser capture microscopy coupled to quantitative PCR showed, in contrast, that *Kiss1* and *Kiss2* were co-expressed in neurons of the hypothalamus, indicating promiscuous Kiss synthesis sites (Zmora et al., 2012). However, the two *Kissr* of the striped bass were expressed in different brain cells, indicating that the kisspeptin systems are not fully redundant (Zmora et al., 2012). All these data underline the importance of investigating the gene diversity, the anatomical organization and the functional properties of the kisspeptin system in various species, regarding the potential high variability of this system among vertebrates.

## CONCLUSION

Kisspeptin system is known to play a role in many physiological processes such as antimetastasis, energy metabolism homeostasis, pregnancy, and puberty onset. Even though this system has been widely studied in the last few years, its diversity and evolutionary history remained unclear. Thanks to the newly published genomes of osteichthyans of key phylogenetical positions, we were able to provide new data on the diversity of *Kiss* and *Kissr* genes, to clarify the classification of these genes and to bring new insights on the evolutionary history of these gene families. Four *Kissr* and four *Kiss* genes may have arisen via the 1R and 2R in early vertebrates. This would have been followed by multiple independent *Kiss* and *Kissr* gene loss events in the sarcopterygian and actinopterygian lineages. In particular, due to massive *Kiss* and *Kissr* gene losses, no impact of the teleost-specific 3R can be recorded on the number of *Kissr* or *Kiss* paralogs in current teleost species. The comparison of both *Kiss* and *Kissr* gene status, in the current vertebrates, supports both parallel and independent evolutionary histories of the *Kiss* and *Kissr* families across vertebrate radiation. It also underlines a large diversity of *Kiss*/*Kissr* possible combinations that needs to be taken into account in future comparative studies.

## ACKNOWLEDGMENTS

We thank Dr. B. Quérat (CNRS, Paris, France) for his helpful advices and discussions concerning phylogeny and synteny. We also thank all the different consortiums at the initiative of sequencing, assembly, annotation, and publication of genomes, in particular the consortiums of the European eel genome, the spotted gar genome, the coelacanth genome, the elephant shark genome, and the sea lamprey genome. Our thanks also include the authors of the Ensembl genome browser web site and all web sites providing free access to their genomic databases. We thank the authors of the Genomicus web site providing a very useful and friendly tool for synteny analysis. Jérémy Pasquier is a recipient of a Ph.D. fellowship from the Ministry of Research and Education. This work was supported by grants from the National Research Agency, PUBERTEEL N ANR-08-BLAN-0173 to Karine Rousseau and Sylvie Dufour, and from the European Community, Seventh Framework Program, PRO-EEL N No. 245257 to Anne-Gaëlle Lafont and Sylvie Dufour.

**Table S1 | Names, references, and locations of the genes used in the *Kiss* synteny analysis.**

## REFERENCES

Amores, A., Catchen, J., Ferrara, A., Fontenot, Q., and Postlethwait, J. H. (2011). Genome evolution and meiotic maps by massively parallel DNA sequencing: spotted gar, an outgroup for the teleost genome duplication. *Genetics* 188, 799–808.

Amores, A., Force, A., Yan, Y. L., Joly, L., Amemiya, C., Fritz, A., et al. (1998). Zebrafish hox clusters and vertebrate genome evolution. *Science* 282, 1711–1714.

Biran, J., Ben-Dor, S., and Levavi-Sivan, B. (2008). Molecular identification and functional characterization of the kisspeptin/kisspeptin receptor system in lower vertebrates. *Biol. Reprod.* 79, 776–786.

Cartwright, J. E., and Williams, P. J. (2012). Altered placental expression of kisspeptin and its receptor in pre-eclampsia. *J. Endocrinol.* 214, 79–85.

Curtis, A. E., Cooke, J. H., Baxter, J. E., Parkinson, J. R., Bataveljic, A., Ghatei, M. A., et al. (2010). A kisspeptin-10 analog with greater in vivo bioactivity than kisspeptin-10. *Am. J. Physiol. Endocrinol. Metab.* 298, E296–E303.

de Roux, N., Genin, E., Carel, J. C., Matsuda, F., Chaussain, J. L., and Milgrom, E. (2003). Hypogonadotropic hypogonadism due to loss of function of the KiSS1-derived peptide receptor GPR54. *Proc. Natl. Acad. Sci. U.S.A.* 100, 10972–10976.

Dehal, P., and Boore, J. L. (2005). Two rounds of whole genome duplication in the ancestral vertebrate. *PLoS Biol.* 3:e314. doi:10.1371/journal.pbio.0030314

Eipper, B. A., Stoffers, D. A., and Mains, R. E. (1992). The biosynthesis of neuropeptides: peptide alpha-amidation. *Annu. Rev. Neurosci.* 15, 57–85.

Felip, A., Zanuy, S., Pineda, R., Pinilla, L., Carrillo, M., Tena-Sempere, M., et al. (2009). Evidence for two distinct KiSS genes in non-placental vertebrates that encode kisspeptins with different gonadotropin-releasing activities in fish and mammals. *Mol. Cell. Endocrinol.* 312, 61–71.

Funes, S., Hedrick, J. A., Vassileva, G., Markowitz, L., Abbondanzo, S., Golovko, A., et al. (2003). The KiSS-1 receptor GPR54 is essential for the development of the murine reproductive system. *Biochem. Biophys. Res. Commun.* 312, 1357–1363.

Gutiérrez-Pascual, E., Leprince, J., Martínez-Fuentes, A. J., Ségalas-Milazzo, I., Pineda, R., Roa, J., et al. (2009). In vivo and in vitro structure-activity relationships and structural conformation of Kisspeptin-10-related peptides. *Mol. Pharmacol.* 76, 58–67.

Henkel, C. V., Burgerhout, E., de Wijze, D. L., Dirks, R. P., Minegishi, Y., Jansen, H. J., et al. (2012). Primitive duplicate Hox clusters in the European eel's genome. *PLoS ONE* 7:e32231. doi:10.1371/journal.pone.0032231

Hultqvist, G., Ocampo Daza, D., Larhammar, D., and Kilimann, M. W. (2012). Evolution of the vertebrate paralemmin gene family: ancient origin of gene duplicates suggests distinct functions. *PLoS ONE* 7:e41850. doi:10.1371/journal.pone.0041850

Inoue, N., Sasagawa, K., Ikai, K., Sasaki, Y., Tomikawa, J., Oishi, S., et al. (2011). Kisspeptin neurons mediate reflex ovulation in the musk shrew (*Suncus murinus*). *Proc. Natl. Acad. Sci. U.S.A.* 108, 17527–17532.

Kasahara, M., Naruse, K., Sasaki, S., Nakatani, Y., Qu, W., Ahsan, B., et al. (2007). The medaka draft genome and insights into vertebrate genome evolution. *Nature* 447, 714–719.

Kim, D. K., Cho, E. B., Moon, M. J., Park, S., Hwang, J. I., Do Rego, J. L., et al. (2012). Molecular coevolution of neuropeptides gonadotropin-releasing hormone and kisspeptin with their cognate G protein-coupled receptors. *Front. Neurosci.* 6:3. doi:10.3389/fnins.2012.00003

Kitahashi, T., Ogawa, S., and Parhar, I. S. (2009). Cloning and expression of kiss2 in the zebrafish and medaka. *Endocrinology* 150, 821–831.

Kotani, M., Detheux, M., Vandenbogaerde, A., Communi, D., Vanderwinden, J. M., Le Poul, E., et al. (2001). The metastasis suppressor gene KiSS-1 encodes kisspeptins, the natural ligands of the orphan G protein-coupled receptor GPR54. *J. Biol. Chem.* 276, 34631–34636.

Lee, J. H., Miele, M. E., Hicks, D. J., Phillips, K. K., Trent, J. M., Weissman, B. E., et al. (1996). KiSS-1, a novel human malignant melanoma metastasis-suppressor gene. *J. Natl. Cancer Inst.* 88, 1731–1737.

Lee, Y. R., Tsunekawa, K., Moon, M. J., Um, H. N., Hwang, J. I., Osugi, T., et al. (2009). Molecular evolution of multiple forms of kisspeptins and GPR54 receptors in vertebrates. *Endocrinology* 150, 2837–2846.

Li, S., Zhang, Y., Liu, Y., Huang, X., Huang, W., Lu, D., et al. (2009). Structural and functional multiplicity of the kisspeptin/GPR54 system in goldfish (*Carassius auratus*). *J. Endocrinol.* 201, 407–418.

Pinilla, L., Aguilar, E., Dieguez, C., Millar, R. P., and Tena-Sempere, M. (2012). Kisspeptins and reproduction: physiological roles and regulatory mechanisms. *Physiol. Rev.* 92, 1235–1316.

Seminara, S. B., Messager, S., Chatzidaki, E. E., Thresher, R. R., Acierno, J. S., Shagoury, J. K., et al. (2003). The GPR54 gene as a regulator of puberty. *N. Engl. J. Med.* 349, 1614–1627.

Servili, A., Le Page, Y., Leprince, J., Caraty, A., Escobar, S., Parhar, I. S., et al. (2011). Organization of two independent kisspeptin systems derived from evolutionary-ancient kiss genes in the brain of zebrafish. *Endocrinology* 152, 1527–1540.

Tena-Sempere, M., Felip, A., Gomez, A., Zanuy, S., and Carrillo, M. (2012). Comparative insights of the kisspeptin/kisspeptin receptor system: lessons from non-mammalian vertebrates. *Gen. Comp. Endocrinol.* 175, 234–243.

Tomikawa, J., Homma, T., Tajima, S., Shibata, T., Inamoto, Y., Takase, K., et al. (2010). Molecular characterization and estrogen regulation of hypothalamic KISS1 gene in the pig. *Biol. Reprod.* 82, 313–319.

Tomikawa, J., Uenoyama, Y., Ozawa, M., Fukanuma, T., Takase, K., Goto, T., et al. (2012). Epigenetic regulation of Kiss1 gene expression mediating estrogen-positive feedback action in the mouse brain. *Proc. Natl. Acad. Sci. U.S.A.* 109, E1294–E1301.

Van de Peer, Y., Maere, S., and Meyer, A. (2010). 2R or not 2R is not the question anymore. *Nat. Rev. Genet.* 11, 166.

Venkatesh, B., Kirkness, E. F., Loh, Y. H., Halpern, A. L., Lee, A. P., Johnson, J., et al. (2007). Survey sequencing and comparative analysis of the elephant shark (*Callorhinchus milii*) genome. *PLoS Biol.* 5:e101. doi:10.1371/journal.pbio.0050101

Zmora, N., Stubblefield, J., Zulperi, Z., Biran, J., Levavi-Sivan, B., Munoz-Cueto, J. A., et al. (2012). Differential and gonad stage-dependent roles of Kisspeptin1 and Kisspeptin2 in reproduction in the modern teleosts, morone species. *Biol. Reprod.* 86:177. doi:10.1095/biolreprod.111.097667

Meyer, A., and Van de Peer, Y. (2005). From 2R to 3R: evidence for a fish-specific genome duplication (FSGD). *Bioessays* 27, 937–945.

Muffato, M., Louis, A., Poisnel, C. E., and Roest Crollius, H. (2010). Genomicus: a database and a browser to study gene synteny in modern and ancestral genomes. *Bioinformatics* 26, 1119–1121.

Muir, A. I., Chamberlain, L., Elshourbagy, N. A., Michalovich, D., Moore, D. J., Calamari, A., et al. (2001). AXOR12, a novel human G protein-coupled receptor, activated by the peptide KiSS-1. *J. Biol. Chem.* 276, 28969–28975.

Nakatani, Y., Takeda, H., Kohara, Y., and Morishita, S. (2007). Reconstruction of the vertebrate ancestral genome reveals dynamic genome reorganization in early vertebrates. *Genome Res.* 17, 1254–1265.

Pasquier, J., Lafont, A.-G., Jeng, S.-R., Morini, M., Dirks, R., van den Thillart, G., et al. (2012). Multiple kisspeptin receptors in early osteichthyans provide new insights into the evolution of this receptor family. *PLoS ONE* 7:e48931. doi:10.1371/journal.pone.0048931

Pasquier, J., Lafont, A. G., Leprince, J., Vaudry, H., Rousseau, K., and Dufour, S. (2011). First evidence for a direct inhibitory effect of kisspeptins on LH expression in the eel, Anguilla anguilla. *Gen. Comp. Endocrinol.* 173, 216–225.

## APPENDIX

**A European eel Kiss1 ORF (Contig 384214.1)**

```
  1 - TCG ACC GAG GCC CCG CCC TAC CCG CAC CGC CCC GCC CAC TGG CCC ACC GCA CTG GCC AAT CCA CTG  -  66
  1 -  S   T   E   A   P   P   Y   P   H   R   P   A   H   W   P   T   A   L   A   N   P   L   -  22

 67 - CCG GGA GGG GCC GGC CTT CCC AGG AGG TCG TGG TGG TGG TAC CCC GAG GTG CCG CCA CAA GCG GCC  - 132
 23 -  P   G   G   A   G   L   P   R   R   S   W   W   W   Y   P   E   V   P   P   Q   A   A   -  44

133 - AAG AAG CGG GAA AAC TTC TCC TCC TAC AAC TGG AAC TCT TTC GGT TTA CGT TAT GGG AAA TGA      - 195
 45 -  K   K   R   E   N   F   S   S   Y   N   W   N   S   F   G   L   R   Y   G   K   *       -  65
```

**B European eel Kiss2 ORF (Scaffold 13.1)**

```
  1 - TTT ATT AAC ATG CTT TGT GTT CAT CGT CTA GGT TCT CTG TAT CCA GAG CGT GCG TCT GCT GGG GTC  -  66
  1 -  F   I   N   M   L   C   V   H   R   L   G   S   L   Y   P   E   R   A   S   A   G   V   -  22

 67 - TGG GAC CGC TCT AAA GTA CTG AGA GAA GTC ACG GGT CCG AAT TAT TCA GAC GAA GCA GAT CTC TGC  - 132
 23 -  W   D   R   S   K   V   L   R   E   V   T   G   P   N   Y   S   D   E   A   D   L   C   -  44

133 - TTC TTC CTG AAA GAC AGT GAA ATC GAG GGC CAC ATT TCC TGC CGA CTC CGA TAC TCT CGA AGC AAA  - 198
 45 -  F   F   L   K   D   S   E   I   E   G   H   I   S   C   R   L   R   Y   S   R   S   K   -  66

199 - TTC AAC CGC AAT CCG TTC GGT CTC CGT TTT GGA AAA CGT GAG TGG AGT TAC CTT CCC AAG AGC AAA  - 264
 67 -  F   N   R   N   P   F   G   L   R   F   G   K   R   E   W   S   Y   L   P   K   S   K   -  88

265 - ACT GCA AAA CCC GGG ACA AGC AAG CTT CTC CCC TAT CTA CTG TAC ATC CAA GAG CGG AAA GCC TGA  - 330
 89 -  T   A   K   P   G   T   S   K   L   L   P   Y   L   L   Y   I   Q   E   R   K   A   *   - 110
```

**FIGURE A1 | Prediction of two *Kiss* ORFs from the European eel genome.** Nucleotide and deduced amino-acid sequences of the ORF encoding the European eel Kp1(10) **(A)** and Kp2(10) **(B)**. Nucleotides (top) are numbered from 5′ to 3′. The amino-acid residues (bottom) are numbered beginning with the first amino-acid residue encoded by the ORF. The asterisk (*) indicates the stop codon. The predicted Kp(10) are underlined. The amino-acids of the C-terminal α-amidation and cleavage site are shaded in gray.

**A Spotted gar Kiss1 ORF (LG3)**

```
  1 - AAC CAG AAC TCG GCA TTA TGG TCA GCC CTG CAT TTG CCA AAT CAC ATG TTT CCG TCC TTT CCA GTG  -  66
  1 -  N   Q   N   S   A   L   W   S   A   L   H   L   P   N   H   M   F   P   S   F   P   V  -  22

 67 - TCG GGG AAG AAG CCG GAG CCC GGC GTG CAG GAC ATC CTG AGA CGG ATG AGC ACC ACG CCC CCG CCA  - 132
 23 -  S   G   K   K   P   E   P   G   V   Q   D   I   L   R   R   M   S   T   T   P   P   P  -  44

133 - GGA GCT CGC CTG ATC CTG CCT GCC GCT GGG AAG ATT CCC CCT GCG CTG GCC AGC CTG CTG TTC GGG  - 198
 45 -  G   A   R   L   I   L   P   A   A   G   K   I   P   P   A   L   A   S   L   L   F   G  -  66

199 - TCT CGG TTC CCC AGG AGG GGC GGG TGG GCT CAG GCG AGA CCC CAG CCC CCC GCT GCG AAA CGA GAG  - 264
 67 -  S   R   F   P   R   R   G   G   W   A   Q   A   R   P   Q   P   P   A   A   K   R   E  -  88

265 - AAG AAC CTT TCC GCC TAC AAC TGG AAT TCC TTC GGG CTC CGT TAC GGA AAA CGC CGG TCA AAC ACC  - 330
 89 -  K   N   L   S   A   Y   N   W   N   S   F   G   L   R   Y   G   K   R   R   S   N   T  - 110

331 - CCG CCG CCG CAG CTC GGC TGA                                                              - 351
111 -  P   P   P   Q   L   G   *                                                               - 117
```

**B Spotted gar Kiss2 ORF (LG8)**

```
  1 - GCA CCT GTG CAC GCA GCC AGC ACA CCT GCC GGT CTC GGA AGC CTG CCC CAC CTG GCG GTG AGG GAG  -  66
  1 -  A   P   V   H   A   A   S   T   P   A   G   L   G   S   L   P   H   L   A   V   R   E  -  22

 67 - GTT GAA GGT CCA AAT TCG GCA GAC CAG GCG AGT CTC TGC TAC TTT GTC CAA GAG AGC GAA GTG GAG  - 132
 23 -  V   E   G   P   N   S   A   D   Q   A   S   L   C   Y   F   V   Q   E   S   E   V   E  -  44

133 - AGT CAG ATC TCC TGC AAA CTC CGT TTC ACC CGG AGT AAA TTT AAC TTC AAT CCG TTT GGA CTT CGC  - 198
 45 -  S   Q   I   S   C   K   L   R   F   T   R   S   K   F   N   F   N   P   F   G   L   R  -  66

199 - TTC GGA AAG CGC AAC AGG AAT ATC GTG GCC AAC GAC AGG AGC GCT ATA CCC AGT GAG CTG TTG CTT  - 264
 67 -  F   G   K   R   N   R   N   I   V   A   N   D   R   S   A   I   P   S   E   L   L   L  -  88

265 - TAC CTG CTG TAC CTC AAA GAG ACG GGC CTG GCC CCT TGA                                      - 303
 89 -  Y   L   L   Y   L   K   E   T   G   L   A   P   *                                       - 101
```

**FIGURE A2 | Prediction of two *Kiss* ORFs from the spotted gar genome.** Nucleotide and deduced amino-acid sequences of the ORF encoding the spotted gar Kp1(10) **(A)** and Kp2(10) **(B)**. Nucleotides (top) are numbered from 5′ to 3′. The amino-acid residues (bottom) are numbered beginning with the first amino-acid residue encoded by the ORF. The asterisk (*) indicates the stop codon. The predicted Kp(10) are underlined. The amino-acids of the C-terminal α-amidation and cleavage site are shaded in gray.

**A Coe a a t Kiss1 ORF ( H126665 1)**

```
  1 - TTT TTA CTG TAT TTC TAT TTT TTT TCC CTT TTT GCT TTA GGT GAA GTT CTG AAA GCT ATC GCC AGT  -  66
  1 -  F   L   L   Y   F   Y   F   F   S   L   F   A   L   G   E   V   L   K   A   I   A   S   -  22

 67 - GGG CTT CTA CAG AAG GAG GAA AGT GCT CCT TGT TTG GTC CAA ACT CCG CAG TCC AGA ACC CAG CAT  - 132
 23 -  G   L   L   Q   K   E   E   S   A   P   C   L   V   Q   T   P   Q   S   R   T   Q   H   -  44

133 - CCA AAA ATG CTG CGT CCC CTC GTC AAG CTG TTT GAT CTC AAG CAC GGG AGT AGA CCT AGG ATT TCA  - 198
 45 -  P   K   M   L   R   P   L   V   K   L   F   D   L   K   H   G   S   R   P   R   I   S   -  66

199 - CGG AAA ATC GGG CTC TCC CTG TGC AAG TTT AAC TCG AGC TCC CTC GGA GTG CAA ACC GTT AAA CGA  - 264
 67 -  R   K   I   G   L   S   L   C   K   F   N   S   S   S   L   G   V   Q   T   V   K   R   -  88

265 - GAA AAT GAC CTC TCC TCC TAC AAC TGG AAC ACT TTT GGA CTG AGA TAT GGG AAA AGG CAA GCA GGA  - 330
 89 -  E   N   D   L   S   S   Y   N   W   N   T   F   G   L   R   Y   G   K   R   Q   A   G   - 110

331 - ACA CTG AAA GCC CAA AGT AAC ATA TGG AAG ATT TGA                                          - 366
111 -  T   L   K   A   Q   S   N   I   W   K   I   *                                           - 122
```

**B Coe a a t Kiss2 ORF ( H127043 1)**

```
  1 - TTA CGC ATA GCT AGT GCT ACC ATT ATT CAC TCT TAT TTT ATT TTT GTC TTG TGT TTA TTC TTC CTT  -  66
  1 -  L   R   I   A   S   A   T   I   I   H   S   Y   F   I   F   V   L   C   L   F   F   L   -  22

 67 - TTG GTT GCA GTT TAC CCA CTC AGT GAA GCA GAA GCC GAA AGA CAG TCC CAC CAC ATG ACC CGA GAT  - 132
 23 -  L   V   A   V   Y   P   L   S   E   A   E   A   E   R   Q   S   H   H   M   T   R   D   -  44

133 - ATA GAT GCC CAG AAC TCC GCA GAA CAT GCT AGT CTC TGC TAC TTT GTC CAG GAG AGT GAA ATC GAG  - 198
 45 -  I   D   A   Q   N   S   A   E   H   A   S   L   C   Y   F   V   Q   E   S   E   I   E   -  66

199 - AGC CAG ATC TCC TGC AGA CTT CGA TTT ACC AGG AGT AAA TTT AAC TTC AAC CCC TTT GGA CTT CGC  - 264
 67 -  S   Q   I   S   C   R   L   R   F   T   R   S   K   F   N   F   N   P   F   G   L   R   -  88

265 - TTT GGA AAA CGT GGT CAG AGC AGC TCC AGC AAC AGG AAT CCT GTT TTG GTT AGC AGG AAA TTA ATA  - 330
 89 -  F   G   K   R   G   Q   S   S   S   S   N   R   N   P   V   L   V   S   R   K   L   I   - 110

331 - CCA CAA TAC CTA CTG AAA CTA AAA GAA AGC AGA ATG CTG GAA TGT GAG GAC TCC AGC GAT TAT TGT  - 396
111 -  P   Q   Y   L   L   K   L   K   E   S   R   M   L   E   C   E   D   S   S   D   Y   C   - 132

397 - TAA                                                                                      - 399
133 -  *                                                                                       - 154
```

**C Coe a a t Kiss3 ORF ( H126891 1)**

```
  1 - TTC AGC AAG AGA GGC AGT AAG TTC AAC TGG AAC TCG TTC GGG CTG CGT TTT GGG AAA AAG CAC CAG  -  66
  1 -  F   S   K   R   G   S   K   F   N   W   N   S   F   G   L   R   F   G   K   K   H   Q   -  22

 67 - ATG CCA TTC CCA CTT TGA                                                                  -  84
 23 -  M   P   F   P   L   *                                                                   -  28
```

**FIGURE A3 | Prediction of three *Kiss* ORFs from the coelacanth genome.** Nucleotide and deduced amino-acid sequences of the ORF encoding the coelacanth Kp1(10) **(A)**, Kp2(10) **(B)**, and Kp3(10) **(C)**. Nucleotides (top) are numbered from 5′ to 3′. The amino-acid residues (bottom) are numbered beginning with the first amino-acid residue encoded by the ORF. The asterisk (*) indicates the stop codon. The predicted Kp(10) are underlined. The amino-acids of the C-terminal α-amidation and cleavage site are shaded in gray.

**E ep a t s ar Kiss3 ORF (AAV 01250489 1)**

```
  1 - ATA CTT TGG GTC CAT TTG TTT TTA GCA GCA GAG GTG AAG AGC GCG GGA CAC CGA GGT GAT GGA AGC  -  66
  1 -  I   L   W   V   H   L   F   L   A   A   E   V   K   S   A   G   H   R   G   D   G   S   -  22

 67 - CTG CTG TCT TGC AGC ACT GCG AAG GGA GCA CTC CTT TGG CTC AGC AGG CCA GAC CCC AAG ACT TCA  - 132
 23 -  L   L   S   C   S   T   A   K   G   A   L   L   W   L   S   R   P   D   P   K   T   S   -  44

133 - GCC CCA CCG AAG CCG AGT GGA CCA CAG AGA GAT TGC ATC AGG AAA ATC CTG ACC AGT TTC CAC ACC  - 198
 45 -  A   P   P   K   P   S   G   P   Q   R   D   C   I   R   K   I   L   T   S   F   H   T   -  66

199 - CAG AGT CGG CCA AAG AAG AAC ACG TGG GCC AGC TAC AAT CTC AAC TCC TTC GGT CTG AAG TTT GGC  - 264
 67 -  Q   S   R   P   K   K   N   T   W   A   S   Y   N   L   N   S   F   G   L   K   F   G   -  88

265 - AAA CGG CTG CCG AGG TCC AAG AGG AAC GGT TGG AGG TTG AGA TTC GGG GAG TAG                  - 318
 89 -  K   R   L   P   R   S   K   R   N   G   W   R   L   R   F   G   E   *                   - 106
```

**FIGURE A4 | Prediction of a third *Kiss* ORF from the elephant shark genome.** Nucleotide and deduced amino-acid sequences of the ORF encoding the elephant shark Kp3(10). Nucleotides (top) are numbered from 5′ to 3′. The amino-acid residues (bottom) are numbered beginning with the first amino-acid residue encoded by the ORF. The asterisk (*) indicates the stop codon. The predicted Kp(10) is underlined. The amino-acids of the C-terminal α-amidation and cleavage site are shaded in gray.

# 20

# Evolution of vertebrate GnRH receptors from the perspective of a basal vertebrate

**_Stacia A. Sower*, Wayne A. Decatur, Nerine T. Joseph and Mihael Freamat_**

*Department of Molecular, Cellular and Biomedical Sciences, Center for Molecular and Comparative Endocrinology, University of New Hampshire, Durham, NH, USA*

***Edited by:***
*Hubert Vaudry, University of Rouen, France*

***Reviewed by:***
*Olivier Kah, CNRS UMR 6026, France*
*Jae Young Seong, Korea University, Korea*

****Correspondence:***
*Stacia A. Sower, Department of Molecular, Cellular and Biomedical Sciences, Center for Molecular and Comparative Endocrinology, University of New Hampshire, 46 College Road, Durham, NH 03824-3544, USA.*
*e-mail: sasower@unh.edu*

This minireview provides the current status on gonadotropin-releasing hormone receptors (GnRH-R) in vertebrates, from the perspective of a basal vertebrate, the sea lamprey, and provides an évolutionary scheme based on the recent advance of whole genome sequencing. In addition, we provide a perspective on the functional divergence and evolution of the receptors. In this review we use the phylogenetic classification of vertebrate GnRH receptors that groups them into three clusters: type I (mammalian and non-mammalian), type II, and type III GnRH receptors. New findings show that the sea lamprey has two type III-like GnRH receptors and an ancestral type GnRH receptor that is more closely related to the type II-like receptors. These two novel GnRH receptors along with lGnRH-R-1 share similar structural features and amino acid motifs common to other known gnathostome type II/III receptors. Recent data analyses of the lamprey genome provide strong evidence that two whole rounds of genome duplication (2R) occurred prior to the gnathostome-agnathan split. Based on our current knowledge, it is proposed that lGnRH-R-1 evolved from an ancestor of the type II receptor following a vertebrate-shared genome duplication and that the two type III receptors resulted from a duplication within lamprey of a gene derived from a lineage shared by many vertebrates.

**Keywords: gonadotropin-releasing hormone receptors, G protein-coupled receptors, evolution, lamprey, basal vertebrate, receptor, hormone, pituitary**

## INTRODUCTION

The study of gonadotropin-releasing hormone (GnRH) receptors in basal and later-evolved vertebrates can provide insight into the evolution and molecular mechanisms of signaling of this receptor family. Numerous full-length GnRH receptor (GnRH-R) sequences have been identified, with more than one receptor isoform identified within a single species. In most vertebrates there are usually two to three forms of GnRH-Rs present (Millar, 2005), although there are fewer GnRH-R genes in mammals compared to protochordates, fish, and amphibians (Morgan and Millar, 2004). To date, there is only a partial understanding of the physiological significance of each receptor type in regards to the spatial expression of GnRH-Rs since more than one receptor type can be expressed in the same tissue.

Of the numerous available forms of GnRH-R nomenclature that have been proposed by several investigators, in this review, we use the phylogenetic classification in which three distinct classes of GnRH-Rs from the vertebrate lineage group into separate clusters: type I (mammalian and non-mammalian), type II, and type III GnRH-Rs (Millar, 2005), with a new slight modification based on partial synteny analysis. Vertebrate type I GnRH-Rs are represented in teleosts, amphibians, reptiles, and avian species and in mammals. The type II GnRH-Rs include receptors from amphibians, reptiles, and mammals; however, type II GnRH-Rs are inactivated in most mammals studied to date (Stewart et al., 2009). Unlike the type II GnRH-Rs, the type III GnRH-Rs include sequences from teleost fish, amphibians, reptiles, and avian species but do not occur in mammals. New findings show that an ancestral extant vertebrate, the lamprey, has two type III-like GnRH-Rs and an ancestral type GnRH-R that is more closely related to the type II-like GnRH-Rs (Joseph et al., 2012). Based on our current knowledge, it is proposed that lGnRH-R-1 evolved from an ancestor of the type II receptor following a vertebrate-shared genome duplication and that the two type III receptors resulted from a duplication within lamprey of a gene derived from a lineage shared by many vertebrates.

Gonadotropin-releasing hormone action is mediated through high affinity binding with the GnRH receptor (GnRH-R), a rhodopsin-like seven transmembrane G protein-coupled receptor (GPCR). Pituitary GnRH receptors are thought to signal primarily through $G\alpha_{q/11}$, resulting in the stimulation of the inositol phosphate (IP) second messenger system; however, $G\alpha_s$ activation and cAMP signaling have been reported as well (Arora et al., 1995; Stanislaus et al., 1998; Grosse et al., 2000; Liu et al., 2002; Oh et al., 2005).

Lampreys along with hagfish are the only living representatives of the agnathans, the most ancient class of vertebrates, whose lineage dates back over 550 million years (Sower et al., 2009). Lampreys, which express three hypothalamic peptides of GnRH, lamprey GnRH-I, -II, and -III are important to our understanding of the reproductive endocrinology of the first vertebrates and are likely to have retained key characteristics of the ancestral GnRH and GnRH receptor from which modern GnRH isoforms and GnRH receptors arose, as reviewed (Sower et al., 2009).

## MOLECULAR EVOLUTION

As a basal vertebrate, the sea lamprey is well positioned to give us insight into the evolution of the GnRH receptors, particularly in reference to the seminal event of the acquisition of the hypothalamic-pituitary-gonadal axis in vertebrates (Sower et al., 2009). In framing this review, it is important to recognize that there are substantial factors acting in this immensely broad and profound transition that started approximately 550 million years ago with the beginnings of the vertebrate lineages. This shift was facilitated by two rounds of whole-genomic duplication (WGD) between the divergence of the protochordates and the lineage leading to modern vertebrates (Putnam et al., 2008; Van de Peer et al., 2010). Up until very recently, the placement of these two rounds of WGD relative to the split of the agnathans and gnathostomes was in question with the prevailing view placing the second round after the branching of the lamprey from the vertebrate lineage (see for example, Andreakis et al., 2011; Dores, 2011; Parmentier et al., 2011). Recent analysis of the numbers of paralogous gene regions and the pattern of shared synteny represented in the current sea lamprey genome assembly provides new evidence supporting two rounds of WGD occurring prior to the split of the agnathans and gnathostomes (Smith et al., submitted).

Recent identification and phylogenetic analysis of the three GnRH receptors in the sea lamprey (Joseph et al., 2012) in tandem with a reasonable-quality genome assembly (Smith et al., submitted) followed by more in-depth synteny analysis will help to elucidate the overall molecular evolution of the GnRH receptor family. Indeed, a similar approach has been most illuminating in the case of the family of vertebrate GnRHs. Shared synteny analysis of the genome (Decatur et al., 2011; Smith et al., submitted) clarified the ancestry of the genes for the lamprey GnRH peptides compared to the previous extensive phylogenetic studies that had been done (Guilgur et al., 2006; Kah et al., 2007; Kavanaugh et al., 2008; Okubo and Nagahama, 2008; Tsai and Zhang, 2008; Zhang et al., 2008). The synteny data provide evidence for an alternate view of the evolution of the GnRH peptide family and suggest that all duplication events that generated the different fish and tetrapod GnRH groups likely took place before the split of the ancestral lamprey and gnathostome lineages (Smith et al., submitted). The lamprey GnRH-I and -III, formerly referred to as group IV (Kavanaugh et al., 2008; Zhang et al., 2008) share a more recent common ancestry with GnRH2 and three paralogs (Decatur et al., 2011).

However, in the case of the GnRH receptors themselves, the state of the lamprey genome assembly precludes full analyses of the shared synteny, and genomic structure (**Figure 1**). Although half of the assembly is in scaffolds of 173 kb or longer (Smith et al., submitted), significant portions of the genome remain incompletely assembled and prevents investigations of many of the neuroendocrine genes in lamprey (Decatur et al., 2011). A similar issue was faced by Meyer and colleagues in their work resolving orthology of vertebrate genes (Qiu et al., 2011). These authors concluded that single exon genes are the best candidates to use given the current state of the assembly (Qiu et al., 2011). The genes for the lamprey GnRH peptides possess introns in the coding region except one (Kavanaugh et al., 2008) and the genes themselves encode small precursors (ca. 90 amino acids) that serendipitously fall on scaffolds of much larger size (95 and 302 kb) than those of the GnRH receptors. The open reading frame for the GnRH receptors in lamprey are substantially larger than those of the GnRH precursor and span three exons and two introns, similar to GnRH receptor genes of gnathostomes and even some genes of the protochordate

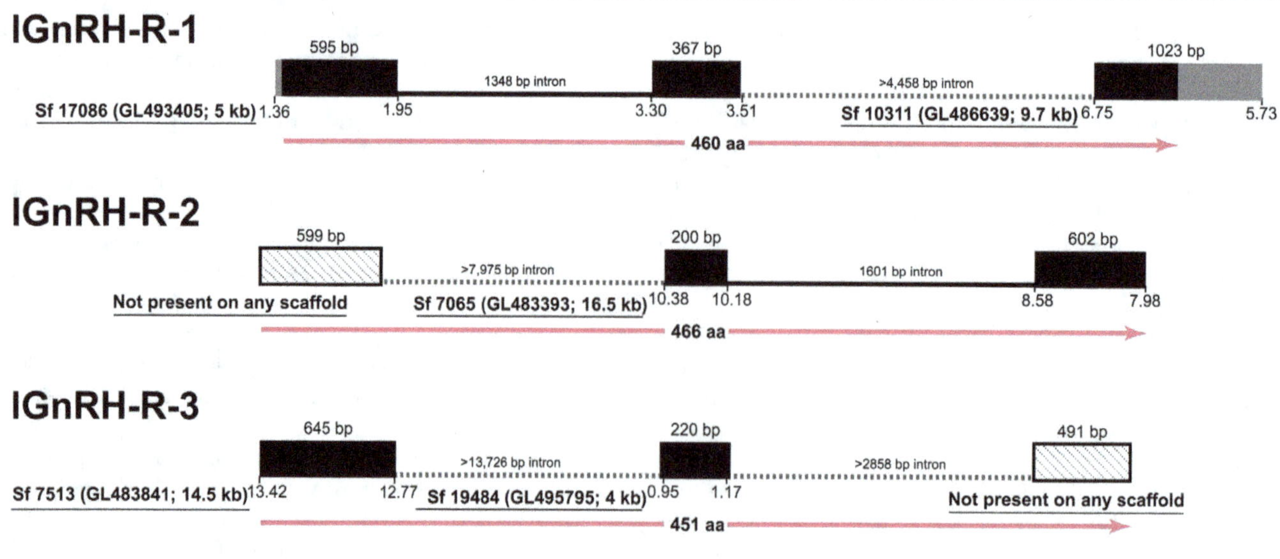


**FIGURE 1 | Gene structure of the three GnRH receptors in lamprey in the context of the current gene assembly.** Exons are represented as black boxes with 5′- and 3′-UTRs in gray. In cases of incomplete data, angled-stippled fill is used for exons identified by cDNA sequencing that are not present among assembled scaffolds, and minimum lengths of the introns are provided based on the available flanking sequences of the scaffolds. Sf, Scaffold from Lamprey genome project consortium; details of the Ensembl scaffold designation are provided in parentheses, along with the size rounded to kilobase (kb). The position on the scaffold corresponding to the transcribed regions is below the boxes. At the bottom of each structure, the length of the deduced protein is given in amino acids with.

amphioxus (Tello and Sherwood, 2009). A number of factors, including the high GC-content, vast numbers of repetitive elements, and dramatic genetic rearrangements that occur during somatic cell development, have been suggested as contributing to the challenge of sequencing and assembling a complete version of the lamprey genome (Smith et al., 2009, submitted).

Accepting these limitations, we can use the initial characterization of the lamprey GnRH receptor evolution proposed by Kim et al. (2011) that was based on shared synteny and provide a new current model on GnRH receptor evolution based on the latest, although limited, synteny from the lamprey genome and our recent phylogenetic analysis (**Figure 2**). Maximum likelihood-based phylogenetic analysis showed a substantial degree of similarity (ca. 55% identity) between lamprey GnRH receptor 2 and 3 suggesting that these genes shared a recent ancestor. We further propose that they arose by local tandem or segmental duplication of one of the receptors within the lamprey lineage (Joseph et al., 2012). Based on this information, we expect lamprey GnRH receptors 2 and 3 are on the lineage shared by the zebrafish type III GnRH receptor, whereas lamprey GnRH receptor 1 is most similar to the lineage on which the mammalian type II receptor occurs. Teleost fish have undergone a third round (3R) of WGD. Following 3R, there was retention of some of these paralogs resulting in a greater number of GnRH receptor genes in teleosts (Kim et al., 2011).

## FUNCTIONAL DIVERGENCE OF GNRH RECEPTORS

As a measure of function, we looked at the binding characteristics of the GnRH receptors using GnRH ligands, and as a measure of receptor activation we looked at the signal transduction (Joseph et al., 2012). In an attempt to decipher the evolutionary lineage of specific motifs in terms of binding ability and signal transduction, we compared the three identified lamprey GnRH receptors (lGnRH-R-1, lGnRH-R-2, and lGnRH-R-3) with GnRH receptors of later vertebrates. Given the limited synteny data, we will describe this functional divergence of the GnRH receptors based solely in phylogenetic analysis, and not incorporate the emerging new current model on GnRH receptor evolution (described above). On the premise that lGnRH-R-1 evolved from a common ancestor of the type II GnRH receptor, we propose that identification of key motifs can assist in the elucidation of these motifs/residues in terms of evolutionary stringency. lGnRH-R-2 and lGnRH-R-3 which likely occurred due to a local gene duplication in the lamprey lineage may provide evidence of plasticity in amino acid residue functionality. The table below summarizes the key motifs of binding kinetics and signal transduction through studies on vertebrates in relation to those of an extant agnathan, the lamprey (**Table 1**).

All three GnRH receptors in the lamprey have similar nonmammalian GnRH receptor characteristics (Zhou et al., 1994; Flanagan et al., 1999; Millar et al., 2004). However in terms of ligand binding, there is less conservation of key residues in lGnRH-R-1 compared to the two type III lGnRH receptors. Of the four ligand binding residues considered, two His residues are substituted in lGnRH-R-1 for Asn (Davidson et al., 1996) and Glu (Flanagan et al., 1994), suggesting there is less conservation of key residues in lGnRH-R-1 when compared to the type III lamprey GnRH receptors. However, lGnRH-R-1 remains as the only lamprey receptor displaying an affinity to lGnRH-I, despite all the lamprey receptors coding for Asp in the helix2/7 microdomain,

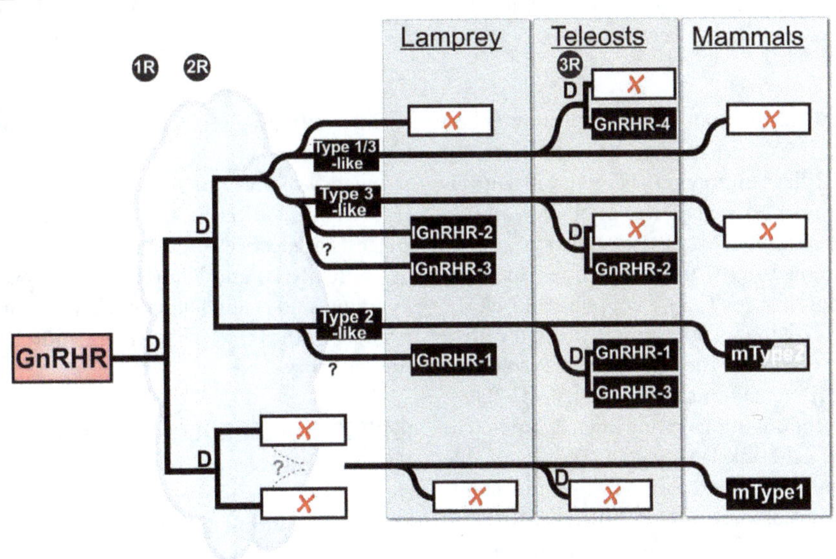


**FIGURE 2 | Working Hypothesis on the evolution of the GnRH receptor gene family in vertebrates with emphasis on placement of the lamprey genes.** "D" represents duplication events for each of the 3 rounds of whole genome duplication in vertebrate evolution (1R, 2R, and 3R), the third being specific to teleosts. Open rectangles with red X's indicate lost loci. Zebrafish are used here as a representative for teleosts. The half-shaded box for mammalian Type2 indicates that there is no functional gene product produced in several mammals, including humans. The cloud suggests the ambiguity concerning the relative time between early events, in particular the duration available for resolution of duplicated paralogs between the last common whole genome duplication event and the split of the agnathans from the gnathostome lineage. The dashed lines specify a proposed gene translocation, see Kim et al. (2011) for details and more vertebrates.

**Table 1 | Comparison of characteristics contributing to non-mammalian receptors and motifs pertaining to ligand binding and receptor activation of GnRH-R types.**

| | **Motif/ residue** | **Mammalian (gnathostome)** | | | **Amphibian (gnathostome)** | | | **Petromyzonids (agnatha)** | |
|---|---|---|---|---|---|---|---|---|---|
| Species | | Human | Mouse | | Bullfrog | | | Sea lamprey | |
| Receptor type | | Type I | Type I | Type I | Type II | Type III | Type III | Type III | Ancestral type |
| Receptor abbreviation | | hGnRH-R | mGnRH-R | bfGnRH-R-2 | bfGnRH-R-3 | bfGnRH-R-1 | lGnRH-R-2 | lGnRH-R-3 | lGnRH-R −1 |
| Non-mammalian characteristic | C-terminal tail<br>Asp, helix 2, and helix 7 MD | No<br>Asn in helix 2, Asp in helix 7 | No<br>Asn in helix 2, Asp in helix 7 | Yes<br>Asp in helix 2 and 7 | Yes<br>Asp in helix 2 and 7 | Yes<br>Asp in helix 2 and 7 | Yes<br>Asp in helix 2 and 7 | Yes<br>Asp in helix 2 and 7 | Yes<br>Asp in helix 2 and 7 |
| Ligand binding | Asp, TMD 2<br>Asn, TMD 2<br>Lys, TMD 3<br>"SE/DP" motif ECL 3 | Asp<br>Asn<br>Lys<br>SDP | Asp<br>Asn<br>Lys<br>SEP | Asp<br>Asn<br>Lys<br>PEY | Asp<br>Asn<br>Lys<br>PPS | Asp<br>Asn<br>Lys<br>SQS | Asp<br>Asn<br>Lys<br>PEA | Asp<br>Asn<br>Lys<br>PEY | Asp<br>His<br>Arg<br>PHF |
| $G\alpha_{q/11}$ coupling motifs | Leu, IL 2, and the Arg cage motif "D/ERY/XXXI/V" | Leu and DRSLAI | Leu and DRSLAI | Leu and DRHWAI | Leu and DRHAAI | Leu and DRQSAI | Leu and DRHAAV | Leu and DRYSAV | Leu and DRHSAI |
| | Ala, ICL3<br>Leu, IL 3 | Ala<br>Leu | Ala<br>Leu | Ala<br>Ile | Ala<br>Ile | Ala<br>Ile | Ala<br>Ile | Ala<br>Ile | Ala<br>Ile |
| cAMP | HFRK motif K71LSR75; L58;L80 | (no C-tail)<br>KLSR; L; L | (no C-tail)<br>KLSR; L; L | SFKE<br>CKSH; C; I | HFRR<br>KKSH; W; I | HFRK<br>KRSH; W; I | PLGP<br>RRSH; W;L | QWDG<br>RGSH; R;L | HVRR motif<br>TKSH; C;I |

*Representative sequences of non-mammalian type I GnRH-Rs (mouse and human) and amphibian type I, II, and III GnRH-Rs (bullfrog) were compared with the three identified GnRH receptors in the lamprey (Flanagan et al., 1994, 1999; Zhou et al., 1994, 1995; Arora et al., 1995, 1997; Davidson et al., 1996; Ballesteros et al., 1998; Myburgh et al., 1998; Chung et al., 1999; Fromme et al., 2001; Kitanovic et al., 2001; Millar et al., 2004; Wang et al., 2004; Li et al., 2005; Oh et al., 2005).*

enabling binding of configured and non-configured ligands (Zhou et al., 1994; Flanagan et al., 1999). Perhaps there are motifs retained within the ancestral type II-like lamprey GnRH receptor (lGnRH-R-1) that were stringently selected for in terms of binding affinity which would need to be determined by mutation analysis.

In relation to the examined signal transduction residues and motifs known to be responsible for $G\alpha_{q/11}$ coupling and cAMP accumulation there are no striking substitutions between the three lamprey GnRH receptors except for the HFRK motif recognized for its attribution for cAMP signal transduction (Oh et al., 2005). lGnRH-R-1 has less substitutions at this motif when compared to the type III lGnRH-Rs and is the only lamprey GnRH receptor able to result in cAMP accumulation when activated by endogenous ligands (Kavanaugh et al., 2008; Joseph et al., 2012). lGnRH-R-1, which is proposed to have arisen from a common ancestor of type II receptors, retained this feature compared to the type III lamprey GnRH receptors that do not have this HRFK-like motif. It is difficult to attribute receptor types to specific signal transduction pathways, although it will be more feasible, when more representative receptors from each vertebrate are examined. However, it may remain that the plasticity in formation of signal transduction complexes drives the retention of specific GnRH receptor types.

Interestingly, given lGnRH-R-1 remains as the only receptor to bind to lGnRH-I (Joseph et al., 2012), investigation of evolutionary stringency of receptor residues/motifs in comparing lGnRH-R-1 (type II-like GnRH receptor) and other type II GnRH receptors suggests a selective co-evolution of cognate ligand/receptor pairing of lGnRH-I and lGnRH-R-1. However, in terms of plasticity in amino acid residue functionality, we surmise that the examined residues of the type III lGnRH receptors are pertinent for receptor functionality.

## PHYSIOLOGICAL ROLES OF GnRH RECEPTORS

Physiological roles of GnRH receptor isoforms are the result of the combined effects of binding and activation of the receptor by one or multiple forms of GnRH at the molecular structural level and the spatio-temporal regulation of its expression in one or multiple tissues of an organism (True and Carroll, 2002). Major mutational events like whole genome duplications as well as local gene duplications generate new input for the evolutionary processes that result in creation of new morphological or functional characteristics. Functional divergence of protein sequences through neo- or sub-functionalization of protein sequences is one of the main mechanisms of the generation of evolutionary novelty.

Consequently, the last decade has seen an increase in the number of research studies dedicated to detection of the traces of purifying or adaptive changes in the coding regions of various proteins as well as to understanding of co-evolutionary mechanisms that link receptors to their ligands. We briefly reviewed here the main sequence determinants of ligand binding and signal transduction in GnRH receptors and their conservation from the perspective of sea lamprey isoforms.

In contrast, much less attention has been given to the other source of adaptive potential generated by duplication events, i.e., the non-coding genomic regions. Investigation of GnRH receptors, of their expression pattern in relation to their role in reproductive or non-reproductive physiological processes has generated a wealth of experimental data regarding these aspects in numerous vertebrate taxa. An overview of these data suggests that the GnRH/GnRH receptor system is a very interesting system to be approached from the perspective of the role of gene expression regulation in its evolution, given the relative promiscuity of GnRH receptors and their wide spectrum of tissue expression (Chen and Fernald, 2008). This is however a considerably more difficult endeavor than modeling the coding sequence evolution. At the DNA level, the regions of particular interest may include not only the *cis*-acting control elements of the target gene but also the *cis* elements of the network of *trans*-acting factors that ultimately determine the expression not only of the receptor but also of its GnRH ligands (Fraser, 2011).

The strength of lamprey as an evolutionary model is that no other organism is better positioned to offer clues in respect to the earliest events in the evolution of the neuroendocrine mechanisms in vertebrates. It has evolved directly from the jawless ancestor of all vertebrates, independently from the gnathostome radiation. Its pituitary (hypophysis) is probably a plesiomorphic character in vertebrates and given the surprising overall morphological similarity of this animal with lamprey-like Devonian fossils (Janvier, 2006), it may also reflect the ancestral organization of this gland. Moreover, the experimental evidence accumulated so far on the function of lamprey pituitary is consistent with its involvement in the endocrine control of reproduction (Sower and Kawauchi, 2001; Sower et al., 2009).

As mentioned before, lamprey receptor isoforms are hypothesized to belong to two paralogous lineages shared with the gnathostomes (type II and III). A likely local duplication event within the type III lineage resulted in subsequent divergence of the lamprey-specific GnRH-R 2 and 3 pair of paralogs. Similarly with their orthologs in a majority of the gnathostome lineages, tissue expression of the lamprey receptors show a diverse, frequently overlapping pattern, connected to their three main functional roles in brain, pituitary, and gonadal physiology. The recently found lGnRH-R-2 precursor transcript was detected in the pituitary as well as in a wide variety of non-reproductive tissues. Interestingly, the expression control of the lGnRH-R-3 precursor transcript seems to have sharply diverged from its more recent paralog, its expression was detected only in the brain and eye of male and female lampreys (Joseph et al., 2012). In addition it seems to exhibit a sexually dimorphic expression pattern, being detected in the ovary but not in the testes. The previously described lGnRH-R-1 showed limited expression, its transcripts being detected only in the pituitary and testes of sea lamprey (Silver et al., 2005). A diverse and often overlapping functionality appears to characterize their interaction with lamprey GnRH isoforms as well: the widely expressed lGnRH-R-2 is activated by hypothalamic lGnRH-III and in a lesser extent by ubiquitous lGnRH-II. lGnRH-R-3 from brain and eyes has lGnRH-II as putative main activator and in a lesser extent lGnRH-III. lGnRH-R-1 in pituitary and gonads is promiscuously activated by GnRH-I, -II and -III but the interaction with hypothalamic GnRH-I seems to be highly selective. An interesting aspect of the evolutionary history of the lamprey isoforms is that their functional diversity was initiated by duplication events that are estimated to have taken place on different scales in the genome, i.e., local gene duplication (2 and 3) versus whole genome duplication (2, 3, and 1). Since the local duplications are more likely to change the regulatory environment of a gene and therefore to induce an immediate major shift in gene expression, this might offer the opportunity to compare the non-coding versus coding sequence roles in influencing the fate of paralogs.

## SUMMARY

The accumulation of more data regarding the GnRH and GnRH receptors both in mammals as well as in more basal groups of vertebrates has started to unravel a more complex picture of their specificity of expression and ligand-receptor interaction. In turn, this leads to a more nuanced understanding of their physiological roles, both in relation to their central role in reproduction as well as outside the hypothalamic-pituitary system. Increase in the number of isoforms of vertebrate GnRH and GnRH receptors raises the question of their origin and of the evolutionary events and mechanisms that contributed to the situation seen in today's vertebrates.

The constant in the convoluted history of GnRH receptor in vertebrates is the organization of the hypothalamo-pituitary axis. Different vertebrate lineages have solved the question of neural control of pituitary gonadotropin secretion using different pieces of the material generated by successive genome and/or gene duplications.

Understanding of the evolutionary mechanisms that molded the GnRH regulation of reproduction in vertebrates by acting at the level of protein expression requires further knowledge on genetic and epigenetic mechanisms and understanding the change in the endocrine, paracrine, and neural pathways that converge into regulating the release of the ligand from the GnRH neurons and expression of receptors in gonadotropes.

## ACKNOWLEDGMENTS

This research was supported by NSF IOS-0849569. Partial funding was provided by the New Hampshire Agricultural Experiment Station. This is scientific contribution number 2489. We thank members of the Sea Lamprey Genome Consortium especially Drs. Weiming Li and Jeramiah Smith for their contributions in the annotation of the sea lamprey genome that provided key information for our synteny data.

## REFERENCES


Andreakis, N., D'Aniello, S., Albalat, R., Patti, F. P., Garcia-Fernandez, J., Procaccini, G., et al. (2011). Evolution of the nitric oxide synthase family in metazoans. *Mol. Biol. Evol.* 28, 163–179.

Arora, K. K., Cheng, Z., and Catt, K. J. (1997). Mutations of the conserved DRS motif in the second intracellular loop of the gonadotropin-releasing hormone receptor affect expression, activation, and internalization. *Mol. Endocrinol.* 11, 1203–1212.

Arora, K. K., Sakai, A., and Catt, K. J. (1995). Effects of second intracellular loop mutations on signal transduction and internalization of the gonadotropin-releasing hormone receptor. *J. Biol. Chem.* 270, 22820–22826.

Ballesteros, J., Kitanovic, S., Guarnieri, F., Davies, P., Fromme, B. J., Konvicka, K., et al. (1998). Functional microdomains in G-protein-coupled receptors. The conserved arginine-cage motif in the gonadotropin-releasing hormone receptor. *J. Biol. Chem.* 273, 10445–10453.

Chen, C. C., and Fernald, R. D. (2008). GnRH and GnRH receptors: distribution, function, and evolution. *J. Fish Biol.* 73, 1099–1120.

Chung, H. O., Yang, Q., Catt, K. J., and Arora, K. K. (1999). Expression and function of the gonadotropin-releasing hormone receptor are dependent on a conserved apolar amino acid in the third intracellular loop. *J. Biol. Chem.* 274, 35756–35762.

Davidson, J. S., McArdle, C. A., Davies, P., Elario, R., Flanagan, C. A., and Millar, R. P. (1996). Asn102 of the gonadotropin-releasing hormone receptor is a critical determinant of potency for agonists containing C-terminal glycinamide. *J. Biol. Chem.* 271, 15510–15514.

Decatur, W. A., Smith, J. J., Hall, J., Li, W., and Sower, S. A. (2011). "Annotation of the neuroendocrine-associated genes of the lamprey petromyzon marinus and the implications for evolution of vertebrate gonadotropin-releasing hormones," in: *Frontiers in Endocrinology Conference Abstract: NASCE 2011: The Inaugural Meeting of the North American Society for Comparative Endocrinology*, Ann Arbor.

Dores, R. M. (2011). Hagfish, genome duplications, and RFamide neuropeptide evolution. *Endocrinology* 152, 4010–4013.

Flanagan, C. A., Becker, I. I., Davidson, J. S., Wakefield, I. K., Zhou, W., Sealfon, S. C., et al. (1994). Glutamate 301 of the mouse gonadotropin-releasing hormone receptor confers specificity for arginine 8 of mammalian gonadotropin-releasing hormone. *J. Biol. Chem.* 269, 22636–22641.

Flanagan, C. A., Zhou, W., Chi, L., Yuen, T., Rodic, V., Robertson, D., et al. (1999). The functional microdomain in transmembrane helices 2 and 7 regulates expression, activation, and coupling pathways of the gonadotropin-releasing hormone receptor. *J. Biol. Chem.* 274, 28880–28886.

Fraser, H. B. (2011). Genome-wide approaches to the study of adaptive gene expression evolution: systematic studies of evolutionary adaptations involving gene expression will allow many fundamental questions in evolutionary biology to be addressed. *Bioessays* 33, 469–477.

Fromme, B. J., Katz, A. A., Roeske, R. W., Millar, R. P., and Flanagan, C. A. (2001). Role of aspartate 7.32(302) of the human gonadotropin-releasing hormone receptor in stabilizing a high-affinity ligand conformation. *Mol. Pharmacol.* 60, 1280–1287.

Grosse, R., Schmid, A., Schoneberg, T., Herrlich, A., Muhn, P., Schultz, G., et al. (2000). Gonadotropin-releasing hormone receptor initiates multiple signaling pathways by exclusively coupling to G(q/11) proteins. *J. Biol. Chem.* 275, 9193–9200.

Guilgur, L. G., Moncaut, N. P., Canario, A. V. M., and Somoza, G. M. (2006). Evolution of GnRH ligands and receptors in gnathostomata. *Comp. Biochem. Physiol. Part A Mol. Integr. Physiol.* 144, 272–283.

Janvier, P. (2006). Palaeontology: modern look for ancient lamprey. *Nature* 443, 921–924.

Joseph, N. T., Aquilina-Beck, A., Macdonald, C., Decatur, W. A., Hall, J. A., Kavanaugh, S. I., et al. (2012). Molecular cloning and pharmacological characterization of two novel GnRH receptors in the lamprey (*Petromyzon marinus*). *Endocrinology* 153, 3345–3356.

Kah, O., Lethimonier, C., Somoza, G., Guilgur, L. G., Vaillant, C., and Lareyre, J. J. (2007). GnRH and GnRH receptors in metazoa: a historical, comparative, and evolutive perspective. *Gen. Comp. Endocrinol.* 153, 346–364.

Kavanaugh, S. I., Nozaki, M., and Sower, S. A. (2008). Origins of gonadotropin-releasing hormone (GnRH) in vertebrates: identification of a novel GnRH in a basal vertebrate, the sea lamprey. *Endocrinology* 149, 3860–3869.

Kim, D. K., Cho, E. B., Moon, M. J., Park, S., Hwang, J. I., Kah, O., et al. (2011). Revisiting the evolution of gonadotropin-releasing hormones and their receptors in vertebrates: secrets hidden in genomes. *Gen. Comp. Endocrinol.* 170, 68–78.

Kitanovic, S., Yuen, T., Flanagan, C. A., Ebersole, B. J., and Sealfon, S. C. (2001). Insertional mutagenesis of the arginine cage domain of the gonadotropin-releasing hormone receptor. *Mol. Endocrinol.* 15, 390–397.

Li, J. H., Choe, H., Wang, A. F., Maiti, K., Wang, C., Salam, A., et al. (2005). Extracellular loop 3 (EL3) and EL3-proximal transmembrane helix 7 of the mammalian type I and type II gonadotropin-releasing hormone (GnRH) receptors determine differential ligand selectivity to GnRH-I and GnRH-II. *Mol. Pharmacol.* 67, 1099–1110.

Liu, F., Usui, I., Evans, L. G., Austin, D. A., Mellon, P. L., Olefsky, J. M., et al. (2002). Involvement of both G(q/11) and G(s) proteins in gonadotropin-releasing hormone receptor-mediated signaling in L beta T2 cells. *J. Biol. Chem.* 277, 32099–32108.

Millar, R. (2005). GnRHs and GnRH receptors. *Anim. Reprod. Sci.* 88, 5–28.

Millar, R. P., Lu, Z. L., Pawson, A. J., Flanagan, C. A., Morgan, K., and Maudsley, S. R. (2004). Gonadotropin-releasing hormone receptors. *Endocr. Rev.* 25, 235–275.

Morgan, K., and Millar, R. P. (2004). Evolution of GnRH ligand precursors and GnRH receptors in protochordate and vertebrate species. *Gen. Comp. Endocrinol.* 139, 191–197.

Myburgh, D. B., Millar, R. P., and Hapgood, J. P. (1998). Alanine-261 in intracellular loop III of the human gonadotropin-releasing hormone receptor is crucial for G-protein coupling and receptor internalization. *Biochem. J.* 331, 893–896.

Oh, D. Y., Song, J. A., Moon, J. S., Moon, M. J., Kim, J. I., Kim, K., et al. (2005). Membrane-proximal region of the carboxyl terminus of the gonadotropin-releasing hormone receptor (GnRHR) confers differential signal transduction between mammalian and nonmammalian GnRHRs. *Mol. Endocrinol.* 19, 722–731.

Okubo, K., and Nagahama, Y. (2008). Structural and functional evolution of gonadotropin-releasing hormone in vertebrates. *Acta Physiol. (Oxf.)* 193, 3–15.

Parmentier, C., Hameury, E., Dubessy, C., Quan, F. B., Habert, D., Calas, A., et al. (2011). Occurrence of two distinct urotensin II-related peptides in zebrafish provides new insight into the evolutionary history of the urotensin II gene family. *Endocrinology* 152, 2330–2341.

Putnam, N. H., Butts, T., Ferrier, D. E., Furlong, R. F., Hellsten, U., Kawashima, T., et al. (2008). The amphioxus genome and the evolution of the chordate karyotype. *Nature* 453, 1064–1071.

Qiu, H., Hildebrand, F., Kuraku, S., and Meyer, A. (2011). Unresolved orthology and peculiar coding sequence properties of lamprey genes: the KCNA gene family as test case. *BMC Genomics* 12, 325. doi:10.1186/1471-2164-12-325

Silver, M. R., Nucci, N. V., Root, A. R., Reed, K. L., and Sower, S. A. (2005). Cloning and characterization of a functional type II gonadotropin-releasing hormone receptor with a lengthy carboxy-terminal tail from an ancestral vertebrate, the sea lamprey. *Endocrinology* 146, 3351–3361.

Smith, J. J., Antonacci, F., Eichler, E. E., and Amemiya, C. T. (2009). Programmed loss of millions of base pairs from a vertebrate genome. *Proc. Natl. Acad. Sci. U.S.A.* 106, 11212–11217.

Sower, S. A., Freamat, M., and Kavanaugh, S. I. (2009). The origins of the vertebrate hypothalamic-pituitary-gonadal (HPG) and hypothalamic-pituitary-thyroid (HPT) endocrine systems: new insights from lampreys. *Gen. Comp. Endocrinol.* 161, 20–29.

Sower, S. A., and Kawauchi, H. (2001). Update: brain and pituitary hormones of lampreys. *Comp. Biochem. Physiol. B Biochem. Mol. Biol.* 129, 291–302.

Stanislaus, D., Ponder, S., Ji, T. H., and Conn, P. M. (1998). Gonadotropin-releasing hormone receptor couples to multiple G proteins in rat gonadotrophs and in GGH3 cells: evidence from palmitoylation and overexpression of G proteins. *Biol. Reprod.* 59, 579–586.

Stewart, A. J., Katz, A. A., Millar, R. P., and Morgan, K. (2009). Retention and silencing of prepro-GnRH-II and type II GnRH receptor genes in mammals. *Neuroendocrinology* 90, 416–432.

Tello, J., and Sherwood, N. (2009). Amphioxus: beginning of vertebrate and end of invertebrate type GnRH receptor lineage. *Endocrinology* 150, 2847–2856.

True, J. R., and Carroll, S. B. (2002). Gene co-option in physiological and morphological evolution. *Annu. Rev. Cell Dev. Biol.* 18, 53–80.

Tsai, P. S., and Zhang, L. (2008). The emergence and loss of gonadotropin-releasing hormone (GnRH) in protostomes: orthology, phylogeny, structure, and function. *Biol. Reprod.* 79, 798–805.

Van de Peer, Y., Maere, S., and Meyer, A. (2010). 2R or not 2R is not the question anymore. *Nat. Rev. Genet.* 11, 166.

Wang, C., Yun, O., Maiti, K., Oh, D. Y., Kim, K. K., Chae, C. H., et al. (2004). Position of Pro and Ser near Glu7.32 in the extracellular loop 3 of mammalian and non-mammalian gonadotropin-releasing hormone (GnRH) receptors is a critical determinant for differential ligand selectivity for mammalian GnRH and chicken GnRH-II. *Mol. Endocrinol.* 18, 105–116.

Zhang, L., Tello, J. A., Zhang, W., and Tsai, P. S. (2008). Molecular cloning, expression pattern, and immunocytochemical localization of a gonadotropin releasing hormone-like molecule in the gastropod mollusk, *Aplysia californica*. *Gen. Comp. Endocrinol.* 156, 201–209.

Zhou, W., Flanagan, C., Ballesteros, J. A., Konvicka, K., Davidson, J. S., Weinstein, H., et al. (1994). A reciprocal mutation supports helix 2 and helix 7 proximity in the gonadotropin-releasing hormone receptor. *Mol. Pharmacol.* 45, 165–170.

Zhou, W., Rodic, V., Kitanovic, S., Flanagan, C. A., Chi, L., Weinstein, H., et al. (1995). A locus of the gonadotropin-releasing hormone receptor that differentiates agonist and antagonist binding sites. *J. Biol. Chem.* 270, 18853–18857.

# 21

# PROK2/PROKR2 signaling and Kallmann syndrome

***Catherine Dodé[1]* and Philippe Rondard[2]***

[1] *INSERM U1016, Institut Cochin, Université Paris-Descartes, Paris, France*
[2] *CNRS UMR5203, INSERM U661, Institut de Génomique Fonctionnelle, Université Montpellier 1, 2, Montpellier, France*

***Edited by:***
*Hubert Vaudry, University of Rouen, France*

***Reviewed by:***
*Ishwar S. Parhar, Monash University, Malaysia*
*Nicolas De Roux, INSERM U676, France*

****Correspondence:***
*Catherine Dodé, INSERM U1016, Institut Cochin, Département de génétique et développement, 24 rue du Faubourg Saint-Jacques, 75014 Paris, France.*
*e-mail: catherine.dode@inserm.fr*

Kallmann syndrome (KS) is a developmental disease that associates hypogonadism and a deficiency of the sense of smell. The reproductive phenotype of KS results from the primary interruption of the olfactory, vomeronasal, and terminal nerve fibers in the frontonasal region, which in turn disrupts the embryonic migration of neuroendocrine gonadotropin-releasing hormone (GnRH) synthesizing cells from the nose to the brain. This is a highly heterogeneous genetic disease, and mutations in any of the nine genes identified so far have been found in approximately 30% of the KS patients. *PROKR2* and *PROK2*, which encode the G protein-coupled prokineticin receptor-2 and its ligand prokineticin-2, respectively, are two of these genes. Homozygous knockout mice for the orthologous genes exhibit a phenotype reminiscent of the KS features, but biallelic mutations in *PROKR2* or *PROK2* (autosomal recessive mode of disease transmission) have been found only in a minority of the patients, whereas most patients carrying mutations in these genes are heterozygotes. The mutations, mainly missense mutations, have deleterious effects on PROKR2 signaling in transfected cells, ranging from defective cell surface-targeting of the receptor to defective coupling to G proteins or impaired receptor-ligand interaction, but the same mutations have also been found in apparently unaffected individuals, which suggests a digenic/oligogenic mode of inheritance of the disease in heterozygous patients. This non-Mendelian mode of inheritance has so far been confirmed only in a few patients. However, it may account for the unusually high proportion of KS sporadic cases compared to familial cases.

**Keywords: PROK2, PROKR2, Kallmann syndrome, hypogonadotropic hypogonadism, anosmia, digenic/oligogenic mode of inheritance**

## INTRODUCTION

Kallmann syndrome (KS) is a developmental disease that associates hypogonadotropic hypogonadism, due to gonadotropin-releasing hormone (GnRH) deficiency, and anosmia, related to the absence or hypoplasia of the olfactory bulbs (Kallmann, 1944; deMorsier, 1954; Naftolin et al., 1971). The degree of the hypogonadism and that of the smell deficiency can vary significantly, not only between unrelated KS patients, but also between patients from the same family. The prevalence of KS has been estimated at one out of 8000 in boys. In girls, the prevalence is thought to be five times lower, but it is probably underestimated because some affected females only have mild hypogonadism, and also because primary amenorrhea in females often remains unexplored (Jones and Kemmann, 1976).

Pathohistological studies of fetuses with olfactory bulb agenesis have shown that the reproductive phenotype of KS results from a pathological sequence in embryonic life, whereby premature interruption of the olfactory, vomeronasal, and terminal nerve fibers in the frontonasal region disrupts the migration of neuroendocrine GnRH cells, which normally migrate from the nose to the brain along these nerve fibers (Schwanzel-Fukuda and Pfaff, 1989; Teixeira et al., 2010). What causes the primary failure of these fibers to establish proper contact with the forebrain is, however, still unknown.

Kallmann syndrome is genetically heterogeneous and involves various modes of transmission, specifically, X-chromosome linked, autosomal recessive, autosomal dominant with incomplete penetrance, and also digenic/oligogenic inheritance (Dodé and Hardelin, 2009; Sykiotis et al., 2010). Because the common infertility in affected individuals and, most importantly, the incomplete penetrance of the disease impede genetic linkage analysis, researchers have used various strategies to identify genes involved in KS, including mutation screening in genes that are disrupted by deletion or translocation breakpoints in chromosomal rearrangements associated with the disease phenotype, and candidate gene approaches. Nine causal genes have been reported to date, namely, by chronological order of discovery, *KAL1* (Franco et al., 1991; Legouis et al., 1991; Hardelin et al., 1992), *FGFR1* (Dodé et al., 2003), *PROKR2* and *PROK2* (Dodé et al., 2006), *FGF8* (Falardeau et al., 2008), *CHD7* (Kim et al., 2008; Jongmans et al., 2009), *WDR11* (Kim et al., 2010), *HS6ST1* (Tornberg et al., 2011), and *SEMA3A* (Hanchate et al., 2012; Young et al., 2012) (**Table 1**). Various loss-of-function mutations in *KAL1*, encoding the extracellular matrix glycoprotein anosmin-1, and in *FGFR1* or *FGF8*, encoding fibroblast growth factor receptor-1 and fibroblast growth factor-8, underlie the X-chromosome linked form and an autosomal dominant form of KS, respectively. Mutations in *KAL1* and *FGFR1/FGF8* account for roughly 8 and 10% of

**Table 1 | KS genes.**

| Genes | *KAL1* | *FGFR1* and *FGF8* | *PROKR2* and *PROK2* | *CHD7* | *WDR11* | *HS6ST1* | *SEMA3A* |
|---|---|---|---|---|---|---|---|
| Mode(s) of transmission | X-linked recessive | Autosomal dominant (incomplete penetrance) or digenic/oligogenic | Autosomal recessive or digenic/oligogenic | ? | ? | digenic/ oligogenic? | digenic/ oligogenic? |
| Strategy for gene identification | Cytogenetics | Cytogenetics and mouse model | Mouse models | Candidate gene | Cytogenetics | *C. elegans* model | Mouse model |
| Prevalence of mutations in KS patients | 8% of male patients | 10 and <1% | 7 and 3% | 1–5% | <1% | <1% | 6% |
| Reference | Legouis et al. (1991), Franco et al. (1991), Hardelin et al. (1992) | Dodé et al. (2003), Falardeau et al. (2008) | Dodé et al. (2006) | Kim et al. (2008), Jongmans et al. (2009) | Kim et al. (2010) | Tornberg et al. (2011) | Hanchate et al. (2012), Young et al. (2012) |

*?, not known.*

all KS cases, respectively. The *KAL1* gene product, anosmin-1, binds to heparan-sulfate glycosaminoglycans, and may act as a co-receptor for FGF signaling through FGFR1, which also requires interaction with heparan-sulfate glycosaminoglycans for receptor activation. Mutations in the genes encoding heparan-sulfate 6-*O*-sulfotransferase 1, an enzyme involved in glycosaminoglycan modifications, WDR11, an intracellular protein that interacts with the transcription factor EMX1, and semaphorin 3A, a secreted protein involved in axonal pathfinding, have also been found in some KS patients. Mutations in the chromodomain helicase DNA-binding protein 7 gene (*CHD7*) are present in approximately 70% of the patients affected by the CHARGE syndrome, which in most patients includes KS (Pinto et al., 2005), and mutations in this gene have been found in some patients who initially presented with KS. Finally, mutations in *PROKR2* and *PROK2*, encoding prokineticin receptor-2 and prokineticin-2, respectively, have been identified in approximately 9% of the KS patients, both in heterozygous and in homozygous or compound heterozygous states.

## PROKINETICINS AND THEIR RECEPTORS

Prokineticins are secreted cysteine-rich proteins that possess diverse biological activities. The first identified member of this family was isolated from the venom of the black mamba snake (Joubert and Strydom, 1980), and was named mamba intestinal toxin 1 (MIT1) owing to its ability to induce intestinal contraction (Schweitz et al., 1999). Then, a small protein of similar size (77 amino acid residues, 8 kDa), with 58% sequence identity with MIT1, was isolated from skin secretions in the amphibian *Bombina variegata,* and called Bv8 (Mollay et al., 1999). Soon after, two mammalian proteins of this family were identified and named prokineticin-1 and -2 (PROK1 and PROK2) (Li et al., 2001; Kaser et al., 2003). PROK1 has 80% sequence identity with MIT1 and 58% identity with PROK2 (Li et al., 2001). The amino-terminal domain of prokineticins contains a sequence of six amino acid residues (AVITGA), which is conserved in all mammalian and non-mammalian orthologs. Substitutions, deletions, or insertions to this hexapeptide result in the loss of agonist activity on prokineticin receptors (Kaser et al., 2003; Bullock et al., 2004). The carboxy-terminal region of prokineticins contains 10 cysteine residues forming five disulfide bonds. Apart from its potent effect on gastrointestinal smooth muscle contraction, PROK1 was also characterized as an angiogenic factor with specific effects on steroidogenic glands, thus earning its initial name EG-VEGF (endocrine gland vascular endothelial growth factor) (LeCouter et al., 2003). Mouse and human orthologs of Bv8, also known as PROK2, have been involved in a variety of biological activities, including effects on neuronal survival, gastrointestinal smooth muscle contraction (Li et al., 2001), circadian locomotor rhythm (Cheng et al., 2002), survival and migration of adrenal cortical capillary endothelial cells (LeCouter et al., 2003). PROK2 also has a role in appetite regulation and its anorectic effect is mediated partly by the melanocortin system (Gardiner et al., 2006).

Prokineticins can bind to two different G protein-coupled receptors, prokineticin receptor-1 and -2 (PROKR1 and PROKR2), which have about 85% sequence identity. These receptors were characterized simultaneously by three different groups (Lin et al., 2002; Masuda et al., 2002; Soga et al., 2002). Both are able to bind to PROK1 and PROK2 with similar nanomolar range affinities. They have a central core formed by seven transmembrane α-helical segments (TM1–TM7) connected by intracellular (i1–i3) and extracellular (e1–e3) loops, an extracellular amino-terminal end, and an intracellular carboxy-terminal end. These plasma membrane receptors operate as molecular switches to relay extracellular ligand-activation to intracellular heterotrimeric G proteins. PROKR1 is mainly expressed in peripheral tissues, including endocrine glands and organs of the reproductive system, the gastrointestinal tract, lungs, and the circulatory system (Soga et al., 2002; Battersby et al., 2004), whereas PROKR2 shows relatively localized distribution in the central nervous system (Cheng et al., 2002; Lin et al., 2002).

The olfactory bulb is one of the few areas in the mammalian brain that produce neurons throughout life. New interneurons originating from progenitors in the subventricular zone (SVZ) are continually added to the olfactory bulbs. The mRNAs of both receptors (PROKR1 and PROKR2) are expressed in the SVZ and the olfactory bulbs. The expression of PROKR1 have been detected in these areas although less abundantly than PROKR2. Whereas PROK1 mRNAs were not detected in any of these brain region (Ng et al., 2005). It was first shown that PROK2 functions as a chemoattractant for these neuronal progenitors, which follow a rostral migratory stream. Accordingly, PROK2 deficiency in mice leads to a loss of normal olfactory bulb architecture, and accumulation of neuronal progenitors in the rostral migratory stream (Ng et al., 2005). Soon after, it was found that *Prokr2*$^{-/-}$ knockout mice exhibit early hypoplasia of the olfactory bulbs and severe atrophy of the reproductive organs in both sexes, a phenotype reminiscent of the KS features. In addition, immunohistochemical analysis of these mice revealed that the neuroendocrine GnRH cells were absent from the hypothalamus (Matsumoto et al., 2006).

*PROK2* is a clock-controlled gene: the level of its messenger RNA shows a circadian oscillation profile in the suprachiasmatic nuclei (Cheng et al., 2002; Li et al., 2006). It has been postulated that PROK2 signaling through PROKR2 is a suprachiasmatic nuclei clock output signal that regulates circadian rhythms (Prosser et al., 2007; Li et al., 2012). PROK2-null mice show accelerated acquisition of food anticipatory activity during a daytime food restriction (Li et al., 2006), exhibit reduced total sleep time predominantly during the light period, and also have an impaired response to sleep disturbance (Hu et al., 2007).

PROK2 is a functional target gene of proneural basic helix-loop-helix (bHLH) factors. Neurogenin-1 (NGN1) and MASH1 activate *PROK2* transcription by binding to E-box motifs on the *PROK2* promoter with the same set of E-boxes critical for another pair of bHLH factors, CLOCK and BMAL1, in the regulation of circadian clock (Cheng et al., 2002; Zhang et al., 2007).

## COMPLEX GENETICS OF KALLMANN SYNDROME CAUSED BY MUTATIONS IN *PROKR2* OR *PROK2*

We first considered that *PROKR2* was a relevant KS candidate because of the KS-like phenotype of PROKR2-null mice (see above). We thus sequenced the two coding exons of *PROKR2* in a cohort of patients affected by KS, and identified 10 different mutations (one frame-shifting and nine missense mutations) in 14 patients, either in heterozygous state (10 cases) or in homozygous or compound heterozygous state (4 cases) (Dodé et al., 2006) (**Table 2**). Notably, most of these mutations were missense mutations, and many were also found in apparently unaffected individuals, thus initially raising some questions regarding their pathogenic role. A deleterious effect on the signaling activity of PROKR2 was, however, confirmed in transfected HEK-293 cells for most of the mutations (Cole et al., 2008; Monnier et al., 2009).

Then, we considered the possibility that mutations in *PROK2* also account for some KS cases, especially since mutant mice defective in PROK2 showed a marked reduction in the size of their olfactory bulbs. *PROK2* contains four coding exons (Bullock et al., 2004), of which exon 3, encoding an arginine- and lysine-rich peptide of 21 amino acid residues, may or may not be included in the mature transcript due to alternative splicing (Wechselberger et al., 1999) (**Figure 1**). We sequenced the entire coding sequence of *PROK2* in the patients, and identified four different point mutations (two missense mutations, one frame-shifting mutation, and one single nucleotide substitution in the translation initiation sequence), all in the heterozygous state (Dodé et al., 2006). *PROK2* mutations in homozygous state were subsequently found in a few patients, and a KS-like phenotype was concomitantly reported in PROK2-null mutant mice (Pitteloud et al., 2007; Leroy et al., 2008). Since then, additional mutations in *PROKR2* and *PROK2* have been reported in KS patients. A list of the mutations, together with the corresponding references, is provided in **Table 2.**

The finding, for given *PROKR2* and *PROK2* mutations, of both heterozygous and homozygous (or compound heterozygous) unrelated patients is quite remarkable, and argues in favor of a digenic or oligogenic mode of inheritance in heterozygous patients. To date, digenic inheritance of KS has been shown in few patients who had monoallelic missense mutations both in *PROKR2* or *PROK2*, and in other KS genes (*KAL1, FGFR1*) or genes underlying normosmic congenital hypogonadotropic hypogonadism (*GNRHR, KISS1R*) (Dodé et al., 2006; Cole et al., 2008; Raivio et al., 2009; Martin et al., 2010; Sarfati et al., 2010). The other patients harboring monoallelic mutations in *PROKR2* or *PROK2* are expected to carry at least one additional pathogenic mutation in as yet uncharacterized genes. Indeed, mutations in any of the currently known KS genes have been identified in only 30% of all KS patients, thus indicating that other disease genes remain to be discovered. Notably, it has been found that patients carrying biallelic mutations in *PROKR2* or *PROK2* consistently have a severe, complete KS phenotype, whereas the phenotype of patients carrying monoallelic mutations in these genes is more variable, and likely depends on the additional genetic hits in these patients (Martin et al., 2010; Sarfati et al., 2010).

Kallmann syndrome patients who carry biallelic mutations in *PROK2* or *PROKR2* do not seem to have any of the non-olfactory, non-reproductive occasional anomalies that have been reported in the previously characterized genetic forms of the disease (i.e., X-linked KAL1 form and autosomal dominant KAL2 form), specifically, bimanual synkinesis, renal agenesis, dental agenesis, and cleft lip or palate, and even though sleep disorders or increased body mass index have been reported in some of these patients, there is so far no evidence that these clinical features can be ascribed to the *PROKR2* and *PROK2* mutations, despite potential roles of these genes in sleep-wake regulation and ingestive behavior (see above). In addition, plasma cortisol levels were measured during 24 h in five patients mutated in *PROK2* or *PROKR2*, including one patient with biallelic *PROKR2* mutations, and normal circadian variation was observed in all cases (Sarfati et al., 2010), which argues against a major contribution of PROK2/PROKR2 signaling to physiological circadian variation of plasma cortisol levels in humans. Of course, this result does not exclude the presence of more subtle defects in the patients.

## CONSEQUENCES OF THE *PROKR2* AND *PROK2* MISSENSE MUTATIONS ON RECEPTOR SIGNALING ACTIVITY

A total of 24 *PROKR2* missense mutations have been identified (Dodé et al., 2006; Cole et al., 2008; Sinisi et al., 2008; Chan et al., 2009; Abreu et al., 2010; Sarfati et al., 2010) in KS patients (**Table 2**;

**Table 2 | *PROKR2* and *PROK2* mutations in Kallmann syndrome.**

| Exon | Nucleotide change | Amino acid change | Localization (domain) | Functional consequence | Reference |
|---|---|---|---|---|---|
| ***PROKR2*** | | | | | |
| 1 | 58del | Frameshift | N-terminal region | NMD or protein truncation | Dodé et al. (2006) |
| | 151G > A | A51T | N-terminal region | None? | Reynaud et al. (2012), Sbai et al. (unpublished) |
| | 238C > T | R80C | First intracellular loop | None? | Abreu et al. (2010), Sbai et al. (unpublished) |
| – | 253C > T | R85C | – | Mild G protein-coupling defect | Cole et al. (2008), Monnier et al. (2009), Sarfati et al. (2010) |
| – | 253C > G | R85G | – | Strong G protein-coupling defect | Sarfati et al. (2010), Raivio et al. (2012) |
| – | 254G > T | R85L | – | Mild protein-coupling defect | Sarfati et al. (2010), Sbai et al. (unpublished) |
| – | 254G > A | R85H | – | Mild G protein-coupling defect | Dodé et al. (2006), Monnier et al. (2009) |
| – | 337T > C | Y113H | First extracellular loop | Strong G protein-coupling defect | Cole et al. (2008), Sbai et al. (unpublished) |
| – | 343G > A | V115M | – | Strong G protein-coupling defect | Cole et al. (2008), Sbai et al. (unpublished) |
| | 349C > T | R117W | – | Strong G protein-coupling defect | Sbai et al. (unpublished) |
| – | 420C > G | Y140X | Third transmembrane domain | NMD or protein truncation | Abreu et al. (2010) |
| 2 | 491G > A | R164Q | Second intracellular loop | Mild G protein-coupling defect | Dodé et al. (2006), Cole et al. (2008), Monnier et al. (2009) |
| – | 518T > G | L173R | Fourth transmembrane domain | Cell surface-targeting defect | Dodé et al. (2006), Abreu et al. (2010), Cole et al. (2008), Monnier et al. (2009) |
| – | 533G > C | W178S | – | Cell surface-targeting defect | Dodé et al. (2006), Cole et al. (2008), Monnier et al. (2009) |
| – | 563C > T | S188L | – | Strong G protein-coupling defect | Cole et al. (2008), Sbai et al. (unpublished) |
| – | 604A > G | S202G | Second extracellular loop | ? | Chan et al. (2009) |
| – | 629A > G | Q210R | – | Ligand-binding defect | Dodé et al. (2006), Monnier et al. (2009) |
| | 701G > A | G234D | Fifth transmembrane domain | Cell surface-targeting defect | Sbai et al. (unpublished) |
| – | 743G > A | R248Q | Third intracellular loop | None? | Cole et al. (2008) |
| – | 752G > T | W251L | – | Strong G protein-coupling defect? | Sarfati et al. (2010), Sbai et al. (unpublished) |
| – | 802C > T | R268C | – | G protein-coupling defect? | Dodé et al. (2006), Abreu et al. (2010), Monnier et al. (2009), Sarfati et al. (2010) |
| – | T820 > A | V274D | Sixth transmembrane domain | Strong G protein-coupling defect | Sinisi et al. (2008), Sbai et al. (unpublished) |
| – | 868C > T | P290S | – | Cell surface-targeting defect | Dodé et al. (2006), Monnier et al. (2009) |
| – | 969G > A | M323I | Seventh transmembrane domain | None? | Dodé et al. (2006), Monnier et al. (2009) |
| – | 989del | Frameshift | – | NMD or protein truncation | Sarfati et al. (2010) |
| – | 991G > A | V331M | – | Mild G protein-coupling defect | Dodé et al. (2006), Cole et al. (2008), Monnier et al. (2009), Sarfati et al. (2010) |
| – | 1069C > T | R357W | C-terminal region | None? | Cole et al. (2008), Sbai et al. (unpublished) |

*(Continued)*

**Table 2 | Continued**

| Exon | Nucleotide change | Amino acid change | Localization (domain) | Functional consequence | Reference |
|---|---|---|---|---|---|
| ***PROK2*** | | | | | |
| 1 | −4C > A | | Translation initiation site | Reduced protein synthesis? | Dodé et al. (2006) |
| – | 70G > C | A24P | Signal peptide | ? | Cole et al. (2008) |
| – | 94G > C | G32R | AVITGA motif | Strongly impaired activity? | Dodé et al. (2006) |
| 2 | 101 G > A | C34Y | Cysteine-rich region | Strongly impaired activity | Cole et al. (2008) |
| – | 137G > A | C46Y | Cysteine-rich region | ? | Dodé et al. (unpublished) |
| – | 150C > G | I50M | – | None? | Cole et al. (2008) |
| – | 161G > A | S54N | – | ? | Sarfati et al. (2010) |
| – | 163del | Frameshift | – | NMD or protein truncation | Pitteloud et al. (2007), Leroy et al. (2008) |
| – | 217C > T | R73C | – | Strongly impaired activity | Dodé et al. (2006), Leroy et al. (2008), Cole et al. (2008) |
| 4 | 297_298insT | Frameshift | – | NMD or protein truncation | Dodé et al. (2006), Abreu et al. (2010) |
| | 301C > T | R101W | – | ? | Dodé et al. (unpublished) |
| – | 302G > A | R101Q | – | ? | Dodé et al. (unpublished) |
| – | 310C > T | H104Y | – | ? | Sarfati et al. (2010) |

*Mutations reported in PROKR2 and PROK2 are mainly missense mutations. In most patients, the mutations have been found in heterozygous state. The R85C, R85H, R164Q, L173R, and P290S PROKR2 mutations, as well as R73C, c.163del, and c.297_298insT PROK2 mutations have, however, been found both in heterozygous and homozygous (or compound heterozygous) states, which suggests that patients heterozygous for PROKR2 or PROK2 mutations carry additional mutations, presumably in other, as yet unidentified Kallmann syndrome genes in most cases. Notably, two such patients have the L173R mutation in PROKR2 together with S396L or R423X mutations in KAL1 (Dodé et al., 2006; Sarfati et al., 2010), another patient has the V115M mutation in PROKR2 together with the A24P mutation in PROK2 (Cole et al., 2008), and still another patient has the R85L mutation in PROKR2 together with a A604T mutation in FGFR1 (Sarfati et al., 2010). In addition, the patient who has the S202G mutation in PROKR2 also has I239T and R31C monoallelic mutations in FGFR1 and GNRH1, respectively (Chan et al., 2009). Finally, two patients who carry R268C and V331M mutations in PROKR2 also carry A189T and R240Q monoallelic mutations in KISS1R and GNRHR, respectively (Sarfati et al., 2010). Abbreviation: NMD, nonsense-mediated mRNA decay.*

*?, not known.*

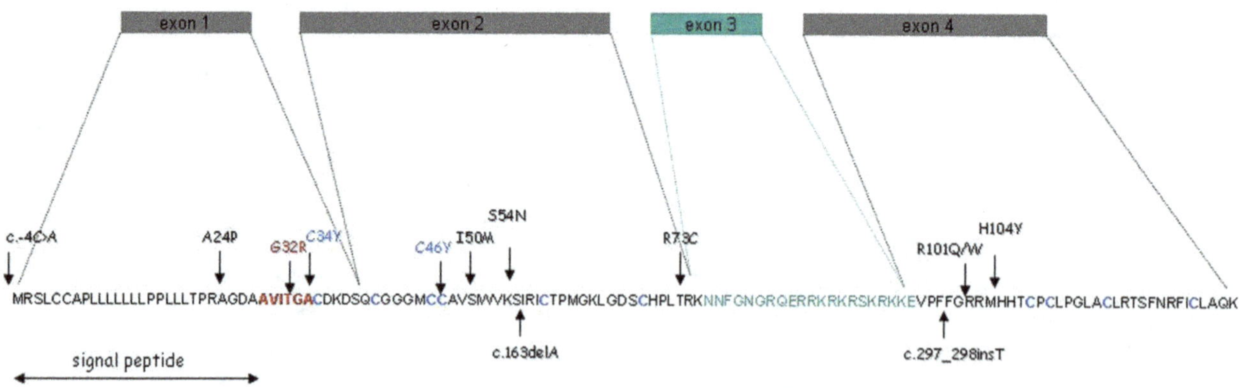


**FIGURE 1 | PROK2 gene structure and amino acid sequence.** The green box and green amino acid sequence denote the alternative exon and encoded peptide, respectively. The AVITGA motif is shown in red, and the 10 cysteinyl residues (forming five disulfide bonds) are in blue. Vertical arrows indicate the positions of the mutations identified in the patients.

**Figure 2**). Most of the mutant receptors have been characterized regarding their ability to induce intracellular release of calcium upon PROK2-stimulation, their cell surface expression, and their PROK2-binding, in mammalian cell lines (Cole et al., 2008; Monnier et al., 2009; Abreu et al., 2012; Raivio et al., 2012; Sbai et al., in preparation). Although PROKR2 can activate different

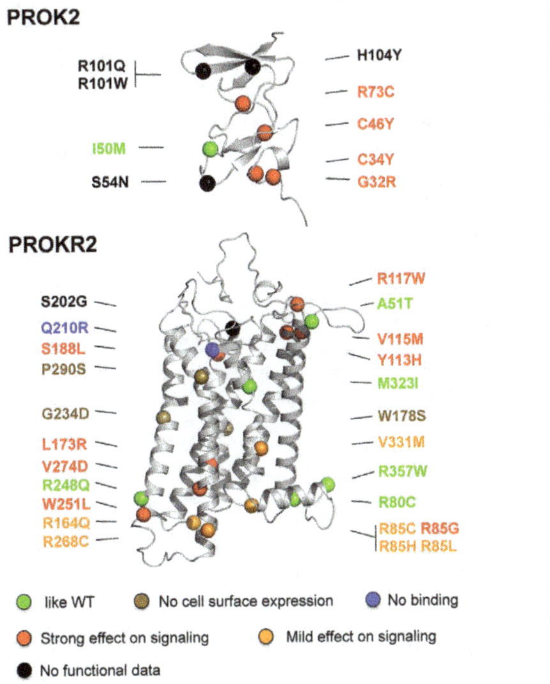


**FIGURE 2 | Positions of missense mutations in PROK2 and PROKR2 in the structural models of the ligand and the receptor.** The mutations are classified in different categories according to their effects on PROKR2 signaling activity: similar to wild-type (green), absence of the receptor at the cell surface (brown), absence of ligand-binding (blue), and strong or mild effect on signaling (red and orange, respectively). The mutations for which functional data are not available are denoted in black. The colored balls indicate the atom of alpha carbon of the polypeptidic chain of the mutated residue. Note that residue R357 is located in the proximal part of the C-terminal region of the receptor.

G protein pathways (Lin et al., 2002; Soga et al., 2002; Chen et al., 2005), its coupling to Gq, leading to intracellular release of calcium, represents the best characterized transduction mechanism. Only five mutants (A51T, R80C, R248Q, M321I, R357W) have properties similar to the wild-type PROKR2, thus calling into question the pathogenic effect of these missense variants. Notably, the R268C mutation has also been found in heterozygous state in a relatively large proportion (174 out of 2203, i.e., 7.9%) of individuals from the African American general population, and in homozygous state in six individuals from the same population (0.3%; see Exome Variant Server website URL: http://evs.gs.washington.edu/EVS/). Moreover, a clear deleterious effect of the R268C mutation on PROKR2 signaling through Gq protein activation could not be found in transfected HEK-293 cells, thus calling into question the pathogenic effect of this missense variant too. Most of the *PROKR2* mutations, however, impair cell surface expression, ligand-binding, or G protein-binding of the receptor (**Figure 2**). Three mutations affecting conserved residues located in the middle of the transmembrane helices, W178S, G234D, and P290S, impede targeting of the receptor to the cell surface. The Q210R mutant receptor is present at the cell surface, but is not able to bind to the ligand. The other mutants impair, either mildly or strongly, intracellular release of calcium in the Gq signaling pathway, and for some of them this effect might be due to the low expression of the mutant at the cell surface. Interestingly, the mutations that mostly impair the signaling are located nearby the extracellular side or the intracellular side of the receptor, and for these mutants, the loss-of-function is associated to a loss of cell surface expression. The mutations that result in a mildly impaired signaling activity are located in the intracellular loops, in agreement with the important role played by these loops in G protein-coupling. In addition, when wild-type and mutant receptors were coexpressed in HEK-293 cells, none of the mutant receptors that were retained within the cells did affect cell surface-targeting of the wild-type receptor, and none of the mutant receptors properly addressed at the plasma membrane did affect wild-type receptor signaling activity. This argues against a dominant negative effect of the mutations *in vivo*.

A total of 10 missense mutations have been identified in PROK2 (**Table 2**, **Figure 2**) (Dodé et al., 2006; Cole et al., 2008; Leroy et al., 2008; Sarfati et al., 2010). A mutation located at the translation initiation site (−4C > A) likely reduced the protein synthesis. Mutations of conserved residues in prokineticins are expected to strongly impair PROK2 activity such as those in the N-terminal conserved region AVITGA important for prokineticin activity (G32R), and those of the conserved cysteines (C34Y and C46Y). In addition, mutations that introduce an additional cysteine (R73C) in the cysteine-rich region of PROK2 may affect folding of the hormone then leading to a loss-of-function. This is consistent with the functional analysis of Cole et al. (2008) who have examined the signaling properties of three PROK2 mutants: the C34Y and R73C mutations totally abolished and strongly impaired the intracellular calcium release activity of PROKR2, respectively, whereas the I50M mutation had an activity similar to that of the wild-type PROK2. The functional consequence of the other mutations (A24P, S54N, R101Q, R101W, and H104Y) are more difficult to predict in the absence of model of the complex between PROK2 and PROKR2. Further studies will be necessary to better analyze whether the mutations in PROK2 affect the process of binding and/or activation of PROKR2 by the hormone.

## CONCLUSION

The characterization of new genes involved in KS is a difficult goal. Because of the hypogonadotropic hypogonadism, sizes of the KS families are small and the mode of inheritance is very often difficult to establish. Animal models in which a gene has been inactivated and involving a KS phenotype are an alternative approach for the identification of new KS genes. The inactivation of *PROK2* or *PROKR2* lead to defective olfactory morphogenesis and hypogonadism in mice and humans. Curiously, *PROK2* and *PROKR2* mutations in homozygous state were found in a few patients and the main part of the KS patients carried only heterozygous mutations. In all of the functional studies done so far, only Gq signaling pathways have been investigated to characterize the PROK2 and PROKR2 mutants and further studies will be necessary to analyze other signaling pathways. Interestingly, few patients who had monoallelic missense mutations both in *PROK2* or *PROKR2*, and in other KS or normosmic congenital hypogonadotropic hypogonadism genes, raising the idea of oligogenism. So far, this hypothesis has been validated only in a few patients suggesting that the second mutation in the other heterozygous patients resides in unexplored regions of the genes or as yet undiscovered KS genes.

## ACKNOWLEDGMENTS

We thank Jean-Pierre Hardelin for critical reading of the manuscript, Oualid Sbai and Carine Monnier for sharing unpublished data, and Guillaume Lebon for his help in preparing the 3D models of PROKR2 and PROK2. This work was supported by ANR-09-GENO-017-01 and GIS maladies rares (Project A09051KS).

## REFERENCES

Abreu, A. P., Kaiser, U. B., and Latronico, A. C. (2010). The role of prokineticins in the pathogenesis of hypogonadotropic hypogonadism. *Neuroendocrinology* 91, 283–290.

Abreu, A. P., Noel, S. D., Xu, S., Carroll, R. S., Latronico, A. C., and Kaiser, U. B. (2012). Evidence of the importance of the first intracellular loop of prokineticin receptor 2 in receptor function. *Mol. Endocrinol.* 26, 1417–1427.

Battersby, S., Critchley, H. O., Morgan, K., Millar, R. P., and Jabbour, H. N. (2004). Expression and regulation of the prokineticins (endocrine gland-derived vascular endothelial growth factor and Bv8) and their receptors in the human endometrium across the menstrual cycle. *J. Clin. Endocrinol. Metab.* 89, 2463–2469.

Bullock, C. M., Li, J.-D., and Zhou, Q.-Y. (2004). Structural determinants required for the bioactivities of prokineticins and identification of prokineticin receptor antagonists. *Mol. Pharmacol.* 65, 582–588.

Chan, Y. M., de Guillebon, A., Lang-Muritano, M., Plummer, L., Cerrato, F., Tsiaras, S., et al. (2009). GNRH1 mutations in patients with idiopathic hypogonadotropic hypogonadism. *Proc. Natl. Acad. Sci. U.S.A.* 106, 11703–11708.

Chen, J., Kuei, C., Sutton, S., Wilson, S., Yu, J., Kamme, F., et al. (2005). Identification and pharmacological characterization of prokineticin 2 β as a selective ligand for prokineticin receptor 1. *Mol. Pharmacol.* 67, 2070–2076.

Cheng, M., Bullock, C. M., Li, C., Lee, A. G., Bermak, J. C., Belluzzi, J., et al. (2002). Prokineticin 2 transmits the behavioural circadian rhythm of the suprachiasmatic nucleus. *Nature* 417, 405–410.

Cole, L. W., Sidis, Y., Zhang, C., Quinton, R., Plummer, L., Pignatelli, D., et al. (2008). Mutations in prokineticin 2 and prokineticin receptor 2 genes in human gonadotrophin-releasing hormone deficiency: molecular genetics and clinical spectrum. *J. Clin. Endocrinol. Metab.* 93, 3551–3559.

deMorsier, G. (1954). Etudes sur les dysraphies crânio-encéphaliques. I. Agénésie des lobes olfactifs (telencéphaloschizis latéral) et des commissures calleuse et antérieure (telencéphaloschizis médian). La dysplasie olfacto-génitale. *Schweiz. Arch. Neurol. Psychiatr.* 74, 309–361.

Dodé, C., and Hardelin, J.-P. (2009). Kallmann syndrome. *Eur. J. Hum. Genet.* 17, 139–146.

Dodé, C., Levilliers, J., Dupont, J.-M., De Paepe, A., Le Dû, N., Soussi-Yanicostas, N., et al. (2003). Loss-of-function mutations in FGFR1 cause autosomal dominant Kallmann syndrome. *Nat. Genet.* 33, 463–465.

Dodé, C., Teixeira, L., Levilliers, J., Fouveaut, C., Bouchard, P., Kottler, M.-L., et al. (2006). Kallmann syndrome: mutations in the genes encoding prokineticin-2 and prokineticin receptor-2. *PLoS Genet.* 2:e175. doi:10.1371/journal.pgen.0020175

Falardeau, J., Chung, W. C., Beenken, A., Raivio, T., Plummer, L., Sidis, Y., et al. (2008). Decreased FGF8 signaling causes deficiency of gonadotropin-releasing hormone in humans and mice. *J. Clin. Invest.* 118, 2822–2831.

Franco, B., Guioli, S., Pragliola, A., Incerti, B., Bardoni, B., Tonlorenzi, R., et al. (1991). A gene deleted in Kallmann's syndrome shares homology with neural cell adhesion and axonal path-finding molecules. *Nature* 353, 529–536.

Gardiner, J. V., Bataveljic, A., Patel, N. A., Bewick, G. A., Roy, D., Campbell, D., et al. (2006). Prokineticin 2 is a hypothalamic neuropeptide that potently inhibits food intake. *Diabetes* 59, 397–406.

Hanchate, N. K., Giacobini, P., Lhuillier, P., Parkash, J., Espy, C., Fouveaut, C., et al. (2012). SEMA3A, a gene involved in axonal pathfinding, is mutated in some patients with Kallmann syndrome. *PLoS Genet.* 8:e1002896. doi:10.1371/journal.pgen.1002896

Hardelin, J.-P., Levilliers, J., del Castillo, I., Cohen-Salmon, M., Legouis, R., Blanchard, S., et al. (1992). X chromosome-linked Kallmann syndrome: stop mutations validate the candidate gene. *Proc. Natl. Acad. Sci. U.S.A.* 89, 8190–8194.

Hu, W. P., Li, J. D., Zhang, C., Boehmer, L., Siegel, J. M., and Zhou, Q. Y. (2007). Altered circadian and homeostatic sleep regulation in prokineticin 2-deficient mice. *Sleep* 30, 247–256.

Jones, J., and Kemmann, E. (1976). Olfacto-genital dysplasia in the female. *Obstet. Gynecol. Annu.* 5, 443.

Jongmans, M. C., van Ravenswaaij-Arts, C. M., Pitteloud, N., Ogata, T., Sato, N., Claahsen-van der Grinten, H. L., et al. (2009). CHD7 mutations in patients initially diagnosed with Kallmann syndrome – the clinical overlap with CHARGE syndrome. *Clin. Genet.* 75, 65–71.

Joubert, F. J., and Strydom, D. J. (1980). Snake venom: the amino acid sequence of protein A from *Dendroaspis polylepis* (black mamba) venom. *Hoppe-Seyler's Z. Physiol. Chem.* 361, 1787–1794.

Kallmann, F. J. (1944). The genetic aspects of primary eunuchoidism. *Am. J. Ment. Defic.* 48, 203–236.

Kaser, A., Winklmayr, M., Lepperdinger, G., and Kreil, G. (2003). The AVIT protein family. *EMBO Rep.* 4, 469–473.

Kim, H. G., Ahn, J.-W., Kurth, I., Ullmann, R., Kim, H.-T., Kulharya, A., et al. (2010). WDR11, a WD protein that interacts with transcription factor EMX1, is mutated in idiopathic hypogonadotropic hypogonadism and Kallmann syndrome. *Am. J. Hum. Genet.* 87, 465–479.

Kim, H. G., Kurth, I., Lan, F., Meliciani, I., Wenzel, W., Eom, S. H., et al. (2008). Mutations in CHD7, encoding a chromatin-remodeling protein, cause idiopathic hypogonadotropic hypogonadism and Kallmann syndrome. *Am. J. Hum. Genet.* 83, 511–519.

LeCouter, J., Lin, R., Tejada, M., Frantz, G., Peale, F., Hillan, K. J., et al. (2003). The endocrine-gland-derived VEGF homologue Bv8 promotes angiogenesis in the testis: localization of Bv8 receptors to endothelial cells. *Proc. Natl. Acad. Sci. U.S.A.* 100, 2685–2690.

Legouis, R., Hardelin, J.-P., Levilliers, J., Claverie, J.-M., Compain, S., Wunderle, V., et al. (1991). The candidate gene for the X-linked Kallmann syndrome encodes a protein related to adhesion molecules. *Cell* 67, 423–435.

Leroy, C., Fouveaut, C., Leclercq, S., Jacquemont, S., Boullay, H. D., Lespinasse, J., et al. (2008). Biallelic mutations in the prokineticin-2 gene in two sporadic cases of Kallmann syndrome. *Eur. J. Hum. Genet.* 16, 865–868.

Li, J. D., Hu, W. P., Boehmer, L., Cheng, M. Y., Lee, A. G., Siegel, J. M., et al. (2006). Attenuated circadian rhythms in mice lacking the prokineticin 2 gene. *J. Neurosci.* 26, 11615–11623.

Li, J. D., Hu, W. P., and Zhou, Q. Y. (2012). The circadian output signals from the suprachiasmatic nuclei. *Prog. Brain Res.* 199, 119–127.

Li, M., Bullock, C. M., Knauer, D. J., Ehlert, F. J., and Zhou, Q. Y. (2001). Identification of two prokineticin cDNAs: recombinant proteins potently contract gastrointestinal smooth muscle. *Mol. Pharmacol.* 59, 692–698.

Lin, D. C., Bullock, C. M., Ehlert, F. J., Tian, H., and Zhou, Q. Y. (2002). Identification and molecular characterization of two closely related G protein-coupled receptors activated by prokineticins/endocrine gland vascular endothelial growth factor. *J. Biol. Chem.* 277, 19276–19280.

Martin, C., Balasubramanian, R., Dwyer, A. A., Au, M. G., Sidis, Y., Kaiser, U. B., et al. (2010). The role of the prokineticin 2 pathway in human reproduction: evidence from the study of human and murine gene mutations. *Endocr. Rev.* 32, 225–246.

Masuda, Y., Takatsu, Y., Terao, Y., Kumano, S., Ishibashi, Y., Suenaga, M., et al. (2002). Isolation and identification of EG-VEGF/prokineticins as cognate ligands for two orphan G-protein-coupled-receptors. *Biochem. Biophys. Res. Commun.* 293, 396–402.

Matsumoto, S.-I., Yamazaki, C., Masumoto, K.-H., Nagano, M., Naito, M., Soga, T., et al. (2006). Abnormal development of the olfactory bulb and reproductive system in mice lacking prokineticin receptor PKR2. *Proc. Natl. Acad. Sci. U.S.A.* 103, 4140–4145.

Mollay, C., Wechselberger, C., Mignogna, G., Negri, L., Melchiorri, P., Barra, D., et al. (1999). Bv8, a small protein from frog skin and its homologue from snake venom induce hyperalgesia in rats. *Eur. J. Pharmacol.* 374, 189–196.

Monnier, C., Dodé, C., Fabre, L., Teixeira, L., Labesse, G., Pin, J.-P., et al. (2009). PROKR2 missense mutations associated with Kallmann syndrome impair receptor signalling activity. *Hum. Mol. Genet.* 18, 75–81.

Naftolin, F., Harris, G. W., and Bobrow, M. (1971). Effect of purified luteinizing hormone releasing factor on normal and hypogonadotropic anosmic men. *Nature* 232, 496–497.

Ng, K. L., Li, J.-D., Cheng, M. Y., Leslie, F. M., Lee, A. G., and Zhou, Q.-Y. (2005). Dependence of olfactory bulb morphogenesis on prokineticin 2 signaling. *Nature* 308, 1923–1927.

Pinto, G., Abadie, V., Mesnage, R., Blustajn, J., Cabrol, S., et al. (2005). CHARGE syndrome includes hypogonadotropic hypogonadism and abnormal olfactory bulb development. *J. Clin. Endocrinol. Metab.* 90, 5621–5626.

Pitteloud, N., Zhang, C., Pignatelli, D., Li, J.-D., Raivio, T., Cole, L. W., et al. (2007). Loss-of-function mutation in the prokineticin 2 gene causes Kallmann syndrome and normosmic idiopathic hypogonadotropic hypogonadism. *Proc. Natl. Acad. Sci. U.S.A.* 104, 17447–17452.

Prosser, H. M., Bradley, A., Chesham, J. E., Ebing, F. J. P., Hastings, M. H., and Maywood, E. S. (2007). Prokineticin receptor 2 (Prokr2) is essential for the regulation of circadian behaviour by suprachiasmatic nuclei. *Proc. Natl. Acad. Sci. U.S.A.* 104, 648–653.

Raivio, T., Avbelj, M., McCabe, M. J., Romero, C. J., Dwyer, A. A., Tommiska, J., et al. (2012). Genetic overlap in Kallmann syndrome, combined pituitary hormone deficiency, and septo-optic dysplasia. *J. Clin. Endocrinol. Metab.* 97, E694–E699.

Raivio, T., Sidis, Y., Plummer, L., Chen, H., Ma, J., Mukherjee, A., et al. (2009). Impaired fibroblast growth factor receptor 1 signaling as a cause of normosmic idiopathic hypogonadotropic hypogonadism. *J. Clin. Endocrinol. Metab.* 94, 4380–4390.

Reynaud, R., Jayakody, S. A., Monnier, C., Saveanu, A., Bouligand, J., Guedj, A. M., et al. (2012). PROKR2 variants in multiple hypopituitarism with pituitary stalk interruption. *J. Clin. Endocrinol. Metab.* 97, 1068–1073.

Sarfati, J., Guiochon-Mantel, A., Rondard, P., Arnulf, I., Garcia-Pineiro, A., Wolczynski, S., et al. (2010). A comparative phenotypic study of Kallmann syndrome patients carrying monoallelic and biallelic mutations in the prokineticin 2 or prokineticin receptor 2 genes. *J. Clin. Endocrinol. Metab.* 95, 659–969.

Schwanzel-Fukuda, M., and Pfaff, D. W. (1989). Origin of luteinizing hormone-releasing hormone neurons. *Nature* 338, 161–164.

Schweitz, H., Pacaud, P., Diochot, S., Moinier, D., and Lazdunski, M. (1999). MIT1, a black mamba toxin with a new and highly potent activity on intestinal contraction. *FEBS Lett.* 461, 183–188.

Sinisi, A. A., Asci, R., Bellastella, G., Maione, L., Esposito, D., Elefante, A., et al. (2008). Homozygous mutation in the prokineticin-receptor 2 gene (Val274Asp) presenting as reversible Kallmann syndrome and persistent oligozoospermia: case report. *Hum. Reprod.* 23, 2380–2384.

Soga, T., Matsumoto, S., Oda, T., Saito, T., Hiyama, H., Takasaki, J., et al. (2002). Molecular cloning and characterization of prokineticin receptors. *Biochim. Biophys. Acta* 1579, 173–179.

Sykiotis, G. P., Plummer, L., Hughes, V. A., Au, M., Durrani, S., Nayak-Young, S., et al. (2010). Oligogenic basis of isolated gonadotropin-releasing hormone deficiency. *Proc. Natl. Acad. Sci. U.S.A.* 107, 15140–15144.

Teixeira, L., Guimiot, F., Dodé, C., Fallet-Bianco, C., Millar, R. P., Delezoide, A.-L., et al. (2010). Defective migration of neuroendocrine GnRH cells in human arrhinencephalic conditions. *J. Clin. Invest.* 120, 3668–3672.

Tornberg, J., Sykiotis, G. P., Keefe, K., Plummer, L., Hoang, X., Hall, J. E., et al. (2011). Heparan sulfate 6-O-sulfotransferase 1, a gene involved in extracellular sugar modifications, is mutated in patients with idiopathic hypogonadotropic hypogonadism. *Proc. Natl. Acad. Sci. U.S.A.* 108, 11524–11529.

Wechselberger, C., Puglisi, R., Engel, E., Lepperdinger, G., Boitani, C., and Kreil, G. (1999). The mammalian homologues of frog Bv8 are mainly expressed in spermatocytes. *FEBS Lett.* 462, 177–181.

Young, J., Metay, C., Bouligand, J., Tou, B., Francou, B., Maione, L., et al. (2012). SEMA3A deletion in a family with Kallmann syndrome validates the role of semaphorin 3A in human puberty and olfactory system development. *Hum. Reprod.* 27, 1460–1465.

Zhang, C., Ng, K. L., Li, J.-D., He, F., Anderson, D. J., Sun, Y. E., et al. (2007). Prokineticin 2 is a target gene of proneural basic helix loop-helix factors for olfactory bulb neurogenesis. *J. Biol. Chem.* 282, 6917–6921.

# 22

# Is it really a matter of simple dualism? Corticotropin-releasing factor receptors in body and mental health

**Donny Janssen[1] and Tamás Kozicz[1,2,3] ***

[1] Department of Cellular Animal Physiology, Donders Institute for Brain, Cognition and Behavior, Nijmegen, Netherlands
[2] Department of Anatomy, Donders Institute for Brain, Cognition and Behavior, Nijmegen, Netherlands
[3] Human Genetics Center, Tulane University, New Orleans, LA, USA

**Edited by:**
Hubert Vaudry, University of Rouen, France

**Reviewed by:**
James A. Carr, Texas Tech University, USA
Rafael Vazquez-Martinez, University of Cordoba, Spain

***Correspondence:**
Tamás Kozicz, Department of Anatomy, Radboud University Nijmegen Medical Centre, P.O. Box 9101, 6500 HB Nijmegen, Netherlands.
e-mail: t.kozicz@anat.umcn.nl

Physiological responses to stress coordinated by the hypothalamo-pituitary-adrenal axis are concerned with maintaining homeostasis in the presence of real or perceived challenges. Regulators of this axis are corticotrophin releasing factor (CRF) and CRF related neuropeptides, including urocortins 1, 2, and 3. They mediate their actions by binding to CRF receptors (CRFR) 1 and 2, which are located in several stress-related brain regions. The prevailing theory has been that the initiation of and the recovery from an elicited stress response is coordinated by two elements, viz. the (mainly) opposing, but well balanced actions of CRFR1 and CRFR2. Such a dualistic view suggests that CRF/CRFR1 controls the initiation of, and urocortins/CRFR2 mediate the recovery from stress to maintain body and mental health. Consequently, failed adaptation to stress can lead to neuropathology, including anxiety and depression. Recent literature, however, challenges such dualistic and complementary actions of CRFR1 and CRFR2, and suggests that stress recruits CRF system components in a brain area and neuron specific manner to promote adaptation as conditions dictate.

**Keywords: CRFR1, CRFR2, CRF, Urocortins, stress, anxiety, depression, HPA-axis**

*"The idea would be not to abolish the CRFR1 receptor's response to the brain's stress hormone but to bring it into the normal range so that it would have appropriate levels of anxiety and stress as conditions dictate."*

*Wylie W. Vale (1941–2012)*

## INTRODUCTION

The concept of stress and adaptation was first observed in 1936 and further defined in 1951 (Selye, 1936, 1951). After exposure to a stressor, corticotrophin releasing factor (CRF) is released by endocrine cells of the paraventricular nucleus (PVN) of the hypothalamus into the portal vessels thereby stimulating the release of adrenocorticotropic hormone (ACTH) by the anterior pituitary. Subsequently, circulating ACTH stimulates secretion of glucocorticoids from the adrenal gland (Vale et al., 1981). In the 1980s, the group of Vale isolated the 41-residue CRF peptide from the ovine hypothalamus (Vale et al., 1981) and throughout the decades, many members of the CRF family have been identified, including urocortin 1 (Ucn1), urocortin 2 (Ucn2), and urocortin 3 (Ucn3). The urocortins differ in their tissue distribution and receptor pharmacology (Vaughan et al., 1995; Hsu and Hsueh, 2001; Lewis et al., 2001; Reyes et al., 2001). First shown to be important regulators of the endocrine stress response, the CRF family of neuropeptides is now known to play a role in diverse roles of homeostatic balance, important in mobilization of resources and behaviors during stress (Bale and Vale, 2004). In addition, members of the CRF peptide family play a role in regulation of food intake and satiety, as well as gastrointestinal tract motility, vascular tone, and development, and also acoustic and cardiac function (Heinrichs et al., 1992; Spina et al., 1996; Parkes et al., 1997; Okosi et al., 1998; Koob and Heinrichs, 1999; Maillot et al., 2000; Terui et al., 2001; Vetter et al., 2002; Inoue et al., 2003).

The actions of these peptides are initiated by binding and activating G-protein coupled receptors, CRFR1 and CRFR2, which display distinct affinity for members of the CRF peptide family, with CRF and Ucn1 binding to both receptors, while Ucn2 and 3 selectively bind to CRFR2 (Vaughan et al., 1995; Lewis et al., 2001). Besides CRF receptors (CRFRs) and their cognate ligands, another peptide that plays an important role in the neurobiology of the CRF family of neuropeptides is CRF binding protein (CRF-BP), a 37 kDa N-linked glycoprotein which binds both CRF and Ucn1 with high affinity (Orth and Mount, 1987; Boorse et al., 2005).

In this review, we highlight evidence supporting the notion of a dualistic action of CRFR1 and CRFR2 in mediating an adequate physiological, endocrine, and behavioral response to stress, followed by recent studies challenging this view. As this function is largely dependent upon structure, we will start with a short summary on the functional neuroanatomy of CRF system components followed by data on the animals' stress (mal)adaptation response.

## DISTRIBUTION OF CRF SYSTEM COMPONENTS

### CRF

The distribution of CRF is consistent with its hypothesized functions of controlling the endocrine, physiological, and behavioral response to stress, and it is abundantly expressed in the mammalian brain, with especially high amounts of the peptide concentrated in the parvocellular division of the hypothalamic PVN, bed nucleus of the stria terminalis, central amygdala, lateral hypothalamus, and locus coeruleus (Merchenthaler et al., 1982; Morin et al., 1999). Dense CRF fibers have been located in the lateral septum, bed nucleus of the stria terminalis, central nucleus of the amygdala, median eminence, the raphe nuclei, and the spinal cord (Merchenthaler et al., 1982; Morin et al., 1999; Korosi et al., 2007).

#### UROCORTIN 1

Urocortin 1 is related to CRF, with a sequence identify of 45% (Vaughan et al., 1995). It binds CRFR2 with 100-fold higher affinity than CRF does, indicating that this peptide might be an endogenous ligand for CRFR2 (Vaughan et al., 1995; Chalmers et al., 1996; Perrin and Vale, 1999). The most dominant sites of Ucn1 expression in the mammalian brain includes the centrally projecting Edinger–Westphal nucleus (EWcp) in the rostroventral midbrain, the supraoptic nucleus in the hypothalamus and the superior lateral olive, which have been confirmed in mammalian and non-mammalian species (Iino et al., 1997; Takahashi et al., 1998; Bittencourt et al., 1999; Kozicz et al., 2002, 2008, 2011a; Ryabinin et al., 2005). Networks of Ucn1 fibers have been identified in the lateral septum, internal layer of the median eminence, dorsal raphe nucleus, and the spinal cord, with scattered fibers located in the hypothalamus, hippocampus, cortex, and posterior pituitary (Kozicz et al., 1998; Bittencourt et al., 1999; Iino et al., 1999; Morin et al., 1999; Korosi et al., 2007).

#### UROCORTIN 2

Urocortin 2 is a 38 amino acid peptide, which selectively binds CRFR2 (Reyes et al., 2001). Ucn2 mRNA shows a distinct subcortical distribution, including regions known to be involved in physiological and behavioral responses to stress, such as the PVN, locus coeruleus, and the arcuate nucleus (Reyes et al., 2001). Ucn2 mRNA partially overlaps with the expression of CRF in the PVN and Ucn1 in the brainstem and spinal motor nuclei (Swanson et al., 1983; Bittencourt et al., 1999; Reyes et al., 2001). To date no reliable Ucn2 immunohistochemistry has been performed (due to lack of reliable and specific antibody against Ucn2), hence the distribution of Ucn2 immunoreactive fiber terminals remains to be mapped.

#### UROCORTIN 3

Urocortin 3 is just like Ucn2 a 38 amino acid peptide which selectively binds CRFR2 (Lewis et al., 2001). Ucn3 expressing neurons have a limited distribution compared to CRF and Ucn1, and the peptide is mostly located in forebrain regions, including the preoptic region, hypothalamus, and amygdala. Two areas of the hypothalamus express Ucn3, the first population being neurons in the preoptic nucleus and the second group of neurons are associated with the fornix ("perifornical" Ucn3 neuron population) near the PVN of the hypothalamus (Lewis et al., 2001; Li et al., 2002). More Ucn3 expressing neurons are located in the medial amygdala and paraolivary nucleus (Lewis et al., 2001; Li et al., 2002). Densest innervation of Ucn3 includes the ventromedial hypothalamus, lateral septum, posterior division of the bed nucleus of the stria terminalis and the medial amygdala, which are areas known to express CRFR2 (Lewis et al., 2001; Li et al., 2002).

#### CRF BINDING PROTEIN

CRF binding protein is relatively widely expressed in the mammalian brain, including the cerebral cortex, subcortical limbic system, various sensory relays, raphe nuclei, hypothalamus, and pituitary (Orth and Mount, 1987; Behan et al., 1989; Potter et al., 1992). In humans, the CRF-BP has been found in the liver and in the circulation, where it inactivates CRF and/or Ucn1. The exact function of the protein is still unknown, but it has been proposed that CRF-BP prevents inappropriate pituitary-adrenal activation, e.g., during pregnancy (Potter et al., 1991). Upon binding to CRF-BP, CRF forms a dimer complex and is thought to modulate the endocrine activity of CRF (Lowry et al., 1996). In rat pituitary cells, recombinant CRF-BP blocks secretion of ACTH (Potter et al., 1991). The binding proteins have also been detected in brain regions not associated with CRF actions, suggesting it may have other functions independent from CRF (Potter et al., 1992; Cortright et al., 1995; Bale and Vale, 2004).

#### CRFR1

CRFR1 is a 415 amino acid peptide in mammals and has a widespread expression in stress-related areas located in the central nervous system (CNS). CRFR1 mRNA has been located in the cortex, cerebellum, hippocampus, amygdala, olfactory bulb, lateral septum, thalamus, basal ganglia, the raphe nuclei, pituitary, brain stem, and spinal cord (Van Pett et al., 2000; Korosi et al., 2006, 2007; Justice et al., 2008; Kuhne et al., 2012). Outside the CNS, the CRFR1 is expressed in the thymus, spleen, skin, ovary, testis, gastrointestinal tissue, and adrenal gland (Dufau et al., 1993; Nappi and Rivest, 1995; Slominski et al., 1995; Baigent and Lowry, 2000; Muller et al., 2001; Chatzaki et al., 2004).

A recent study, which aimed at accurately determining the presence of CRFR1 in the brain, revealed that this receptor is present in glutamatergic neurons of the cortex and hippocampus, in gamma-aminobutyric acid containing neurons of the reticular thalamic nucleus, globus pallidus, and septum, and in dopaminergic neurons of the substantia nigra pars compacta and ventral tegmental area. It is also expressed in few serotonergic neurons of the dorsal and media raphe nuclei (Refojo et al., 2011).

#### CRF RECEPTOR 2

CRF receptor 2 is a 397–437 amino acid protein in mammals and it is abundantly expressed in both the CNS and in the periphery (Kishimoto et al., 1995; Lovenberg et al., 1995b; Kostich et al., 1998; Palchaudhuri et al., 1999; Van Pett et al., 2000; Korosi et al., 2007; Justice et al., 2008; Kuhne et al., 2012). In the CNS, CRFR2 is expressed in the olfactory bulb, hippocampus, amygdala, septum, the dorsal and median raphe nuclei, cortex, pituitary, and spinal cord (Palchaudhuri et al., 1999; Bittencourt and Sawchenko, 2000; Van Pett et al., 2000; Korosi et al., 2006, 2007; Lukkes et al., 2011). In the periphery, the receptor has been identified in the retina, heart, skeletal muscle, vasculature, adrenal gland, and gastrointestinal tissue (Lovenberg et al., 1995a; Palchaudhuri et al., 1999; Muller et al., 2001; Chatzaki et al., 2004).

Despite the fact that the distribution of CRFR1 and CRFR2 overlaps in the brain, clear distinctions can be made among brain subregions. For example, the CRFR1 receptor is expressed in the basolateral nucleus of the amygdala, while both CRFR1 and CRFR2 are present in the medial nucleus of the amygdala (Bittencourt and Sawchenko, 2000; Van Pett et al., 2000). Interestingly, mRNA of CRFR2 has been discovered in non-neuronal structures as well, like the choroid plexus and cerebral arterioles (Lovenberg et al., 1995a). In the cerebral arteries and arterioles, stimulation of CRFR2 leads to an increased cerebral blood flow (De Michele et al., 2005).

## EVIDENCE SUPPORTING A DUALISTIC ACTION OF CRFR1 AND CRFR2 DURING STRESS (MAL)ADAPTATION

### STRESS

Stress has been defined as various physiologic alterations, including misbalance of homeostasis and activation of the hypothalamo-pituitary-adrenal (HPA)-axis (Selye, 1936, 1951; Dallman et al., 1987). Upon exposure to a stressor, the HPA-axis is activated by the release of CRF into portal vessels and subsequently acts upon the CRFR1 located in the anterior pituitary (Turnbull and Rivier, 1997; Vale et al., 1997). The initial understanding on the biological significance of CRF system components governing the endocrine stress response has come from various genetically modified animal models. As follows we will overview these animal models.

#### *CRF knockout*

In order to assess the central physiological role of CRF a knockout model was created (Muglia et al., 1995). Mice lacking CRF show decreased glucocorticoid levels after exposure to stress, showing the importance of CRF in regulating the HPA-axis (Muglia et al., 1995; Venihaki and Majzoub, 1999). However, interpretation of data from this animal model is significantly hampered/influenced by compensatory changes in other members of the CRF system. For example, in the absence of CRF, Ucn1 levels in the EWcp are elevated, while distribution remains unchanged (Weninger et al., 1999, 2000).

#### *CRF overexpression*

In order to study chronic activation of the HPA-axis, two independent CRF overexpressing mouse lines were created (Stenzel-Poore et al., 1992; Groenink et al., 2002). Both lines revealed elevated basal plasma corticosterone levels in response to stress. Delayed and attenuated HPA-axis hormone responses to stress, which might be the result of HPA-axis desensitization, were reported in the mice created by Stenzel-Poore et al. (Coste et al., 2001).

#### *Ucn1 knockout*

Two independent Ucn1 knockout models were generated by two groups (Vetter et al., 2002; Wang et al., 2002). Both lines have normal endocrine stress responses, supporting the notion that Ucn1 has a minor or no role in stress induced activation of the HPA-axis. It has been proposed that Ucn1 plays a role in adaptation to stress, rather than initiating the stress response. The fact that Ucn1 KO mice have impaired adaptation to repeated stress supports this notion (Zalutskaya et al., 2007).

#### *Ucn2 knockout*

Ucn2 knockout model showed that HPA-axis activity was normal in male and female mice deficient for Ucn2 (Breu et al., 2012). Stress induced release of corticosterone was equal between knockout and wild type animals. Interestingly, a gender specific phenotype was detected in Ucn2 deficient mice. Females, but not males, lacking Ucn2 show a significant increase in basal daily rhythms of ACTH and corticosterone (Chen et al., 2006). It is known that CRFR2 can modulate the HPA-axis, however, Ucn2 deficiency does not seem to have an impact on the stress induced activation of the axis (Breu et al., 2012).

#### *Ucn3 knockout*

Ucn3 knockout mouse model recently showed that absence of Ucn3 does not have an impact on basal activity of the HPA-axis, as corticosterone levels remained unchanged when compared to wild type littermates (Deussing et al., 2010). After exposure to stress, the corticosterone levels in Ucn3 knockout and wild type mice were equal, which resulted in an operational negative feedback loop of corticosterone on the HPA-axis (Deussing et al., 2010).

#### *Multiple Ucn knockouts*

The importance of the urocortins in the stress system was confirmed by multiple urocortin knockout studies. A double knockout of Ucn1 and 2 in mice showed equal basal corticosterone, but elevated levels after exposure to stress (Neufeld-Cohen et al., 2010a). However, the elevated corticosterone levels after exposure to stress were not observed in an urocortin 1, 2, and 3 triple knockout (Neufeld-Cohen et al., 2010b). These mice deficient for the urocortins were unable to recover properly and this was paired with dysregulated serotonergic function in stress-related neuronal circuits (Neufeld-Cohen et al., 2010b).

#### *CRFR1 knockout*

Two independent lines of CRFR1 knockout lines have demonstrated the importance of CRFR1 in regulation of the HPA-axis in response to stress. KO mice in both lines show an attenuated response to restraint stress by a minimal increase in ACTH and corticosterone. However, basal levels in the CRFR1 null mice are equal between KO and wild type littermates (Smith et al., 1998; Timpl et al., 1998).

#### *CRFR2 knockout*

CRFR2 knockout mice reveal a role for CRFR2 in regulating HPA-axis activation in response to stress, but it appears initiation of the response seems to be normal. These null mice show an early termination of ACTH release, suggesting a role for CRFR2 in maintaining activation of the HPA-axis (Coste et al., 2000). Furthermore, coping with stressors seems to be reduced in CRFR2 KO mice (Coste et al., 2000). Mice deficient for CRFR2 are also hypersensitive to stress, which leads to increased anxiety-like behaviors (Bale et al., 2000; Gammie et al., 2005). Mutant CRFR2 mice have increased CRF mRNA in the central amygdala and increased Ucn-1 and -3 in the EWcp and lateral perifornical region, respectively suggesting a compensatory activation of extrahypothalamic CRF and Ucn systems (Bale et al., 2000, 2002a; Kozicz, 2009). Chronic activation of CRFR2 also promotes an anxiety-like state, with attenuated behavioral and HPA-axis responses to stress (Neufeld-Cohen et al., 2012).

#### *CRFR1 and 2 double knockout*

CRFR1 and CRFR2 double knockout mice show the central role of these receptors in the stress response system. In the absence of both receptors, the double knockout mice show an impaired HPA-axis activation in response to stress (Preil et al., 2001; Bale et al., 2002b). Further, ACTH and corticosterone levels after exposure to stress are lowered in the double knockout mice compared to CRFR1 deficient mice, suggesting a role for CRFR2 in mediating HPA-axis sensitivity (Coste et al., 2000; Bale et al., 2002b).

### ANXIETY

The CRF system has been proposed to be involved in the development of anxiety-related disorders. Cumulative evidence relates dysregulation of CRF systems to the etiology and pathobiology of stress-associated diseases, including anxiety. The following studies which are related to anxiety- and depressive-like behaviors are summarized in **Table 1**.

#### *CRF knockout*

Surprisingly, no behavioral abnormalities have been reported with the CRF knockouts generated by Muglia et al. (1995). Similarly, anxiety-like behavior is the same between knockout and wild type animals under normal and stressful conditions in another CRF deficient mouse created by Weninger et al. (1999). Interestingly, CRFR antagonists have an anxiolytic effect in CRF knockout animals, suggesting that CRFR1 activation is crucial to induce anxiety, while CRF itself may not. These data point toward the significance of another CRFR ligand, like Ucn1, or a yet unidentified neuropeptide, compensating for CRF deficiency in the brain (Weninger et al., 1999; Kozicz, 2007; Kozicz et al., 2011b).

#### *CRF overexpression*

In the model created by Stenzel-Poore et al. (1992), increased anxiety-like and decreased exploratory behavior was observed (Heinrichs et al., 1997; van Gaalen et al., 2002). This increase in anxiety-like behavior could be reversed by administration of CRF antagonist alpha-helical CRF (Stenzel-Poore et al., 1994). Removing the adrenal gland in these animals did not inhibit the anxiogenic effects of CRF overexpression, although corticosterone levels were normalized. This suggests that behavioral effects caused by CRF overexpression are mediated by CRF and CRFRs, rather than being affected by corticosterone (Heinrichs et al., 1997). Along these lines, Refojo et al. (2011) demonstrated that overexpression of limbic CRF in CRF-COE$^{\mathrm{Camk2aCre}}$ mice (Camk2aCre, Cre driven by the calcium/calmodulin-dependent protein kinase type II alpha chain promoter) resulted in increased anxiety-like behavior too, suggesting that limbic CRF in particular would be instrumental in mediating anxiety-like behavior. To date, no data is available on anxiety-like behavior of the CRF overexpressing mice created by Groenink et al. (2002).

#### *Ucn1 knockout*

The behavioral phenotype of Ucn1 KO mice is controversial. The group of Wang et al. (2002) have shown no differences in anxiety-like behavior, whereas Vetter et al. (2002) have demonstrated that Ucn1 deficient animals display increased anxiety-like behavior.

#### *Ucn2 knockout*

Ucn2 knockout mice have revealed no significant changes in anxiety-like behavior. However, when investigating social activities, it was seen that male Ucn2 deficient mice had more passive social interactions and reduced aggressiveness compared to wild type littermates, suggesting that Ucn2 may rather modulate aggressive behavior in male mice (Breu et al., 2012).

#### *Ucn3 knockout*

Ucn3 knockout mice created by Deussing et al. (2010) showed unchanged anxiety-related behaviors compared to wild type mice. However, based on the prevalent expression of Ucn3 throughout the accessory olfactory bulb and altered social discrimination abilities of male and female Ucn3 knockout mice, it has been suggested that Ucn3 plays a role in processing of social cues and establishment of social memories (Deussing et al., 2010).

#### *Multiple Ucn knockout*

Urocortin 1 and 2 double knockout mouse model has demonstrated an anxiolytic phenotype (Neufeld-Cohen et al., 2010a). A further reduction in anxiety-like behavior was observed after double Ucn1/Ucn2 deficient mice were exposed to acute stress, and this reduction in anxiety was correlated with levels of serotonin in anxiety-related brain regions (Neufeld-Cohen et al., 2010a). Remarkably, the triple urocortin knockout mouse showed an increase in anxiety-like behavior 24 h post-stress. This increase in anxiety in triple urocortin knockout mice was also associated with serotonergic function in stress-linked neurocircuits. It has been suggested that Ucn3 is pivotal to the observed phenotype of the triple knockout model (Neufeld-Cohen et al., 2010b).

#### *CRFR1 knockout*

Three studies reported that mice deficient for CRFR1 exhibited, what seemed to be, reduced anxiety-like behavior. In different tests of spontaneous anxiety, open field (a measure of exploratory behavior and general activity), light-dark box (based on the aversion of mice to well illuminated areas and on exploratory behavior in response to stressors), defensive withdrawal (a measure of conflict between exploratory behavior and retreat), and elevated plus maze (based on the aversion for open and elevated areas and on exploratory behavior in novel areas), which normally inhibit behavioral activity, CRFR1 deficient mice showed heightened levels of locomotion consistent with anxiety-like behavior (Smith et al., 1998; Timpl et al., 1998; Contarino et al., 1999). The anxiolytic effect of CRFR1 deficient mice seems to be mediated by reduced CRFR1 expression in the basolateral amygdala (Sztainberg et al., 2010). Furthermore, stress induced hormone secretion showed that CRFR1 knockout mice had reduced levels of ACTH and corticosterone, providing evidence that CRFR1 mediates anxiety and stress induced-hormone activation (Smith et al., 1998; Timpl et al., 1998). Opposite effects were found in CRFR1$^{\mathrm{Camk2aCre}}$ mice generated by Muller et al. (2003) in which Cre mediated deletion of CRFR1 starts in the second week of postnatal life. After

**Table 1 | Summary of animal models targeting CRF system components.**

| Experimental procedure | Specificity | Anxiety | Depression | Reference |
|---|---|---|---|---|
| **CRF KNOCKOUT** | | | | |
| Targeted mutation of mice embryonic stem cells | Developmental | = | No data | Muglia et al. (1995) |
| **CRF OVEREXPRESSION** | | | | |
| Transgenic CRF-OE mice under metallothionein promoter | Developmental | ↑ | No data | Stenzel-Poore et al. (1992) |
| Transgenic CRF-$OE_{2122}$ mice C57BL/6J background | Developmental | No data | No data | Groenink et al. (2002) |
| Lentiviral based overexpression in mice | Central amygdala (1); bed nucleus of the stria terminalis (2) | (1) ↑<br>(2) = | (1) =<br>(2) ↑ | Regev et al. (2011) |
| Lentiviral based overexpression in mice | Central amygdala | ↑ | ↑ | Keen-Rhinehart et al. (2009) |
| **Ucn1 KNOCKOUT** | | | | |
| Ucn1 gene replacement with neomycin-resistant gene cascette on C57BL/6 background (mice) | Developmental | ↑ | No data | Vetter et al. (2002) |
| Mice embryonic stem cell technology | Developmental | = | No data | Wang et al. (2002) |
| Mice embryonic stem cell technology | Developmental | No data | No data | Zalutskaya et al. (2007) |
| **Ucn2 KNOCKOUT** | | | | |
| Replacement Ucn2 open reading frame by a tau-lacZ reporter gene in mice | Developmental | = | ↓ | Breu et al. (2012) |
| Ucn2 gene replacement with neomycin-resistant gene cascette on C57BL/6 background in mice | Developmental | = | ↓ | Chen et al. (2006) |
| **Ucn3 KNOCKOUT** | | | | |
| Replacement Ucn3 open reading frame by a tau-lacZ reporter gene in mice | Developmental | = | = | Deussing et al. (2010) |
| **Ucn1 AND 2 DOUBLE KNOCKOUT** | | | | |
| Crossbreeding Ucn1 and Ucn2 single knockout mice on mixed C57BL/6 × 129 background (mice) | Developmental | ↓ | No data | Neufeld-Cohen et al. (2010a) |
| **Ucn1, 2, AND 3 TRIPLE KNOCKOUT** | | | | |
| Crossbreeding Ucn1, Ucn2, and Ucn3 single knockout mice on mixed C57BL/6 × 129 background (mice) | Developmental | ↑ | No data | Neufeld-Cohen et al. (2010b) |
| **CRFR1 KNOCKOUT** | | | | |
| Deletion of CRFR1 locus in mice embryonic stem cells | Developmental | ↓ | No data | Timpl et al. (1998) |
| Replacement of CRFR1 gene exons by PGK-neo cascette (mice) | Developmental | ↓ | No data | Smith et al. (1998) |
| Lentiviral-based CRFR1 interference (mice) | Basolateral amygdala | ↓ | No data | Sztainberg et al. (2010) |
| Cre mediated deletion of CRFR1 (mice) | Anterior forebrain and limbic system | ↓ | No data | Muller et al. (2003) |
| Cre mediated deletion of CRFR1 in mice | Site specific knockouts in forebrain glutamatergic neurons (1); forebrain GABAergic neurons (2); midbrain dopaminergic neurons (3); brainstem serotonergic neurons (4) | (1) ↓<br>(2) =<br>(3) ↑<br>(4) = | No data | Refojo et al. (2011) |
| Lentiviral based system of RNA interference in mice | Globus pallidus | ↑ | No data | Sztainberg et al. (2011) |

*(Continued)*

**Table 1 | Continued**

| Experimental procedure | Specificity | Anxiety | Depression | Reference |
|---|---|---|---|---|
| **CRFR2 KNOCKOUT** | | | | |
| Homologous recombination in mice embryonic stem cells | Developmental | = | No data | Coste et al. (2000) |
| Targeted deletion of CRFR2 locus in mice embryonic stem cells | Developmental | ↑ | ↑ | Bale et al. (2000) |
| CRFR2 exon replacement with neomycin-resistant gene cascette in mice | Developmental | ↑ | No data | Kishimoto et al. (2000) |
| Lentiviral based system of RNA interference in mice | Bed nucleus of the stria terminalis | ↑ | No data | Lebow et al. (2012) |
| **CRFR 1 AND 2 DOUBLE KNOCKOUT** | | | | |
| CRFR2 knockout mice bred to CRFR1 knockout mice on mixed 129:C57BL/6 background | Developmental | ↑ | No data | Bale et al. (2002b) |
| CRFR2 knockout mice bred to CRFR1 knockout mice | Developmental | No data | No data | Preil et al. (2001) |

*↑, indicates an increase; ↓, indicates a decrease; =, indicates no difference in anxiety- or depressive-like behavior as comparing mutant and wildtype animals.*

exposure to restraint stress, these mice exhibited elevated levels of ACTH and corticosterone, while showing reduced anxiety-like behavior.

#### *CRFR2 knockout*

In contrast to CRFR1 deficient mice, CRFR2 deficient mice do not show a consistent change in anxiety-like behavior. One study has shown that CRFR2 knockouts produced no significant effects on anxiety responses in the elevated plus maze or in an open field test (Coste et al., 2000). Another study has demonstrated no behavioral changes in the light-dark test, but appealingly, the CRFR2 knockout mice have increased anxiety in the elevated plus maze and open field test (Kishimoto et al., 2000). These anxiogenic-like effects may be influenced by the reported increase in CRF mRNA in the central amygdala of the CRFR2 knockout mice (Bale et al., 2000). This brain region is associated in the activation of diverse responses induced by stress (Davis, 1992). However, some data suggests a sex effect of emotional behavior mediated by CRFR2. Female knockout mice seem to have behavior comparable to wild type littermates, while the male knockouts exhibit more anxiogenic-like behavior (Kishimoto et al., 2000).

#### *CRFR 1 and 2 double knockout*

CRFR 1 and 2 double knockout mice, in terms on anxiety-like behavior, displayed a sexually dichotomous phenotype (Preil et al., 2001; Bale et al., 2002b). Female double mutant mice showed reduced levels of anxiety-like behavior, while male double knockouts did not, compared to their wild type littermates (Bale et al., 2002b). The behavioral phenotype of the double knockout model generated by Preil et al. (2001) has not been researched yet.

### DEPRESSION

Strong evidence links the stress response, and the sensitivity to stressful encounters, to the development of depression (e.g., Nestler et al., 2002; de Kloet et al., 2005; McEwen et al., 2012). While the stress response is essential for successful adaptation, chronic stress can accelerate disease processes, and lead to depression or other mood disorders (Nestler et al., 2002). As follows we will highlight some of the available large body of evidence linking CRF family of neuropeptides and their receptors to the development of depression.

#### *CRF*

Elevated CRF levels and decreased receptor expression have been found in post-mortem examination of suicide victims. In addition, disproportionate activation of the HPA-axis has been reported in more than one-half of patients diagnosed with depression, and these symptoms can be corrected by treatment with antidepressants (Holsboer, 1999). CRF was also found to be elevated in cerebrospinal fluid of depressed patients, which was reversed in patients treated with antidepressants (De Bellis et al., 1993; Heuser et al., 1998). Reduced CRF binding sites in the frontal cortex of suicide victims have also been identified (Nemeroff et al., 1984, 1988). This was interpreted as central CRF overabundance leading to CRFR desensitization, a common phenomenon for G-protein coupled receptors (Holsboer and Ising, 2010). Furthermore, hypercortisolemia and impairment of negative feedback by cortisol on the HPA-axis have also been attributed to elevated CRF levels (Reul and Holsboer, 2002; Keck, 2006). In support for a role for CRF overexpression in the pathobiology of depression, a recent study performed by Keen-Rhinehart et al. (2009), in which CRF was chronically overexpressed in the central nucleus of the amygdala in female rats revealed an amplified CRF concentration in the PVN and a decreased glucocorticoid negative feedback, both markers which have previously been associated with the pathophysiology of depression (Nemeroff et al., 1984, 1988). Depressive-like behavior was further confirmed in the forced swim test (FST; measures escape behavior and behavioral despair), as mutant rats overexpressing CRF showed increased floating times and reduced escape behavior (Keen-Rhinehart et al., 2009).

No behavioral tests were performed on the CRF null mice created by Muglia et al. (1995) and Weninger et al. (1999) to assess depressive-like behavior.

#### *Urocortins*

A study where urocortin peptides have been injected i.c.v. into mice (Tanaka and Telegdy, 2008) revealed that while Ucn1 had no effect on the animal's behavior, both Ucn2 and 3 displayed strong antidepressant-like activity by decreasing immobility time and increased climbing and swimming behavior in a FST (Tanaka and Telegdy, 2008). Moreover, single nucleotide polymorphisms (SNP) located in the gene for Ucn3 have also been associated with the antidepressant response (Wong et al., 2008). While a study assessing levels of Ucn1 and 2 has not found any significantly changes in patients suffering from major depressive disorder vs. controls (Kang et al., 2007), Ucn1 mRNA is markedly upregulated in the EWcp in depressed male suicide victims, compared to healthy males (Kozicz et al., 2008). This upregulation was not observed in female suicide victims, suggesting a gender specific neuropathology (Kozicz et al., 2008).

In animal models for depression, Ucn2 knockout mice showed a significant decrease in depressive-like behavior as assessed by the FST. These effects were only evident in the female null mice, suggesting a role for Ucn2 in mediating the sex differences observed in the stress response (Wang et al., 2002; Chen et al., 2006) albeit in an opposite direction as Ucn1 may (Kozicz et al., 2008). In contrast, mice deficient for Ucn3 have unchanged depressive-like behavior compared to wild type mice (Deussing et al., 2010).

#### *CRFR1*

CRFR1 activation of CRFR1 has been associated with anxiety or depressive-like behaviors, which could be treated by administrating CRFR antagonists in patients suffering from major depression (Kehne and Cain, 2010). Furthermore, quantitative PCR analyses have shown that mRNA for CRFR1, but not CRFR2, is reduced in the frontopolar cortex in suicide brains, which might be secondary to high CRF or Ucn1 levels (Merali et al., 2004; Kozicz et al., 2008). These data suggests that at least for CRFR1, dysregulation in the forebrain may contribute to the neuropathology of depression. To date, major pharmaceutical companies are focusing on CRFR1 as the primary target for antidepressant development. However, limited phase 2/3 clinical trial results with two CRFR1 antagonists, suggest a lack of efficacy in patients suffering from major depressive disorder (Kehne and Cain, 2010). This suggests that an overall inhibition of CRFR1 does not inhibit depressive-like behavior, which could mean a more complex role for CRFR1 in mediating mood disorders (see later in text).

#### *CRFR2*

The role of CRFR2 is more complex, as the receptor has been associated with enhancement as well as inhibition of stress responsivity (Kehne and Cain, 2010). More specifically, CRFR2 deficient mice tested in the FST displayed increased immobility which indicates depressive-like behavior (Bale and Vale, 2003; Todorovic et al., 2005) which could be effectively reversed by the CRFR1 antagonist antalarmin (Bale and Vale, 2003).

Taken together, the findings listed above have led to the notion that activation of CRFR1 is responsible for the initiation of the stress response and mediates a rather pro anxiety/depression behavior (**Table 1**). In contrast, CRFR2 is involved in the recovery phase of the stress response, and exhibit a more anxiolytic anti-depression function (**Table 1**). Although a great deal of experimental evidence supported this dualistic action of CRFR1 and CRFR2 in health and disease, not all data are in favor of this notion. Consequently, the fundamental question has recently been raised; are the endocrine, physiological and behavioral changes controlled/mediated by CRFR1 and CRFR2 the consequence of a balanced, dualistic function of these receptors or in a broader sense that of CRF system components? Or can we possibly identify specific brain regions and/or neuron populations responsible for the endocrine, physiological and behavioral stress response? Recent technical developments have allowed us to directly address this issue by creating unique animal models.

### FINDINGS THAT CHALLENGE THE DUALISTIC ACTION OF CRFR1 AND CRFR2 IN STRESS (MAL)ADAPTATION

Conditional mutagenesis of CRFR1 using a *Cre-Lox* system has led to the development of various conditional knockouts were CRFR1 has been deleted in specific neuron populations previously implicated in stress and stress-associated anxiety and depression: (a) $CRFR1^{GLU\text{-}CKO}$, where CRFR1 is deleted in forebrain glutamatergic neurons; (b) $CRFR1^{GABA\text{-}CKO}$, deleting the receptor in forebrain GABAergic neurons; (c) $CRFR1^{DA\text{-}CKO}$, carrying CRFR1 deletion in midbrain dopaminergic neurons; and (d) $CRFR1^{5HT\text{-}CKO}$, deleting CRFR1 in brainstem serotonergic neurons (Refojo et al., 2011) (**Figure 2**). The roles of the different neuronal populations expressing CRFR1 on emotional behavior, these knockouts were subjected to a series of tests. $CRFR1^{GLU\text{-}CKO}$ mice showed reduced anxiety-like behavior pointing toward a central role of glutamate neurotransmission in stress induced anxiety. These mice lack CRFR1 expression in glutamatergic neurons in the hippocampus and amygdala, two important limbic regions in the neuropathology of mood disorders (Refojo et al., 2005; Sanacora et al., 2008). In line with these data, $CRFR1^{Glu\text{-}CKO}$ animals also show impairments in CRF-induced changes on excitatory neurotransmission in these limbic regions (Refojo et al., 2011). It was also shown that CRFR1 facilitates neuronal activity propagation from the classical hippocampal input region (dentate gyrus) to the CA1 output area. In conclusion, activation of CRFR1 in limbic glutamatergic neurons, as it would in response to a stressor, modulates glutamatergic neurotransmission, giving rise to neuronal excitation in the hippocampal network, and consequently anxiogenesis (Refojo et al., 2011).

Unexpectedly, for $CRFR1^{DA\text{-}CKO}$, an increase in anxiety-like behavior was found, whereas for $CRFR1^{GABA\text{-}CKO}$ and $CRFR1^{5HT\text{-}CKO}$ no anxiety-related behavioral changes were observed (Refojo et al., 2011). As to the $CRFR1^{DA\text{-}CKO}$, the deletion of CRFR1 in dopaminergic neurons in the midbrain ventral tegmental area and substantia nigra pars compacta (VTA/SNpc), together with the fact that CRF increases the action potential

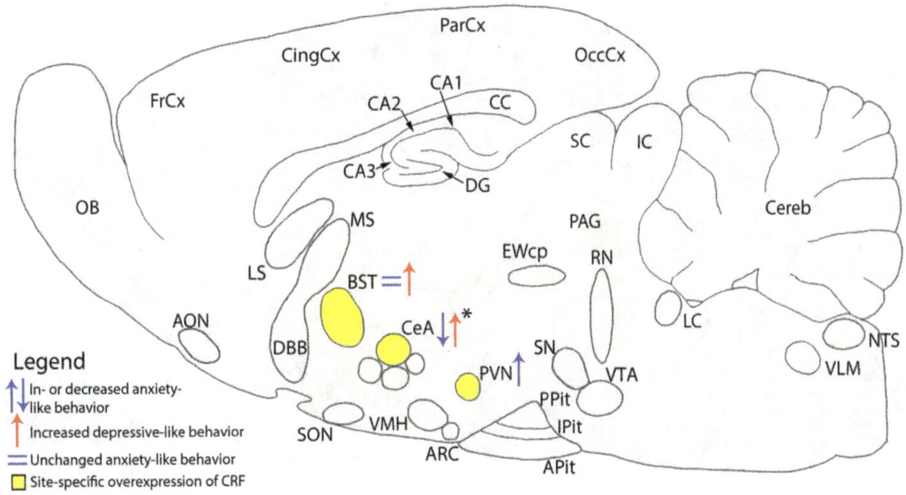


**FIGURE 1 | Schematic cross-section of the mouse brain showing site specific overexpression of CRF and the resulting change on anxiety- or depressive-like behavior.** Areas of interest are the Bed nucleus of the Stria Terminalis (BST) (Regev et al., 2011), central nucleus of the Amygdala (CeA) (Keen-Rhinehart et al., 2009; Regev et al., 2011), and the paraventricular nucleus (PVN) (Elliott et al., 2010). *Change in anxiety- or depressive-like behavior is dependent on the conditions the mice were subjected to. AON, anterior olfactory nucleus; Apit, anterior pituitary; ARC, arcuate nucleus; BLA, basolateral amygdala; BST, bed nucleus of the stria terminalis; CA1-3, fields CA1-3 of Ammon's horn; CC, corpus callosum; CeA, central nucleus of the amygdala; Cereb, cerebellum; CingCx, cingulate cortex; DBB, diagonal band of Broca; DG, dentate gyrus; EWcp, centrally projecting Edinger–Westphal nucleus; FrCx, frontal cortex; IC, inferior colliculus; IPit, intermediate pituitary; LC, locus coeruleus; LS, lateral septum; MS, medial septum; NTS, nucleus tractus solitarii; OB, olfactory bulb; OccCx, occipital cortex; PAG, periaqueductal gray; ParCx, parietal cortex; PPit, posterior pituitary; PVN, paraventricular nucleus; RN, raphe nuclei; SC, superior colliculus; SN, substantia nigra; SON, supraoptic nucleus; VLM, ventrolateral medulla; VMH, ventromedial hypothalamus; VTA, ventral tegmental area.

firing of dopamine neurons in the VTA (Wanat et al., 2008) are important to control the animal's mood. It was also shown that $CRFR1^{DA\text{-}CKO}$ displayed a decreased response to stress induced dopamine release in the prefrontal cortex (PFC), indicating that CRFR1 targets dopamine cells to control dopamine release into the PFC under stressful conditions (Refojo et al., 2011). The findings mentioned above strongly imply that stress-associated anxiety-like behavior might be a consequence of an imbalance between CRFR1 controlled glutamatergic and dopaminergic neuronal populations involved in mediating emotional behavior (Refojo et al., 2011).

In addition, the contrasting roles for CRFR1 expressed by dopaminergic vs. glutamatergic neurons suggest that under physiological conditions, CRF and CRFR1 controlled glutamatergic and dopaminergic systems might function in an antagonistic manner to maintain adaptive anxiety responses during periods of stress (Refojo et al., 2011). The fact that simultaneous deletion of CRFR1 in both glutamatergic and dopaminergic neurons do not show alterations in anxiety-like behavior, supports this notion.

A neuron population specific role for CRF system components in mediating stress-associated emotional response is further supported by a study by Sztainberg et al. (2011). These authors have demonstrated that a viral-mediated specific knock-down (KD) of CRFR1 in the globus pallidus results in increased anxiety-like behavior in mice (Sztainberg et al., 2011) (**Figure 2**). Earlier studies have demonstrated that this region is a key mediator of anxiety behavior, as it is associated with motor and associative functions (Baumann et al., 1999; Critchley et al., 2001; Kita, 2007; Sztainberg et al., 2011). In contrast CRFR1 expressed in the basolateral amygdala mediates anxiogenic behaviors in mice, further substantiating the view that the very same receptor can mediate opposing behavioral responses depending on the brain site of action (Sztainberg et al., 2010) (**Figure 2**).

To date there is only one study examining a site specific action of CRFR2. A lentiviral KD of CRFR2 specifically in the bed nucleus of the stria terminalis reduces susceptibility to stress induced anxiety in an animal model for post-traumatic stress disorder, suggesting an important role for CRFR2 in stress coping (Lebow et al., 2012) (**Figure 2**).

With regard to CRF, a site specific action can also been proposed. More specifically, prolonged and site specific overexpression of CRF in the central amygdala attenuates stress induced anxiety-like behaviors without effecting depression-like behavior, whereas CRF overexpression in the bed nucleus of the stria terminalis increased depressive-like behavior, without affecting anxiety levels in male mice (Regev et al., 2011) (**Figure 1**). Somewhat conflicting data were reported in a mouse model, in which unrestrained CRF synthesis in CeA produced a dysregulation of the HPA-axis, depression-like behavior, as well as physiological and reproductive consequences associated with stress-related disorders (Keen-Rhinehart et al., 2009) (**Figure 1**).

Using two lentiviral-based approaches to specifically KD or conditionally overexpress (OE) CRF in the CeA of adult mice anxiety- and depression-like behaviors were evaluated under basal and stressful conditions. Intriguingly, changing CeA-CRF levels mildly affected anxiety-like behaviors under basal conditions. In contrast, following exposure to an acute stressor, CeA-CRF-KD

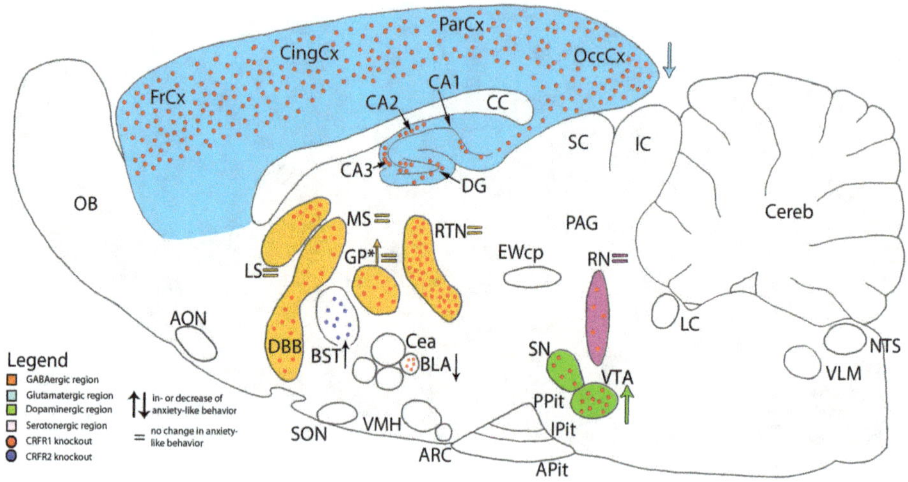


**FIGURE 2 | Schematic cross-section of the mouse brain showing site specific knockouts of either CRF receptor 1 or 2 and the associated neurotransmitter specificity.** Colored arrows show the direction of change on anxiety-like behavior in mice which lack CRFR1 in specific brain areas (Refojo et al., 2011). *In one study, CRFR1 was deleted in only the GP (Sztainberg et al., 2011), while in another study CRFR1 was deleted in all areas expressing GABA (Refojo et al., 2011). Other areas of interest are the basolateral Amygdala (BLA) (Sztainberg et al., 2010) and Bed nucleus of the Stria Terminalis (BST) (Lebow et al., 2012). AON, anterior olfactory nucleus; Apit, anterior pituitary; ARC, arcuate nucleus; BLA, basolateral amygdala; BST, bed nucleus of the stria terminalis; CA1-3, fields CA1-3 of Ammon's horn; CC, corpus callosum; CeA, central nucleus of the amygdala; Cereb, cerebellum; CingCx, cingulate cortex; DBB, diagonal band of Broca; DG, dentate gyrus; EWcp, centrally projecting Edinger–Westphal nucleus; FrCx, frontal cortex; GP, globus pallidus; IC, inferior colliculus; IPit, intermediate pituitary; LC, locus coeruleus; LS, lateral septum; MS, medial septum; NTS, nucleus tractus solitarii; OB, olfactory bulb; OccCx, occipital cortex; PAG, periaqueductal gray; ParCx, parietal cortex; PPit, posterior pituitary; RN, raphe nuclei; RTN, reticular thalamic nucleus; SC, superior colliculus; SN, substantia nigra; SON, supraoptic nucleus; VLM, ventrolateral medulla; VMH, ventromedial hypothalamus; VTA, ventral tegmental area.

strongly attenuated stress induced anxiety-like behaviors, whereas a short-term CeA-CRF-OE enhanced the stress induced effects on these behaviors (Regev et al., 2012). This study suggests that an adequate behavioral response to stress is not only determined by the level and site of expression of CRF system components, but depends also on the condition an animal is exposed to.

Based on the pioneering studies discussed above (for overview see **Table 1** as well as **Figures 1** and **2**), a picture is emerging that the roles of CRF system components in the animal's stress response and mood cannot be simplified to a dualistic model of action, but are rather linked to the recruitment of specific brain areas and neuron populations. Therefore, researches in the field must embark on a long journey to systematically and comprehensively exploring the significance of the many brain areas and neuron populations expressing one or several of the CRF system components, before we can conclude on the role(s) of CRFR1 and CRFR2 in health and disease.

## CONCLUSION

Taken together, recent studies using conditional mutagenesis or viral knock-down or overexpression of CRF system components strongly indicate that the involvement of CRF system components in stress-associated anxiety and depression-like behavior cannot be explained by a universal and brain wide mechanisms, and therefore the earlier proposed dualistic action of CRFR1 and CRFR2 in stress may not hold. Rather, CRF system components would be specifically recruited in particular functional neuronal circuits, which in turn would allow the expression of the necessary and sufficient endocrine, physiological, and behavioral responses to stress as conditions dictate.

## REFERENCES


Baigent, S. M., and Lowry, P. J. (2000). mRNA expression profiles for corticotrophin-releasing factor (CRF), urocortin, CRF receptors and CRF-binding protein in peripheral rat tissues. *J. Mol. Endocrinol.* 25, 43–52.

Bale, T. L., Contarino, A., Smith, G. W., Chan, R., Gold, L. H., Sawchenko, P. E., et al. (2000). Mice deficient for corticotropin-releasing hormone receptor-2 display anxiety-like behaviour and are hypersensitive to stress. *Nat. Genet.* 24, 410–414.

Bale, T. L., Lee, K. F., and Vale, W. W. (2002a). The role of corticotropin-releasing factor receptors in stress and anxiety. *Integr. Comp. Biol.* 42, 552–555.

Bale, T. L., Picetti, R., Contarino, A., Koob, G. F., Vale, W. W., and Lee, K. F. (2002b). Mice deficient for both corticotropin-releasing factor receptor 1 (CRFR1) and CRFR2 have an impaired stress response and display sexually dichotomous anxiety-like behavior. *J. Neurosci.* 22, 193–199.

Bale, T. L., and Vale, W. W. (2003). Increased depression-like behaviors in corticotropin-releasing factor receptor-2-deficient mice: sexually dichotomous responses. *J. Neurosci.* 23, 5295–5301.

Bale, T. L., and Vale, W. W. (2004). CRF and CRF receptors: role in stress responsivity and other behaviors. *Annu. Rev. Pharmacol. Toxicol.* 44, 525–557.

Baumann, B., Danos, P., Krell, D., Diekmann, S., Leschinger, A., Stauch, R., et al. (1999). Reduced volume of limbic system-affiliated basal ganglia in mood disorders: preliminary data from a postmortem study. *J. Neuropsychiatry Clin. Neurosci.* 11, 71–78.

Behan, D. P., Linton, E. A., and Lowry, P. J. (1989). Isolation of the human plasma corticotrophin-releasing factor-binding protein. *J. Endocrinol.* 122, 23–31.

Bittencourt, J. C., and Sawchenko, P. E. (2000). Do centrally administered neuropeptides access cognate receptors? An analysis in the central corticotropin-releasing factor system. *J. Neurosci.* 20, 1142–1156.

Bittencourt, J. C., Vaughan, J., Arias, C., Rissman, R. A., Vale, W. W., and Sawchenko, P. E. (1999). Urocortin expression in rat brain: evidence against a pervasive relationship of urocortin-containing projections with targets bearing type 2 CRF receptors. *J. Comp. Neurol.* 415, 285–312.

Boorse, G. C., Crespi, E. J., Dautzenberg, F. M., and Denver, R. J. (2005). Urocortins of the South African clawed frog, *Xenopus laevis*: conservation of structure and function in tetrapod evolution. *Endocrinology* 146, 4851–4860.

Breu, J., Touma, C., Holter, S. M., Knapman, A., Wurst, W., and Deussing, J. M. (2012). Urocortin 2 modulates aspects of social behaviour in mice. *Behav. Brain Res.* 233, 331–336.

Chalmers, D. T., Lovenberg, T. W., Grigoriadis, D. E., Behan, D. P., and De Souza, E. B. (1996). Corticotrophin-releasing factor receptors: from molecular biology to drug design. *Trends Pharmacol. Sci.* 17, 166–172.

Chatzaki, E., Murphy, B. J., Wang, L., Million, M., Ohning, G. V., Crowe, P. D., et al. (2004). Differential profile of CRF receptor distribution in the rat stomach and duodenum assessed by newly developed CRF receptor antibodies. *J. Neurochem.* 88, 1–11.

Chen, A., Zorrilla, E., Smith, S., Rousso, D., Levy, C., Vaughan, J., et al. (2006). Urocortin 2-deficient mice exhibit gender-specific alterations in circadian hypothalamus-pituitary-adrenal axis and depressive-like behavior. *J. Neurosci.* 26, 5500–5510.

Contarino, A., Dellu, F., Koob, G. F., Smith, G. W., Lee, K. F., Vale, W., et al. (1999). Reduced anxiety-like and cognitive performance in mice lacking the corticotropin-releasing factor receptor 1. *Brain Res.* 835, 1–9.

Cortright, D. N., Nicoletti, A., and Seasholtz, A. F. (1995). Molecular and biochemical characterization of the mouse brain corticotropin-releasing hormone-binding protein. *Mol. Cell. Endocrinol.* 111, 147–157.

Coste, S. C., Kesterson, R. A., Heldwein, K. A., Stevens, S. L., Heard, A. D., Hollis, J. H., et al. (2000). Abnormal adaptations to stress and impaired cardiovascular function in mice lacking corticotropin-releasing hormone receptor-2. *Nat. Genet.* 24, 403–409.

Coste, S. C., Murray, S. E., and Stenzel-Poore, M. P. (2001). Animal models of CRH excess and CRH receptor deficiency display altered adaptations to stress. *Peptides* 22, 733–741.

Critchley, H. D., Melmed, R. N., Featherstone, E., Mathias, C. J., and Dolan, R. J. (2001). Brain activity during biofeedback relaxation: a functional neuroimaging investigation. *Brain* 124, 1003–1012.

Dallman, M. F., Akana, S. F., Cascio, C. S., Darlington, D. N., Jacobson, L., and Levin, N. (1987). Regulation of ACTH secretion: variations on a theme of B. *Recent Prog. Horm. Res.* 43, 113–173.

Davis, M. (1992). The role of the amygdala in fear and anxiety. *Annu. Rev. Neurosci.* 15, 353–375.

De Bellis, M. D., Gold, P. W., Geracioti, T. D. Jr., Listwak, S. J., and Kling, M. A. (1993). Association of fluoxetine treatment with reductions in CSF concentrations of corticotropin-releasing hormone and arginine vasopressin in patients with major depression. *Am. J. Psychiatry* 150, 656–657.

de Kloet, E. R., Joels, M., and Holsboer, F. (2005). Stress and the brain: from adaptation to disease. *Nat. Rev. Neurosci.* 6, 463–475.

De Michele, M., Touzani, O., Foster, A. C., Fieschi, C., Sette, G., and McCulloch, J. (2005). Corticotropin-releasing factor: effect on cerebral blood flow in physiologic and ischaemic conditions. *Exp. Brain Res.* 165, 375–382.

Deussing, J. M., Breu, J., Kuhne, C., Kallnik, M., Bunck, M., Glasl, L., et al. (2010). Urocortin 3 modulates social discrimination abilities via corticotropin-releasing hormone receptor type 2. *J. Neurosci.* 30, 9103–9116.

Dufau, M. L., Tinajero, J. C., and Fabbri, A. (1993). Corticotropin-releasing factor: an antireproductive hormone of the testis. *FASEB J.* 7, 299–307.

Elliott, E., Ezra-Nevo, G., Regev, L., Neufeld-Cohen, A., and Chen, A. (2010). Resilience to social stress coincides with functional DNA methylation of the Crf gene in adult mice. *Nat. Neurosci.* 13, 1351–1353.

Gammie, S. C., Hasen, N. S., Stevenson, S. A., Bale, T. L., and D'Anna, K. L. (2005). Elevated stress sensitivity in corticotropin-releasing factor receptor 2 deficient mice decreases maternal, but not intermale aggression. *Behav. Brain Res.* 160, 169–177.

Groenink, L., Dirks, A., Verdouw, P. M., Schipholt, M., Veening, J. G., van der Gugten, J., et al. (2002). HPA axis dysregulation in mice overexpressing corticotropin releasing hormone. *Biol. Psychiatry* 51, 875–881.

Heinrichs, S. C., Cole, B. J., Pich, E. M., Menzaghi, F., Koob, G. F., and Hauger, R. L. (1992). Endogenous corticotropin-releasing factor modulates feeding induced by neuropeptide Y or a tail-pinch stressor. *Peptides* 13, 879–884.

Heinrichs, S. C., Min, H., Tamraz, S., Carmouche, M., Boehme, S. A., and Vale, W. W. (1997). Anti-sexual and anxiogenic behavioral consequences of corticotropin-releasing factor overexpression are centrally mediated. *Psychoneuroendocrinology* 22, 215–224.

Heuser, I., Bissette, G., Dettling, M., Schweiger, U., Gotthardt, U., Schmider, J., et al. (1998). Cerebrospinal fluid concentrations of corticotropin-releasing hormone, vasopressin, and somatostatin in depressed patients and healthy controls: response to amitriptyline treatment. *Depress. Anxiety* 8, 71–79.

Holsboer, F. (1999). The rationale for corticotropin-releasing hormone receptor (CRH-R) antagonists to treat depression and anxiety. *J. Psychiatr. Res.* 33, 181–214.

Holsboer, F., and Ising, M. (2010). Stress hormone regulation: biological role and translation into therapy. *Annu. Rev. Psychol.* 61, 81–109, C1–C11.

Hsu, S. Y., and Hsueh, A. J. (2001). Human stresscopin and stresscopin-related peptide are selective ligands for the type 2 corticotropin-releasing hormone receptor. *Nat. Med.* 7, 605–611.

Iino, K., Sasano, H., Oki, Y., Andoh, N., Shin, R. W., Kitamoto, T., et al. (1997). Urocortin expression in human pituitary gland and pituitary adenoma. *J. Clin. Endocrinol. Metab.* 82, 3842–3850.

Iino, K., Sasano, H., Oki, Y., Andoh, N., Shin, R. W., Kitamoto, T., et al. (1999). Urocortin expression in the human central nervous system. *Clin. Endocrinol. (Oxf.)* 50, 107–114.

Inoue, K., Valdez, G. R., Reyes, T. M., Reinhardt, L. E., Tabarin, A., Rivier, J., et al. (2003). Human urocortin II, a selective agonist for the type 2 corticotropin-releasing factor receptor, decreases feeding and drinking in the rat. *J. Pharmacol. Exp. Ther.* 305, 385–393.

Justice, N. J., Yuan, Z. F., Sawchenko, P. E., and Vale, W. (2008). Type 1 corticotropin-releasing factor receptor expression reported in BAC transgenic mice: implications for reconciling ligand-receptor mismatch in the central corticotropin-releasing factor system. *J. Comp. Neurol.* 511, 479–496.

Kang, H. J., Adams, D. H., Simen, A., Simen, B. B., Rajkowska, G., Stockmeier, C. A., et al. (2007). Gene expression profiling in postmortem prefrontal cortex of major depressive disorder. *J. Neurosci.* 27, 13329–13340.

Keck, M. E. (2006). Corticotropin-releasing factor, vasopressin and receptor systems in depression and anxiety. *Amino Acids* 31, 241–250.

Keen-Rhinehart, E., Michopoulos, V., Toufexis, D. J., Martin, E. I., Nair, H., Ressler, K. J., et al. (2009). Continuous expression of corticotropin-releasing factor in the central nucleus of the amygdala emulates the dysregulation of the stress and reproductive axes. *Mol. Psychiatry* 14, 37–50.

Kehne, J. H., and Cain, C. K. (2010). Therapeutic utility of non-peptidic CRF1 receptor antagonists in anxiety, depression, and stress-related disorders: evidence from animal models. *Pharmacol. Ther.* 128, 460–487.

Kishimoto, T., Pearse, R. V. II, Lin, C. R., and Rosenfeld, M. G. (1995). A sauvagine/corticotropin-releasing factor receptor expressed in heart and skeletal muscle. *Proc. Natl. Acad. Sci. U.S.A.* 92, 1108–1112.

Kishimoto, T., Radulovic, J., Radulovic, M., Lin, C. R., Schrick, C., Hooshmand, F., et al. (2000). Deletion of crhr2 reveals an anxiolytic role for corticotropin-releasing hormone receptor-2. *Nat. Genet.* 24, 415–419.

Kita, H. (2007). Globus pallidus external segment. *Prog. Brain Res.* 160, 111–133.

Koob, G. F., and Heinrichs, S. C. (1999). A role for corticotropin releasing factor and urocortin in behavioral responses to stressors. *Brain Res.* 848, 141–152.

Korosi, A., Kozicz, T., Richter, J., Veening, J. G., Olivier, B., and Roubos, E. W. (2007). Corticotropin-releasing factor, urocortin 1, and their receptors in the mouse spinal cord. *J. Comp. Neurol.* 502, 973–989.

Korosi, A., Veening, J. G., Kozicz, T., Henckens, M., Dederen, J., Groenink, L., et al. (2006). Distribution and expression of CRF receptor 1 and 2 mRNAs in the CRF over-expressing mouse brain. *Brain Res.* 1072, 46–54.

Kostich, W. A., Chen, A., Sperle, K., and Largent, B. L. (1998). Molecular identification and analysis of a novel human corticotropin-releasing factor (CRF) receptor: the CRF2gamma receptor. *Mol. Endocrinol.* 12, 1077–1085.

Kozicz, T. (2007). On the role of urocortin 1 in the non-preganglionic Edinger-Westphal nucleus in stress adaptation. *Gen. Comp. Endocrinol.* 153, 235–240.

Kozicz, T. (2009). "Neurobiology of corticotrophin-releasing factor system components in stress; from adaptation to maladaptation," in *Neuropeptides and Peptide Analogs*, eds M. Kovacs and I. Merchenthaler (Kerala: Research Signpost), 59–90.

Kozicz, T., Arimura, A., Maderdrut, J. L., and Lazar, G. (2002). Distribution of urocortin-like immunoreactivity in the central nervous system of the frog *Rana esculenta*. *J. Comp. Neurol.* 453, 185–198.

Kozicz, T., Bittencourt, J. C., May, P. J., Reiner, A., Gamlin, P. D., Palkovits, M., et al. (2011a). The Edinger-Westphal nucleus: a historical, structural, and functional perspective on a dichotomous terminology. *J. Comp. Neurol.* 519, 1413–1434.

Kozicz, T., Sterrenburg, L., and Xu, L. (2011b). Does midbrain urocortin 1 matter? A 15-year journey from stress (mal)adaptation to energy metabolism. *Stress* 14, 376–383.

Kozicz, T., Tilburg-Ouwens, D., Faludi, G., Palkovits, M., and Roubos, E. (2008). Gender-related urocortin 1 and brain-derived neurotrophic factor expression in the adult human midbrain of suicide victims with major depression. *Neuroscience* 152, 1015–1023.

Kozicz, T., Yanaihara, H., and Arimura, A. (1998). Distribution of urocortin-like immunoreactivity in the central nervous system of the rat. *J. Comp. Neurol.* 391, 1–10.

Kuhne, C., Puk, O., Graw, J., Hrabe de Angelis, M., Schutz, G., Wurst, W., et al. (2012). Visualizing corticotropin-releasing hormone receptor type 1 expression and neuronal connectivities in the mouse using a novel multifunctional allele. *J. Comp. Neurol.* 520, 3150–3180.

Lebow, M., Neufeld-Cohen, A., Kuperman, Y., Tsoory, M., Gil, S., and Chen, A. (2012). Susceptibility to PTSD-like behavior is mediated by corticotropin-releasing factor receptor type 2 levels in the bed nucleus of the stria terminalis. *J. Neurosci.* 32, 6906–6916.

Lewis, K., Li, C., Perrin, M. H., Blount, A., Kunitake, K., Donaldson, C., et al. (2001). Identification of urocortin III, an additional member of the corticotropin-releasing factor (CRF) family with high affinity for the CRF2 receptor. *Proc. Natl. Acad. Sci. U.S.A.* 98, 7570–7575.

Li, C., Vaughan, J., Sawchenko, P. E., and Vale, W. W. (2002). Urocortin III-immunoreactive projections in rat brain: partial overlap with sites of type 2 corticotrophin-releasing factor receptor expression. *J. Neurosci.* 22, 991–1001.

Lovenberg, T. W., Chalmers, D. T., Liu, C., and De Souza, E. B. (1995a). CRF2 alpha and CRF2 beta receptor mRNAs are differentially distributed between the rat central nervous system and peripheral tissues. *Endocrinology* 136, 4139–4142.

Lovenberg, T. W., Liaw, C. W., Grigoriadis, D. E., Clevenger, W., Chalmers, D. T., De Souza, E. B., et al. (1995b). Cloning and characterization of a functionally distinct corticotropin-releasing factor receptor subtype from rat brain. *Proc. Natl. Acad. Sci. U.S.A.* 92, 836–840.

Lowry, P. J., Koerber, S. C., Woods, R. J., Baigent, S., Sutton, S., Behan, D. P., et al. (1996). Nature of ligand affinity and dimerization of corticotrophin-releasing factor-binding protein may be detected by circular dichroism. *J. Mol. Endocrinol.* 16, 39–44.

Lukkes, J. L., Staub, D. R., Dietrich, A., Truitt, W., Neufeld-Cohen, A., Chen, A., et al. (2011). Topographical distribution of corticotropin-releasing factor type 2 receptor-like immunoreactivity in the rat dorsal raphe nucleus: co-localization with tryptophan hydroxylase. *Neuroscience* 183, 47–63.

Maillot, C., Million, M., Wei, J. Y., Gauthier, A., and Tache, Y. (2000). Peripheral corticotropin-releasing factor and stress-stimulated colonic motor activity involve type 1 receptor in rats. *Gastroenterology* 119, 1569–1579.

McEwen, B. S., Eiland, L., Hunter, R. G., and Miller, M. M. (2012). Stress and anxiety: structural plasticity and epigenetic regulation as a consequence of stress. *Neuropharmacology* 62, 3–12.

Merali, Z., Du, L., Hrdina, P., Palkovits, M., Faludi, G., Poulter, M. O., et al. (2004). Dysregulation in the suicide brain: mRNA expression of corticotropin-releasing hormone receptors and GABA(A) receptor subunits in frontal cortical brain region. *J. Neurosci.* 24, 1478–1485.

Merchenthaler, I., Vigh, S., Petrusz, P., and Schally, A. V. (1982). Immunocytochemical localization of corticotropin-releasing factor (CRF) in the rat brain. *Am. J. Anat.* 165, 385–396.

Morin, S. M., Ling, N., Liu, X. J., Kahl, S. D., and Gehlert, D. R. (1999). Differential distribution of urocortin- and corticotropin-releasing factor-like immunoreactivities in the rat brain. *Neuroscience* 92, 281–291.

Muglia, L., Jacobson, L., Dikkes, P., and Majzoub, J. A. (1995). Corticotropin-releasing hormone deficiency reveals major fetal but not adult glucocorticoid need. *Nature* 373, 427–432.

Muller, M. B., Preil, J., Renner, U., Zimmermann, S., Kresse, A. E., Stalla, G. K., et al. (2001). Expression of CRHR1 and CRHR2 in mouse pituitary and adrenal gland: implications for HPA system regulation. *Endocrinology* 142, 4150–4153.

Muller, M. B., Zimmermann, S., Sillaber, I., Hagemeyer, T. P., Deussing, J. M., Timpl, P., et al. (2003). Limbic corticotropin-releasing hormone receptor 1 mediates anxiety-related behavior and hormonal adaptation to stress. *Nat. Neurosci.* 6, 1100–1107.

Nappi, R. E., and Rivest, S. (1995). Stress-induced genetic expression of a selective corticotropin-releasing factor-receptor subtype within the rat ovaries: an effect dependent on the ovulatory cycle. *Biol. Reprod.* 53, 1417–1428.

Nemeroff, C. B., Widerlov, E., Bissette, G., Walleus, H., Karlsson, I., Eklund, K., et al. (1984). Elevated concentrations of CSF corticotropin-releasing factor-like immunoreactivity in depressed patients. *Science* 226, 1342–1344.

Nemeroff, C. B., Owens, M. J., Bissette, G, Andorn, A. C., and Stanley, M. (1988). Postmortem study with brains of suicide victims revealing reduced CRH-binding sites in the frontal cortex as result of chronic CRH overexpression. *Arch. Gen. Psychiatry* 45, 577–579.

Nestler, E. J., Barrot, M., DiLeone, R. J., Eisch, A. J., Gold, S. J., and Monteggia, L. M. (2002). Neurobiology of depression. *Neuron* 34, 13–25.

Neufeld-Cohen, A., Evans, A. K., Getselter, D., Spyroglou, A., Hill, A., Gil, S., et al. (2010a). Urocortin-1 and -2 double-deficient mice show robust anxiolytic phenotype and modified serotonergic activity in anxiety circuits. *Mol. Psychiatry* 15, 426–441, 339.

Neufeld-Cohen, A., Tsoory, M. M., Evans, A. K., Getselter, D., Gil, S., Lowry, C. A., et al. (2010b). A triple urocortin knockout mouse model reveals an essential role for urocortins in stress recovery. *Proc. Natl. Acad. Sci. U.S.A.* 107, 19020–19025.

Neufeld-Cohen, A., Kelly, P. A., Paul, E. D., Carter, R. N., Skinner, E., Olverman, H. J., et al. (2012). Chronic activation of corticotropin-releasing factor type 2 receptors reveals a key role for 5-HT1A receptor responsiveness in mediating behavioral and serotonergic responses to stressful challenge. *Biol. Psychiatry* 72, 437–447.

Okosi, A., Brar, B. K., Chan, M., D'Souza, L., Smith, E., Stephanou, A., et al. (1998). Expression and protective effects of urocortin in cardiac myocytes. *Neuropeptides* 32, 167–171.

Orth, D. N., and Mount, C. D. (1987). Specific high-affinity binding protein for human corticotropin-releasing hormone in normal human plasma. *Biochem. Biophys. Res. Commun.* 143, 411–417.

Palchaudhuri, M. R., Hauger, R. L., Wille, S., Fuchs, E., and Dautzenberg, F. M. (1999). Isolation and pharmacological characterization of two functional splice variants of corticotropin-releasing factor type 2 receptor from *Tupaia belangeri*. *J. Neuroendocrinol.* 11, 419–428.

Parkes, D. G., Vaughan, J., Rivier, J., Vale, W., and May, C. N. (1997). Cardiac inotropic actions of urocortin in conscious sheep. *Am. J. Physiol.* 272, H2115–H222.

Perrin, M. H., and Vale, W. W. (1999). Corticotropin releasing factor receptors and their ligand family. *Ann. N. Y. Acad. Sci.* 885, 312–328.

Potter, E., Behan, D. P., Fischer, W. H., Linton, E. A., Lowry, P. J., and Vale, W. W. (1991). Cloning and characterization of the cDNAs for human and rat corticotropin releasing factor-binding proteins. *Nature* 349, 423–426.

Potter, E., Behan, D. P., Linton, E. A., Lowry, P. J., Sawchenko, P. E., and Vale, W. W. (1992). The central distribution of a corticotropin-releasing factor (CRF)-binding protein predicts multiple sites and modes of interaction with CRF. *Proc. Natl. Acad. Sci. U.S.A.* 89, 4192–4196.

Preil, J., Muller, M. B., Gesing, A., Reul, J. M., Sillaber, I., van Gaalen, M. M., et al. (2001). Regulation of the hypothalamic-pituitary-adrenocortical system in mice deficient for CRH receptors 1 and 2. *Endocrinology* 142, 4946–4955.

Refojo, D., Echenique, C., Muller, M. B., Reul, J. M., Deussing, J. M., Wurst, W., et al. (2005). Corticotropin-releasing hormone activates ERK1/2 MAPK in specific brain areas.

*Proc. Natl. Acad. Sci. U.S.A.* 102, 6183–6188.

Refojo, D., Schweizer, M., Kuehne, C., Ehrenberg, S., Thoeringer, C., Vogl, A. M., et al. (2011). Glutamatergic and dopaminergic neurons mediate anxiogenic and anxiolytic effects of CRHR1. *Science* 333, 1903–1907.

Regev, L., Neufeld-Cohen, A., Tsoory, M., Kuperman, Y., Getselter, D., Gil, S., et al. (2011). Prolonged and site-specific over-expression of corticotropin-releasing factor reveals differential roles for extended amygdala nuclei in emotional regulation. *Mol. Psychiatry* 16, 714–728.

Regev, L., Tsoory, M., Gil, S., and Chen, A. (2012). Site-specific genetic manipulation of amygdala corticotropin-releasing factor reveals its imperative role in mediating behavioral response to challenge. *Biol. Psychiatry* 71, 317–326.

Reul, J. M., and Holsboer, F. (2002). Corticotropin-releasing factor receptors 1 and 2 in anxiety and depression. *Curr. Opin. Pharmacol.* 2, 23–33.

Reyes, T. M., Lewis, K., Perrin, M. H., Kunitake, K. S., Vaughan, J., Arias, C. A., et al. (2001). Urocortin II: a member of the corticotropin-releasing factor (CRF) neuropeptide family that is selectively bound by type 2 CRF receptors. *Proc. Natl. Acad. Sci. U.S.A.* 98, 2843–2848.

Ryabinin, A. E., Tsivkovskaia, N. O., and Ryabinin, S. A. (2005). Urocortin 1-containing neurons in the human Edinger-Westphal nucleus. *Neuroscience* 134, 1317–1323.

Sanacora, G., Zarate, C. A., Krystal, J. H., and Manji, H. K. (2008). Targeting the glutamatergic system to develop novel, improved therapeutics for mood disorders. *Nat. Rev. Drug Discov.* 7, 426–437.

Selye, H. (1936). A syndrome produced by diverse nocuous agents. *Nature* 138, 32.

Selye, H. (1951). The general adaptation syndrome and the diseases of adaptation. *Am. J. Med.* 10, 549–555.

Slominski, A., Ermak, G., Hwang, J., Chakraborty, A., Mazurkiewicz, J. E., and Mihm, M. (1995). Proopiomelanocortin, corticotropin releasing hormone and corticotropin releasing hormone receptor genes are expressed in human skin. *FEBS Lett.* 374, 113–116.

Smith, G. W., Aubry, J. M., Dellu, F., Contarino, A., Bilezikjian, L. M., Gold, L. H., et al. (1998). Corticotropin releasing factor receptor 1-deficient mice display decreased anxiety, impaired stress response, and aberrant neuroendocrine development. *Neuron* 20, 1093–1102.

Spina, M., Merlo-Pich, E., Chan, R. K., Basso, A. M., Rivier, J., Vale, W., et al. (1996). Appetite-suppressing effects of urocortin, a CRF-related neuropeptide. *Science* 273, 1561–1564.

Stenzel-Poore, M. P., Cameron, V. A., Vaughan, J., Sawchenko, P. E., and Vale, W. (1992). Development of Cushing's syndrome in corticotropin-releasing factor transgenic mice. *Endocrinology* 130, 3378–3386.

Stenzel-Poore, M. P., Heinrichs, S. C., Rivest, S., Koob, G. F., and Vale, W. W. (1994). Overproduction of corticotropin-releasing factor in transgenic mice: a genetic model of anxiogenic behavior. *J. Neurosci.* 14, 2579–2584.

Swanson, L. W., Sawchenko, P. E., Rivier, J., and Vale, W. W. (1983). Organization of ovine corticotropin-releasing factor immunoreactive cells and fibers in the rat brain: an immunohistochemical study. *Neuroendocrinology* 36, 165–186.

Sztainberg, Y., Kuperman, Y., Justice, N., and Chen, A. (2011). An anxiolytic role for CRF receptor type 1 in the globus pallidus. *J. Neurosci.* 31, 17416–17424.

Sztainberg, Y., Kuperman, Y., Tsoory, M., Lebow, M., and Chen, A. (2010). The anxiolytic effect of environmental enrichment is mediated via amygdalar CRF receptor type 1. *Mol. Psychiatry* 15, 905–917.

Takahashi, K., Totsune, K., Sone, M., Murakami, O., Satoh, F., Arihara, Z., et al. (1998). Regional distribution of urocortin-like immunoreactivity and expression of urocortin mRNA in the human brain. *Peptides* 19, 643–647.

Tanaka, M., and Telegdy, G. (2008). Antidepressant-like effects of the CRF family peptides, urocortin 1, urocortin 2 and urocortin 3 in a modified forced swimming test in mice. *Brain Res. Bull.* 75, 509–512.

Terui, K., Higashiyama, A., Horiba, N., Furukawa, K. I., Motomura, S., and Suda, T. (2001). Coronary vasodilation and positive inotropism by urocortin in the isolated rat heart. *J. Endocrinol.* 169, 177–183.

Timpl, P., Spanagel, R., Sillaber, I., Kresse, A., Reul, J. M., Stalla, G. K., et al. (1998). Impaired stress response and reduced anxiety in mice lacking a functional corticotropin-releasing hormone receptor 1. *Nat. Genet.* 19, 162–166.

Todorovic, C., Jahn, O., Tezval, H., Hippel, C., and Spiess, J. (2005). The role of CRF receptors in anxiety and depression: implications of the novel CRF1 agonist cortagine. *Neurosci. Biobehav. Rev.* 29, 1323–1333.

Turnbull, A. V., and Rivier, C. (1997). Corticotropin-releasing factor (CRF) and endocrine responses to stress: CRF receptors, binding protein, and related peptides. *Proc. Soc. Exp. Biol. Med.* 215, 1–10.

Vale, W., Spiess, J., Rivier, C., and Rivier, J. (1981). Characterization of a 41-residue ovine hypothalamic peptide that stimulates secretion of corticotropin and beta-endorphin. *Science* 213, 1394–1397.

Vale, W., Vaughan, J., and Perrin, M. H. (1997). Corticotropin-releasing factor (CRF) family of ligands and their receptors. *Endocrinologist* 7, 3S–9S.

van Gaalen, M. M., Stenzel-Poore, M. P., Holsboer, F., and Steckler, T. (2002). Effects of transgenic overproduction of CRH on anxiety-like behaviour. *Eur. J. Neurosci.* 15, 2007–2015.

Van Pett, K., Viau, V., Bittencourt, J. C., Chan, R. K., Li, H. Y., Arias, C., et al. (2000). Distribution of mRNAs encoding CRF receptors in brain and pituitary of rat and mouse. *J. Comp. Neurol.* 428, 191–212.

Vaughan, J., Donaldson, C., Bittencourt, J., Perrin, M. H., Lewis, K., Sutton, S., et al. (1995). Urocortin, a mammalian neuropeptide related to fish urotensin I and to corticotropin-releasing factor. *Nature* 378, 287–292.

Venihaki, M., and Majzoub, J. A. (1999). Animal models of CRH deficiency. *Front. Neuroendocrinol.* 20, 122–145.

Vetter, D. E., Li, C., Zhao, L., Contarino, A., Liberman, M. C., Smith, G. W., et al. (2002). Urocortin-deficient mice show hearing impairment and increased anxiety-like behavior. *Nat. Genet.* 31, 363–369.

Wanat, M. J., Hopf, F. W., Stuber, G. D., Phillips, P. E., and Bonci, A. (2008). Corticotropin-releasing factor increases mouse ventral tegmental area dopamine neuron firing through a protein kinase C-dependent enhancement of Ih. *J. Physiol. (Lond.)* 586, 2157–2170.

Wang, X., Su, H., Copenhagen, L. D., Vaishnav, S., Pieri, F., Shope, C. D., et al. (2002). Urocortin-deficient mice display normal stress-induced anxiety behavior and autonomic control but an impaired acoustic startle response. *Mol. Cell. Biol.* 22, 6605–6610.

Weninger, S. C., Dunn, A. J., Muglia, L. J., Dikkes, P., Miczek, K. A., Swiergiel, A. H., et al. (1999). Stress-induced behaviors require the corticotropin-releasing hormone (CRH) receptor, but not CRH. *Proc. Natl. Acad. Sci. U.S.A.* 96, 8283–8288.

Weninger, S. C., Peters, L. L., and Majzoub, J. A. (2000). Urocortin expression in the Edinger-Westphal nucleus is up-regulated by stress and corticotropin-releasing hormone deficiency. *Endocrinology* 141, 256–263.

Wong, M. L., Dong, C., Maestre-Mesa, J., and Licinio, J. (2008). Polymorphisms in inflammation-related genes are associated with susceptibility to major depression and antidepressant response. *Mol. Psychiatry* 13, 800–812.

Zalutskaya, A. A., Arai, M., Bounoutas, G. S., and Abou-Samra, A. B. (2007). Impaired adaptation to repeated restraint and decreased response to cold in urocortin 1 knockout mice. *Am. J. Physiol. Endocrinol. Metab.* 293, E259–E263.

# Permissions

All chapters in this book were first published in NGPCRSN, by Frontiers; hereby published with permission under the Creative Commons Attribution License or equivalent. Every chapter published in this book has been scrutinized by our experts. Their significance has been extensively debated. The topics covered herein carry significant findings which will fuel the growth of the discipline. They may even be implemented as practical applications or may be referred to as a beginning point for another development.

The contributors of this book come from diverse backgrounds, making this book a truly international effort. This book will bring forth new frontiers with its revolutionizing research information and detailed analysis of the nascent developments around the world.

We would like to thank all the contributing authors for lending their expertise to make the book truly unique. They have played a crucial role in the development of this book. Without their invaluable contributions this book wouldn't have been possible. They have made vital efforts to compile up to date information on the varied aspects of this subject to make this book a valuable addition to the collection of many professionals and students.

This book was conceptualized with the vision of imparting up-to-date information and advanced data in this field. To ensure the same, a matchless editorial board was set up. Every individual on the board went through rigorous rounds of assessment to prove their worth. After which they invested a large part of their time researching and compiling the most relevant data for our readers.

The editorial board has been involved in producing this book since its inception. They have spent rigorous hours researching and exploring the diverse topics which have resulted in the successful publishing of this book. They have passed on their knowledge of decades through this book. To expedite this challenging task, the publisher supported the team at every step. A small team of assistant editors was also appointed to further simplify the editing procedure and attain best results for the readers.

Apart from the editorial board, the designing team has also invested a significant amount of their time in understanding the subject and creating the most relevant covers. They scrutinized every image to scout for the most suitable representation of the subject and create an appropriate cover for the book.

The publishing team has been an ardent support to the editorial, designing and production team. Their endless efforts to recruit the best for this project, has resulted in the accomplishment of this book. They are a veteran in the field of academics and their pool of knowledge is as vast as their experience in printing. Their expertise and guidance has proved useful at every step. Their uncompromising quality standards have made this book an exceptional effort. Their encouragement from time to time has been an inspiration for everyone.

The publisher and the editorial board hope that this book will prove to be a valuable piece of knowledge for researchers, students, practitioners and scholars across the globe.

# List of Contributors

**Ayumu Inutsuka and Akihiro Yamanaka**
Department of Neuroscience II, Research Institute of Environmental Medicine, Nagoya University, Nagoya, Japan

**Nadezhda D. Goncharova**
Research Institute of Medical Primatology of Russian Academy of Medical Sciences, Sochi, Russia
Sochi State University, Sochi, Russia

**Kazunori Kageyama**
Department of Endocrinology and Metabolism, Hirosaki University Graduate School of Medicine, Hirosaki, Aomori, Japan

**Ludwik K. Malen dowicz, Agnieszka Ziolkowska and Marcin Rucinski**
Department of Histology and Embryology, Poznan University of Medical Sciences, Poznan, Poland

**Marie-Odile Guimond and Nicole Gallo-Payet**
Divisio of Endocrinology, Department of Medicine, Faculté de Médecine et des Sciences de la Santé, Université de Sherbrooke, Sherbrooke, QC, Canada

**Jean-Claude Le Mével, Frédéric Lancien and Nagi Mimassi**
INSERM UMR 1101, Laboratoire de Traitement de l'Information Médicale, Laboratoire de Neurophysiologie, SFR ScInBioS, Faculté de Médecine et des Sciences de la Santé, Université Européenne de Bretagne, Université de Brest, CHUde Brest, Brest, France

**J. Michael Conlon**
Department Of Biochemistry Faculty Of Medicine and Health Sciences, United Arab Emirates University, Al Ain, United Arab Emirates

**Yosra Hamdi, Hadhemi Kaddour, Salma Douiri, Seyma Bahdoudi, Mohamed Amri and Olfa Masmoudi-Kouki**
Laboratory of Functional Neurophysiology and Pathology, Research UnitUR/11ES09
Department of Biological Sciences, Faculty of Science of Tunis, University Tunis ElManar, Tunis, Tunisia

**David Vaudry, Jérôme Leprince and Hubert Vaudry**
Inserm U982, Laboratory of Neuronal and Neuroendocrine Communication and Differentiation, University of Rouen, Mont-Saint-Aignan, France
International Associated Laboratory Samuelde Champlain, Mont-Saint-Aignan, France
Regional Platform for Cell Imaging of Haute Normandie, Institute for Medical Research and Innovation, University of Rouen, Mont-Saint-Aignan, France

**Hélène Castel and Marie-Christine Tonon**
Inserm U982, Laboratory of Neuronal and Neuroendocrine Communication and Differentiation, University of Rouen, Mont-Saint-Aignan, France
Regional Platform for Cell Imaging Of Haute Normandie, Institute For Medical Research and Innovation, University of Rouen, Mont-Saint-Aignan, France

**Magali Basille-Dugay, Hubert Vaudry and David Vaudry**
INSERMU982, Laboratory of Neuronal and Neuroendocrine Differentiation and Communication, University of Rouen, Mont-Saint-Aignan, France
Institute for Research and Innovation in Biomedicine, University of Rouen, Mont-Saint-Aignan, France
PRIMACEN, University of Rouen, Mont-Saint-Aignan, France
International Associated Laboratory Samuelde Champlain, University of Rouen, Mont-Saint-Aignan, France

**Alain Fournier**
International Associated Laboratory Samuelde Champlain, University of Rouen, Mont-Saint-Aignan, France
Institut National dela Recherch eScienti ique Institut Armand Frappier, University of Québec, Laval, QC, Canada

**Bruno Gonzalez**
Institute for Research and Innovation in Biomedicine, University of Rouen, Mont-Saint-Aignan, France
Région INSERM ERI28, Laboratory of Microvascular Endothelium and Neonate Lesions, University of Rouen, Rouen, France

**Stelios Kokkoris**
Intensive Care Unit, Western General Hospital, Edinburgh, UK

**Peter Andrews**
Centre for Clinical Brain Sciences, University of Edinburgh, Edinburgh, UK

**David J. Webb**
Clinical Pharmacology Unit, British Heart Foundation Centre for Cardiovascular Science, Queen's Medical Research Institute, University of Edinburgh, Edinburgh, UK

**Mona Boules, Zhimin Li, Kristin Smith, Paul Fredrickson and Elliott Richelson**
Neuropsycho pharmacology Laboratory, Department of Neuroscience, Mayo Clinic Florida, Jacksonville, FL, USA

**Rafael Roesler**
Laboratory of Neuropharmacology and Neural Tumor Biology
Department of Pharmacology, Institute for Basic Health Sciences, Federal University of Rio Grande do Sul, Porto Alegre, Brazil
Cancer Research Laboratory, University Hospital Research Center (CPEHCPA), Federal University of Rio Grande do Sul, Porto Alegre, Brazil
National Institute for Translational Medicine, Porto Alegre, Brazil

**Gilberto Schwartsmann**
Laboratory of Neuropharmacology and Neural Tumor Biology
Department of Pharmacology, Institute for Basic Health Sciences, Federal University of Rio Grande do Sul, Porto Alegre, Brazil
Cancer Research Laboratory, University Hospital Research Center (CPEHCPA), Federal University of Rio Grande do Sul, Porto Alegre, Brazil
National Institute for Translational Medicine, Porto Alegre, Brazil
Department of Internal Medicine, School of Medicine, Federal University of Rio Grande do Sul, Porto Alegre, Brazil

**Illana Gozes**
The Lily and Avraham Gildor Chair for the Investigation of Growth Factors, Department of Human Molecular Genetic sand Biochemistry, Sagol School of Neuroscience, Adams Super Center for Brain Studies, Sackler Faculty of Medicine, Tel Aviv University, Tel Aviv, Israel

**Guillaume Martel, Patrick Dutar, Jacques Epelbaum and Cécile Viollet**
Inserm UMR894 Center for Psychiatry and Neuroscience, Université Paris Descartes, Sorbonne Paris Cité, Paris, France

**Jack H. Jhamandas**
Division of Neurology, Department of Medicine, Centre for Neuroscience, University of Alberta, Edmonton, AB, Canada

**Valeri Goncharuk**
Division of Neurology, Department of Medicine, Centre for Neuro science, University of Alberta, Edmonton, AB, Canada
Russian Cardiology Research Center, Moscow, Russia

**Miwa Mori, Kenji Mori, Mikiya Miyazato and Kenji Kangawa**
Department of Biochemistry, National Cerebral and Cardiovascular Center Research Institute, Osaka, Japan

**Takanori Ida**
Interdisciplinary Research Organization, University of Miyazaki, Miyazaki, Japan

**Takahiro Sato and Masayasu Kojima,**
Molecular Genetics, Institute of Life Sciences Kurume University, Fukuoka, Japan

**Takeshi Sakurai**
Kanazawa University, Kanazawa, Japan

**Seiji Shioda**
Department of Anatomy, Showa University School of Medicine, Tokyo, Japan

**Tomoya Nakamachi**
Department of Anatomy, Showa University School of Medicine, Tokyo, Japan
Center for Biotechnology, Showa University, Tokyo, Japan

**Attila Matkovits**
Department of Anatomy, Showa University School of Medicine, Tokyo, Japan
Department of Anatomy, University of Pécs, Pécs, Hungary

**Tamotsu Seki**
Department of Anatomy, Showa University School of Medicine, Tokyo, Japan
Department of Ophthalmology, Showa University School of Medicine, Tokyo, Japan

**Robert M. Dores**
Department of Biological Sciences, University of Denver, Denver, CO, USA

**Jérémy Pasquier, Anne-Gaëlle Lafont, Karine Rousseau and Sylvie Dufour**
Research Unit BOREA, Biology of Aquatic Organisms and Ecosystems, Centre National de la Recherche Scientifique 7208, Institutde Recherch epourle Développement 207, Université Pierreet Marie Curie, Muséum National d'Histoire Naturelle, Paris, France

**Hervé Tostivint**
UMR 7221CNRS/MNHN Evolution des Régulations Endocriniennes, Muséum Nationald 'Histoire Naturelle, Paris, France

**Hubert Vaudry**
Laboratory of Cellular and Molecular Neuroen docrinology, INSERM U982, European Institute for Peptide Research (IFRMP 23), University of Rouen, Mont-Saint-Aignan, France

**Stacia A. Sower, Wayne A. Decatur, Nerine T. Joseph and Mihael Freamat**
Department of Molecular, Cellular and Biomedical Sciences, Center for Molecular and Comparative Endocrinology, University of New Hampshire, Durham, NH, USA

**Catherine Dodé**
INSERM U1016, Institut Cochin, Université Paris-Descartes, Paris, France

**Philippe Rondard**
CNRSUMR 5203, INSERMU 661, Institut de Génomique Fonctionnelle, Université Montpellier, Montpellier, France

**Donny Janssen**
Department of Cellular Animal Physiology, Donders Institute for Brain, Cognition and Behavior, Nijmegen, Netherlands

**Tamás Kozicz**
Department of Anatomy, Donders Institute for Brain, Cognition and Behavior, Nijmegen, Netherlands
Department ofAnatomy, Donders Institute for Brain, Cognition and Behavior, Nijmegen, Netherlands
Human Genetics Center, Tulane University, New Orleans, LA, USA

# Index

www.ingramcontent.com/pod-product-compliance
Lightning Source LLC
LaVergne TN
LVHW081021210926
848485LV00004B/921